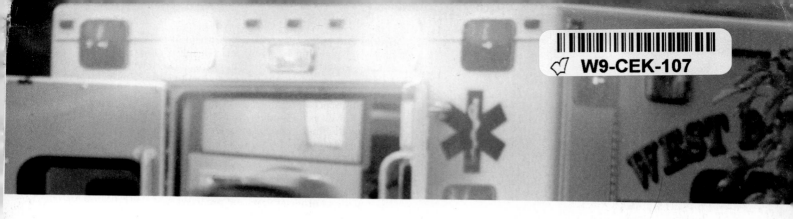

FIRST
RESPONDER

7th Edition

J. David Bergeron

Gloria Bizjak

George W. Krause

Chris Le Baudour

Medical Reviewer

Howard A. Werman, M.D.

PEARSON
Prentice Hall

Upper Saddle River, New Jersey 07458

Library of Congress Cataloging-in-Publication Data

First responder / J. David Bergeron . . . [et al.]; medical reviewer,
Howard A. Werman. — 7th ed.
   p. ; cm.
   Rev. ed. of: First responder / J. David Bergeron, Gloria Bizjak. c2001.
   Includes bibliographical references and index.
   ISBN 0-13-108990-0
    1. Medical emergencies. 2. Emergency medical technicians.
   [DNLM: 1. Emergency Medical Services. 2. Emergencies. 3.
Emergency Medical Technicians. 4. Emergency Treatment. WX 215
B496f 2005] I. Bergeron, J. David II. Bergeron, J. David. First responder.
RC86.7.B47 2005
616.02′5—dc22

2004009260

Publisher: Julie Levin Alexander
Publisher's Assistant: Regina Bruno
Executive Editor: Marlene McHugh Pratt
Assistant Editor: Monica Moosang
Senior Editor: Tiffany Price Salter
Editorial Assistant: Joanna Rodzen-Hickey
Senior Managing Editor: Lois Berlowitz
Development Editor: Josephine Cepeda
Director of Production & Manufacturing: Bruce Johnson
Managing Editor: Patrick Walsh
Production Liaison: Julie Li
Media Editor: John Jordan
Manager of New Media Production: Amy Peltier
New Media Project Manager: Stephen Hartner
Manufacturing Manager: Ilene Sanford
Manufacturing Buyer: Pat Brown
Director of Marketing: Karen Allman
Senior Marketing Manager: Katrin Beacom
Channel Marketing Manager: Rachele Strober
Managing Photography Editor: Michal Heron
Photographers: Michael Gallitelli, Michal Heron, Richard
  Logan, Maria A. H. Lyle
Design Director: Cheryl Asherman
Design Coordinator: Christopher Weigand
Cover Design: Blair Brown
Cover Photo: Mark Ide
Interior Design: Mary Siener
Composition: Pine Tree Composition, Inc.
Printing and Binding: Von Hoffman Press, Inc.

Pearson Education, Ltd., *London*
Pearson Education Australia Pty. Limited, *Sydney*
Pearson Education Singapore Pte. Ltd.
Pearson Education North Asia Ltd., *Hong Kong*
Pearson Education Canada, Ltd., *Toronto*
Pearson Educación de Mexico, S.A. de C.V.
Pearson Education—Japan, *Tokyo*
Pearson Education Malaysia, Pte. Ltd.
Pearson Education, Upper Saddle River, New Jersey

Studentaid.ed.gov, the U.S. Department of Education's website on college planning assistance, is a valuable tool for anyone intending to pursue higher education. Designed to help students at all stages of schooling, including international students, returning students, and parents, it is a guide to the financial aid process. The website presents information on applying to and attending college as well as on funding your education and repaying loans. It also provides links to useful resources, such as state education agency contact information, assistance in filling out financial aid forms, and an introduction to various forms of student aid.

Notice on Care Procedures
It is the intent of the authors and publisher that this textbook be used as part of a formal First Responder education program taught by qualified instructors and supervised by a licensed physician. The procedures described in this textbook are based upon consultation with First Responder and medical authorities. The authors and publisher have taken care to make certain that these procedures reflect currently accepted clinical practice; however, they cannot be considered absolute recommendations.

The material in this textbook contains the most current information available at the time of publication. However, federal, state, and local guidelines concerning clinical practices, including, without limitation, those governing infection control and universal precautions, change rapidly. The reader should note, therefore, that new regulations may require changes in some procedures.

It is the responsibility of the reader to familiarize himself or herself with the policies and procedures set by federal, state, and local agencies as well as the institution or agency where the reader is employed. The authors and the publisher of this textbook and the supplements written to accompany it disclaim any liability, loss, or risk resulting directly or indirectly from the suggested procedures and theory, from any undetected errors, or from the reader's responsibility to stay informed of any new changes or recommendations made by any federal, state, and local agency as well as by his or her employing institution or agency.

Notice on Gender Usage
The English language has historically given preference to the male gender. Among many words, the pronouns "he" and "his" are commonly used to describe both genders. Society evolves faster than language, and the male pronouns still predominate our speech. The authors have made great effort to treat the two genders equally, recognizing that a significant percentage of First Responders are female. However, in some instances, male pronouns may be used to describe both males and females solely for the purpose of brevity. This is not intended to offend any readers.

Brief Contents

Appendices

Contents

Unit 1 Preparatory   1

Unit 7 EMS Operations   497

Photo Scans

Algorithms

Letter to Students

Congratulations as you begin your training to become a First Responder. First Responder programs were developed to provide highly trained individuals with the skills necessary to begin assessing and caring for patients at the scene of injury or illness. In many areas of the nation, First Responders now are able to reach patients in less than 10 minutes from the onset of the emergency. This quick response and the quality of care save thousands of lives each year.

First Responder programs are growing in number and complexity. This commitment has allowed the First Responder to become an important part of the EMS system in the United States. Other nations also are developing similar programs.

The first six editions of this textbook have been used by several hundred thousand students as part of their training. This new 7th edition retains what was found to be successful in the previous editions and also includes some new topics and concepts that have recently become a part of most First Responder courses. The text bases its format on the U.S. Department of Transportation's First Responder National Standard Curriculum, as well as on projections made by the National Association of EMS Educators (NAEMSE). The 7th Edition includes EMT-Basic national program terminology and assessment and care procedures, uses current American Heart Association (AHA) guidelines, and includes automated external defibrillation (AED) procedures in the CPR chapter.

Changes occur because medicine and the EMS system are dynamic, technology improves, and different care procedures develop as new techniques are found to be effective. This textbook responds to those changes. Because each jurisdiction has somewhat different requirements, First Responder students should check with their instructor, who is the authority for their course. With frequent medical discoveries and changing procedures, it is not always possible for jurisdictions and publishers to keep every protocol or publication 100 percent current on a daily basis. However, your instructor will learn of protocol and procedure changes and inform you of new requirements and responsibilities.

We welcome you to EMS!

Preface

THE FIRST RESPONDER PROGRAM

First Responder courses are designed to meet training needs in local communities. While all First Responder courses meet the same National Standard Curriculum objectives, jurisdictions may require that prerequisites be met before enrolling in the course. For the most part, emergency care procedures remain the same from EMS system to EMS system. However, many EMS programs may require completion of American Heart Association (AHA) CPR, or basic life support, before entering a First Responder program. While CPR guidelines are undergoing changes for the layperson, this textbook includes the most recent AHA guidelines for the emergency care provider at the time of printing. AED procedures are also included in the CPR chapter. AED has become an important part of basic life support, and many public facilities are beginning to place them on the premises and train their personnel in their use.

The content of the 7th edition is summarized below, with emphasis on "what's new" in each unit of this edition:

UNIT 1, PREPARATORY: CHAPTERS 1–5

The first unit sets a framework for all the units that follow by introducing essential concepts, information, and skills. The EMS system and the role of the First Responder within the system are introduced. Issues of First Responder safety, well-being, and legal and ethical issues are covered. So are basic anatomy and physiology and techniques of safe lifting and moving.

What's New in the Preparatory Unit?

- In Chapter 1, *Introduction to EMS Systems:*
  - "First Responder" is defined in relation to other rescue personnel who may be among the first on the scene of an emergency.
  - List of patient-related duties has been expanded to include confidentiality and patient advocacy.
  - Using an AED and working under direction of Incident Commander has been added to the list of First Responder skills.
  - Appropriate barriers (masks and gloves) is now included in the list of DOT-recommended equipment.
  - N-95 respirator has been added to the list of personal protective equipment.

- In Chapter 2, *Legal and Ethical Issues:*
  - Difference between scope of care and standard of care is explained more fully.
  - Documentation of refusal of care has been given more emphasis.
  - "Vial of Life" is included as an example of a medical identification device.

- In Chapter 3, *Well-Being of the First Responder:*
  - Information on stress has been folded into this chapter. It includes discussion of stressors, burnout, and long- and short-term stress.
  - The term "critical incident stress management" has been added.

- In Chapter 4, *The Human Body:*
  - Supine, prone, and lateral recumbent positions are now included in the discussion of terms.

- In Chapter 5, *Lifting, Moving, and Positioning Patients:*
  - Full-body spinal immobilization devices and pedi-boards are included in the list of equipment used to move patients.

UNIT 2, AIRWAY MANAGEMENT: CHAPTER 6

There is only one chapter in Unit 2, but it may be considered the most important one in the text, because no patient will survive without an open airway. Basic airway management techniques are covered in detail.

What's New in the Airway Management Unit?

- In Chapter 6, *Airway Management:*
  - Discussion of barrier devices has been expanded.
  - Section on mouth-to-barrier ventilation is now included.

UNIT 3, PATIENT ASSESSMENT: CHAPTER 7

This unit explains and illustrates some of the most important skills of a First Responder. All the steps of the assessment and their application to different types of trauma and medical patients, plus the skills of measuring vital signs, taking a patient history, communication, and hand-off to EMTs are discussed.

What's New in the Patient Assessment Unit?

- In Chapter 7, *Assessment of the Patient:*
  - Discussions of a stable vs. unstable scene and a stable vs. unstable patient have been added.
  - New algorithm for patient assessment is now included.

UNIT 4, CIRCULATION: CHAPTER 8

This unit discusses one- and two-rescuer CPR, the chain of survival, the responsibilities of the First Responder, and using automated defibrillators.

What's New in the Circulation Unit?

- In Chapter 8, *CPR and Automated External Defibrillators (AEDs):*
  - The new AHA guidelines have been incorporated.
  - New AHA information on pediatric defibrillation is now included.
  - The "newly born" category is now part of the discussion of pediatric CPR.

UNIT 5, ILLNESS AND INJURY: CHAPTERS 9–11

The Illness and Injury unit covers medical emergencies such as chest pain and respiratory emergencies, environmental emergencies such as heat and cold emergencies, behavioral emergencies, emergencies related to alcohol and other drugs, and poisoning, bites, and stings. Also contained in this unit are a chapter on bleeding and soft-tissue injuries, which covers types of bleeding, shock, and burns; and a chapter on muscle and bone injuries, which discusses the musculoskeletal system, injuries to the extremities, injuries to the head, spine, and chest, and helmet removal.

What's New in the Illness and Injury Unit?

- In Chapter 9, *Medical Emergencies:*
  - Nitroglycerin patches (called transdermal patches) have been added.

- In Chapter 10, *Bleeding, Shock, and Soft-Tissue Injuries:*
  - Hemorrhagic shock is now included in the list of types of shock.

UNIT 6, CHILDBIRTH AND CHILDREN: CHAPTERS 12–13

This unit offers an understanding of childbirth and the complications and emergencies that may arise from delivery. Also discussed are the characteristics of infants and children and providing emergency care to pediatric patients.

What's New in the Childbirth and Children Unit?

- Chapter 13, *Infants and Children:*
  - Algorithms for the START and JumpSTART systems have been added.

UNIT 7, EMS OPERATIONS: CHAPTERS 14–15

This unit deals with nonmedical operations and special situations, including gaining access in motor-vehicle collisions and buildings, hazards such as fire, hazardous materials, and radiation accidents, multiple-casualty incidents, triage, and the Incident Management System.

What's New in the EMS Operations Unit?

- Chapter 14, *Gaining Access and Hazards on Scene:*
  - Above-ground transformers have been added to the section on electrical hazards.
  - Material Safety Data Sheet (MSDS) have been included in the hazmat section.
- Chapter 15, *Multiple-Casualty Incidents, Triage, and the Incident Management System:*
  - Incident Management System is introduced.
  - The JumpSTART Pediatric MCI Triage system has been added.

APPENDICES

Six appendices cover determining blood pressure, breathing aids and oxygen therapy, pharmacology, swimming and diving accidents, response to terrorism and weapons of mass destruction, and First Responder roles and responsibilities.

What's New in the Appendices?

- Appendix 1, *Determining Blood Pressure:*
  - The term "trending" is introduced.
- Appendix 3, *Pharmacology:*
  - Transdermal patch has been added to the routes of medication administration.
- Appendix 5, *Response to Terrorism and Weapons of Mass Destruction:*
  - ALL NEW

Our Goal: Improving Future Training and Education
Some of the best ideas for better training and education methods come from instructors who can tell us what areas of study caused their students the most trouble. Other sound ideas come from practicing First Responders and from students

who are new to the field. We welcome any of your suggestions. Please write to us at:

Brady/Prentice Hall Health
c/o EMS Editor
Pearson Education
One Lake Street
Upper Saddle River, NJ 07458

Visit Brady's website at www.bradybooks.com

If you experience a problem with the companion CD, please write to technical support at media.support@pearsoned.com or call 800 677-6337.

Acknowledgments

MEDICAL REVIEWER

Our special thanks to Dr. Howard A. Werman, Professor, Department of Emergency Medicine, The Ohio State University College of Medicine and Public Health, Columbus, Ohio, Medical Director, Medflight of Ohio. Dr. Werman's reviews were carefully prepared, and we appreciate the thoughtful advice and keen insight offered.

CONTRIBUTORS

Our appreciation to the contributors below for the ideas and advice given.

Bob Elling, MPA, REMT-P
Clinical Instructor, Albany Medical Center
Instructor, EMT-Basic and Paramedic courses,
    Hudson Valley Community College's Institute of
    Prehospital Emergency Medicine
Professor of Management, American College of
    Prehospital Medicine
Regional Faculty, NYS Dept.of Health EMS Bureau
Regional Faculty, American Heart Association
Paramedic, Colonie, NY

Donny Boyd
Firefighter, Montgomery County, MD
Montgomery County Urban Search and Rescue Team
Engineering Technician and Fire Instructor
Maryland Fire and Rescue Institute
College Park, MD

James L. Jenkins, Jr., BA, NREMT-P
Tuckahoe Volunteer Rescue Squad
LifeNet
Richmond, VA

Craig Edward Smith
Fire Service Instructor
Prince George's County Fire/EMS Department
Fire/EMS Training Academy
Prince George's County, MD

REVIEWERS

We wish to thank the following EMS professionals who reviewed material for the 7th Edition of *First Responder*. The quality of their reviews has been outstanding, and their assistance is deeply appreciated.

Vicki Bacidore, RN, MS
EMS Instructor
Loyola University Medical Center
Maywood, IL

Billy Murray, NREMT-P
Nags Head Fire and Rescue
Nags Head, NC

Nikhil Natarajan, NREMT-P, CCEMT-P, I/C
Adjunct Instructor
Ulster Community College
Ulster, NY

Attila Hertelendy BHSc, CCEMT-P,
    NREMT-P, ACP
University of Mississippi Medical Center
Jackson, MS

Stephen Garrison, RN, NREMT-P
EMS Manager
Memorial Hospital
South Bend, IN

William H. Clark
Paramedic, ACLS Instructor
Chief and EMS Coordinator
Escatawpa Volunteer Fire Department
Escatawpa, MS

Robert Hancock, B.S., L.P., MS-IV
University of North Texas Health Science
    Center
Fort Worth, TX

Tony Crystal
Director, EMS
Lake Land College
Mattoon, IL

Willard Wright, EMT-B, eic SIEMT
Staten Island EMT
Staten Island, NY

Larry Thompson, FAE./Paramedic
EMT Program Coordinator
College of Marin
Marin County Fire Department
Kentfield, CA

We also wish to express appreciation to the following EMS professionals who reviewed earlier editions of First Responder. Their suggestions and insights helped to make this program a successful teaching tool.

Chad D. Andrews, BA, EMT-P, EMS-I
Program Director of Emergency Medical
  Services
Kirkwood Community College
Cedar Rapids, IA

Sgt. Charles Angello
Essex County Police Academy
Cedar Grove, NJ

John L. Beckman, FF/EMT-P
Affiliated with Addison Fire Protection
  District
Highland Park Hospital
Highland Park, IL

Kenneth O. Bradford, EMT-P.
Santa Rosa Jr. College
Emergency Medical Care Programs
Petaluma, CA

Steven M. Carlo, BS, FNAEMD, EMT-I,
  EMD
Erie Community College-North
Emergency Medical Technology Dept.
Williamsville, NY

Patricia A. Ciara, B.S., EMT-P
Assistant Deputy Chief Paramedic
EMS/CME Supervisor
Chicago Fire Department
Chicago, IL

Jo Ann Cobble, M.A., NREMT-P, R.N.
Chair, Dept EMS
University of Arkansas for Medical Sci-
  ences
Little Rock, AR

Captain Dale A. Crutchley, NREMT-P
EMS Administrator/Training
  Coordinator
Annapolis Fire Department
Annapolis, MD

Jeff Daleske, NREMT-P
Program Coordinator
Mercy School of EMS
Des Moines, IA

Gary Dean
Education Coordinator
East Texas Medical Center EMS
Tyler, TX

Garry L. DeJong, NREMT-P
EMS Training Coordinator
Captain, Albuquerque Fire Department
Albuquerque, NM

Jerry Domaschk, NREMT-P
Instructor
Louisiana Technical Colleges
Schriever, LA

T.J. Feldman, MA, EMT-B
West Hartford, CT

Alejandro Garcia, EMT-P
EMS Coordinator
Wichita Falls Fire Department
Wichita Falls, TX

Donald Graesser
Bergen County EMS Training Center
Paramus, NJ

Jaime S. Greene, BA, EMT-B
EMT Education Program Director
Palm Beach County Schools
West Palm Beach, FL

Steve Harrell, EMT-P
Associate Professor
Daytona Beach Community College
Daytona Beach, FL

Glenn R. Henry, NREMT-P
Transport Coordinator-Rainbow Response
Egleston Children's Hospital
Atlanta, GA

Sgt. David M. Johnson, NREMT-P
Emergency Services Unit
Montville Township Police
Montville, NJ

Jerry W. Jones, MPA, BA, EMT-IV
Paramedic Program
Columbia State Community College
Shelbyville, TN

Kathleen M. King, BA, MS, EMT-B
Instructor
Northampton County EMS Training In-
  stitute
Northampton Community College
Bethlehem, PA

Barbara L. Klingensmith, MS, NREMT-P
Director, Public Services Programs
Edison Community College
Fort Myers, FL

Doug Lawson
Devil Lake, ND

Tom LeGros, NREMT
Fire District 12
St. Tammany, LA

Jon F. Levine
Medical Director
Boston Emergency Medical Services
Boston, MA

John A, Lewin, EMT-P
EMS Coordinator
Illinois State Police Academy
Springfield, IL

Glenn H. Luedtke, NREMT-P
Director
Cape & Islands Emergency Medical Ser-
  vices System
Cape Cod, MA

Sergeant David M. Magnino, EMT-P
Paramedic: California Highway Patrol
  Academy
Emergency Medical Services
West Sacramento, CA

William D. McElhiney
Massachusetts State Police, Medical Unit
New Braintree, MA

Geoffrey T. Miller
Assistant Professor
Institute of Public Safety
Santa Fe Community College
Gainesville, FL

Ronold Morton
EMS Coordinator
Marshall Fire/EMS
Marshall, TX

Ronald A. Olson
Milwaukee Police Department Training
  Bureau
Milwaukee, WI

Ham Robbins
Rent-A-Medic
Eastport, ME

Bryan Scyphers
Chairperson, Public Safety Services
Davidson County Community College
Winston-Salem, NC

Mark Slettum
North EMS Education
Division of North Memorial Health Care
Robbinsdale, MN

E.A. Sowinski, BSN, RN, NREMT-B
Delaware State Fire School
Dover, DE

Michael Strong, FF/EMT-P
Public Safety Training Associates
Paw Paw, MI

Jack L. Taylor, BA, EMT-P, I/C
EMS Program Director
Kalamazoo Valley Community College
Kalamazoo, MI.

Tim Taylor, NREMT-P
Captain, Department of Fire and
  Rescue
Prince William County
Woodbridge, VA

Ronald C. Thomas, Jr.
Training and Research Manager
Florida State Fire College
Ocala, FL

Pat D. Trevathan, MS., EMT-Instructor/Coordinator
Kentucky Tech Fire/Rescue Training
West Kentucky State Technical Institute
Paducah, KY

James E. Walker
Special Projects Coordinator
Northeastern University
Burlington, MA

Holly Weber, NREMT-B, I/C
Stonehearth Open Learning Opportunities, Inc. (SOLO)
Conway, NH

Jeff Zuckernick
EMS Department
Kapiolani Community College
Honolulu, HI

PHOTO ACKNOWLEDGMENTS

All photographs not credited adjacent to the photograph or in the photo credit section below were photographed on assignment for Brady/Prentice Hall Health/Pearson Education.

ORGANIZATIONS

We wish to thank the following organizations for their valuable assistance in creating the photo program for the 7th Edition:

Dave Casey, Bureau Chief
Division of State Fire Marshal
Florida Bureau of Fire Standards and Training
Florida State Fire College
Ocala, FL

Bob White, Sheriff
Corporal Dan Dede
Pasco County Sheriff's Office
Pasco County, FL

Transeastern Homes Corporation
Tampa Bay Golf and Tennis Club
San Antonio, FL

TBGCC First Responders Group
San Antonio, FL

Chief John R. Leahy, Jr.
Pinellas Suncoast Fire & Rescue
Indian Rocks Beach, FL

Richard T. Walker, REMT
District Chief
Pinellas Suncoast Fire & Rescue
Indian Rocks Beach, FL

Robert A. Walley, REMTP
District Chief, EMS
Pinellas Suncoast Fire & Rescue
Indian Rocks Beach, FL

Marshall Eiss, REMT
Special Events Coordinator
Indian Rocks Volunteer Firemen's Association
Indian Rocks Beach, FL

Rev. Robert A. Wagenseil, Jr.
Chaplain—Pinellas Suncoast Fire & Rescue
Rector—Calvary Episcopal Church
Indian Rocks Beach, FL

C. T. "Chuck" Kearns, MBA, EMT-P
Director,
Pinellas County EMS/Sunstar
Largo, FL

Steve Fravel, NREMT-P
Pinellas County EMS & Fire Administration
Largo, FL

TECHNICAL ADVISORS

Thanks to the following people for providing valuable technical support during the photo shoots for the 7th Edition:

Barbara L. Klingensmith, NREMTP, PhD
Division of State Fire Marshal
Florida Bureau of Fire Standards and Training
Florida State Fire College, Ocala FL

Michael Cox, Instructor
Division of State Fire Marshal
Florida Bureau of Fire Standards and Training

Florida State Fire College
Ocala, FL

Richard T. Walker, EMTP
District Chief
Pinellas Suncoast Fire & Rescue
Indian Rocks Beach, FL

Corporal Dan Dede
Corporal Julie A. Satre

Deputies: Gennis Folsom, Rodney Philon, Wendy Penna
Pasco County Sheriff's Office
Pasco County, FL

Photo Assistant: Brigette Hein
Assistant model coordinator: Ritchel G. Klingensmith
Digital post-production: Richard Carter, Tampa, FL

We wish to thank the following who have provided assistance with photography on previous editions:

Chief Brian Gorski, Captain Paul Dezzi
Sarasota County Fire Department
Sarasota, FL

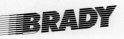

ONE LAKE STREET
UPPER SADDLE RIVER, NJ 07458

Dear Instructor:

Brady, your partner in education, is pleased to bring you the 7th Edition of the classic text *First Responder*. This new edition contains a wealth of tools to make your job easier and to enhance the learning process, making it more interesting and fun for students.

More instructors use *First Responder* than any other First Responder text on the market. Our authors, editors, marketers, and salespeople regularly receive comments from customers who tell us what they like, what they don't like, what works, what doesn't, what's new, what's obsolete, and what they would change. One message comes through clearly: you lead a busy life, juggling multiple roles, and you need all the help and support you can get. You need a solid book you can rely on and a supplements package that helps you to easily and quickly prepare for an engaging class.

The following walkthrough outlines the tried-and-true features in the text and covers the student and instructor supplements that make this the most complete learning system for First Responders. We also introduce several related products that can be used to make your program the best it can be. We are truly proud to be able to offer you a complete set of resources for education.

First Responder continues to offer the high-quality content and instructor support that you have come to know and trust. We are proud of our tradition of bringing to First Responder education the highest standards of writing, development, production, and service that our customers expect and deserve.

Sincerely,

Julie Levin Alexander
VP/Publisher

Tiffany Price Salter
Senior Acquisitions Editor

Lois Berlowitz
Senior Managing Editor

Katrin Beacom
Senior Marketing Manager

Thomas Kennally
National Sales Manager

WELCOME TO THE 7th EDITION OF

FIRST RESPONDER

Bergeron   Bizjak   Krause   Le Baudour

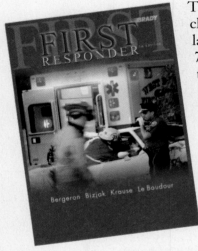

The leader in the field, this easy-to-understand text provides clear First Responder-level training for fire service, emergency, law enforcement, military, civil, and industrial personnel. The 7th Edition of **FIRST RESPONDER** retains the hallmark that has made it the best-selling First Responder book on the market—solid, with thorough coverage of the U.S. DOT First Responder National Standard Curriculum.

FULL TEACHING AND LEARNING PACKAGE

Setting the standard for instructor resources! **FIRST RESPONDER** has a comprehensive **Teaching/Learning Package** that includes:

- **Companion Website** (www.prenhall.com/bergeron) Contains chapter-by-chapter interactive review quizzes with immediate scoring and feedback, A&P matching exercises, a Trauma Gallery, and annotated links to appropriate EMS resources. In addition to resources for the student, you will find our Syllabus Manager feature, which allows you to create your own online syllabus.

- **First Responder PowerPoint Slides** (0-13-118080-0) A brand new Power-Point Slide set provides you with everything you need for a dynamic presentation. This set contains over 700 easy-to-use PowerPoint Slides that are book-specific and follow the U.S. DOT curriculum.

- **Instructor's Resource Manual** (0-13-118087-8) Contains lecture outlines, suggested lesson plans, additional classroom activities, and assignments.

- **TestGen** (0-13-118082-7) This computerized test manager contains more than 500 text-specific questions on disk in a customizable format that contains an electronic grade book and allows for online testing using a LAN.

- **Certificates of Completion** (0-13-118079-7) Call your Brady Representative for more details.

You have always relied on **FIRST RESPONDER** to provide the content you need in a manner that students can easily understand.

NEW TO THIS EDITION

■ **New and Updated Flow-of-Care Diagrams**—Provide students with visual schematics to help them learn and apply patient assessment and other skills critical to First Responders.

Assessment of a Heat Emergency

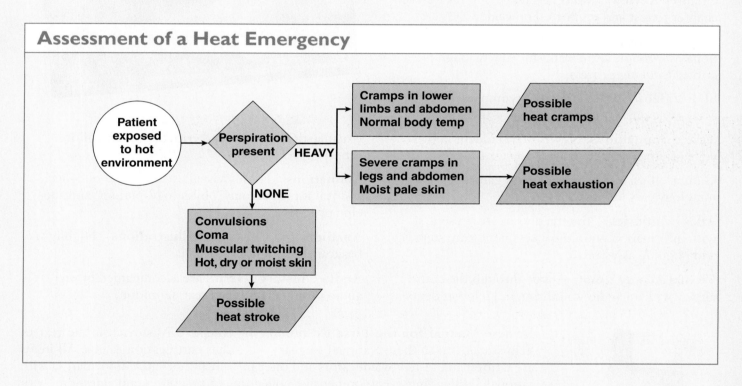

■ **New and Updated Content**—Includes a new chapter on MCI, Triage, and IMS; expanded coverage of barrier devices; and new information on pediatric defibrillation.

■ **New Appendix on Response to Terrorism and Weapons of Mass Destruction**—Presents information on the role of First Responders in patient care should a terrorist event occur.

■ **Updated to Meet AHA Guidelines**

In today's fast-paced learning environment, training takes place beyond the printed page. **FIRST RESPONDER'S** rich supplemental resources expand upon the book content to provide additional learning opportunities.

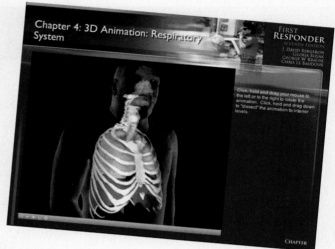

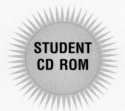

STUDENT CD ROM

An exciting multimedia tool that helps reinforce key concepts. Ideal for the way today's students learn. The CD ROM includes:

Chapter Review   Multiple-choice quizzes for each chapter to test and reinforce knowledge.

Making it Real   Scenarios with questions and rationales throughout to walk students through the critical thinking process.

Skill Videos   Video clips are accompanied by essay-style questions to encourage critical thinking.

Triage Simulations. New!   Test student knowledge of proper triage in MCI scenarios.

Games   Basketball and hangman games make terminology easy and fun.

Atlas of Injuries   Trauma photos are presented with information on initial assessment, care steps, and ongoing assessment.

Virtual Airway Tour   A tour through the entire airway with an audio walkthrough. Helps students

visualize this complex and critical component of care.

Animations   Highly visual exercises that enhance and reinforce anatomy, physiology, biology, and specific processes.

Anatomy and Physiology Illustrations   Highlight basic anatomy and physiology.

Audio Glossary   Terms are accompanied by an audio pronunciation and text definition.

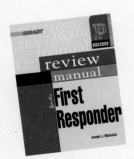

Review Manual for the First Responder by Joseph J. Mistovich is the text to help students pass their National Registry and other certification exams. All items are written and tested by educators and offer proven authoritative information with rationales. Blending a comprehensive collection of practice exam questions with helpful test-taking tips and student hints, all items reference the Department of Transportation's objectives. As you build confidence by digging into this rich content review, you'll find that the Brady/Prentice Hall Health test preparation system is a blueprint for success across the boards.

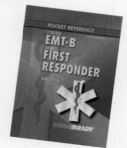

Pocket Reference for the EMT-B and First Responder by Bob Elling is written specifically for EMT-Bs and First Responders. A must-have for every EMT-B and First Responder, this handy, easy-to-carry pocketsize field reference complements all Brady First Responder and EMT-Basic textbooks and includes patient assessment flow charts and skills sequences .

MISSION OF THE AMERICAN SAFETY & HEALTH INSTITUTE

ASHI is a non-profit association of professional educators providing nationally recognized training programs across the United States and in several foreign countries. ASHI's mission is to continually improve safety and health education by promoting high standards for members, principles of sound research for curriculum development, and the professional development of safety and health instructors worldwide.

ASHI FIRST RESPONDER COURSE

This education program is designed to provide students with the core knowledge, skills, and attitudes to function as First Responders. The curriculum includes skills necessary for students to provide emergency medical care with a limited amount of equipment. Approximately 40 hours in length, the course does not require clinical time by students prior to successful completion.

PROGRAM RECOGNITION, GUIDELINES & ACCREDITATION

ASHI works on a regular and ongoing basis with hundreds of federal and state authorities to ensure regulatory compliance. ASHI programs have been reviewed by and/or satisfy the requirements of the Department of Labor, Occupational Safety & Health Administration (DOL/OSHA), and the Department of Homeland Security, United States Coast Guard (DHS/USGC). ASHI programs are also recognized, endorsed, accepted or approved by state regulatory agencies, including those licensing Emergency Medical Services, child care, education, public health, labor, and other programs. ASHI programs enjoy widespread recognition and meet requirements established by many professional associations, councils, academies, and boards. Should an issue arise regarding acceptance, please contact ASHI's Regulatory Affairs Department for assistance.

American Safety & Health Institute
4148 Louis Avenue
Holiday, FL 34691 USA
800-682-5067

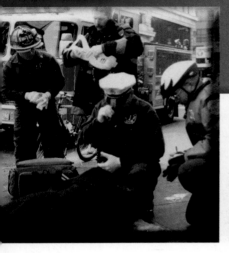
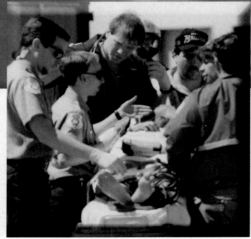
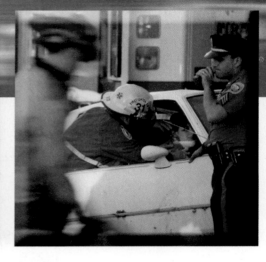

Introduction to EMS Systems

CHAPTER

1

Thousands of people become ill or are injured every day. Unfortunately, physicians are seldom close by when those emergencies occur. In fact, some time usually passes between the onset of injury or illness and a physician's medical care. That is why emergency medical services (EMS) systems have been developed. Their purpose is to get trained medical personnel to the patient as quickly as possible and to provide emergency care on scene, en route to the hospital, and at the hospital. First Responders are essential members of the EMS team.

Realizing that so many people depend on you to provide assistance when they need it may cause you to feel overwhelmed. To gain confidence in your knowledge and skills, you can learn the steps for providing appropriate care by participating in an emergency care training program. To begin, this chapter will introduce you to emergency medical services (EMS) systems and to the roles and responsibilities of the First Responder.

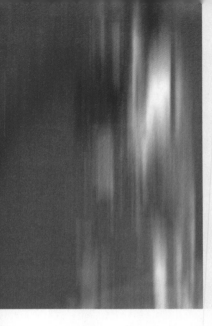

NATIONAL STANDARD OBJECTIVES

This chapter focuses on the objectives of Module 1, Lesson 1–1, of the U.S. DOT's First Responder National Standard Curriculum and serves as an instructional aid to help you meet any specific objectives added to the course by your local EMS system.

By the end of this chapter, you will be able to (from cognitive or knowledge information):

1–1.1 Define the components of Emergency Medical Services (EMS) systems. (pp. 2–3)

1–1.2 Differentiate the roles and responsibilities of the First Responder from other out-of-hospital care providers. (pp. 5, 6–14)

1–1.3 Define medical oversight and discuss the First Responder's role in the process. (pp. 5–6)

1–1.4 Discuss the types of medical oversight that may affect the medical care of a First Responder. (pp. 5–6)

1–1.5 State the specific statutes and regulations in your state regarding the EMS system. (pp. 6, 14, 16)

LEARNING TASKS

It is very important that you learn and understand just what is expected of you as a First Responder. When you do, you can act more quickly to provide effective emergency care. As you participate in this program and practice your skills, think about the six major duties of First Responders and be able to:

✔ Apply these duties directly to patients.

It is also important to know exactly what your responsibilities are as a First Responder when responding to an emergency. First Responders have specific responsibilities that are somewhat different from those of other levels of emergency care certification. Being aware of your responsibilities and providing care at your level means no one needlessly duplicates tasks and you perform within your scope of training. Be able to:

✔ Demonstrate a knowledge of and be able to perform the tasks that fall within the First Responder scope of care.

THE EMS SYSTEM

Emergency medical care saves millions of lives each year. The advances made in medicine during the last 50 years are startling. Highly trained health-care teams use advanced methods of detecting illness, complex medical procedures, elaborate equipment, and new wonder drugs to provide the best of care for patients. Before the twentieth century, most patients who entered hospitals did so to die. Today, we fully expect the majority of hospitalized patients to recover and lead normal lives.

COMPONENTS OF THE EMS SYSTEM

emergency medical services (EMS) system the chain of human resources and services linked together to provide continuous emergency care from the onset of care at the prehospital scene, during transport, and on arrival at the medical facility. In some localities, multiple EMS agencies work together as an EMS network.

If hospital personnel waited for patients to come to them, many individuals would die before getting medical care. Fortunately, it is possible to extend care from hospitals out to the patient through a chain of human resources known as the **emergency medical services (EMS) system** (Scan 1-1). Once the system is activated, care begins at the emergency scene and continues during transport to a medical facility. At the hospital, an orderly transfer to the emergency department (ED) staff at the medical facility ensures continued care. Note that the ED may still be commonly referred to as the emergency room or ER.

**Feel comfortable enough to
(by changing attitudes, values, and beliefs):**

1–1.6 Accept and uphold the responsibilities of a First Responder in accordance with the standards of an EMS professional. (pp. 8–10)

1–1.7 Explain the rationale for maintaining a professional appearance when on duty or when responding to calls. (pp. 10–11)

1–1.8 Describe why it is inappropriate to judge a patient based on a cultural, gender, age, or socioeconomic model, and to vary the standard of care rendered as a result of that judgment. (p. 10)

The events that occurred on September 11, 2001, increased public awareness of EMS systems, their personnel, and others who may be involved with security, rescue, and other types of response to emergency scenes. In the media, however, all of those individuals were referred to as *first responders*. In this textbook, only personnel who are EMS providers trained to a specific level of care are called (note the capital letters) *First Responders*. When possible, all other emergency personnel—even those first on the emergency scene—will be referred to by their proper titles (firefighters, law enforcement officers, and so on).

Activating the EMS System

Once an emergency occurs and is recognized, the EMS system must be activated. Most citizens activate it by way of a 9-1-1 phone call to an emergency dispatcher, who then sends available responders—**First Responders** and Emergency Medical Technicians (EMTs)—to the scene. Refer to Table 1-1 to compare the roles and responsibilities of four types of EMS responders.

Some areas may not have a 9-1-1 activation system, and the caller may need to seek initial help through fire, police, or rescue personnel. The most desirable EMS activation is the *enhanced* 9-1-1 service that enables the communications center to receive caller information (for example, phone number and address) electronically. In some 9-1-1 services, the dispatchers are trained as Emergency Medical Dispatchers, who can provide pre-arrival care instructions to the caller in an attempt to help and instruct bystanders to protect the patient and initiate certain aspects of emergency care.

No matter which way the EMS system is activated, after EMS personnel arrive on scene and provide the proper emergency care, the patient is transported to a medical facility.

First Responder a member of the EMS system who has been trained to render first care for a patient and to help EMTs at the emergency scene.

In-Hospital Care System

From the ambulance, the emergency department receives the patient. There the patient is further evaluated using advanced technology such as laboratory tests, diagnostic exams, and further treatment. The emergency department is the gateway to the rest of the services that the hospital offers. If a patient has a serious injury or illness, the role of emergency department personnel is to stabilize all immediate life threats and transfer care to the most appropriate in-hospital resources, such as the medical/surgical or intensive care unit, or to another more specialized hospital.

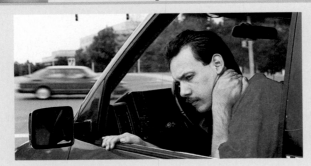

1. Emergency scene.

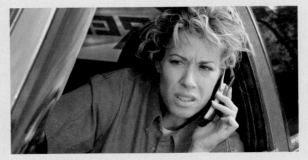

2. Recognition of the crash scene and activation of EMS.

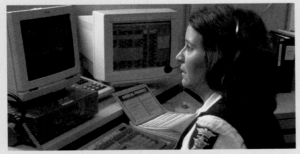

3. Emergency Medical Dispatcher (EMD).

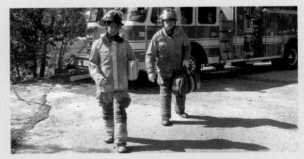

4. Arrival of First Responders.

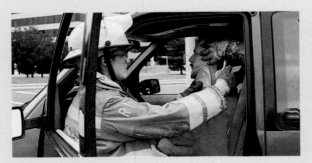

5. Care given at the scene.

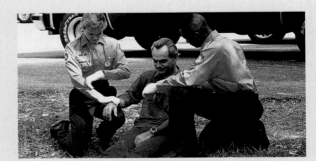

6. Arrival of additional EMS personnel.

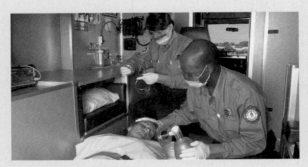

7. Care during transport.

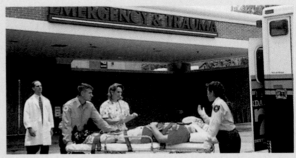

8. Transfer to hospital emergency department (ED).

TABLE 1-1 LEVELS OF EMS TRAINING

- *First Responder*—This level of EMS training is designed specifically for the person who is often first to arrive at the scene. Many police officers, firefighters, industrial workers, and other public service providers are certified as First Responders. This training emphasizes how to activate the EMS system and provide immediate care for life-threatening injuries and illnesses, control the scene, and prepare for the arrival of the ambulance.

- *EMT-Basic*—In most areas, an EMT-B is considered the minimum level of certification for ambulance personnel. The training emphasizes assessment and care of the ill or injured patient. The EMT-B may assist with the administration of certain common medications.

- *EMT-Intermediate*—An EMT-I is a basic-level EMT who has passed specific additional training programs, allowing the individual to provide some level of advanced life support. Some of the additional skills an EMT-I may be able to perform are starting IV (intravenous) lines, using advanced airway techniques, and administering medications classified above those that EMT-Bs are permitted to administer.

- *EMT-Paramedic*—Paramedics are trained to perform invasive patient care, such as inserting endotracheal (ET) tubes and starting IV lines. They also administer medications, interpret electrocardiograms, monitor cardiac rhythms, and perform cardiac defibrillation.

NOTE: The four levels of EMS training are based on the U.S. Department of Transportation's national standard curricula but vary slightly from state to state. Your instructor will explain variations in your area.

Some hospitals handle all routine and emergency cases but have a specialty that sets them apart from other hospitals. One specialty hospital is the trauma center, in which surgery teams are available 24 hours a day. Some hospitals have centers that specialize in the care of certain conditions and patients, such as burn centers, pediatric centers, perinatal (the period before, during, and after birth) centers, and poison control centers.

There are many key members in the hospital portion of the EMS system, including physicians, nurses, physician assistants, respiratory and physical therapists, technicians, aides, and more.

MEDICAL OVERSIGHT

FIRST➤ Each EMS system has a Medical Director. The Medical Director is a physician who assumes the ultimate responsibility for direction, or oversight, of the patient care aspects of the EMS system. The Medical Director also oversees training and develops *protocols* (lists of steps, such as for assessment, care, and interventions in different situations). First Responders and EMTs act as designated agents of the Medical Director. This means that their authority to give medications and provide emergency care is actually an extension of the Medical Director's license to practice medicine. ■

The physician obviously cannot physically be present at every emergency, so the EMS system develops *standing orders*. These standing orders are in the form of protocols that authorize rescuers to perform particular skills in certain situations without actually speaking to the Medical Director (Figure 1.1). This kind of "behind the scenes" medical direction is called **off-line medical direction** (or *indirect medical direction*). Procedures not covered by standing orders or protocols require the rescuer to contact the on-duty physician by radio or telephone prior to performing a particular skill or administering care. Orders from the on-duty physician

off-line (indirect) medical direction standing orders and protocols developed by an EMS system that authorize rescuers to perform particular skills in certain situations without actually speaking to the Medical Director.

FIGURE 1.1
Medical direction given by on-line (direct) orders.

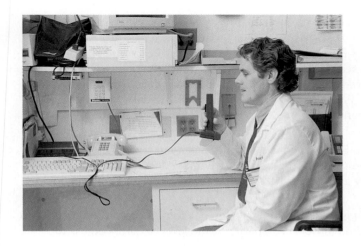

on-line (direct) medical direction orders to perform a skill or administer care from the on-duty physician given by radio or phone to a rescuer.

given in this manner—by radio or phone—are called **on-line medical direction** (or *direct medical direction*).

As a First Responder at the scene of an emergency, you may have limited access to the Medical Director. It will be necessary for you to adhere to the training you receive or to follow the orders of on-scene EMS providers who have a higher level of certification. All EMS personnel, however, must provide care only within their scope of care. The *scope of care* is what a First Responder is allowed and supposed to do according to the National Standard Curriculum. The *standard of care* includes protocols and guidelines set in place by the local jurisdiction. The scope of care is the same nationwide; the standard of care will vary depending on your jurisdiction.

Your instructor will inform you of your local policies. Always follow your local protocols. There are specific statutes and regulations regarding EMS in every state and in local jurisdictions. Your instructor will explain these to you.

THE FIRST RESPONDER

The lack of people with enough training to provide care before more highly skilled EMS providers arrive at a scene is the weakest link in the chain of the EMS system. Training First Responders may help correct this problem.

emergency care the prehospital assessment and basic care for the sick or injured patient. The physical and emotional needs of the patient are considered and attended to during care.

FIRST▷ First Responders are trained to reach patients, find out what is wrong, provide **emergency care** and, only when necessary, move patients without causing further injury. These individuals are usually the first trained personnel to reach the patient. A First Responder may be a law enforcement officer, a member of the fire service, an office coworker, or a private citizen (Scan 1-2). In all cases, a First Responder is trained and has successfully completed a First Responder course. Many police officers and firefighters are trained to the First Responder level. Industrial companies are beginning to train employees as First Responders. The more private citizens who are willing to be trained as First Responders, the stronger the EMS system becomes. ■

Since the beginning of First Responder training programs, hundreds of thousands of people have completed formal courses, with many going on to provide essential care. In most areas of the United States, First Responders are now an important part of the EMS system. The care they provide reduces suffering, prevents additional injuries, and saves many lives.

First Responders

First Responders work in many different fields and environments.

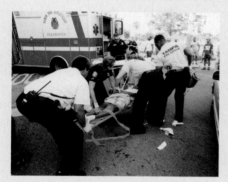

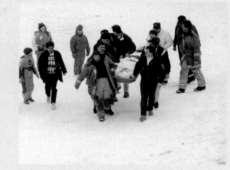

1. Fire department personnel or firefighter volunteers (may be required to have EMT-Basic certification).

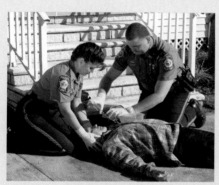

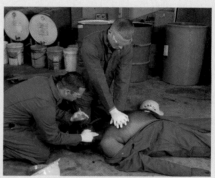

2. Law enforcement personnel, public safety officers, state troopers, ATF, DEA, FBI, and other federal law enforcement and homeland defense personnel, campus security police, shopping mall and factory security personnel.

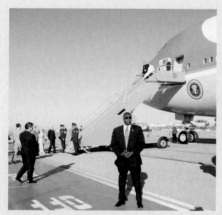

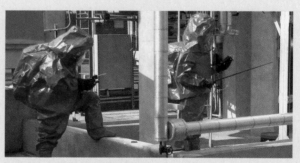

4. Rescue team specialists for specific disciplines, such as hazardous materials, confined space, swift water, ice, trench, high angle, cave, and urban rescues.

3. Executive protection personnel, such as Secret Service agents; rescuers in recreational environments, such as park rangers, lifeguards, athletic trainers; military combat life savers (CLS); and industrial safety officers and safety response teams.

ROLES AND RESPONSIBILITIES

Personal Safety

FIRST➤ Your primary concern as a First Responder at an emergency scene is *personal safety*. The desire to help those who are in need of care may tempt you to ignore the hazards at the scene. You must make certain that you can safely reach the patient and that you will remain safe while providing care. ■

Part of a First Responder's concern for personal safety must include the proper protection from infectious diseases. All First Responders who assess or provide care for patients *must* avoid direct contact with patient blood or other body fluids, membranes, wounds, and burns. Personal protection items that minimize contact with infectious agents include:

● Latex, vinyl, or other synthetic gloves.

● Barrier devices such as pocket face masks with one-way valves and special filters for rescue-breathing procedures.

● Protective eye wear such as goggles or face shields to avoid contact with droplets expelled during certain care procedures (for example, assisting with childbirth).

● Special face masks to avoid contact with airborne microorganisms.

● Gowns or aprons to avoid being splashed by blood or other body fluids and having direct contact with contaminated items.

Typically, you will only need protective gloves and possibly face masks for most patient care situations. However, all the items listed above should be on hand so that you can protect yourself and provide care safely. More will be said about infectious diseases and personal protection in Chapter 3.

First Responders who are in law enforcement, the fire service, or industry may be required to carry out their specific job tasks before they provide patient care (controlling traffic, stabilizing vehicles, shutting down machinery). If this applies to you, always follow your department's standard operating procedures.

FIRST➤ The EMS system responds to an emergency scene to provide care for the patient. Remember, as a First Responder, you are part of the EMS system. Your activities at the scene and the care you provide until more highly trained personnel arrive will help to save lives, prevent additional injury, and give comfort to patients. ■

Patient-Related Duties

Before care begins for someone, that person is a *victim*. Once you start to carry out your duties as a First Responder, the victim becomes a *patient*. Your presence at the scene means that the EMS system has begun its first phase of care. True, the patient may need a physician at the hospital to survive, but the patient's chances of reaching the hospital alive are greatly improved because a First Responder has initiated emergency care.

FIRST➤ As a First Responder, you have six main patient-related duties to carry out at the emergency scene. These duties are (Figure 1.2):

1. *Size up the scene.* Scene safety is your first concern, even before patient care. Evaluate how to protect yourself and the patient, try to determine what caused the injury or illness, how many patients you have, and what kind of assistance

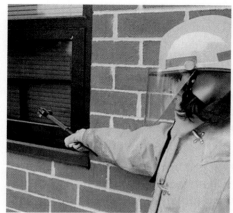

A. Size up the scene and safely gain access.

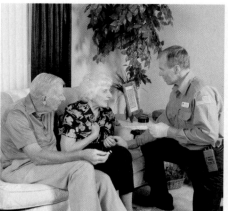

B. Find out what is wrong with the patient.

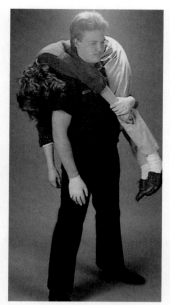

C. Lift or move the patient when necessary and without further injury.

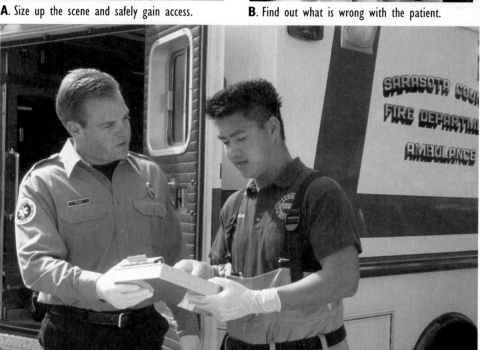

D. Transfer the patient and patient information.

FIGURE 1.2
First Responders carry out patient-related duties.

you will need. Then safely gain access to the patient, using simple hand tools when necessary. You must gain access, whether patients are surrounded by a crowd or trapped in a vehicle or inside a building. You must control the scene to protect yourself and the patients and to minimize additional injuries. At the same time, make sure that the dispatcher is alerted so more highly trained personnel can be sent. Should you need the police, fire department, rescue squad, power company, or others at the scene, you must make sure that the dispatcher is aware of this need. If your system trains dispatchers in emergency medical dispatch procedures, EMDs may provide pre-arrival care instructions by phone or radio until more highly trained personnel arrive.

2. *Find out what is wrong with the patient* by gathering information from the scene, from bystanders, and from the patient, and by assessing the patient. Using

what limited supplies you have, provide emergency care to the level of your training. Remember, emergency care deals with both illness and injury. Emergency care can be as simple as providing emotional support to someone who is frightened because of a crash or mishap. Or it can be more complex, requiring you to deal with life-threatening emergencies, such as starting basic life support (BLS) measures for a heart attack victim. In later chapters, you will learn how to provide a combination of emotional support and physical care skills to help the patient until more highly trained personnel arrive.

3. *Lift or move the patient only when it is necessary.* You need to judge when safety or care requires you to move or reposition patients and to use techniques that minimize additional injury. Remember, when moving patients do so without causing additional harm.

4. *Transfer the patient and patient information.* Provide for an orderly transfer of patients and patient information to more highly trained personnel. You may also be asked to assist them and work under their direction.

5. *Protect the patient's privacy and maintain confidentiality.* You must also provide a high level of privacy and confidentiality concerning the patient and the care that you provide to him.

6. *Be the patient's advocate.* You must be willing to be an advocate for the patient and do what is best for him at all times, so long as it is safe to do so. ■

TRAITS

To be a First Responder, you must be willing to take on certain duties and responsibilities. It takes hard work and study to be a First Responder. This effort does not end with your course, since you must keep your emergency care skills sharp and current (Figure 1.3). You also may be required to recertify periodically.

If you want to be a First Responder, you have to be willing to deal with people. Individuals who are sick or injured are not at their best. You must be able to overlook rude behavior and unreasonable demands, realizing that patients may act this way because of fear, uncertainty, or pain. Dealing with patient reactions is often the hardest part of the job. To do so in a professional manner is sometimes very difficult.

FIRST➤ All patients have the same right to the very best of care. Your respect for others and acceptance of their rights are essential parts of the total patient care that you provide as a First Responder. You cannot modify the care you provide according to your view of religious beliefs, cultural expression, age, gender, social behavior, socioeconomic background, or geographic origin. Likewise, you must take a realistic view. That is, not all care can be identical for all patients of all ages. For example, assessment and care for an infant with burns is not the same as care for a burn patient who is over 35 years of age. Nor can you ignore the observation that low-income families may have a history of inadequate health care and improper diet. Every patient is unique and deserves to have his or her needs met by a consistent standard of care. ■

To be a First Responder, you must be honest and realistic. When helping patients, you cannot tell them they are okay if they are sick or hurt. You cannot tell them that everything is all right, when they know that something is wrong. Telling someone not to worry is not realistic. When an emergency occurs, there is truly something to worry about. Your conversations with patients can help relax them, if

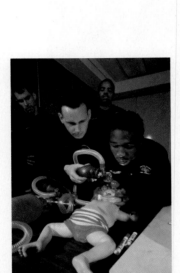

FIGURE 1.3

As a First Responder, you must focus on keeping your skills sharp and current.

you are honest. By telling patients that you are trained in emergency care and that you will help them, you ease their fears and gain their confidence. Letting patients know that additional aid is on the way also will help them relax.

As a First Responder, there may be limits to what you can say to a patient or a patient's loved ones. Telling a patient that a loved one is dead may not be appropriate if you are still providing care to the patient. In such circumstances, it is often necessary for you to be tactful. By saying that someone is taking care of the loved one, you may be able to put the patient at ease. Remember, people under the stress of illness or injury often cannot tolerate any additional stress.

Being a First Responder requires that you control your own feelings at the emergency scene. You must learn how to become involved with caring for patients, while controlling your emotional reactions to their injuries or serious illnesses. Patients do not need sympathy and tears. They need your professional care.

Providing First Responder care requires you to admit that crashes and other emergency scenes will affect you. You may have to speak with other EMS care providers or a specialist within the EMS system to resolve the stress and emotional problems caused by providing care.

As a First Responder, you have to be a highly disciplined professional at the emergency scene. Watch your language in front of patients and bystanders. Do not make comments about patients or the horror of the incident. Concentrate on patients and avoid unnecessary distractions. Something as simple as smoking a cigarette at the scene shows that you are not willing to discipline yourself to the level required.

No one can demand that you change your lifestyle to be a First Responder. However, since you may be called on to provide care almost anywhere anytime, you should consider the following few points. Your appearance earns a patient's confidence. Putting on a clean shirt before running out to the store may not seem to be a reasonable request. Having one less drink or even not drinking at a party may sound unimportant. Yet the significance of these actions may be very important if you have to provide emergency care at the scene of an illness or injury.

In addition, to be a First Responder, you must keep yourself in reasonably good physical condition. You may be of little help to the patient if you are unable to bend over or catch your breath. So watch your diet, exercise regularly, and be sure to get a yearly check up with your doctor. You do not want to become another patient on the scene.

When you complete your training and become a First Responder, you are someone special, filling a very important need in your community.

SKILLS

In addition to learning facts and information, you will be required to perform certain skills as part of your First Responder training. These skills vary from course to course. The list below is an example of the skills learned by the typical First Responder. You are not expected to memorize this list. Read the list and check off each skill as you learn it in your course.

As a First Responder, you should be able to:

- Assess and control the scene of a simple incident.

- Gain access to patients in vehicles by way of doors and windows.

- Gain access to patients in buildings by way of doors and windows.

- Evaluate a scene for safety and the possible cause of an illness or injury.

- Gather information from patients and bystanders.
- Properly use all items of personal safety.
- Conduct a patient assessment.
- Determine vital signs (pulse, respiration, skin signs, pupils).
- Document assessment signs.
- Relate signs and symptoms to illnesses and injuries.
- Open a patient's airway, provide airway care, perform pulmonary resuscitation for adults, infants, and children, and ventilate patients who breathe through surgical openings in their necks (stomas).
- Use a barrier device such as a pocket face mask with one-way valve and HEPA filter to provide ventilations.
- Identify cardiac arrest in a patient and perform one- and two-rescuer cardiopulmonary resuscitation (CPR).
- Set up and use the automated external defibrillator (AED) on patients in cardiac arrest.
- Control bleeding by using direct pressure, elevation, pressure dressings, pressure points and, as a last resort, tourniquets.
- Assess for shock (including allergy shock) and care for patients who develop shock.
- Assess and provide care for closed injuries and open injuries, including face and scalp wounds, nosebleeds, eye injuries, neck wounds, chest injuries (including rib fractures, flail chest, and penetrating chest wounds), abdominal injuries, and injuries to the genitalia.
- Carry out basic dressing and bandaging techniques.
- Assess and care for painful, swollen, deformed extremities—including possible fractures, dislocations, sprains, and strains—using soft splints and/or commercial and noncommercial rigid splints.
- Assess and care for possible injuries to the cranium (skull) and face.
- Assess and care for possible injuries to the neck and spine.
- Assess and care for possible heart attacks and other serious heart problems, strokes, blood pressure-related events, seizures, and diabetic emergencies.
- Identify and care for poisoning cases.
- Classify and provide care for burns.
- Identify and care for smoke inhalation.
- Assess and care for heat emergencies, including heat exhaustion, heat cramps, and heat stroke, and assess and care for cold injuries, including frostbite and hypothermia.
- Assist a mother in delivering her baby.
- Provide initial care for the newborn.
- Identify and care for drug-abuse and alcohol-abuse patients.
- Perform non-emergency and emergency patient moves when required.
- Perform triage at a multiple-patient emergency scene.

- Work under the direction of an Incident Commander in an incident command or incident management system (ICS or IMS) operation.

- Work under the direction of EMTs to help them provide patient care, doing what you have been trained to do at your level of care as a First Responder.

In some systems that have very special needs, First Responders may be required to perform all or any of the following:

- Provide for the patient's airway.

- Determine blood pressure.

- Use a bag-valve-mask resuscitator (ventilator).

- Deliver oxygen using devices appropriate for the patient's age and condition, such as respiratory emergencies, cardiac emergencies, and allergy shock.

- Apply or assist in applying a traction splint.

- Apply or assist in applying an extrication collar.

- Assist in securing a patient to a long spine board (backboard) or other device used to immobilize the patient's spine.

EQUIPMENT, TOOLS, AND SUPPLIES

Most First Responders carry very little equipment, tools, and supplies. Some First Responders may carry special or separate kits for trauma and medical emergencies and childbirth. It is easier to grab a small kit containing the items needed for the incident than to pick up and carry a large kit with everything in it. If you are assigned to a special event, such as a ball game or a carnival, you may want to include items that will meet the needs of that event (ice packs and hydration packs) in addition to dressings and bandages. Even if you are provided with an emergency care kit, you may find yourself providing care when you do not have the kit. The typical First Responder course explains how to use items found at the emergency scene and how to make items for emergency use.

The DOT has recommended that First Responders know how to use, and have available whenever possible, the following items (Figure 1.4):

- Appropriate barriers (masks and gloves).

- Triangular bandages.

- Roller-type bandages.

- Gauze pads and trauma dressings.

- Occlusive dressings (for airtight seals).

- Adhesive tape.

- Bandage shears.

- Eye protector (paper cup or cone).

- Stick (for tourniquet).

- Blanket and pillow.

- Upper and lower extremity splint sets.

In some localities, First Responders are expected to take a patient's blood pressure. In those areas, the kit would include a blood pressure cuff and a stethoscope. Some jurisdictions may have First Responders administer oxygen and also suction

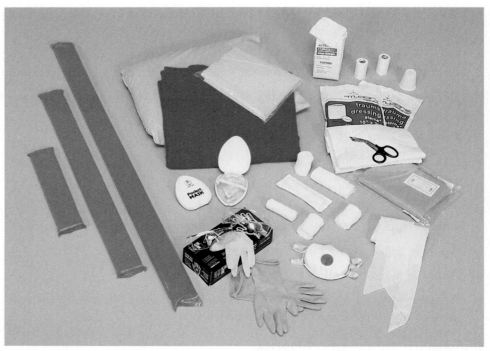

FIGURE 1.4
Emergency medical care equipment and supplies.

the patient's mouth and nose when needed. In those jurisdictions, First Responders carry oxygen delivery systems and suctioning equipment.

First Responders must carry equipment and supplies to protect them from disease-causing agents (infectious and contagious diseases). Typically, the First Responder should have:

- Latex, vinyl, or other synthetic gloves.
- Eye protection (goggles or face shields).
- Masks and barrier devices for ventilating patients, including high-efficiency particulate air (HEPA) or N-95 masks and respirators..
- Gowns.

You may be required to know how to use and improvise other emergency care items. Your instructor may add to the above list, including those items needed for personal safety.

The DOT has suggested that all First Responders should be able to use the following tools and equipment for gaining access to patients (your course may include other items):

- Jack and jack handle.
- Pliers, screwdriver, hammer, and knife.
- Rope.

Chapter Review

The **emergency medical services (EMS) system** is a chain of human services established to provide care to the patient at the scene and during transport to the hospital emergency department (ED). There are four levels of EMS training: First Responder, EMT-Basic, EMT-Intermediate, and EMT-Paramedic. EMS personnel respond to the scene when an emergency dispatcher receives incident information from a 9-1-1 call. Dispatchers may be specially trained as Emergency Medical Dispatchers (EMDs) who offer pre-arrival care instructions to bystanders at the scene.

Each EMS system has a Medical Director, a physician who assumes the ultimate responsibility for **medical direction** or oversight of the patient care aspects of the EMS system. Medical direction can be **off-line** (indirect), including protocols established by the Medical Director that authorize rescuers to perform particular skills in certain situations without actually speaking to the Medical Director. Medical direction also can be **on-line** (direct) via radio or phone contact with the on-duty physician prior to performing a skill or administering care.

The weakest link in the EMS chain is the care provided by untrained individuals who arrive before the EMTs. Training First Responders will help to solve this problem.

First Responders are an important part of the EMS system and are usually the first trained personnel to arrive at the emergency scene. The EMS system's primary goal is personal safety, which must begin with the First Responders themselves. No one should enter or approach an emergency scene until it is found to be safe. No one should begin patient assessment and care without first donning personal protective equipment.

A First Responder's main duties are: sizing up the scene to ensure the scene is safe to enter, gaining access to the patient, finding out what is wrong with the patient and providing emergency care, moving patients (when necessary), transferring the patient and any patient information to more highly trained personnel when they arrive at the scene, protecting the patient's privacy and maintaining confidentiality, and being the patient's advocate.

Included in those duties are responsibilities such as controlling the scene, calling the emergency dispatcher, obtaining help from bystanders, and assisting more highly trained personnel when they arrive.

First Responder emergency care deals with both injury and illness. Care can range from emotional support to basic life support (BLS) measures. First Responders have to maintain skills, keep up to date, and deal with people. They also must know what they should and should not say to patients and their families. Performing as professionals is an important First Responder responsibility.

The decision to become a First Responder is an important one. You should give full consideration to all aspects of emergency care and the training program before taking the step to become a First Responder. Once you have decided, however, you will find it to be very rewarding.

✔ Remember the levels of EMS training and the level of care each member can perform. When you turn over care of a patient to another member of the EMS system, be sure he or she is certified and is able to provide adequate care for the patient. If someone tells you that he or she is an EMT, you have the right, even the responsibility, to request proof of certification if the person is unknown to you.

✔ Keep the roles and responsibilities as well as the traits of the First Responder in mind. Go over a mental checklist occasionally to make sure you are maintaining the necessary level of competency.

✔ Think about the qualities you would like to see in a First Responder who renders care to you or your loved ones. Do you have those qualities? If not, think about how you can come closer to being that kind of First Responder. If possible, talk to someone who is a First Responder or EMT-B to get additional insight.

☑ Determine the locations of medical facilities in your area and the level of care or special services they provide. Also find out where specialty centers are located and how patients are transported to them if they are not in the immediate area.

☑ Learn what you must do to refresh your knowledge and maintain your certification. Find and attend continuing education classes whenever possible.

☑ Investigate the specific statutes and regulations in your state or province regarding the EMS system.

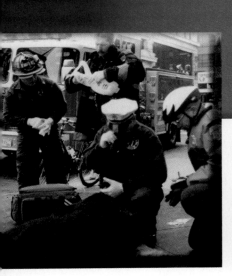
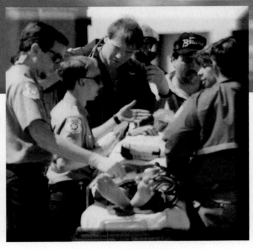
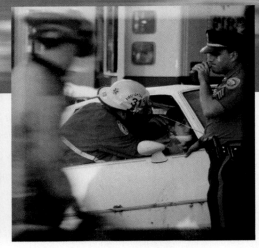

Legal and Ethical Issues

A First Responder must make many decisions in relation to patient care. Understanding the legalities and ethics of a situation will aid in making those decisions better ones.

You may already have concerns about some legal and ethical issues. For example: Should an off-duty First Responder stop to aid victims of an automobile crash? Should the First Responder release patient information to an attorney over the telephone? May a child with a broken arm be treated, even if a parent is not present? What should happen when a patient who needs emergency medical care refuses it?

This chapter will provide you with information and guidance that will be of assistance to you in answering just such important questions.

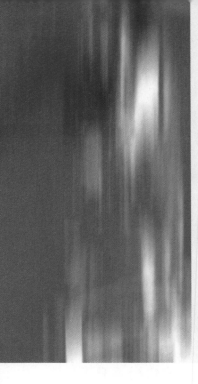

NATIONAL STANDARD OBJECTIVES

This chapter focuses on the objectives of Module 1, Lesson 1–3, of the U.S. DOT's First Responder National Standard Curriculum and serves as an instructional aid to help you meet any specific objectives added to the course by your local EMS system.

By the end of this chapter, you will know how to (from cognitive or knowledge information):

1–3.1 Define the First Responder scope of care. (p. 19)

1–3.2 Discuss the importance of Do Not Resuscitate [DNR] (advance directives) and local or state provisions regarding EMS application. (pp. 23–25)

1–3.3 Define consent and discuss the methods of obtaining consent. (pp. 21–23)

1–3.4 Differentiate between expressed and implied consent. (pp. 21–23)

1–3.5 Explain the role of consent of minors in providing care. (pp. 22–23)

1–3.6 Discuss the implications for the First Responder in patient refusal of transport. (pp. 21–22)

1–3.7 Discuss the issues of abandonment, negligence, and battery, and their implications to the First Responder. (pp. 25–28)

LEARNING TASKS

Good Samaritan laws have been developed in most states to encourage passersby to stop and assist someone who needs emergency care. These laws minimize exposure to civil liability.

✔ Find out if your state has Good Samaritan laws and who they protect and to what extent.

✔ Find out how the Good Samaritan laws relate to you when you are on duty and when you are off duty.

Do Not Resuscitate (DNR) orders are different for each state. It is necessary for the First Responder to become familiar with the legal DNR orders for his or her region or state and the laws and rules governing their implementation. Situations for which DNR orders have been written are always stressful for both the patient's family and EMS personnel.

✔ Become familiar with the forms and policies pertaining to DNR orders in your state or jurisdiction.

LEGAL DUTIES

FIRST➤ Most of us have heard about people being sued because of something they did or did not do when they stopped to help someone at the scene of an emergency. Successful suits of this type are not very common. Most states have established laws that minimize exposure to liability and encourage passersby to provide emergency care to those in need. These laws require the individual who is providing care to be doing so without promise of or actual compensation and to remain within a specified *scope of care* (sometimes called *scope of practice*). ■

I–3.8 State the conditions necessary for the First Responder to have a duty to act. (pp. 25–27)

I–3.9 Explain the importance, necessity, and legality of patient confidentiality. (p. 28)

I–3.10 List the actions that a First Responder should take to assist in the preservation of a crime scene. (pp. 29–31)

I–3.11 State the conditions that require a First Responder to notify local law enforcement officials. (pp. 28–29)

I–3.12 Discuss issues concerning the fundamental components of documentation. (p. 31)

Feel comfortable enough to
(by changing attitudes, values, and beliefs):

I–3.13 Explain the rationale for the needs, benefits, and usage of advance directives. (pp. 23–25)

I–3.14 Explain the rationale for the concept of varying degrees of DNR. (pp. 23–25)

SCOPE OF CARE

The term **scope of care** (or *scope of practice*) refers to the level at which a particular individual has been trained to provide emergency medical care. The scope of care for a layperson is somewhat subjective and might be based on nothing more than common sense or an eight-hour first-aid class taken many years ago. However, the scope of care for First Responders and other EMS care providers is clearly defined by the U.S. Department of Transportation's (DOT's) national standard curricula.

scope of care the level at which a particular individual has been trained to provide emergency medical care. Also called *scope of practice*.

STANDARD OF CARE

The term **standard of care** refers to something more regional. It is based on local laws, administrative orders, and guidelines and protocols established by the local EMS system. It refers to the way prehospital care is practiced in a given jurisdiction and reflects the unique characteristics of that region (Figure 2.1).

standard of care the care provided based on local laws, administrative orders, and guidelines and protocols established by the local EMS system.

In any given region, the standard of care may differ from the scope of care. For instance, the scope of care for an EMT-Basic includes the use of endotracheal intubation, which is the placing of a specialized tube into the trachea of a nonbreathing patient. While this skill is included in the EMT-Basic curriculum, most EMS systems do not allow EMT-Basics to perform it as part of their local standard of care.

The standard of care allows you to be judged based on what is expected of someone with your training and experience working under similar conditions. Your First Responder course follows guidelines proposed by the U.S. Department of Transportation (DOT) or another authority that has studied what is needed to provide the standard of care required at the First Responder level in your region. You will be trained so that you can provide this standard of care. If the care you provide is not up to the standard of care, you may be held liable for your actions.

There may also be medical direction available in your locality. You may be required to communicate with your Medical Director by telephone or radio or there may be approved standing orders or protocols for you to follow.

Keep written notes of what you do at the emergency scene, especially if a crime has occurred. You may be called on to provide this information at a later date. If your EMS system requires you to complete forms, submit reports, or sign patient

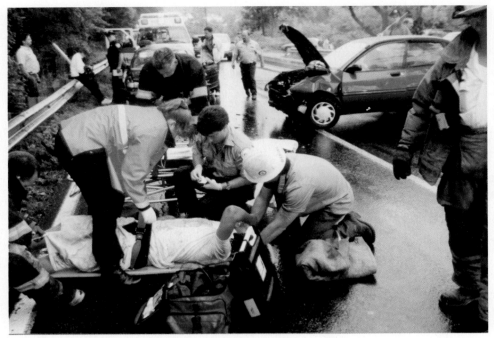

FIGURE 2.1
Different emergency personnel may be assisting during an emergency, including police, firefighters, and EMTs. Each must practice the standard of care expected of his own level of training.

transfer papers, do so at the proper time. You must be able to show that you provided an appropriate standard of care.

ETHICAL RESPONSIBILITIES

There are also ethical responsibilities that the First Responder must be aware of. Your primary ethical consideration is to make the physical and emotional needs of the patient a priority (Figure 2.2). An example would be turning up the heat if the patient feels cold, even if you are feeling overheated. Another ethical responsibility is maintaining your skills and knowledge. This includes practicing until you have obtained confidence and mastery of the skills. You also must attend continuing education and refresher programs. Every patient deserves the best care possible, and it is necessary to keep yourself ready to perform at your level of training at all times.

It is also important that you demonstrate honesty in reporting care that was provided to a patient, even if a mistake was made. While all EMS providers should

FIGURE 2.2
Ethical conduct means that First Responders give all patients respectful and considerate care.

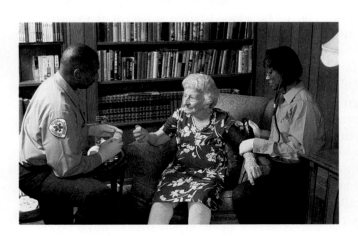

attempt at all times to provide the appropriate care, mistakes do happen. Errors should be reported immediately so any corrective procedures necessary may be instituted as soon as possible.

CONSENT

COMPETENCE

Competence is the patient's ability to understand a First Responder's questions and the implications of decisions made. In order for a First Responder to get consent or a refusal of care, the First Responder should establish if the patient is competent to make such decisions. The patient is not competent to make medical decisions in certain cases, such as intoxication, drug ingestion, serious injury, or mental incompetence. In order to determine competency, the First Responder may ask questions that a competent adult should be able to answer, such as where the patient is at the time, what season of the year it is, and so on. Answering these questions, however, does not always establish competence, as in the case of suicidal patients.

REFUSAL OF CARE

FIRST➤ When alert and competent, adults have the right to refuse care. Their refusal may be based on a variety of reasons, including economic or religious ones. They may even base it on a lack of trust. In fact, they may have reasons that you find senseless. For whatever reason, competent adults may refuse care. You cannot force care on them, nor can you restrain them until EMTs arrive. Restraining a competent adult against his or her wishes could result in a charge of battery for the First Responder. Your only course of action is to try to gain a patient's confidence through conversation.

The courts recognize implied refusal of care. In other words, the patient does not have to speak to refuse your care. If the patient shakes his head to signal "no," or if he holds up his hand to signal you to stop, the patient has refused your help. Should the patient pull away from you, this also may be viewed as refusal of care. ■

When your services are refused:

- Do *not* argue with a patient.

- Do *not* question a patient's reasons if they are based on religious beliefs.

- Do *not* touch a patient. If you do, this could be considered battery and a civil rights violation.

- Stay calm and professional. Any added stress to a patient because of your actions could cause serious complications.

- Make certain that dispatch is alerted, even if a patient has stated he does not want anyone's help.

- Talk with the patient. Let him know that you are concerned. Tell him that you respect his right to refuse care, but that you think he should reconsider your offer to help.

- Carefully document the refusal of care. Document your offer of help, your explanation of your level of training, why you think care is needed, the consequences for not accepting care, and the patient's refusal to accept your care.

Also document the names of anyone who witnessed your efforts to assist the patient. If your EMS system provides you with release forms, ask the patient to please read and sign the form. Make certain that you ask him if he understands what he has read before signing the form.

A parent or legal guardian can refuse to let you care for a child. If the reason is fear or lack of confidence, simple conversation may change the individual's mind. In cases involving children, if the adult takes the child from the scene before EMTs arrive, you must report the incident to the EMTs or to the police. Some states have special laws protecting the welfare of children. In these states, such information may have to be passed on to the courts in order to find out if the child eventually received needed care. Know the laws in your state and jurisdiction regarding reporting such events. In all cases know and follow local protocols.

EXPRESSED CONSENT

expressed consent consent to emergency care that is given to a First Responder by a competent adult who has made an informed decision.

FIRST➤ An adult patient of legal age, when alert and competent, can give you consent to provide care. In First Responder care, a patient's consent is usually oral and commonly referred to as **expressed consent** or *informed consent*. To qualify as expressed consent, the patient must be making an informed decision (Figure 2.3).

To make an informed decision, you need to advise the patient that you are a First Responder, trained in emergency care. You also must tell the patient:

● Your level of training.
● Why you think care may be necessary.
● What you are going to do.
● If there is any risk to the care you offer or risk related to refusing care. ■

There are occasions when a child refuses care. By law only a parent or guardian of the child may give consent or refuse your care. Of course, gaining the child's confidence and easing any fears should be part of your care.

FIGURE 2.3
Obtaining consent from an adult patient.

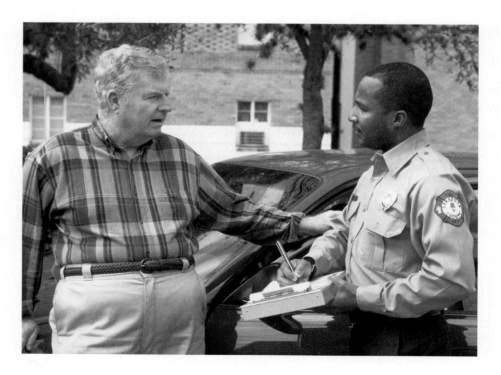

IMPLIED CONSENT

In emergency situations in which a patient is **unresponsive**, confused, or so severely injured that a clear decision cannot be made, you have the right to provide care based on **implied consent**. The law assumes that the patient, if able to do so, would want to receive care and treatment. Since children and mentally incompetent adults are not legally allowed to provide consent or to refuse medical care, a form of implied consent is used in most states when a minor is involved and the parents or guardians are not on the scene and cannot be reached quickly. The law assumes that they would want care to be provided for their child (Figure 2.4). The same holds true in cases of mentally ill people who are hallucinating or having homicidal or suicidal thoughts or in cases of emotionally disturbed or retarded individuals. It is assumed that their parents or legal guardians would give consent for treatment.

unresponsive no reaction to verbal or painful stimuli; previously referred to as *unconscious*.

implied consent a legal position that assumes an unresponsive or incompetent adult patient would consent to receiving emergency care if he could. This form of consent may apply to other types of patients (for example, the mentally ill).

DO NOT RESUSCITATE (DNR) ORDERS

FIRST➤ At some time, you will come upon a patient who has a Do Not Resuscitate (DNR) order. This may be a legal document, usually signed by the patient and his or her physician, which states that the patient has a terminal illness and does not wish to prolong life through resuscitative efforts. A DNR order is one type of *advance directive*, because it is written and signed in advance of any event where resuscitation might be undertaken (Figure 2.5). A DNR order is more than the expressed wishes of the patient or family. It is an actual legal document. In some cases, the patient will be wearing a DNR bracelet. This should not be mistaken for a medical identification bracelet, which gives information about medical conditions and/or allergies. ■

There are varying degrees of DNR orders, expressed through a variety of detailed instructions. For example, an instruction might stipulate that resuscitation be

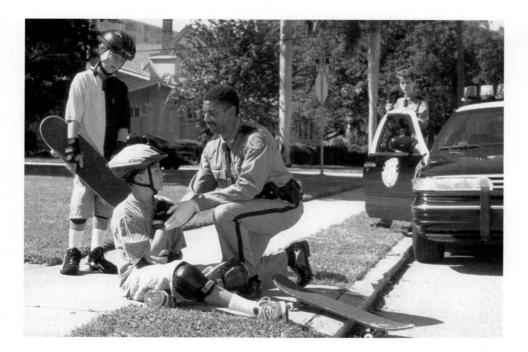

FIGURE 2.4
Use implied consent to provide care to a minor when a parent or guardian is not available.

PREHOSPITAL DO NOT RESUSCITATE ORDERS

ATTENDING PHYSICIAN

In completing this prehospital DNR form, please check part A if no intervention by prehospital personnel is indicated. Please check Part A and options from Part B if specific interventions by prehospital personnel are indicated. To give a valid prehospital DNR order, this form must be completed by the patient's attending physician and must be provided to prehospital personnel.

A) _____ **Do Not Resuscitate (DNR):**
No Cardiopulmonary Resuscitation or Advanced Cardiac Life Support be performed by prehospital personnel

B) _____ **Modified Support:**
Prehospital personnel administer the following checked options:
_____ Oxygen administration
_____ Full airway support: intubation, airways, bag/valve/mask
_____ Venipuncture: IV crystalloids and/or blood draw
_____ External cardiac pacing
_____ Cardiopulmonary resuscitation
_____ Cardiac defibrillator
_____ Pneumatic anti-shock garment
_____ Ventilator
_____ ACLS meds
_____ Other interventions/medications (physician specify)
_____

Prehospital personnel are informed that (print patient name)_____
should receive no resuscitation (DNR) or should receive Modified Support as indicated. This directive is medically appropriate and is further documented by a physician's order and a progress note on the patient's permanent medical record. Informed consent from the capacitated patient or the incapacitated patient's legitimate surrogate is documented on the patient's permanent medical record. The DNR order is in full force and effect as of the date indicated below.

_____   _____
Attending Physician's Signature

_____   _____
Print Attending Physician's Name   Print Patient's Name and Location
                                          (Home Address or Health Care Facility)

_____
Attending Physician's Telephone

_____   _____
Date   Expiration Date (6 Mos from Signature)

FIGURE 2.5
A DNR order is one example of an advance directive. Other examples include health-care proxies and living wills.

attempted only if cardiac or respiratory arrest is observed, but not attempted if the patient is found already in arrest. (This degree of DNR order is meant to avoid the possibility of resuscitating a patient who may already have sustained brain damage.)

Many states also have laws governing living wills. These are statements signed by the patient, usually about use of long-term life support and comfort measures such as respirators, intravenous feedings, and pain medications.

If a patient refuses care, then becomes unresponsive, implied consent usually takes over and care can begin. This is a legal and ethical dilemma that is usually best resolved by providing care. It is better to be criticized or sued for saving a life than for letting a patient die. A legal DNR order prevents these unwanted resuscitation efforts and other situations where cardiac arrest is anticipated. In most cases, the oral requests of a family member are *not* reason to withhold care.

NEGLIGENCE

FIRST➤ The basis for most lawsuits involving prehospital emergency care is **negligence**. This is a term often used to indicate that either a care provider did not do what was expected or did something carelessly. However, from a legal standpoint, negligence is a more complicated concept than that.

negligence a failure to provide the expected standard of care.

In order for a lawsuit alleging negligence to be successful, the following four elements must be established:

- *Duty*—The First Responder had a legal duty to provide care.
- *Breach of duty*—Care for the patient was not provided to an acceptable standard of care.
- *Damages*—The patient was injured (damaged) in some way as a result of improper care or the lack thereof.
- *Causation*—A direct link can be established between the damages and the breach of duty on the part of the First Responder. ■

First Responders in the police and fire service have a **duty to act**. This means that they are required, at least while on duty, to provide care according to their department's standard operating procedures. In some localities, this duty to act may also apply to paid First Responders when they are on their day off (Figure 2.6).

duty to act a requirement that First Responders in the police and fire service, at least while on duty, must provide care according to their department's standard operating procedures.

The duty to act is not so clear in the case of volunteer First Responders. What is expected when they are off duty is unclear because many states do not have specific laws concerning First Responders. Most laws provide direction for physicians and nurses only, while some legislation deals with allied health specialists and EMTs. Several states are now in the process of considering more specific laws for their EMS systems.

Since the laws governing the duty to act vary from state to state, and what is implied in laws that cover the emergency services also varies, your instructor or local EMS system will tell you the specifics as to when you are required to respond and provide care. Your duties will be spelled out and include consideration for your level of training and your safety at the emergency scene.

A First Responder is considered to have a duty to act once help is offered to a patient. If care is offered and then accepted by the patient, it could be assumed that the First Responder has established a legal duty to act. A court might decide that this meets the first requirement for negligence in cases where the standard of care was not met and the patient suffered injury due to this improper care.

After a duty to act has been established, the second condition for negligence would be applicable if care was substandard for the First Responder's level of training and experience under the conditions of the emergency scene. The same would apply if the care rendered was beyond his scope of practice. In either case, the care provided was not to an acceptable standard of care.

Finally, if there was a duty to act and the standard of care was not met, a suit for negligence may be successful if the patient was injured (damaged) in some way due directly to the inappropriate actions of the First Responder. This is a complex legal idea, made more difficult by the fact that the damage may be physical, emotional, or psychological.

FIGURE 2.6
First Responders may have a duty
to act at an emergency scene.

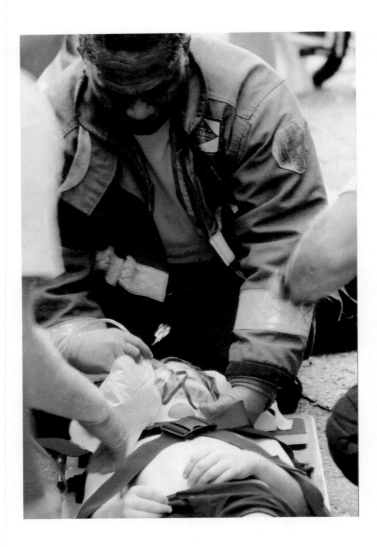

Physical damage is the easiest to understand. For example, if a First Responder moved a patient's injured leg before applying a splint and the standard of care states that the First Responder should have suspected a fracture and splinted the limb, then the First Responder may be negligent if this action worsened the existing injury.

The same case becomes much more involved when the patient claims that the First Responder's inappropriate action caused emotional or psychological problems. The court could decide that the patient has been damaged and establish the third requirement for negligence.

Inappropriate care does not always involve splinting, bandaging, or some other physical skill. As a general rule, you should always advise a patient to seek treatment by EMTs and to go to the hospital. If you tell an ill or injured patient that he does not need to be seen by EMTs or other more highly trained personnel, you could be negligent if you had a duty to act and the patient accepted your care, but:

● Standard of care stated that you should have alerted or had someone activate the EMS system to request an EMT response, and you failed to do so.

● Delay in care caused complications that led to additional injury.

FIRST➤ As stated above, a requirement for proof of negligence is the failure of the First Responder to provide care to a recognized and acceptable standard of care. There is no guarantee that you will not be sued, but a successful suit is unlikely if you provide care to an acceptable standard. ■

If your state has **Good Samaritan laws**, you may be protected from civil liability if you act in good faith to provide care to the level of your training and to the best of your ability. You will be trained to deliver the standard of care expected of First Responders. Your instructor will explain any differences in the laws of your state.

Another factor you must consider is how the Good Samaritan laws of your state affect your liability if you are a paid provider of emergency care. In some states, special laws apply to paid providers, while the Good Samaritan laws apply only to unpaid volunteers. Again, your instructor or local EMS system can provide you with the needed information.

ABANDONMENT

FIRST➤ Once you begin to help someone who is sick or injured, you have established a legal duty and must continue to provide care until you turn over patient care to someone of equal or higher training (such as an EMT or physician). If you leave the scene before more highly trained personnel arrive, you have abandoned the patient and are subject to legal action under specific laws of **abandonment** (Figure 2.7).

Since you are not trained in medical diagnosis or how to predict the stability of a patient, you should not leave a patient if someone with training equal to your own arrives at the scene. The patient may develop more serious problems that would be better handled by two First Responders.

Some legal authorities consider abandonment to include the failure to turn over patient information during the transfer of the patient to more highly trained

> **NOTE**
>
> A requirement for proof of negligence is the First Responder's failure to provide the recognized standard of care.

Good Samaritan laws a series of state laws designed to protect certain care providers if they deliver the standard of care in good faith, to the level of their training, and to the best of their abilities.

abandonment to leave a sick or injured patient before equal or more highly trained personnel can assume responsibility for care.

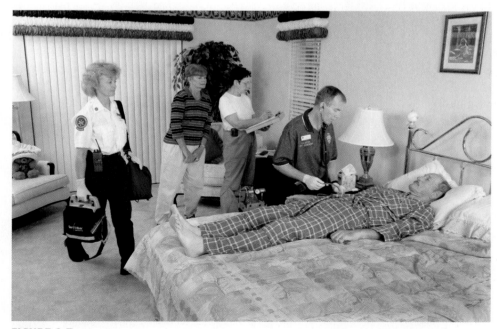

FIGURE 2.7
Once care is initiated, the First Responder assumes responsibility of the patient until relieved by more highly trained personnel.

personnel. You must inform those providers of the facts that you gathered, the assessment made, and the care rendered. ■

CONFIDENTIALITY

You should not speak to your friends, family, and other members of the public (including the press and media) about the details of care you have provided to a patient. You should not name the individuals who received your care. If you speak of the emergency, you should not relate specifics about what a patient may have said, any unusual aspects of behavior, or any descriptions of personal appearance. To do so invades the privacy of the patient. Your state may not have specific laws stating the above, but most individuals in emergency care feel very strongly about protecting the patient's right to privacy. Information about an emergency and patient care should only be released if the patient has authorized you to do so in writing.

Authorization is not required for you to pass on patient information to other health-care providers who arrive to transport and continue care for the patient (Figure 2.8). This pertinent information should also be passed on to emergency department personnel who will be caring for the patient.

REPORTABLE EVENTS

First Responders cannot limit their activities to the assessment and care of patients. Some additional activities are required specific to state guidelines or industrial or military protocols; others are required universally. For example, all First Responders must report certain events or conditions that they know or suspect have occurred. In fact, federal and state agencies require that certain events be re-

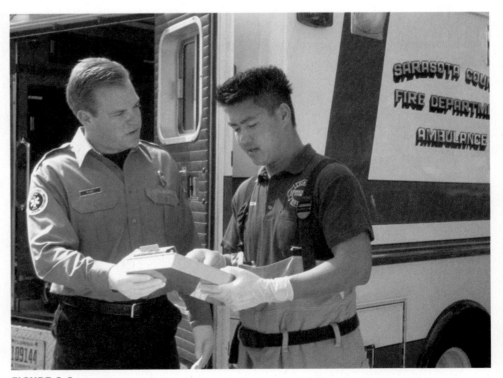

FIGURE 2.8
To maintain patient confidentiality, discuss your patient only with those who will be continuing patient care.

ported. These events include exposures to certain infectious diseases, suspicious burns, vehicle crashes, drug-related injuries, and crimes that result in knife or gunshot wounds, child and elder abuse, domestic violence, and rape. Check with your chief officer, EMS division chief, or with state and federal agencies to learn which incidents are reportable in your area and to whom or to which agency you should report them. Crimes, vehicle crashes, and drug injuries are reported to the police; exposures to infectious disease are usually first reported to your supervisor.

SPECIAL SITUATIONS

ORGAN DONORS

You may respond to a call where a critically injured patient is near death and has been identified as an organ donor. An organ donor is a patient who has completed a legal document that allows for donation of organs and tissues in the event of his or her death. A family member may give you this information, or you may find an organ donor card in a patient's personal effects. Sometimes this information is indicated on the patient's driver license. Ideally, a family member or police officer should go through the patient's effects, but you may look for this document without consent of the patient or his family.

Emergency care of a patient who is an organ donor must not differ in any way from the care of a patient who is not a donor. All emergency care measures must be taken, including performing CPR on a patient you might not normally resuscitate due to the extent of fatal injuries. The oxygen delivered to body cells by CPR will help preserve the organs until they can be harvested for implantation in another person.

MEDICAL IDENTIFICATION DEVICES

Another special situation involves the patient who wears a medical identification device (Figure 2.9). This device—necklace, arm or ankle bracelet, or card—is meant to alert EMS personnel that the patient has a particular medical condition, such as a heart problem, allergies, diabetes, or epilepsy. If the patient is unresponsive or unable to answer questions, this device may provide important medical information.

In some areas of the country the "Vial of Life" program is currently in use. This program offers specific documentation and a special vial where it is stored. The vial is then kept in the patient's refrigerator where it can be found easily by rescuers. Members of the "Vial of Life" program often display a sticker in the front window of their home alerting rescuers to the vial in the refrigerator.

CRIME SCENES

A crime scene is defined as the location where a crime has been committed or any place where evidence relating to a crime may be found. Many crime scenes involve crimes against people, which may cause injuries that are serious. Once the scene has been made safe by police, providing patient care is a priority.

When the First Responder is providing care at a crime scene, certain actions should be taken to preserve evidence. Make as little impact on the scene as possible, only moving items necessary for patient care. Remember the position of the patient and preserve any clothing you may remove or damage. Try not to cut through holes in clothing from gunshot wounds or stabbings. Remember and report any items you move or touch. If you arrived at the scene before the police, remember if doors were ajar or windows open. These signs indicate danger for you

remember

Patient confidentiality does *not* apply if you are required by law to report certain incidents (such as rape, abuse, or gunshot wounds), if you are asked to provide information to the police, or if you receive a subpoena to testify in court. Maintain notes about each incident to which you respond, and keep a copy of any official documents filled out by you or responding EMTs.

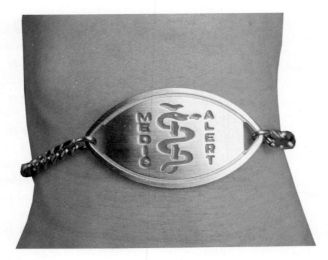
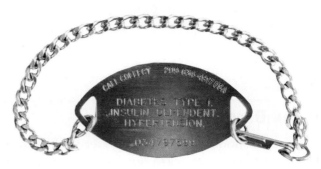

as well. If you have any reason to suspect that a scene is not safe, you should go no farther until police say it is safe to do so.

It is important that EMS personnel and police work together. Sometimes the police may be unfamiliar with EMS procedures and request that you delay patient care in order for them to take pictures or interview the patient. It does not help if tempers are allowed to flare in situations such as this. Explain to the officers as calmly and quickly as possible that delay may cause serious problems in this case and continue your care. It is not appropriate for either of you to engage in an argument while patient care is being performed. This is best handled after the event, perhaps at a joint critique of the incident. As you become familiar with the police officials in your community, and they with you, knowledge of and respect for your

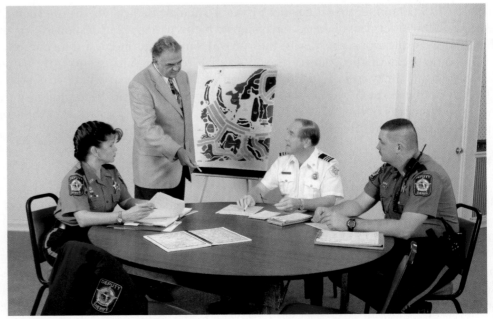

FIGURE 2.10
Police and fire department personnel can meet and establish in advance how to handle emergencies so that there are no conflicts.

respective jobs will grow between you, making you a more effective team in emergency situations. It may be a good idea to establish in advance how these situations will be handled so that there are no conflicts on scene (Figure 2.10).

DOCUMENTATION

Documentation is an important part of the patient care process and may last long after the call is over. Some states do not require First Responders to complete specific types of documentation, but you would be wise to keep records of all calls to which you respond (Figure 2.11). They may be needed in the event of subpoena or lawsuit. Your instructor will inform you of legal requirements in your area.

In special situations, you may be required by law to make written or verbal reports. Special situations include child, elder, or spouse abuse; wounds sustained or potentially sustained by violent crime; sexual assault; or infectious-disease exposure. Again, your instructor will inform you of requirements in your area.

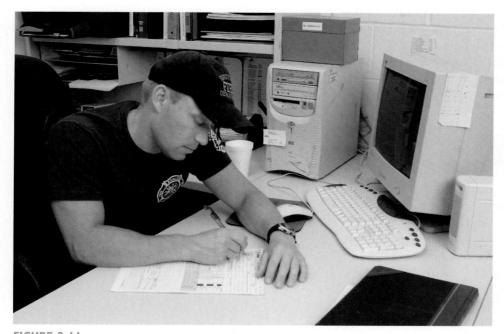

FIGURE 2.11

Even if you are not required to do so, keep records of all calls to which you respond in case they are needed as evidence in court.

Chapter Review

SUMMARY

First Responders have to learn and maintain their skills and knowledge to a level where they can perform patient care to the expected standard of care. In many states, specific laws have been written to allow you to provide emergency care to patients without fear of successful civil legal action being taken against you. Under the Good Samaritan laws, you may be protected from liability. That is, you may be protected if you act in good faith, not for compensation, to a **standard of care** at your level of training and to the best of your abilities.

A patient may refuse your care. You must have **expressed consent** from a responsive, competent adult patient before you may provide care. This consent is usually oral. It must be **informed consent**, with the patient knowing your level of training and what you are going to do. In cases in which the patient is unable to give consent, you may care for the patient under the law of **implied consent**. Implied consent also applies to children and emotionally or mentally disturbed or retarded patients when their parents or legal guardians are not present.

A First Responder may be guilty of **negligence** if it can be established that he had a legal duty to provide care, did not provide care to an acceptable standard of care, and the inappropriate care caused damage (injury) to the patient. When you stop to provide care, you are responsible for the patient until someone more highly trained takes over. If you start to care for a patient and then leave the scene, you can be charged with **abandonment**.

Keep in mind that patients have a right to privacy, so you must respect patient confidentiality. Also remember that care for organ donors should not differ from care given to any other patient, that medical identification devices worn or carried by a patient can provide important medical information, and that you should try to preserve evidence when caring for a patient at a crime scene.

Documentation is part of the patient care process. Keep records!

REMEMBER AND CONSIDER

Every time you respond to a call, you will be faced with some aspect of legal or ethical issues. It may be as simple as making sure the patient is willing to accept your help or as complex as a terminally ill patient who refuses your care. You may have to decide whether or not to stop and help even though you are off duty. You may worry about being sued.

✓ Make sure you are aware of legal requirements and are comfortable with ethical decisions in order to reduce your stress in these situations.

INVESTIGATE

Knowledge is your best protection. Each state enacts laws that protect citizens, but state laws vary. Be sure you are familiar with the laws of your state that guide the actions of First Responders. Check with your department's legal office or with your supervising officers on the legal details of patient consent and care.

✓ Find out what types of consent forms and run sheets for documentation are used in your jurisdiction.

✓ Obtain and review a sample DNR order from the library or a lawyer. Find out if DNR bracelets are used in your jurisdiction.

✓ Learn the different types of evidence and ways you may help to preserve them at a crime scene.

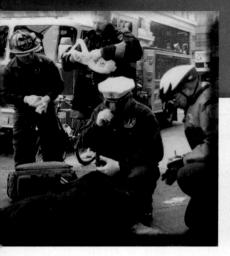
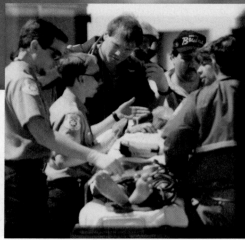
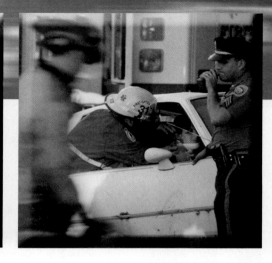

Well-Being of the First Responder

Learning how to take care of yourself in emergency situations is critical. If you do not make personal safety your first priority, you will likely become another victim and part of the problem, further stressing the EMS system. First Responders face challenges—emotional and physical—when acting as part of the EMS team. Knowing about these dangers beforehand can help prepare you to handle them when they arise.

This chapter will help you to learn what to expect and describes how you can assist yourself, the patient, the patient's family, your own family, and other First Responders in dealing with stress. Aspects of personal safety, including how you can protect yourself from infectious diseases, are also presented.

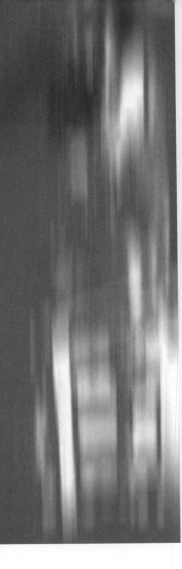

NATIONAL STANDARD OBJECTIVES

This chapter focuses on the objectives of Module 1, Lesson 1–2, of the U.S. DOT's First Responder National Standard Curriculum and serves as an instructional aid to help you meet any specific objectives added to the course by your local EMS system.

By the end of this chapter, you will be able to (from cognitive or knowledge information):

1–2.1 List possible emotional reactions that the First Responder may experience when faced with trauma, illness, death, and dying. (pp. 35–41)

1–2.2 Discuss the possible reactions that a family member may exhibit when confronted with death and dying. (pp. 38–39)

1–2.3 State the steps in the First Responder's approach to the family confronted with death and dying. (pp. 38–39)

1–2.4 State the possible reactions that the family of the First Responder may exhibit. (p. 40)

1–2.5 Recognize the signs and symptoms of critical incident stress. (pp. 36–37, 39)

1–2.6 State possible steps that the First Responder may take to help reduce/alleviate stress. (pp. 40–41)

1–2.7 Explain the need to determine scene safety. (pp. 48–50)

1–2.8 Discuss the importance of body substance isolation (BSI). (pp. 42–48)

1–2.9 Describe the steps the First Responder should take for personal protection from airborne and bloodborne pathogens. (pp. 43–48)

1–2.10 List the personal protective equipment necessary for each of the following situations: (pp. 43–50)

    Hazardous materials

    Rescue operation

    Exposure to bloodborne pathogens

    Violent scenes

LEARNING TASKS

Many states have a crisis intervention or critical incident stress management (CISM) team in place to help responders deal with the stress of a difficult emergency. Talk with your agency and find out about crisis intervention resources. Be able to:

✔ Identify the crisis intervention or CISM team in your region and determine how to access its services.

Protecting yourself—and your patients—from infectious diseases is very important. You must wear protective equipment when responding to emergencies and you should use special disinfectants to clean equipment. As a First Responder, you must be able to:

✔ Put on all personal protective equipment and use it in appropriate situations.
✔ Take off and appropriately discard or dispose of all personal protective equipment.
✔ Disinfect or clean all non-disposable equipment used in patient care.
✔ Properly dispose of all disposable equipment used in patient care.

One of your most important jobs is to stay safe, both physically and emotionally. If you become a victim, you will be of little or no use to a patient, and you may actually put other rescuers in danger. Safeguard yourself by doing the following:

✔ Learn about stressors and understand how to deal with them, especially those that accompany critical incidents.

Crime scenes

Exposure to airborne pathogens

Electricity

Feel comfortable enough to
(by changing attitudes, values, and beliefs):

1–2.11 Explain the importance of serving as an advocate for the use of appropriate protective equipment. (pp. 46–48)

1–2.12 Explain the importance of understanding the response to death and dying and communicating effectively with the patient's family. (pp. 38–39)

1–2.13 Demonstrate a caring attitude toward any patient with illness or injury who requests emergency medical services. (pp. 39, 48)

1–2.14 Show compassion when caring for the physical and mental needs of patients. (pp. 38–39)

1–2.15 Participate willingly in the care of all patients. (p. 48)

1–2.16 Communicate with empathy to patients being cared for, as well as with family members and friends of the patient. (pp. 38–39)

Show how to
(through psychomotor skills):

1–2.17 Given a scenario with potential infectious exposure, the First Responder will use appropriate personal protective equipment. At the completion of the scenario, the First Responder will properly remove and discard the protective garments. (pp. 44, 46–48)

1–2.18 Given the above scenario, the First Responder will complete disinfection/cleaning and all reporting documentation. (pp. 43–48)

✔ Constantly evaluate scene safety.

✔ Before providing emergency care to a patient, always use appropriate body substance isolation (BSI) precautions. That includes wearing gloves at a minimum, and eye protection or face mask and gown as necessary.

EMOTIONAL ASPECTS OF EMERGENCY MEDICAL CARE

FIRST RESPONDERS AND STRESS

Almost everyone must face and deal with some type of **stress** on a daily basis, whether driving in traffic, coping with work and family problems or schedules, meeting school and office deadlines, or waiting for an appointment. Surveys and research reports over the past two decades have revealed that 43% of all adults suffer adverse health effects from stress. In fact, stress may be a factor in 80% of all nontraumatic deaths. Recent research confirms that stress contributes to cardiovascular disease, stroke, diabetes, cancer, arthritis, as well as to gastrointestinal, skin, neurological, and emotional disorders.

For First Responders, stress is a concern for several reasons. The job makes intense physical and psychological demands on emotional and physical well-being. Police officers, firefighters, and disaster response personnel must respond quickly to emergencies and react instantly to situations where lives are at risk. Their need

stress the emotional strain placed on an individual by a situation or a specific element of a situation.

to make immediate decisions about patient care is a big responsibility, and First Responders realize that making a mistake may mean that a patient dies.

Death is not the only fear associated with mistakes in providing care. A mistake can cause an injury to become more serious or pain to become more intense. Care that is delayed at the scene or done improperly may cause a problem that might become chronic for the patient or lead to loss of function.

Another Side of Personal Safety

A threat to the First Responder's well-being is not always as obvious as a burning car or contaminated needle. Sometimes the threat is the emotional reaction to an emergency. Often, providers depend on professional training to put aside their own emotions in order to help patients (Figure 3.1). But patients will suffer and some may die. The result often is a delayed emotional response. We now know that delayed responses are normal and even important to the provider's well-being.

Emergency experiences are stressful and cause a range of reactions. Though First Responders are trained to handle difficult situations, they are not untouched by what they see and do on the job. You must find ways to cope with job-related stressors, keeping in mind that a **stressor** is any factor that causes wear and tear on the body's physical or mental resources. Those who do not find ways to cope with stress can become depressed, suffer physical disorders, experience burnout, and may have to leave the field permanently or suffer personal difficulties that may affect family relationships, work, or school. Though others may appear to be better able to battle the same events, they may be delaying the effects longer, which will eventually take its toll.

First Responders have a duty to confront the psychological effects of the work they do. Ignoring stress does not make it go away. Instead, the stress may crop up in unexpected forms, such as insomnia, fatigue, irritability, high blood pressure, heart disease, alcohol use, increased incidence of illnesses or other disruptive responses.

Causes of Stress

Emergencies are very stressful events, some more than others. The following are examples of very stressful situations, or **critical incidents**, encountered in EMS. The stress of any of these events can continue long after the event is over:

stressor the part of a situation or the situation that causes stress.

critical incident any situation that causes a rescuer to experience unusually strong emotions that interfere with the ability to function either during the incident or after; a highly stressful incident.

FIGURE 3.1
Emergencies can be stressful to all responders and care providers.

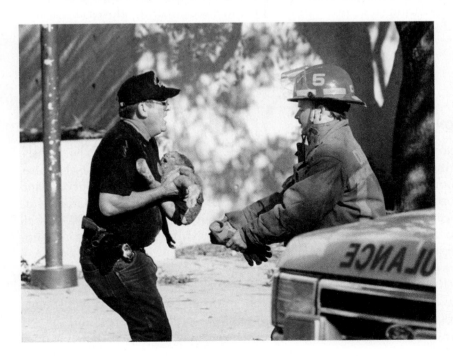

- *Multiple-casualty incidents*—An emergency that involves multiple patients is referred to as a **multiple-casualty incident (MCI)**. MCIs may range from a motor-vehicle crash that injures two drivers and a passenger to a large tropical storm that causes injury to hundreds of people (Figure 3.2).

multiple-casualty incident (MCI) a single incident that involves multiple patients. Also called a *mass-casualty incident*.

- *Pediatric patients*—Emergencies involving infants or children are considered some of the most stressful that EMS providers—even the most experienced ones—are required to handle.

- *Death*—It is can be difficult for a health-care provider to deal with the death of a patient, but even more so if the patient is young or known to the provider.

- *Violence*—Not only is it difficult to witness violence against others, it is also a dangerous situation for the First Responder to be in. Take steps to protect yourself when responding to a violent situation or in a situation that suddenly becomes violent.

- *Abuse and neglect*—As a First Responder, you may be called upon to provide care for an infant, child, adult, or elderly patient who exhibits signs of abuse or neglect. Remember that abuse and neglect occur in all social and economic levels of society.

- *Death or injury of a coworker*—Bonds are formed between members of EMS. The death or injury of another provider, even if you do not personally know that person, can cause a stressful response (Figure 3.3).

Burnout

Stress can be triggered by a single incident, but some First Responders suffer from *burnout*, a reaction to cumulative stress or exposure to multiple critical incidents. First Responders are at increased risk for burnout because of the demands and activities of the job. The signs of burnout include a loss of enthusiasm and energy, replaced by feelings of frustration, hopelessness, low self-esteem, isolation, and mistrust. Many factors contribute to burnout, such as multiple or back-to-back emergency events involving serious medical problems, injuries, or death, facing public hostility, struggling with bureaucratic obstacles, earning low pay, putting up with poor working conditions, dealing with sexism, and a public who cares only when they need EMS.

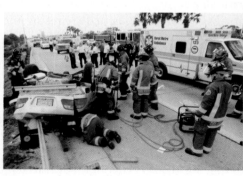

A.

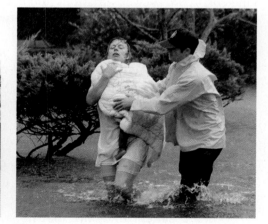

B.

FIGURE 3.2

A range of stressful reactions can result from working at emergency scenes such as (A) a multiple-vehicle collision or (B) storm-related disaster.

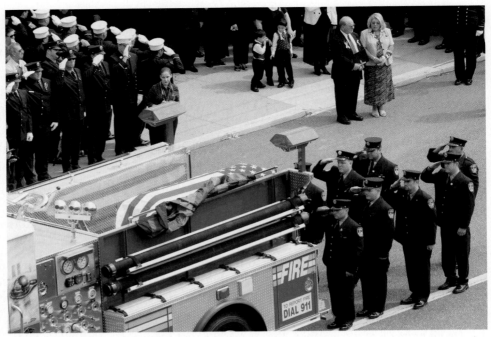

FIGURE 3.3
The death of a member of the emergency services is an emotional event.

Shift work, a disruption accepted by our society for generations, may be a significant source of stress, particularly when combined with other factors. This pattern of work is common in EMS and is found to be even more stressful now that so many families have husbands and wives working, missing meals together and time shared with their children and with each other. Continuing education needs also strain schedules that add additional problems to those in EMS compared to people who do not work shifts. Evening meals that could be restful times, even for those dining by themselves, are too often replaced with coffee and fast, high-fat food, all consumed on the run. A healthier diet and lifestyle can help First Responders combat the stressors that are an unavoidable part of the job.

Both short-term and long-term stresses are occupational hazards for First Responders. Fortunately, research in the past 15 years has found ways to reduce both kinds of stress. Newer variations and combinations of stress are being seen as people attempt to compensate for lost time and shared activities. Many individuals find that they suffer a crossover of job stress and recreational stress as they try to compensate for time lost with others or in a particular activity. The old saying of "work hard and play hard" may not be a useful expression for some, actually causing more difficulties by trying to solve a complex problem with too simple a solution.

DEATH AND DYING

As a First Responder, you will at some time have to deal with a patient who has a terminal illness. Such patients and their families will have many different reactions to the illness. A basic understanding of what they are going through will help you deal with their stress and your own.

When a patient finds out that he is dying, he will go through several stages, each varying in duration and magnitude. Sometimes these stages are not experienced in the same order given below, and sometimes the stages overlap one another. Whatever the length or order of these stages, they all affect both the patient and his family. The stages include the following:

- *Denial, or "not me"*—The patient denies that he is dying and puts off having to deal with the situation.

- *Anger, or "why me?"*—The patient is angry about the situation. This anger is often vented upon family members or even EMS personnel.

- *Bargaining, or "OK, but first let me ..."*—The patient feels that making bargains will postpone the inevitable.

- *Depression, or "OK, but I haven't ..."*—The patient becomes sad, depressed, and often mourns things that he has not accomplished. He then may become unwilling to communicate with others.

- *Acceptance, or "OK, I'm not afraid"*—The patient works through all the stages and finally is able to accept death, even though he may not welcome it. Frequently, the patient will reach this stage before family members do, in which case he may find himself comforting them.

First Responders may also encounter a patient's sudden, unexpected death, in which case the patient's family members are likely to react with a wide range of emotions. You may use several approaches when dealing with a patient who is confronted with death or dying. Most just want someone to listen to them as they express their feelings. First Responders may simply offer them the following courtesies:

- *Recognize the patients' needs.* Treat them with respect and do whatever is possible to preserve their dignity and sense of control. Speak directly to the patients and avoid talking about them to family members or friends in their presence. Try to respond to their choices about how to handle the situation. Allow patients to talk about their feelings, although it may make you feel uncomfortable. Respect their privacy if they do not want to express personal feelings.

- *Be tolerant of angry reactions* from the patient or his family members. Sometimes they will direct their anger at you, but do not take it personally. The patient and family need a chance to vent, and they will often choose whoever is nearby as a target.

- *Listen empathetically.* That is, try to understand the feelings of the patient or family member. There is seldom anything you can do to fix the situation, but sometimes just listening is very helpful.

- *Do not give false hope or reassurance.* Avoid saying things like "everything will be all right" or "there must be some good reason for this to happen." The family knows things will not be all right, and they do not want to try to justify what is happening. A simple "I'm sorry" is sufficient.

- *Offer comfort.* Let both the patient and the family know that you will do everything you can to help or that you will help them to find assistance from other sources if needed. Remember, a gentle tone of voice and possibly a reassuring touch can be very helpful.

SIGNS AND SYMPTOMS OF STRESS

The way you handle stress can affect both your emotional health and the way you respond to emergencies. Recognize the signs and symptoms of stress when they appear. They include irritability with family, friends, and coworkers; inability to concentrate; changes in daily activities, such as difficulty sleeping or nightmares, loss of appetite, and loss of interest in sexual activity; anxiety; indecisiveness; guilt; isolation; and loss of interest in work or poor performance. In addition, you might experience constipation, diarrhea, headache, nausea, and hypertension.

DEALING WITH STRESS

Stress may be caused by a single event, or it may result from the combined effects of several incidents. It is important to remember that any incident can cause different reactions in different health-care providers. Stress may also be caused from a combination of factors, including personal problems, such as friends and family members who just do not understand the job. It is frequently necessary for health-care providers to work on holidays, weekends, and during important family events. This can be frustrating to friends and family members, which may cause stress in the provider. It can also be difficult when family and friends do not understand the strong emotions involved in responding to a serious incident.

Ways in which a First Responder can deal with stress include making lifestyle changes and counseling.

Lifestyle Changes

It is often difficult to make changes in the habits or the lifestyle you have developed, but it is essential to consider the effects that current conditions are having on your well-being. Remember that your health is of primary importance. Look carefully at your life habits and consider making adjustments.

FIRST➤ There are several ways you can change your lifestyle when trying to deal with stress (Figure 3.4). They include the following:

- *Develop more healthful and positive dietary habits.* Avoid fatty foods and increase your carbohydrate intake. Also reduce your consumption of alcohol, sugar, and caffeine, which can negatively affect sleep patterns and cause irritability.

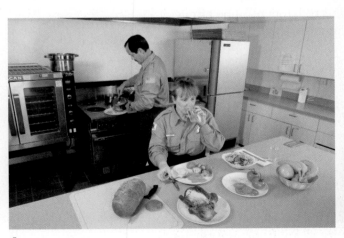

A.

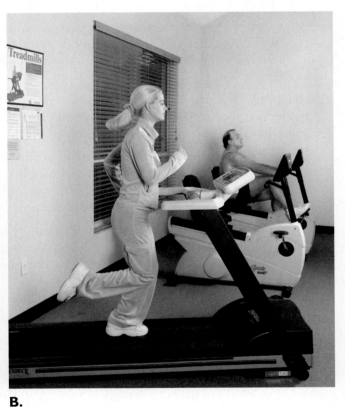

B.

FIGURE 3.4
Making lifestyle changes includes (A) eating a healthy diet and (B) exercising regularly.

- *Exercise.* Properly performed exercise helps reduce stress. It also can help you to deal with the physical aspects of your responsibilities, such as carrying equipment and performing other physically demanding emergency procedures.
- *Devote time to relaxing.* Consider trying relaxation techniques, such as deep-breathing exercises and meditation.
- *Change your work environment or shifts,* if possible, in order to allow more time to relax with family or friends, or ask for a rotation to a less stressful assignment for a brief time.
- *Seek professional help* from a mental-health professional, a social worker, or a member of the clergy. ■

Critical Incident Stress Management

FIRST➤ **Critical incident stress management (CISM)** is an in-depth, broad plan designed to help the First Responder cope with job-related stress. Part of that plan includes the **critical incident stress debriefing (CISD).** CISD is a process in which teams of trained peer counselors and mental-health professionals meet with rescuers and health-care providers who have been involved in a major incident (Figure 3.5). These meetings are usually held within 24 to 72 hours after the incident, thus making the CISD part of the CISM. The goal is to assist the providers in dealing with the stress related to that incident. ■

Participation in a CISD is strictly voluntary. No one should ever be forced or coerced to attend. Participants are encouraged to talk about their fears or their reactions to the incident. It is NOT a critique, and all participants should be made aware that whatever is said during a debriefing will be held in the strictest confidence, both by the participants themselves and the debriefing team. CISDs are usually very helpful in assisting EMS personnel to better understand their reactions and feelings both during and after an incident. They will also come to understand that other members of the team were very likely experiencing similar reactions.

After the open discussion during which everyone is encouraged to share but not forced to do so, the debriefing teams offer suggestions on how to deal with and prevent further stress. It is important to realize that stress after a major incident is both normal and to be expected. The CISD process can be very helpful in speeding up the recovery process.

Your instructor will inform you of situations in which CISD should be requested and how to access the local system.

critical incident stress management (CISM) an in-depth, broad plan designed to help rescue personnel cope with the stress resulting from a highly stressful incident.

critical incident stress debriefing (CISD) a process in which teams of professional and peer counselors provide emotional and psychological support to EMS personnel who are or have been involved in a critical (highly stressful) incident.

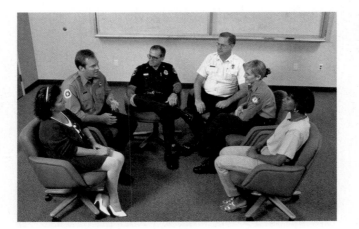

FIGURE 3.5
First Responders at a critical incident stress debriefing.

BODY SUBSTANCE ISOLATION (BSI)

FIRST RESPONDERS AT RISK

body substance isolation (BSI) practice of using specific barriers to minimize contact with a patient's blood and body fluids.

FIRST➤ As a First Responder, you will deal with emergencies involving illness and injury. Therefore, you will need to protect yourself against exposure to infectious diseases. In order to do that, you must take **body substance isolation (BSI) precautions**, which are specific steps that help to minimize exposure to a patient's blood and body fluids. Examples of BSI precautions include wearing protective gloves, masks, gowns, and eyewear. ■

Consider the following situations:

- A police officer puts handcuffs on a suspect who has a small but open wound on his hand.
- A firefighter finds his leather gloves soaked with blood after extricating a patient from a wrecked car.
- A corrections officer touches dried blood in a prison cell.
- A sheriff's deputy is searching the front seat of a suspect's car and is stuck by a needle that the suspect dropped the night before.
- A firefighter, who is checking his equipment, handles a tool covered with blood from an earlier call.
- The firefighters who arrive first at the shopping center to care for a patient who has suddenly become ill are exposed to the patient's heavy coughing spell.

In each situation, the First Responder may be at risk of exposure to an infectious disease. What BSI precautions could be taken in each case? At the start of each shift, First Responders should check their hands for breaks in the skin and cover areas that are not intact. If their unprotected hands come in contact with blood (dry or not) or any other body fluids, they should promptly wash them with soap and water or a commercially produced antiseptic hand cleanser (Figure 3.6). Make sure you wear latex, vinyl, or other synthetic gloves before touching any patient and before handling equipment that may have been exposed to blood and body fluids (Figure 3.7).

To provide care to a patient who is coughing, sneezing, spitting, or otherwise spraying body fluids into the air, wear a mask and eye protection in addition to gloves. If you must search an individual or a vehicle, use a flashlight, mirror, or probe to search in areas that are not visible, such as in pockets or between seat

warning

Liquid or droplet exposure to skin, hair, gloves, clothing, and equipment requires you to find out from medical direction how to proceed. Washing with soap may not be enough. Contact with any unknown microbe or potential pathogen may require being seen by a physician.

FIGURE 3.6
Handwashing is one of the most effective infection-control measures.

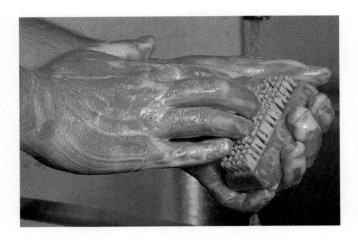

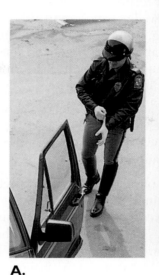
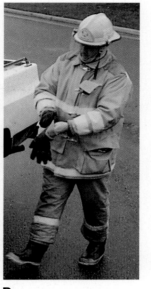

A.   **B.**

FIGURE 3.7
A. Law enforcement officers need to take precautions when dealing with injured individuals in unknown situations. **B.** In non-fire situations involving injury, firefighters should wear synthetic gloves under their leather gloves.

cushions (Figure 3.8). Finally, to dispose of blood-soaked gloves or any other disposable equipment that has blood or body fluids on it, follow the guidelines published by the U.S. Occupational Safety and Health Administration (OSHA).

First Responders frequently face unpredictable, uncontrollable, dangerous, and life-threatening circumstances. Anything can happen in an emergency. Making an arrest, helping a heart-attack victim, carrying a child from a burning building, stopping a brawl, helping deliver a baby—each situation has the potential to expose a First Responder to infectious diseases. Use good judgment. Follow OSHA guidelines.

DEALING WITH RISK

First Responders are familiar with handling risk. Yet some emergency personnel worry more about getting AIDS than they do about going into a burning building. The fact is that the disease feared most—AIDS—is the one a First Responder is least likely to get. As a member of EMS, your chances of being infected with HIV, the virus that causes AIDS, are very slight, even if you come in direct contact with infected blood or body fluids. You are at a much greater risk of contracting hepatitis B. An estimated 250 health-care workers die each year from hepatitis B or its complications, more than from any other infectious disease.

Regardless of the risk of infection, all EMS personnel must follow the rules for their own safety and the safety of others. Keep in mind that an organism that can cause disease may not always do so and that it may affect different people in different ways. An organism that you transfer from one patient to another may cause disease in the second patient, but not the first. In other words, the way disease is spread and develops is a subject that is so complicated that its study is a specialty unto itself. Do not guess at which precautions are necessary or assume that you can easily determine on your own how to prevent disease. You have entered this course prepared to help care for illness and injury. You can begin by not becoming a patient at the scene and by not spreading infections.

Infections are caused by organisms such as *viruses* (which cause illnesses such as colds, flu, HIV, and hepatitis) and *bacteria* (which cause sore throats, food poisoning, rheumatic fever, gonorrhea, Legionnaire's disease, and tuberculosis, to name a few). There are both viral and bacterial forms of pneumonia and meningitis. These organ-

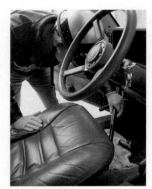

FIGURE 3.8
To avoid accidental needle sticks or other injuries, a police officer can use a probe to search beneath a car seat.

pathogens organisms such as viruses and bacteria that cause infection and disease.

isms are also called **pathogens**. The term *pathogen* means to generate suffering (*patho-*, suffering; *-gen*, create or form). Pathogens are spread by exposure to body fluids such as blood and semen, as well as exposure to airborne droplets such as those that come from coughing, sneezing, spitting, or even breathing close to someone's face.

Infectious diseases are a real danger to First Responders. However, if you follow safety procedures and use the personal protective equipment provided by your agency, the risks can be minimized.

FIRST➤ OSHA has issued strict guidelines about the precautions to take to reduce exposure to infectious disease. You can transmit pathogens to the patient and the patient can transmit them to you unless you use **personal protective equipment (PPE)** (Figure 3.9):

personal protective equipment (PPE) equipment such as gloves, mask, eyewear, gown, turnout gear, and helmet, which protect rescuers from infection and/or from exposure to hazardous materials and the dangers of rescue operations.

- *Gloves*—latex, vinyl, or other synthetic. Inspect your hands before donning and cover any broken skin. Put on your gloves before contact with the patient. Put on a second pair of gloves if you are working around sharp objects, such as broken glass and metal edges at a collision scene. If the outer gloves are torn, the gloves underneath still provide a layer of protection. Wash hands and change gloves between patients. OSHA has stated that handwashing is one of the most important steps to take for infection control.

- *Face shields or masks*—Wear surgical-type masks for blood or fluid splatter. For fine particles of airborne droplets (coughing), wear a high-efficiency particulate air (HEPA) or N-95 respirator. In addition, a surgical-type mask may be placed on the patient if he is alert and cooperates (monitor respirations).

- *Eye protection*—The mucous membranes of your eyes can absorb fluids and are a route for infection. Use eyewear that protects them from both the front and sides.

- *Gowns*—Protect your clothing and bare skin when there is spurting blood, childbirth, or multiple injuries with heavy bleeding. ■

Since you cannot tell if patients have infectious diseases just by looking at them, and you do not know if you are ill until signs and symptoms appear, it is important to wear personal protective equipment (PPE) for any contact with a patient. This includes wearing gloves at all times, plus face shields and eye protection whenever you may be exposed to splattering fluids or airborne droplets. This protection builds a barrier between you and the patient.

FIGURE 3.9
Personal protective equipment (PPE).

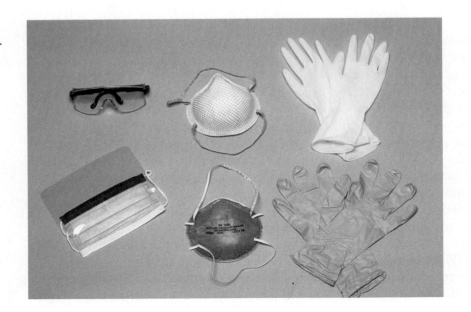

BLOODBORNE AND AIRBORNE PATHOGENS

FIRST➤ Infectious diseases range from such generally mild conditions as influenza to life-threatening diseases such as tuberculosis. The four diseases of most concern to First Responders are (Table 3-1):

- HIV (human immunodeficiency virus).
- Hepatitis.
- Tuberculosis.
- Meningitis. ■

HIV is the pathogen that causes AIDS. As yet, there is no cure, but there are newly developed medications that help reduce the patient's symptoms. However, new medical developments should not prevent you from using personal protective equipment while caring for every patient. Keep in mind several facts about HIV. First, HIV does not survive well outside the body. It also is not as concentrated in body fluids as the hepatitis B virus. HIV also is much more difficult to transmit than hepatitis B. The routes of exposure to HIV are limited to direct contact with non-intact (open) skin or mucous membranes and with blood, semen, or other body fluids. Thus, it is very unlikely that a rescuer taking proper BSI precautions will get the disease on the job.

In contrast to HIV, the hepatitis B virus (HBV) is a very tough virus. It can survive on clothing, newspaper, or other objects for days after infected blood has dried. HBV causes permanent liver damage in many cases and can be fatal. Several other forms of the disease, including hepatitis C, are less common than HBV but still present a risk to First Responders.

Tuberculosis (TB), a disease most often affecting the lungs, can also be fatal. Thought to have been nearly eradicated as recently as 1985, TB has had a resurgence. Even worse, new strains of the disease are resistant to treatment with traditional medication. Unlike HIV and HBV, TB is spread by aerosolized droplets in the air, usually the result of coughing and sneezing. Thus, TB can be contracted even without direct physical contact with a carrier. Use face masks with one-way valves for rescue breathing. Use a high-efficiency particulate air (HEPA) respirator or N-95 respirator when TB is suspected (Figure 3.10). These respirators greatly reduce the risk of exposure to this airborne disease.

Meningitis, an inflammation of the lining of the brain and spinal cord, is also a serious disease, especially for children. The most infectious varieties of meningitis are caused by bacteria. Meningitis is transmitted by respiratory droplets, like TB,

remember

Even dried body fluids are potentially infectious. Take the appropriate measures to prevent contact.

TABLE 3-1 DISEASES OF CONCERN TO FIRST RESPONDERS

DISEASE	HOW TRANSMITTED	VACCINE
AIDS/HIV (Acquired Immune Deficiency Syndrome)	Needle sticks, blood splash on mucous membranes (eye, mouth), or blood contact with open skin	No
Hepatitis B Virus (HBV)	Needle sticks, blood splash on mucous membranes (eye, mouth), or blood contact with open skin; some risk during mouth-to-mouth CPR	Yes
Tuberculosis (TB)	Airborne aerosolized droplets	No
Meningitis	Respiratory secretions or saliva	Yes, for one strain

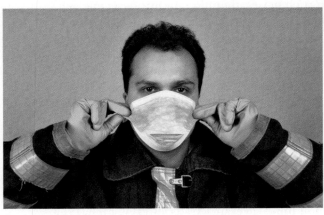

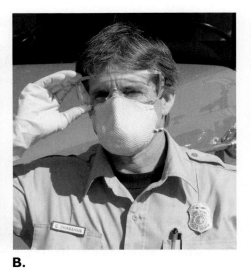

A.

B.

FIGURE 3.10

Wear either (A) a high-efficiency particulate air (HEPA) mask or (B) an N-95 respirator when you suspect a patient may have tuberculosis.

but is far easier to contract. The disease may have a rapid onset (several hours to a few days) and needs quick treatment with antibiotics. First Responders should make sure that EMS and hospital staffs inform them if they have been in contact with a patient infected with meningitis or a scene that may be contaminated with it. Antibiotics taken after exposure to bacterial meningitis may prevent acquiring the disease.

PROTECTING FIRST RESPONDERS

Today, governments at the local, state, and federal levels are taking steps to protect First Responders from exposure to infectious diseases. The Centers for Disease Control and Prevention (CDC) recommended universal precautions, BSI precautions, and now Standard Precautions, which are based on the assumption that all blood and body fluids are potentially hazardous and must be treated as infectious.

FIGURE 3.11

The OSHA-mandated infectious disease program includes immunizations against certain diseases.

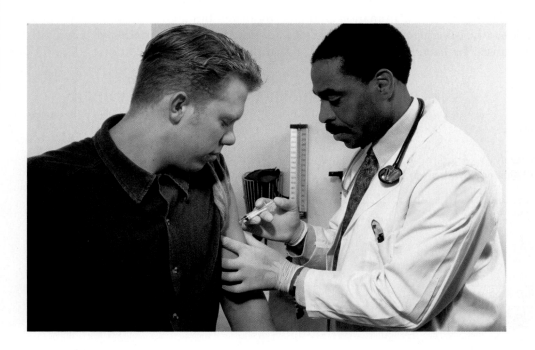

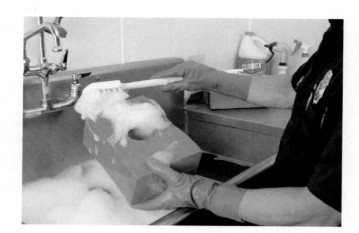

In 1992, OSHA issued guidelines for employers whose workers run a risk of occupational exposure to bloodborne diseases. All such agencies are required to implement plans to meet the OSHA standards. The following list summarizes the main features of an OSHA-mandated infectious disease program:

1. Provide a free hepatitis B vaccination—a safe, routine procedure that protects against HBV infection (Figure 3.11).

2. Educate employees about bloodborne diseases and train employees in safe work practices, including use of personal protective equipment. Training should include questions and answers about individual work sites, hands-on practice with protective gear, and information on reporting exposures.

3. Establish safe workplace procedures, including appropriate personal protective equipment, changes of uniform, and safe facilities for cleaning or disposing of contaminated gear (sometimes through local hospitals) (Figure 3.12).

4. Supply personal protective equipment such as gloves, gowns, masks, eye shields of the correct fit, and resuscitation equipment including pocket masks with one-way valves.

5. Set up engineering controls, such as special containers for needles, alternative handwashing when soap and water are not available, and labels for containers with contaminated items.

6. Provide an equipment-cleaning site separate from food preparation areas where contaminated tools, equipment, and so on can be cleaned.

7. Ensure proper waste disposal according to local regulations, so that used synthetic gloves and dressings are not left at emergency scenes or around agency facilities (Figure 3.13).

8. Implement post-exposure follow-up to determine the significance of an exposure incident, to document the event, and to test the employee.

This outline of exposure-control procedures is not comprehensive. Actual programs vary by state, jurisdiction, and agency. Your employer is required to make infection-control procedures a part of job training. Do not hesitate to suggest changes or improvements that you feel are necessary.

Your instructor will show you how to properly put on and use your protective equipment in a way that maintains its cleanliness. You will also learn how and where to properly dispose of all used materials. In addition, it is important that all reusable equipment is cleaned or disinfected with soap and water and/or a bleach solution. You must learn, understand the need for, and practice these infection-control procedures to reduce your risk of infection. These procedures are based on

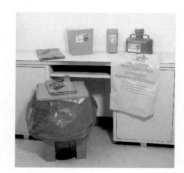

FIGURE 3.13
Examples of biohazard containers.

guidelines from OSHA and the CDC, and practicing them is a part of your responsibility as a First Responder.

EMPLOYEE RESPONSIBILITIES

An infection-control program will only work if First Responders learn and follow correct procedures. As a First Responder, you have an obligation to adhere to safe work practices in order to protect yourself, your family, and the public. Washing hands regularly, using gloves and other personal protective equipment, and making safe work practices a habit are good ways to start.

Note that you may not withhold emergency care from a patient who you think may have an infectious disease. With the proper precautions, you can provide emergency care to people infected with HIV or HBV without putting yourself at risk. To date, there are no known cases of emergency workers contracting HIV or HBV during routine patient care using gloves and appropriate personal protective equipment. First Responders who practice infection control should feel confident that they are not risking their lives.

SCENE SAFETY

Ensuring scene safety starts before First Responders actually arrive at the scene. En route to the scene, it is important to get as much information from dispatch about the emergency as possible. The nature of the call will help to determine what type of BSI precautions and equipment may be needed and what type of approach precautions to take. Dispatchers will not always have complete or accurate details about the incident. Often, those who report an emergency are excited, nervous, confused, in pain, or in a panic. They may even hang up before they finish giving all the details. Become familiar with your response area and the types of calls typical to it, so you can be prepared for the expected as well as the unusual.

When approaching an emergency scene, look around for hazards and listen for noises in the area. Is it quiet, and is that normal for the area? Is there yelling, screaming, gunshots, dogs barking? Decide where to place the vehicle: before the scene to provide lighting, or beyond it to provide quick and easy supply access and patient loading; on the street to block traffic and protect the scene, or off the street to protect EMS personnel. When deciding where to position the vehicle, consider that placement must provide for access to equipment, efficient loading of the patient, and continued traffic flow where possible or at least rerouting of traffic around the scene. As a part of approaching the scene and deciding where to place the vehicle, you will also be sizing up the scene for a variety of hazards ranging from inconvenient to critically dangerous.

Before approaching the patient, you must ensure the safety of not only yourself and the patient but bystanders as well. There may be hazardous materials, toxic substances, downed power lines and broken poles, or unstable vehicles at the scene. Environmental conditions such as icy and slippery roads, steep grades, rocky terrain, or heavy traffic and a crowd of onlookers must all be considered in your approach, placement of your vehicle, and care of your patient.

Violent situations may involve weapons—not just guns but knives or bats, boards, chains, and other items (Figure 3.14). All of these can be used to harm you, just as they harmed the victim. You may also be responding to a crime scene where you want to be aware of the potential for violence, where you do not want to approach until it is clear, and where you do not want to disturb evidence any more than you must while caring for the patient.

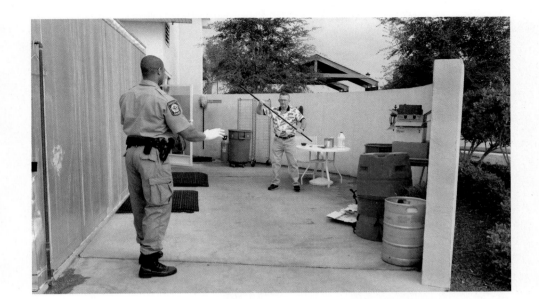

Crowds can also be potentially dangerous. When necessary, notify dispatch that you need assistance for crowd control and law enforcement for protection and scene security.

Keeping yourself safe is your first responsibility. Once you can assure your own safety, approach and take care of the patient. Following are specific types of unsafe incidents where First Responders must take special precautions.

HAZARDOUS MATERIALS INCIDENTS

Some chemicals can cause serious illness or death, even if your exposure is brief. Some of these chemicals are being transported by truck or rail, and some may be stored in warehouses or used in local industries. If there is a collision in which transported chemicals are spilled or if stored containers begin to leak, the spilled chemicals are likely to be considered a hazard to the community and to responding EMS personnel.

First Responders should maintain a safe distance from the source of the hazard and treat it as a **hazardous materials incident**. Placards may help with identifying materials in motor-vehicle collisions. These placards use coded colors and identification numbers that are listed in the *Emergency Response Guidebook* published by the U.S. Department of Transportation (DOT). This book should be placed in every emergency response vehicle. It can provide important information about a hazardous substance, as well as information on safe distances, emergency care, and suggested procedures in the event of spills or fire.

It also is always wise to carry a pair of binoculars in your vehicle. This way, you can identify hazardous materials placards from a safe distance, thus ensuring your own safety.

As a First Responder, your most important duty in a hazardous materials incident is to recognize potential problems and take action to preserve your own safety and that of others. (See Chapter 14 for a more detailed discussion of the First Responder's responsibilities at a hazardous materials incident.) You should also make sure an appropriately trained hazardous materials response team is notified (Figure 3.15). These teams have special training and equipment to handle such incidents, so it is important that you not take any action other than protecting yourself, patients, and bystanders. An inappropriate action could cause a larger problem than the already existing one.

hazardous materials incident the release of a harmful substance into the environment. Also called a *hazmat incident.*

FIGURE 3.15
First Responders should wait for hazmat teams to arrive at the scene of any hazardous materials incident.

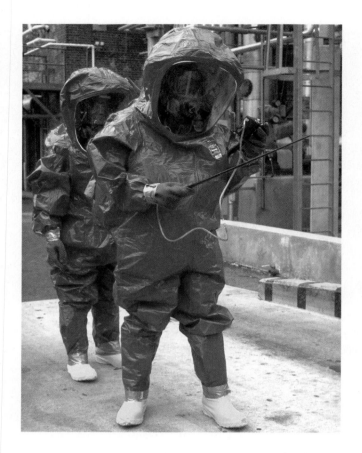

Many emergency response agencies require hazardous materials training at the awareness level. Your instructor can inform you of the requirements in your area.

Rescue Operations

First Responders may be first on the scene of an emergency involving rescue. Rescue scenes may include dangers from electricity, fire, explosion, hazardous materials, traffic, or water and ice. It is important to evaluate each situation and request the appropriately trained teams to assist in handling these incidents. You may need the police, fire department, power company, or other specialized personnel. Never perform acts that you are not properly trained to do. You should secure the scene to the best of your ability, and then wait for the help you have requested to arrive. Remember that whenever you are working at a rescue operation, you must use personal protective equipment, which may include turnout gear, protective eyewear, helmet, puncture-proof gloves, and latex, vinyl, or other synthetic gloves.

Violence and Crime Scenes

First Responders may also respond to scenes involving victims of violence or crimes. Your first priority—even before patient care—is to be certain the scene is safe before you enter it. Dangerous people or pets, people with weapons, intoxicated people, and others may present problems that you are not prepared to handle. Recognize these situations and request the necessary help. Wait until help arrives to secure the scene and make it safe for you to perform your duties. Remember that your first consideration is your own safety. Always wear the appropriate personal protective equipment. In some areas, EMS providers are issued bulletproof vests for their protection.

Chapter Review

Stress is a daily part of a First Responder's job. The initial steps taken at every scene are performed, in large part, to **ensure rescuer safety.** Not as obvious as physical hazards are those factors that affect the **emotional health** of the rescuer. The source may be a single terrible event or a series of events that, when combined, will overload the ability of the rescuer to cope with stress.

Emergencies that produce excess stress include those that involve multiple casualties, pediatric patients, death, violence, abuse and neglect, and the death or injury of another rescuer. First Responders may find themselves reacting unexpectedly and immediately or experiencing a delayed reaction days or weeks following an event. Exposure to critical events can cause what is known as **critical incident stress.** Typically, a rescuer will recover from an acute stress reaction in a few days or weeks. Cumulative stress may lead to **burnout** that may require professional counseling. To help reduce the stress associated with responding to emergency situations, make lifestyle changes or adjustments. In more severe cases, professional help or counseling may be of importance in ensuring emotional well-being.

Taking the steps necessary to deal adequately with stress associated with a critical incident may be best accomplished by following your EMS system's **critical incident stress management (CISM)** recommendations, including peer counseling through **critical incident stress debriefing (CISD).**

One way a First Responder can help cope with death and with terminal patients is to understand the **stages of death and dying,** which include denial, anger, bargaining, depression, and acceptance.

Safeguarding your well-being is critical. Dealing with risk is often a part of the rescuer's roles and responsibilities. Many situations put the First Responder at risk of exposure to infectious disease. It is important for the First Responder to be familiar with and follow OSHA guidelines for infection control. To protect yourself from pathogens, use **personal protective equipment** such as gloves (always), and face shields or masks, eye protection, and gowns when necessary. These protective barriers between you and the patient are called **body substance isolation (BSI) precautions.** Dispose of personal protective equipment appropriately.

Four **pathogens** present especially significant risks to First Responders. They are HIV, hepatitis (typically bloodborne), tuberculosis, and meningitis (typically airborne). Do not limit your thinking to just these four, and do not believe that an outbreak must be reported for there to be a danger.

It is the responsibility of the First Responder to provide emergency care to all patients regardless of their real or potential level of infection. Ensure your personal safety by being alert to the potential for danger at every emergency call.

Remember that your safety has to come first. In order for you to help others, you must first take care of yourself. Keep in mind that your emotional safety is also important in order to prevent burnout, which often causes a loss of personnel to emergency response services.

✔ Identify a network of family or friends who may be able to assist you in handling stress.

✔ Make sure you have the necessary personal protective equipment available whenever you may be responding to an emergency. Use it every time, on every call. If you do this, you will never have to wonder if you were protected on "that" call.

✔ Learn how and when to access the CISM in your local area.

✔ Practice putting on personal protective equipment and determine what equipment is necessary for different types of emergency responses. Learn how to properly dispose of items after use.

✔ Learn what types of specialized assistance or specially trained personnel are available in your area and how to establish contact in case of an emergency.

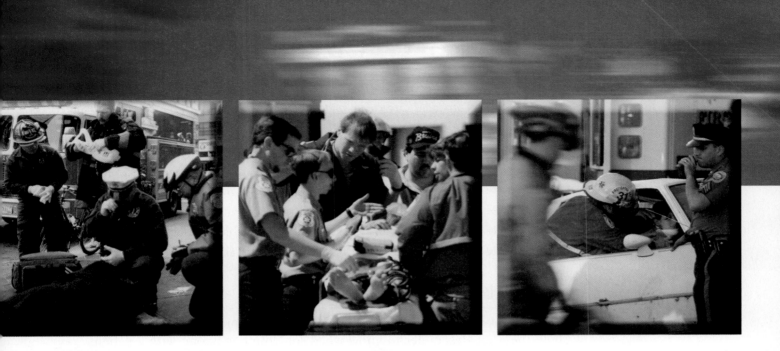

The Human Body

4

As a First Responder, you will not be able to provide care for an ill or injured patient unless you have an idea of where the problem lies. This requires a patient assessment. To assess a patient adequately, you must be familiar with normal anatomy and the terms used to describe it. In addition, this knowledge will make it possible for you to give an accurate patient report, even over a telephone or radio.

This chapter introduces you to the anatomy of the human body, including its major systems and their basic functions. It also introduces you to terms used to describe a patient's position and condition. You know much of this information already. Practice what is new to you often. The more you practice, the more comfortable you will be using it when the need arises.

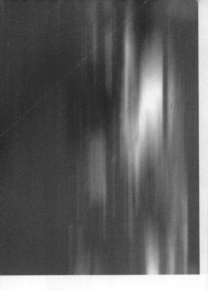

NATIONAL STANDARD OBJECTIVES

This chapter focuses on the objectives of Module 1, Lesson 1–4, of the U.S. DOT's First Responder National Standard Curriculum and serves as an instructional aid to help you meet any specific objectives added to the course by your local EMS system.

By the end of this chapter, you will be able to (from cognitive or knowledge information):

1–4.1 Describe the anatomy and function of the respiratory system. (p. 61; also see Chapter 6)

1–4.2 Describe the anatomy and function of the circulatory system. (p. 61; also see Chapters 8 and 10)

1–4.3 Describe the anatomy and function of the musculoskeletal system. (p. 61; also see Chapter 11)

1–4.4 Describe the components and function of the nervous system. (p. 61; also see Chapter 11)

LEARNING TASKS

A basic understanding of the normal anatomy and function of the human body will help the First Responder to know when something is wrong with a patient. Your instructor will help you to:

✔ Learn ways in which First Responders may be able apply their knowledge.

Topical, positional, and directional terms help you to report patient problems more accurately. Practice using them and be able to:

✔ Describe the anatomical position.
✔ Define and properly apply the terms *anterior, posterior, midline, medial, lateral, proximal, distal, superior, inferior, patient's right and left, prone, supine,* and *right and left lateral recumbent positions.*

It is also helpful to know the five major regions of the body and the contents of the four major body cavities. Be sure you are able to:

✔ Use common terms to list the five major regions of the body and the subdivisions of each region.
✔ Name and locate the four major body cavities.
✔ Name and locate the organs contained in each of the body cavities.
✔ Identify the four abdominal quadrants.
✔ Name two types of structures that are found in every location in the body.
✔ List and define the eleven major body systems.

OVERVIEW OF THE HUMAN BODY

Students beginning training in First Responder courses are often a little worried about having to learn human **anatomy**. Don't be. As a First Responder, you will not need to be as precise as other medical personnel are when they consider the human body. However, you will need to know the basic body structures and their locations.

You might be surprised to find where some of those structures are located, since few of us have an accurate idea of the exact location of them all. But no one will be asking you to take a stethoscope and outline the borders of the heart. You already know, generally, where the heart is located in the chest. When you study CPR, or cardiopulmonary resuscitation (KAR-de-o-PUL-mo-ner-e re-SUS-si-TAY-shun), you will learn to be more specific about its location.

You probably know the general location of the lungs, too, but you may be a little off in locating the stomach and the liver. Odds are you will be less accurate in

anatomy the study of body structure.

locating the uterus (womb), and even less accurate in locating the ovaries. The main thing to keep in mind as you begin your studies is that you know all these structures exist and you have a general idea of where they are located.

Do not become too concerned with trying to learn a lot of medical terms. A head is still a head, and feet are still feet. Most of the terms relating to human anatomy are so important to us that they have been a part of our vocabulary for years. Brain, eyes, ears, teeth, heart, lungs, liver, stomach, bladder, and spinal cord are all valid terms in emergency medicine.

You will learn a few new terms. You also will take a few terms that you have heard before (such as carotid artery) and make them as much a part of your vocabulary as heart and lungs.

FIRST➤ To be a First Responder, you must be able to look at a person's body and know the major internal structures and the general location of each one. Your concern is not how the body looks dissected or how the body looks on an anatomical wall chart. You must be concerned with living bodies and knowing where things are located as you look from the outside.

You know about blood vessels and nerves. As you look at any region of the body, remember that for your purposes:

- Blood vessels go everywhere in the body, to every structure.
- Nerves go everywhere in the body, to every structure. ■

When you look at an arm, you must see something that is alive and part of a living organism. You know that an arm is made of muscles, bones, blood vessels, nerves, and other tissues. When you assess injuries, never forget that there could be internal bleeding and that damaged nerves may be causing pain, loss of feeling, or even loss of function.

POSITIONAL AND DIRECTIONAL TERMS

FIRST➤ The following is a set of very basic terms that can be used to refer to the human body (Figure 4.1):

- *Anatomical position*—Consider the human body, standing erect, facing you. The arms are down at the sides, and the palms of the hands are forward. This is the **anatomical position**. References to all body structures describe the body in this position.
- *Right and left*—Always refer to the patient's right and the patient's left. Even though you may think this is very simple, many students find it difficult. Practice until you can use these terms correctly every time.
- *Anterior and posterior*—The term **anterior** refers to the front of the body, and the term **posterior** refers to the back of the body. The rest of the body can be divided easily into anterior and posterior by following the side seams of your clothing.
- *Midline*—The **midline** is an imaginary vertical line that can be used to divide the body into right and left halves. Anything toward the midline is said to be **medial**, while anything away from the midline is said to be **lateral**. Remember the anatomical position, which places the thumb on the lateral side of the hand and the little finger on the medial side. ■

There are other directional terms that can be useful. **Superior** means toward the top of the head, as in "the eyes are superior to the nose." **Inferior** means toward the feet, as in "the mouth is inferior to the nose." You cannot say something is superior or inferior unless you are comparing at least two structures. The heart

anatomical (AN-ah-TOM-i-kal) **position** the standard reference position for the body in the study of anatomy. The body is standing erect, facing the observer. The arms are down at the sides, and the palms of the hands are forward.

anterior the front of the body or body part.

posterior the back of the body or body part.

midline an imaginary vertical line used to divide the body into right and left halves.

medial toward the midline of the body.

lateral to the side, away from the midline of the body.

superior toward the head (for example, the chest is superior to the abdomen).

inferior away from the head; usually compared with another structure that is closer to the head (for example, the lips are inferior to the nose).

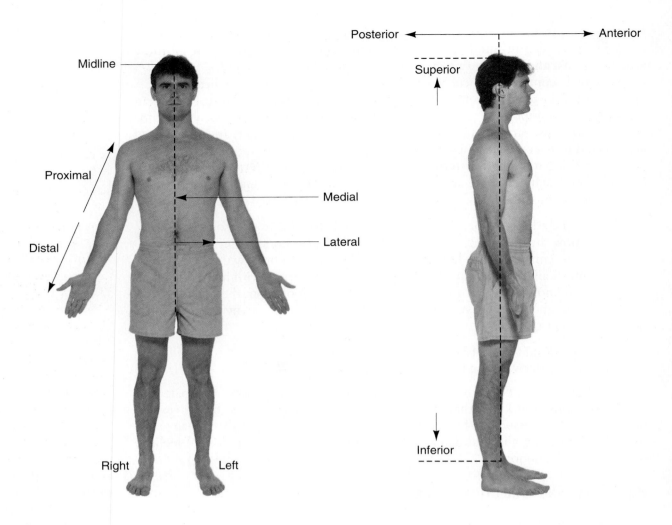

FIGURE 4.1
Directional terms.

proximal closer to the torso.

distal farther away from the torso.

is not superior, it is superior to the stomach. Since you are using the anatomical position for all your references to the body, any medical professional will know what you mean when you say a wound is just above the eye. For this reason, superior and inferior may be optional terms in your course. Superior and inferior are usually reserved for structures in the head, neck, and torso.

Proximal and distal also may be optional. These two terms are often used incorrectly and should be avoided unless you are certain of their correct usage. To use the terms correctly, there must be a point of reference and two structures being compared. The structure closest to the point of reference is said to be proximal, while the structure farthest away is distal. It helps to think that the close structure is in the proximity of the reference, while the far structure is some distance away.

These two terms—proximal and distal—usually replace superior and inferior on the limbs. Proximal and distal also may be used for the torso when referring to vessels and tubes that have an origin and an end. An example would be the pancreatic duct, which delivers digestive enzymes into the small intestine. It starts in the pancreas (proximal) and ends in the small intestine (distal).

The most commonly used points of reference are the shoulder joint and the hip joint. Thus, the elbow is said to be proximal when compared to the wrist, which is distal. The knee is proximal when compared to the ankle. Most medical professionals only use proximal and distal in reference to the arms and legs. Thus, a structure closer to the shoulder is called proximal; another structure near the wrist is called distal. Do not refer to a structure close to the shoulder as superior or one near the elbow as inferior. Keep in mind that superior and inferior are usually used for the head, neck, and torso.

Trying to remember all this in an emergency situation could lead to some confusion. Practice these and other directional terms with your classmates.

There are some other specific positional terms you might use when the patient is not in the anatomical position (Figure 4.2). These terms include **supine** or lying face up, **prone** or lying face down, and **lateral recumbent** for those times when a patient is lying on his or her side. Since lateral recumbent can be used for lying on the right or left, it is proper to state either right lateral recumbent or left lateral recumbent. The correct recording of the patient's position may be of medical significance and also may become part of the legal record of how a patient was first seen. As with directional terms, positional terms need practice to become part of your professional vocabulary.

Most First Responders do not deal with mishaps, motor-vehicle collisions, crashes, or medical emergencies on a daily basis. Unless you review and use related terms often, you may forget them over time. Be aware that medical and rescue personnel are trained to take your information. They will not be confused if you say front, back, above, and below. Do not let terminology stand in the way of clear communication with EMS providers, physicians, and other medical professionals.

BODY REGIONS

FIRST➤ The human body can be divided into five regions (Figure 4.3). These regions have the common, everyday names of head, neck, torso, upper extremities (shoulders, arms, and hands), and lower extremities (hip joint, legs, and feet). Later in this text, you will be asked to study specific areas within each of these regions. For example, you will have to understand the pelvic girdle and how the legs join the torso of the body so that you can relate certain injuries to specific types of emergencies. For now, in

supine the patient is lying face up.

prone the patient is lying face down.

lateral recumbent the patient is lying on his side. Use left or right lateral recumbent.

NOTE

In an emergency, if you are not certain about the correct usage of a medical term, use the common term. You can damage your credibility by using the wrong medical term or delay the EMTs as they try to determine the actual meaning of what you have said.

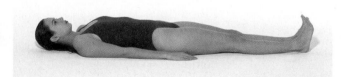

Supine

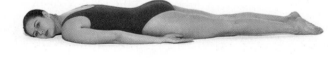

Prone

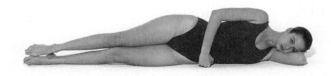

Lateral recumbent position

FIGURE 4.2
Positional terms.

FIGURE 4.3
Body regions.

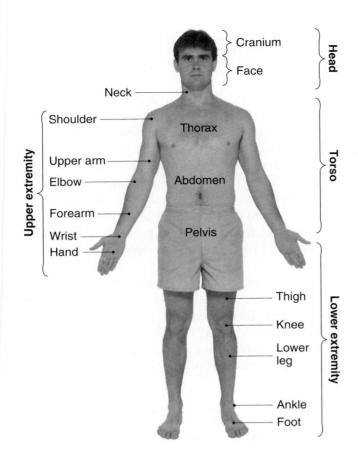

Cranium
Face
Head
Neck
Shoulder
Thorax
Upper arm
Elbow
Abdomen
Forearm
Wrist
Pelvis
Hand
Upper extremity
Torso
Thigh
Knee
Lower
leg
Lower extremity
Ankle
Foot

order to begin your new approach to viewing the body, start with the simplest of subdivisions:

Head
Cranium—housing the brain
Face
Mandible (MAN-di-bl)— the lower jaw

Neck

Torso
Chest—the thorax (THO-raks)
Abdomen—extending from the lower ribs to the pelvic girdle
Pelvic cavity—protected by the bones of the pelvic girdle

Upper Extremities
Shoulder joint
Arm
Elbow
Forearm
Wrist
Hand

Lower Extremities
Hip joint
Thigh
Knee
Leg
Ankle
Foot ■

The terms *cranium*, *thorax*, and *mandible* may not be used in most daily conversations, but all the other terms are already part of your vocabulary. The significant thing is to begin looking for these simple subdivisions each time you consider possible diseases and injuries. As stated earlier, more specifics will be covered throughout this text.

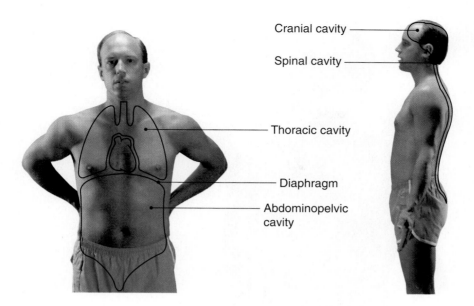

FIGURE 4.4
Body cavities.

Cranial cavity

Spinal cavity

Thoracic cavity

Diaphragm

Abdominopelvic cavity

BODY CAVITIES

FIRST➤ There are four major body cavities—two anterior and two posterior (Figure 4.4). Housed in these cavities are the vital organs, glands, blood vessels, and nerves. ■

Anterior Cavities

● *Chest cavity*—Also known as the **thoracic cavity**, the chest cavity is enclosed by the rib cage. It protects the lungs, heart, great blood vessels, part of the windpipe (trachea), and part of the esophagus (e-SOF-ah-gus), which is the tube leading from the throat to the stomach. The lower border of the chest cavity is the **diaphragm**, a dome-shaped muscle used in breathing. (Remember its location.) The diaphragm separates the chest cavity from the abdominopelvic (ab-DOM-i-no-PEL-vik) cavity (Figure 4.5).

● *Abdominopelvic cavity*—This is the anterior body cavity below the diaphragm. Most people use the terms **abdominal cavity** and **pelvic cavity** to describe the two portions of the abdominopelvic cavity.

   –*Abdominal cavity* lies between the thorax and the pelvis. It is separated from the chest (thoracic) cavity by the diaphragm. The stomach, liver, gallbladder, pancreas, spleen, small intestine, and most of the large intestine can be found in the abdominal cavity. Unlike the other body cavities, the abdominal cavity is not surrounded by bones. If you consider all the organs in this cavity and the lack of bony protection, it is easy to see why blows to the abdomen can cause severe injury.

   –*Pelvic cavity* is protected by the bones of the pelvic girdle. This cavity houses the urinary bladder, portions of the large intestine, and the internal reproductive organs.

Posterior Cavities

● *Cranial cavity*—This is the braincase of the skull, housing the brain and its specialized membranes.

● *Spinal cavity*—This cavity runs through the center of the backbone, protecting the spinal cord and its specialized membranes.

thoracic (tho-RAS-ik) **cavity** the anterior body cavity that is above (superior to) the diaphragm. Also called *chest cavity*.

diaphragm (DI-uh-fram) the muscular structure that divides the chest cavity from the abdominal cavity.

abdominal cavity the anterior body cavity that extends from the diaphragm to the region protected by the pelvic bones.

pelvic cavity the anterior body cavity surrounded by the bones of the pelvis.

FIGURE 4.5
Location of diaphragm and abdominal quadrants.

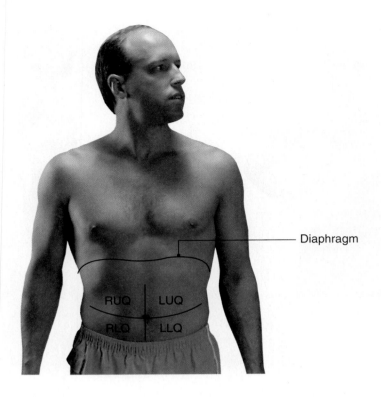

Diaphragm

RUQ | LUQ
RLQ | LLQ

ABDOMINAL QUADRANTS

FIRST➤ The abdomen is a large body region, and the abdominal cavity contains many vital organs. In other body regions, bones may be used for reference (by counting the ribs, for example). This is not the case when trying to be specific about the abdomen. The navel, or umbilicus (um-BIL-i-kus), is the only quick point of reference available to the First Responder. To improve this situation, the abdominal wall has been divided into four **abdominal quadrants** (Figure 4.5). These quadrants are:

- *Right upper quadrant (RUQ)*—containing most of the liver, the gallbladder, and part of the small and large intestine.
- *Left upper quadrant (LUQ)*—containing most of the stomach, the spleen, and part of the small and large intestine.
- *Right lower quadrant (RLQ)*—containing the appendix and part of the small and large intestine.
- *Left lower quadrant (LLQ)*—containing part of the small and large intestine. ■

Some organs and glands are located in more than one quadrant. As you can see from the above list, parts of the large intestine are found in all four quadrants. The same is true for the small intestine. Part of the stomach can be found in the right upper quadrant. The left lobe of the liver extends into the left upper quadrant. Pelvic organs are included in these quadrants, with the urinary bladder being assigned to both lower quadrants.

The kidneys are a special case. They are not part of the abdominal cavity, since they are located behind the cavity's membrane lining. Consider one kidney to be RUQ and the other to be LUQ. However, do not let this abdominal classification make you think that the kidneys are in the abdominal cavity. The location of the kidneys makes them subject to injury from blows to the mid-back. Any pain or ache in the back may involve the kidneys. Most of the pancreas and the aorta are

abdominal quadrants four divisions of the abdomen used to pinpoint the location of a pain or an injury: right upper quadrant, left upper quadrant, right lower quadrant, and left lower quadrant.

remember

"Right" and "left" always refer to the patient's right and the patient's left.

also located behind the abdominal cavity membrane. The pancreas is mostly in the right upper quadrant, and the aorta lies just in front of the spinal column.

BODY SYSTEMS

Knowing the body systems and their functions can prove to be of value to the First Responder. However, most training courses do not have the time to go into great detail in terms of anatomy and physiology. Throughout this text, specific anatomy and some basic functions will be covered as they apply to illness and injury and First Responder-level care.

Remembering the different body functions can be useful when trying to determine the extent of injury or the nature of an illness. The following is a list of the major body systems and their primary functions:

- *Circulatory system*—moves blood, carries oxygen and nutrients to the body's cells, and removes wastes and carbon dioxide from these cells. It includes the heart, blood vessels, and blood.

- *Respiratory system*—exchanges air to bring in oxygen and expel carbon dioxide. Oxygen is placed into the bloodstream while carbon dioxide is being removed. It includes the nose, mouth, structures in the throat, lungs, and associated muscles.

- *Digestive system*—digests and absorbs food and removes certain wastes.

- *Urinary system*—removes chemical wastes from the blood and helps to balance water and salt levels of the blood.

- *Reproductive system*—produces all structures and hormones needed for sexual reproduction. Sometimes it is classified with the urinary system as the genitourinary (jen-e-to-U-re-NER-e) system.

- *Nervous system*—controls movement, interprets sensations, regulates body activities, and generates memory and thought. It includes the brain, spinal cord, and nerves.

- *Endocrine (EN-do-krin) system*—produces the chemicals called hormones that help regulate most body activities and functions.

- *Musculoskeletal (MUS-kyu-lo-SKEL-et-l) system*—provides protection and support for the body and internal organs and permits body movement. It is made up of bones and skeletal muscles, tendons, and ligaments.

- *Special senses*—provide sight, hearing, taste, smell, and the sensations of pain, cold, heat, and tactile responses, such as smoothness, roughness, softness, and the like.

- *Skin*—protects the body from heat, cold, and pollution of the environment; bacteria; and other foreign organisms. It is the largest organ of the body, which covers and protects the body's many tissues, organs, and systems. It regulates body temperature and senses heat, cold, touch, pain, and pressure. It also regulates body fluids and chemical balance.

  The skin is actually part of the integumentary (in-teg-u-MEN-tah-ree) system, which includes all the layers of the skin, nails, hair, sweat glands, oil glands, and mammary glands. Some classifications have all the coverings of any body part listed as structures within the integumentary system.

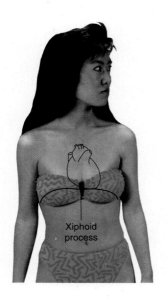

FIGURE 4.6
Position of the heart.

xiphoid (ZI-foid) **process** the inferior portion of the sternum.

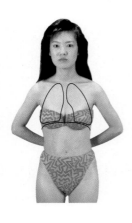

FIGURE 4.7
Position of the lungs.

• *Immune (MYOON) system*—protects the body from disease-causing organisms with white blood cells, microorganism-attacking cells, and antibody-producing cells and the antibodies they produce. It also helps to control allergies and the body's reactions to certain diseases. Some immune-system reactions include the body attacking itself (autoimmune diseases).

RELATING STRUCTURES TO THE BODY

FIRST▶ In this section, a series of illustrations show what you should be able to recognize as a First Responder considering the human body. Your task is a complex one, requiring much thought and practice before you will be comfortable with your new knowledge. As stated earlier, you must know the general location of structures as you view the external body. On many of these illustrations, you will see a line representing the diaphragm. Being able to visualize the position of the diaphragm will greatly help you understand how the various organs and glands fit into the body. ■

Begin with Figure 4.6. Note the position of the heart in the chest cavity. As a quick point of reference, use your fingers to find a small, hard spot just below your breastbone (sternum). This is the **xiphoid process**, a major body landmark. You can find a point directly over the inferior (lower) border of the heart by measuring two finger-widths up from this point. Look at yourself in a mirror and find this point. Each time you look in the mirror during your training, try to visualize where your heart is located.

Figure 4.7 shows the position of the lungs in the chest cavity. The lungs are protected by the rib cage. By studying this figure, you will have a good idea of the size, shape, and position of the lungs.

The two illustrations in Figure 4.8 show the position of the stomach, liver, and the first portion of the small intestine, which is called the duodenum (du-o-DE-num). The lower ribs protect the stomach and liver. The level of the xiphoid process is where the esophagus enters the stomach, immediately after passing through the diaphragm. If this makes sense to you, then you are gaining a firm grasp of human anatomy. If it does not, then you need to set aside time to review the first part of this chapter.

The first portion of the small intestine is important in emergency medicine because it is held in a more rigid position than the rest of the small intestine. Forceful blows to the abdomen, often received in automobile collisions, may injure the first portion of the small intestine without causing any significant damage to the rest of the intestine.

Using Figure 4.9, you can quickly add the positions of three other structures based on what you have already learned. Think of the gallbladder as being behind the liver, the pancreas as behind the lower part of the stomach, and the spleen behind the left side of the stomach. These descriptions would not be good enough if you were a student of anatomy, but they are very useful to a First Responder in an emergency situation. Knowing these general locations will improve your chances of correctly assessing the nature of many injuries to the abdomen.

Figure 4.10 shows the space occupied by the small intestine. As you can see, it fills most of the abdominal cavity. You also can see the space occupied by the large intestine. Note how it passes through each of the four abdominal quadrants as it "frames" the small intestine.

The kidneys and the urinary bladder are shown in Figure 4.11. Remember, the kidneys are behind the abdominal cavity, and the bladder is in the pelvic cavity. Al-

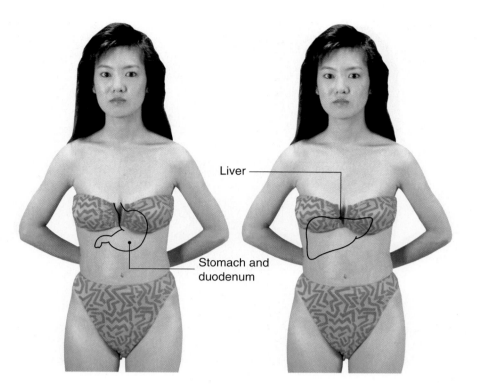

FIGURE 4.8
Position of the stomach, liver, and duodenum.

Liver

Stomach and
duodenum

though they appear well protected, injuries to these structures are common in motor-vehicle collisions. This is particularly true when occupants who are not wearing seat belts are thrown about in the passenger compartment. Internal organs may also be injured by gunshots, stabbings, severe blows to the abdomen or back, and forces or weights that cause crushing.

Scan 4-1 sums up all this material with an internal view of the locations of the major body organs. It shows you all that you have covered so far. Study the drawings and spend the time to relate the positions of these organs to the body's exterior.

FIGURE 4.9
Position of gallbladder, pancreas, and spleen.

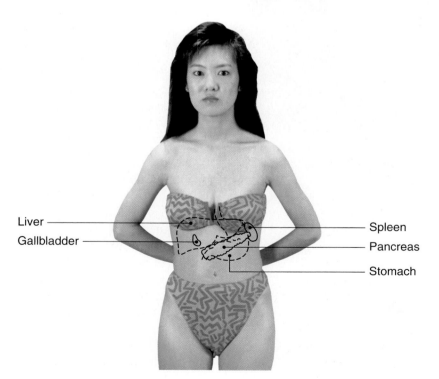

Liver

Gallbladder

Spleen

Pancreas

Stomach

FIGURE 4.10
Position of the small and large intestine.

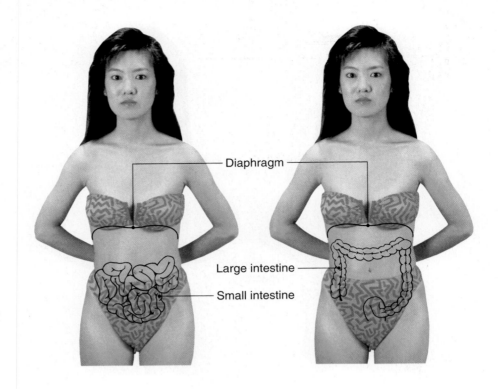

FIGURE 4.11
Position of the urinary system.

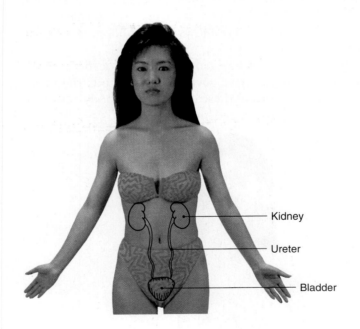

Major Body Organs

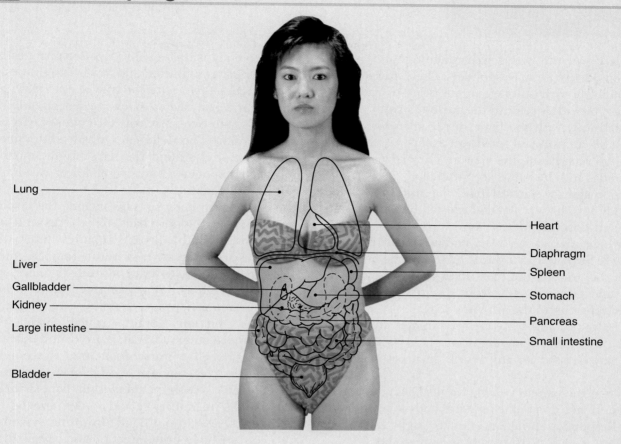

Lung

Heart

Diaphragm

Liver

Spleen

Gallbladder

Stomach

Kidney

Pancreas

Large intestine

Small intestine

Bladder

SOLID ORGANS

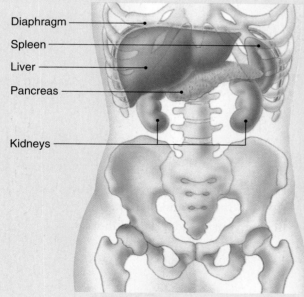

Diaphragm

Spleen

Liver

Pancreas

Kidneys

HOLLOW ORGANS

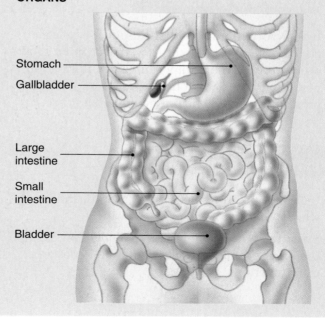

Stomach

Gallbladder

Large intestine

Small intestine

Bladder

Chapter Review

Knowledge of the body's basic anatomy and general functions helps First Responders assess patients and communicate with other emergency care providers.

Care providers refer to the **patient's right** and the **patient's left,** with the body in the anatomical position. The **anatomical position** refers to the body standing erect, facing the viewer. The arms are down at the sides and the palms are forward.

An imaginary vertical line, the **midline,** divides the body into halves. **Medial** means toward the midline, and **lateral** means away from the midline. **Anterior** is toward the front, and **posterior** is toward the back. **Superior** is toward the top of the head, and **inferior** is toward the feet. **Proximal** is toward the torso, and **distal** is away from the torso, both terms usually referring to the arms and legs.

The terms *anterior, posterior, superior,* and *inferior* may be used for a body organ or gland. *Proximal* and *distal* may be used for any vessel, duct, or tube in the body.

When the patient is lying on his back, the body is **supine.** If face down, the patient's body is **prone.** The First Responder should use left or right **lateral recumbent** for when the patient is lying on his side.

The body is divided into five regions: head, neck, torso, upper extremities, and lower extremities. It has four cavities—two anterior (the chest cavity and the abdominopelvic cavity, which are separated by the diaphragm) and two posterior (the cranial cavity and the spinal cavity). The abdomen is divided into four quadrants, centered around the navel: right upper quadrant, left upper quadrant, right lower quadrant, and left lower quadrant.

The eleven body systems include the **circulatory system** (heart, blood vessels, blood), **respiratory system** (nose, mouth, throat structures, lungs, respiratory muscles), **digestive system** (stomach, intestines, liver, gallbladder), **urinary system** (kidneys, ureters, bladder, urethra), **reproductive system** (uterus, ovaries, fallopian tubes, testicles, external genitalia), **nervous system** (brain, spinal cord, nerves), **endocrine system** (adrenal, thyroid, and other special glands and cells), **musculoskeletal system** (bones, skeletal muscles, tendons and ligaments), **skin** (or integumentary system including skin, hair, sweat glands, oil glands, mammary glands), the **special senses** (eyes, ears, nose, mouth), and **immune system** which protects the body from infection and certain diseases.

- It is important for the First Responder to learn and be able to use the terms in this chapter. However, it is even more important that information pertaining to a patient be passed on to other EMS personnel who will be providing patient care. So, if you are unable to remember the appropriate term in an emergency situation, use terms that are familiar to you and others.
- Use the terms *anterior, posterior, medial,* and *lateral.*

- Outline your own major body cavities, and list what is found in each.
- Point to each of your abdominal quadrants. Name the organs found in each quadrant and describe their functions.
- Look in a mirror. Locate your heart, lungs, xiphoid process, and diaphragm.
- Locate your bladder and kidneys.

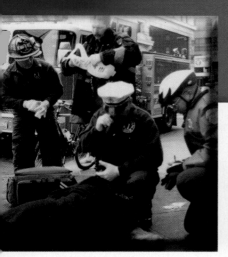
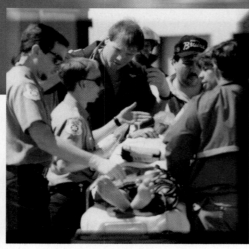
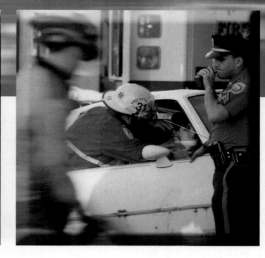

Lifting, Moving, and Positioning Patients

Many First Responders are injured every year because they attempt to lift or move patients or equipment improperly. Avoid making careless mistakes. They can injure your patient. They can also injure you. Back injuries are serious and have the potential to end a career in EMS, as well as cause life-long problems. So one of the most important things you can do for yourself, your coworkers, and any patients you may help is to learn how to lift and move objects and patients properly.

It is also important to know when a patient may be moved. There are many factors to consider, including scene safety and the patient's condition.

This chapter will describe when a First Responder is allowed to move a patient. It also will describe some simple techniques for lifting and moving that will make it possible for you to be an effective First Responder for many years to come.

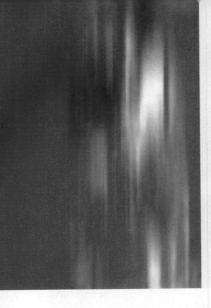

NATIONAL STANDARD OBJECTIVES

This chapter focuses on the objectives of Module 1, Lesson 1–5, of the U.S. DOT's First Responder National Standard Curriculum and serves as an instructional aid to help you meet any specific objectives added to the course by your local EMS system.

By the end of this chapter, you will be able to (from cognitive or knowledge information):

1–5.1 Define body mechanics. (p. 69)

1–5.2 Discuss the guidelines and safety precautions that need to be followed when lifting a patient. (p. 68)

1–5.3 Describe the indications for an emergency move. (pp. 70–71)

1–5.4 Describe the indications for assisting in nonemergency moves. (pp. 71, 74–75)

1–5.5 Discuss the various devices associated with moving a patient in the out-of-hospital arena. (pp. 82–89)

LEARNING TASKS

In an emergency situation, it is important to know how to safely move a patient in the most expedient way.

✔ Learn the most common emergency moves to be used by First Responders and be able to demonstrate them.

There are also nonemergency moves for which you can use equipment and/or additional people.

✔ Learn the most common nonemergency moves to be used by First Responders and be able to demonstrate them.

✔ Demonstrate proper use of the recovery position.

PRINCIPLES OF MOVING PATIENTS

WHEN TO MOVE A PATIENT

FIRST➤ In general, a First Responder should not move a patient. Your role is to assess the patient, provide emergency care, and monitor the patient's condition. Move him only when a dangerous environment presents a life threat or further injury, when you must check airway and breathing to start CPR, or when you are unable to gain access to other patients who need life-saving care. You may also be called upon to assist other EMS responders in lifting and moving patients. With the proper techniques, this can be done safely. ■

Whenever possible, keep the patient at rest, even when the patient appears to be able to move about. Remember that not all signs and symptoms show themselves immediately. Sometimes patients do not consider certain symptoms to be important and do not report them. In addition, some patients may not be straightforward in answering your questions or may even deny having an illness or injury.

Feel comfortable enough to
(by changing attitudes, values, and beliefs):

1–5.6 Explain the rationale for properly lifting and moving patients. (p. 69)

1–5.7 Explain the rationale for an emergency move. (pp. 70–71)

Show how to
(through psychomotor skills):

1–5.8 Demonstrate an emergency move. (pp. 70–71, 72)

1–5.9 Demonstrate a nonemergency move. (pp. 71, 73–81)

1–5.10 Demonstrate the use of equipment utilized to move patients in the out-of-hospital arena. (pp. 82–89)

BODY MECHANICS AND LIFTING TECHNIQUES

FIRST➤ **Body mechanics** is the proper use of your body to facilitate lifting and moving. There are important steps that First Responders must follow to lift efficiently and to prevent injury. ■

body mechanics the proper use of the body to facilitate lifting and moving and to prevent injury.

Before you lift or move a patient or an object, it is important to first plan what you will do and how you will do it (Figure 5.1). Estimate the weight of the patient or object and then, if needed, request additional help. It is also important to consider any physical limitations that may make lifting difficult or unsafe for you.

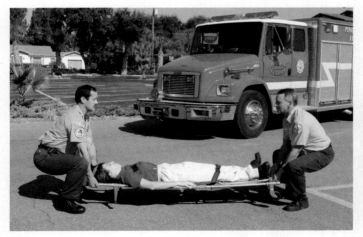

A.

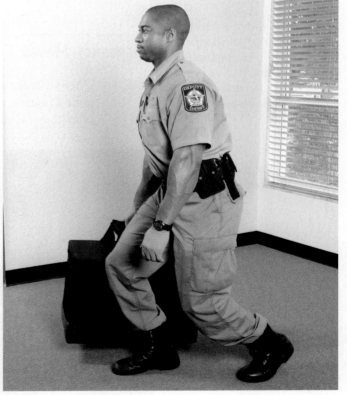

B.

FIGURE 5.1
Plan how you will lift a patient or an object using proper body mechanics.

Whenever possible, lift with a partner whose strength and height are similar to yours. Communicate with your partner and with the patient when you are ready to lift and continue to communicate throughout the process.

When you are ready to lift, follow these rules to prevent injury:

- *Position your feet properly.* They should be on a firm, level surface and positioned shoulder-width apart. Take extra care if the surface is slippery or may be unstable. It may be necessary to postpone the move until more help and equipment are on hand.

- *Use your legs, not your back, to do the lifting.* Keep your back straight and bend your knees.

- *Minimize twisting during a lift.* Attempts to turn or twist while you are lifting can result in serious injury.

- *When lifting with one hand, avoid leaning to either side.* Bend your knees to grasp the object and keep your back straight.

- *Keep the weight as close to your body as possible.* The farther the weight is from your body, the greater your chance of injury.

- *When carrying a patient on stairways, use a chair or commercial stair chair instead of a wheeled stretcher whenever possible.* Keep your back straight. Flex your knees and lean forward from your hips, not your waist. If you are walking backward down stairs, ask someone to "spot" you, by walking behind you and placing a hand on your back to help guide and steady you (Figure 5.2).

With the proper techniques, moving a patient can be done safely. Remember, perform proper lifting and moving techniques on every call.

Moving and Positioning Patients

Emergency Moves

FIRST➤ There are times when a patient must be moved immediately. These urgent situations call for emergency moves. An **emergency move** should take place when:

emergency move a patient move that is carried out quickly when the scene is hazardous, care of the patient requires repositioning, or you must reach another patient who needs life-saving care.

FIGURE 5.2
Have someone spot you as you walk backwards downstairs.

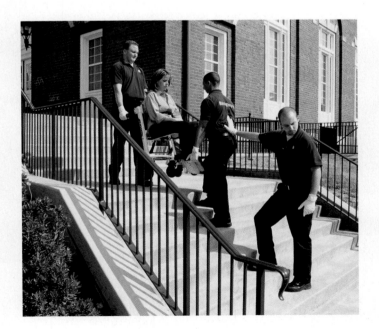

- *There is immediate danger to the patient if not moved.* Problems with the airway, breathing, or circulation (ABCs), or uncontrolled traffic, fire or threat of fire, possible explosions, impending structural collapse, possible electrical hazards, toxic gases, and other such dangers may make it necessary to move a patient quickly in order to protect both you and the patient.
- *Life-saving care cannot be given because of the patient's location or position.* You may have to move a patient to a hard, flat surface to provide CPR, or you may have to move a patient in order to reach a profusely bleeding wound.
- *You are unable to gain access to other patients who need life-saving care.* You may have to quickly move a patient in order to reach another patient who needs immediate care. This is seen most often in motor-vehicle crashes. ■

Emergency moves rarely provide any protection for a patient's injuries, and they may cause great pain for the patient. But because of the reasons listed above, an emergency move is justified; that is, the situation is too dangerous for you and the patient or life-saving care cannot be provided unless the patient is moved quickly.

The greatest danger in moving a patient quickly is the possibility of making a spinal injury worse. It is impossible to remove a patient from a vehicle quickly and at the same time provide complete protection to the spine. But if the patient is on the floor or ground, it is important to make every effort to pull the patient in the direction of the long axis of the body, which will provide as much protection to the spine as possible. The long axis of the body is the line that runs down the center of the body from the top of the head and along the spine.

Drags

There are several emergency moves called *drags*. In this type of move, the patient is dragged by the clothes, feet, shoulders, or a blanket (Scan 5-1). These moves are reserved for urgent situations, when the patient needs to be moved as rapidly and as safely as possible. Note that drags do not provide protection for the neck and spine.

Most commonly, a long-axis drag is made from the area of the shoulders. This causes the remainder of the body to fall into its natural anatomical position, with the spine and all limbs in normal alignment. Never drag a patient sideways. A sideways drag can cause twisting motions and aggravation of injuries. Always drag in the direction of the long axis of the body.

When you are using a drag method and you have to take the patient down stairs or down an incline, go first and use a shoulder drag to pull the patient head-first by lifting under the arms. If possible, try to cradle the patient's head in your forearms as you drag.

Other Emergency Moves

There are many other techniques that can be used to move a patient quickly. Some require only one rescuer (Scan 5-2); others require two rescuers (Scan 5-3). Remember that any emergency move must be justified and that it should be carried out as quickly as possible.

NONEMERGENCY MOVES

FIRST> **Nonemergency moves** are used when there is no immediate threat to life. The situation is not urgent. Unless you are alone, all nonemergency moves should be carried out with the help of other trained personnel or bystanders. Take care to prevent additional injury to the patient, as well as to avoid patient discomfort and pain. ■

nonemergency move a patient move that is carried out if there are other factors at the scene causing the patient to decline, you must reach other patients, part of the care required forces you to move the patient, or the patient insists on being moved.

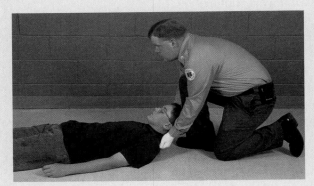

Clothes Drag.

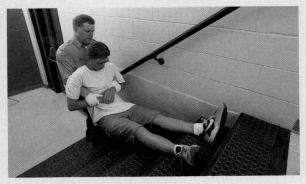

Incline Drag. Always head first.

CAUTION: Always pull in the direction of the long axis of patient's body. Do not pull a patient sideways. Avoid bending or twisting the patient's trunk.

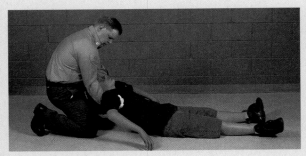

Shoulder Drag.

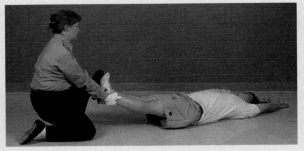

Foot Drag.

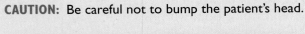

CAUTION: Be careful not to bump the patient's head.

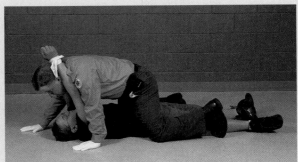

Firefighter's Drag. Place patient on his back and tie hands together. Straddle patient, facing his head. Crouch, pass your head through his trussed arms, and raise your body. Crawl on your hands and knees. Keep patient's head as low as possible.

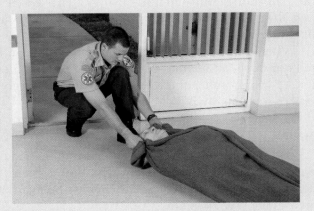

Blanket Drag. Gather half of the blanket material up against patient's side. Roll patient toward your knees so that you can place the blanket under him. Gently roll patient back onto the blanket. During the drag, keep patient's head as low as possible.

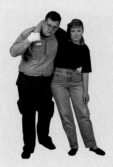

One-Rescuer Assist. Place patient's arm around your neck, grasping her hand in yours. Place your other arm around patient's waist. Help her walk to safety. Be prepared to change technique if level of danger increases. Be sure to communicate with patient about obstacles, uneven terrain, and so on. (Michael A. Gallitelli)

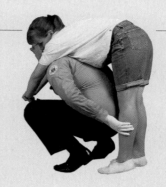

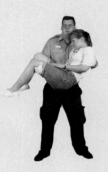

Cradle Carry. Place one arm across patient's back with your hand under her arm. Place your other arm under her knees and lift. If your patient is conscious, have her place her near arm over your shoulder. (Michael A. Gallitelli)

NOTE: This carry places a lot of weight on the carrier's back. It is usually appropriate only for very light patients.

Piggy Back Carry. Assist patient to stand. Place her arms over your shoulder so they cross your chest. Bend over and lift her. While she holds on with her arms, crouch and grasp each thigh. Use a lifting motion to move her onto your back. Pass your forearms under her knees and grasp her wrists. (Michael A. Gallitelli)

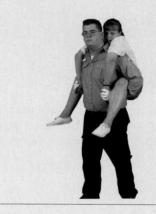

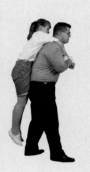

Pack Strap Carry. Have patient stand. Turn your back to her, bringing her arms over your shoulders to cross your chest. Keep her arms as straight as possible, with her armpits over your shoulders. Hold patient's wrists, bend, and pull her onto your back. (Michael A. Gallitelli)

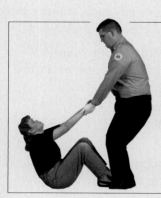

Firefighter's Carry. Place your feet against patient's feet and pull her toward you. Bend at waist and flex knees. Duck and pull her across your shoulders, keeping hold of one of her wrists. Use your free arm to reach between her legs and grasp her thigh. Allow her weight to fall onto your shoulders. Stand up. Transfer your grip on her thigh to her wrist. (Michael A. Gallitelli)

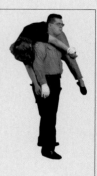

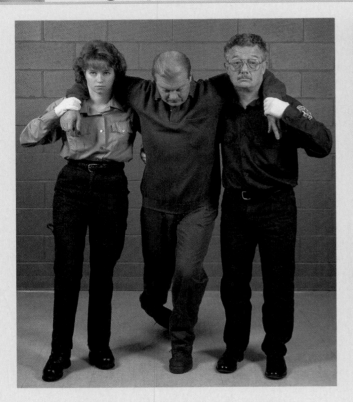

Two-Rescuer Assist. Patient's arms are placed around shoulders of both rescuers. Each rescuer grips one of the patient's hands, places free arm around the patient's waist, and helps him walk to safety.

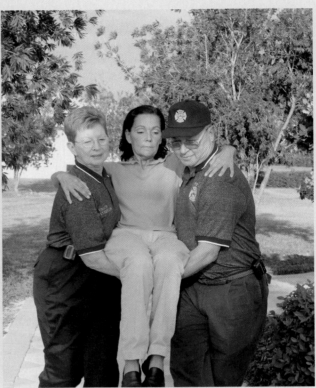

Two-Rescuer Cradle Carry. The rescuers' arms are clasped beneath the patient's legs and behind the back to support the patient in a seated position.

Follow these rules for a nonemergency move:

- Initial assessment should be completed, and the patient's airway, breathing, and circulation (ABCs) should be intact.

- Vital signs should be stable.

- There should be no uncontrolled external bleeding or any indication of internal bleeding.

- Care must be taken to avoid compromising a possible neck or spine injury. Avoid moving a patient who has neck pain, numbness, or weakness.

- All suspected fractures should be splinted.

Even when there is no immediate danger to you or to the patient, a nonemergency move could be justified if:

- *Factors at the scene cause patient decline.* If a patient's condition is rapidly declining due to heat, cold, or an allergic reaction, moving may be necessary.

- *You must reach other patients.* When there are other patients at the scene, you may need to move one in order to reach another to provide care.

- *Care requires moving the patient.* This is usually seen in cases in which there are no suspected spinal injuries. Problems due to extreme heat or cold, such as heat cramps, heat exhaustion, hypothermia, and local cold injuries (frostbite and freezing) are good examples. Reaching a source of water for washing in cases of serious chemical burns also may be a reason to move a patient.

- *Patient insists on being moved.* You are not allowed to restrain patients. If a patient will not listen to the reasons why he should not be moved and tries to move on his own, you may have to assist him. Sometimes a patient becomes so upset that stress worsens his condition. If this type of patient can be moved, and the move is short, you may have to make the move in order to keep him calm and relieve his stress. However, be cautious if the patient is intoxicated.

If one of these situations exists, you may consider using one of the following nonemergency moves.

Direct Ground Lift

FIRST➤ The direct ground lift (three-rescuer lift) is a nonemergency move and is not recommended for use on patients with possible neck or spine injuries. While this procedure can be carried out by two people, at least three are recommended. Additional rescuers may be used for the move by having them position themselves opposite the three main participants in the move. ■

To perform a direct ground lift (see Scan 5-4), the patient should be lying face up (supine) and the arms should be placed on the chest. You and your helpers should line up on one side of the patient. One rescuer should be at the patient's head, another should be positioned at her midsection, and another at the lower legs. Each of you should drop to the knee closest to the patient's feet.

The rescuer at the head should place one arm under the patient's neck and grasp the far shoulder in order to cradle the head. The other arm should be placed under her back, just above the waist. The rescuer at her midsection should place one arm above and one arm below the buttocks. The rescuer at the patient's lower legs should place one arm under her knees and the other arm under her ankles.

First, on the signal of the rescuer at the head, everyone should lift the patient up to the level of their knees.

Second, on signal, the rescuers should roll the patient toward their chests.

Third, on signal, everyone should stand while holding the patient. You can now move her, reversing the process when it is time to place her in a supine position.

Extremity Lift

FIRST➤ An extremity lift requires two people (Figure 5.3). This lift should not be performed if there is a possibility of head, neck, spine, shoulder, hip, or knee injury, or any suspected fractures to the extremities that have not been immobilized. The patient should be alert. If not, you may have incorrectly assessed neck and spine injuries. ■

The patient should be placed face up, with knees flexed. You should kneel at the head of the patient, placing your hands under her shoulders. Have your helper stand at the patient's feet and grasp her wrists. Direct your helper to pull the patient into a sitting position, while you push the patient from the shoulders. (Do not have your helper pull the patient by the arms if there are any signs of suspected fractures.) Slip your arms under the patient's armpits and grasp the wrists. Once the patient is in a semi-sitting position, have your helper turn his back to the patient, crouch down, and grasp the patient's legs behind the knees.

NOTE

It is poor practice to use only two rescuers for a ground lift. A two-rescuer direct ground lift would not allow enough support for the patient or control during the move. However, if you must perform it, position your helper at the patient's thigh so one arm can be placed on her back above her buttocks and the other arm under her knees.

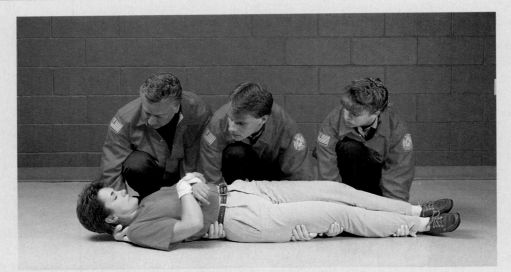

1. Rescuers kneel on one side of the patient and position their hands to support and lift.

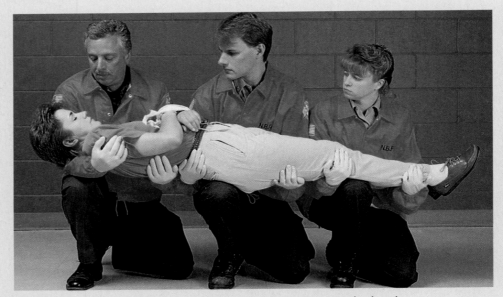

2. Rescuers lift the patient to knee level at the direction of the rescuer at the head.

continued...

Direct your helper so that you both stand at the same time. For example: "Ready? Lift on three. 1 . . . 2 . . . 3 . . . lift" and move as a unit when carrying the patient. Try to walk out of step with your partner to avoid swinging the patient. Direct your helper as to when to stop the carry and when to place the patient down in a supine or seated position.

TRANSFER OF PATIENT FROM BED TO STRETCHER

Once EMS arrives at the scene, they may require your assistance in moving the patient from a bed to a stretcher. This may be accomplished using either the direct carry or draw sheet method.

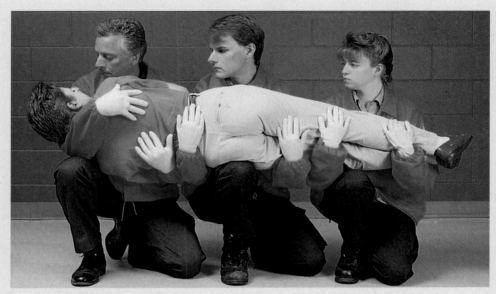

3. Rescuers curl the patient to their chests.

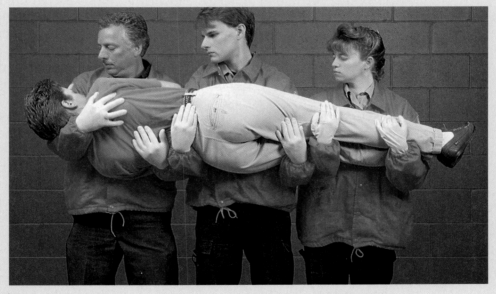

4. Rescuers stand.

Direct Carry Method

The direct carry is performed in order to move a patient with no suspected spine injury from a bed or from a bed-level position to a stretcher (Scan 5-5). First, position the stretcher perpendicular to the bed with the head end of the stretcher at the foot of the bed. Prepare the stretcher by unbuckling straps and removing other items. Then, two rescuers should stand between the bed and the stretcher, facing the patient. The first rescuer should slide an arm under the patient's neck and cup his shoulder while the second rescuer slides a hand under the patient's hip and lifts slightly. The first rescuer then slides his other arm under the patient's back while the second rescuer places his arms underneath the patient's hips and

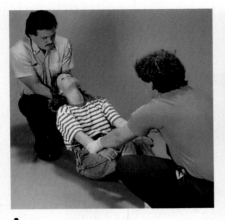

A.

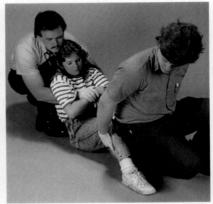

B.

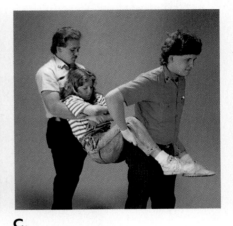

C.

FIGURE 5.3
Extremity lift.

calves. Finally, both rescuers should slide the patient to the edge of the bed, lift/curl him towards their chests, and then rotate and place him gently onto the stretcher.

Draw Sheet Method

The other method of moving a patient with no suspected spine injury from a bed to a stretcher is the draw sheet method. It may be performed from the side of the bed or from either the head or the foot of the bed. Select a method that gives you the easiest access to the patient. Figure 5.4 illustrates how to do it from the side of the bed. To use the draw sheet method from the head or the foot of the bed, one rescuer must make sure the stretcher does not move while transferring the patient.

To perform the draw sheet method from the side of the bed, begin by loosening the bottom sheet of the bed and positioning the stretcher next to the bed. Then, adjust the height of the stretcher, lower the rails, and unbuckle the straps. Both rescuers should reach across the stretcher and roll the sheet against the patient. Grasp the sheet firmly at the patient's head, chest, hips, and knees. Finally, draw the patient onto the stretcher, sliding him in one smooth motion.

PATIENT POSITIONING

Recovery Position

Positioning the patient is also a very important part of your care. Unresponsive patients with no suspected spine injury should be placed in the recovery position, which helps them to maintain an open and clear airway. Place patients on their left side whenever possible to aid drainage of fluids and vomitus. Remember that patients with injuries, especially a suspected spine injury, should not be moved until additional EMS resources arrive to evaluate and stabilize them.

To place an unresponsive but uninjured patient in the recovery position (Figure 5.5), perform the following steps:

1. Kneel beside the patient on the left side. Raise the patient's left arm straight out above his head.

2. Cross the patient's right arm over his chest, placing his right hand next to his left cheek.

3. Raise the right knee until it is completely flexed.

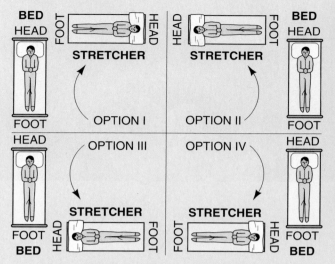

Stretcher is placed at 90° angle to bed, depending on room configuration. Prepare stretcher by lowering rails, unbuckling straps, and removing other items. Both First Responders stand between stretcher and bed, facing patient.

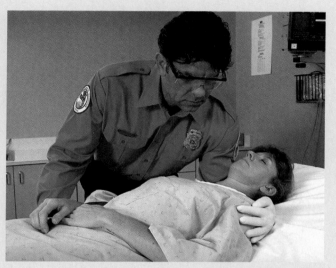

1. The head-end First Responder cradles the patient's head and neck by sliding one arm under her neck and grasping her shoulder.

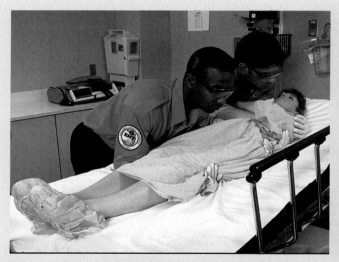

2. The foot-end First Responder slides hand under the patient's hips and lifts slightly. Head-end First Responder slides other arm under patient's back. Foot-end First Responder places arms under hips and calves.

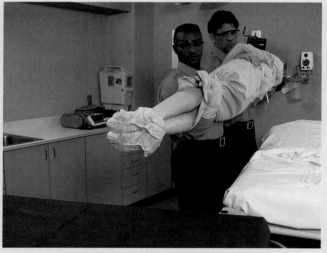

3. First Responders slide patient to edge of bed and bend toward her with their knees slightly bent. They lift and curl patient to their chests and return to a standing position. They rotate and slide patient gently onto stretcher.

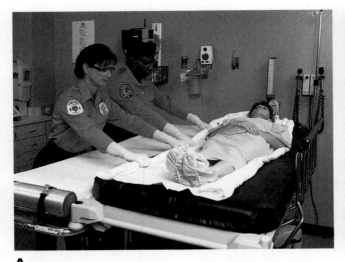
A.

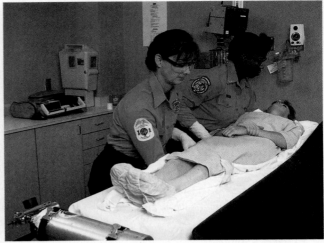
B.

FIGURE 5.4
Draw sheet method.

4. Place your right hand on the patient's right shoulder and your left hand on the patient's flexed right knee. Using the flexed knee as a lever, pull toward you, guiding the patient's torso in a smooth rolling motion onto his side. The patient's head will rest on his left arm.

5. As best as you can, position the patient's right elbow and knee on the floor so that they act like a kickstand, preventing the patient from rolling completely onto his stomach. Place the right hand under the side of his face. The arm will support the patient in this position. The hand will cushion his face and allow the head to angle slightly downward for airway drainage.

Many patients who do not have suspected spine injuries may be placed in a position of comfort. They may include patients with medical complaints such as chest pain, nausea, or difficulty breathing. Breathing is often aided by placing the patient in a semi-sitting (semi-Fowler's) position, which is about a 45° angle. This position of comfort must be used cautiously in case the patient vomits.

Always position yourself appropriately to manage the patient's airway and monitor his mental status. Place the patient in the recovery position at the first sign of a decreased level of responsiveness.

FIGURE 5.5
Patient in the recovery position.

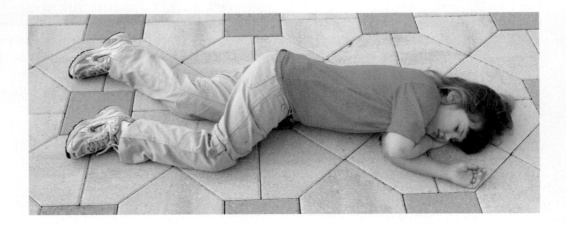

Log Roll

When an unresponsive patient is face down (prone), you must assess breathing differently. Place your hand in front of the patient's mouth and nose to feel for breathing. If you feel breath on your hand, the patient has an airway and is breathing. The patient's condition may worsen, however, and ideally, you want him on his back (supine) for further assessment, proper airway maintenance and care, and basic life support if it becomes necessary.

To move a prone patient to a supine position and ensure stability of the head and spine where a trauma injury is suspected, perform a *log roll*. This move can be done with two rescuers, but three and four rescuers can minimize twisting of the patient's spine during the procedure. Perform the following steps:

1. One rescuer should kneel at the top of patient's head and hold or stabilize the head and neck in a neutral (anatomical) position in line with her spine.

2. A second rescuer should kneel at the patient's side and position her arms. (Note that there are two methods of arm positioning. Each has a specific advantage. One method is to raise and extend the patient's arm above her head. This allows for easy rolling to that side and provides support for the head during the roll, which is helpful if you must do the log roll alone. A second method is to place the patient's arm along her side. It will help splint, support, and maintain alignment of the spine during the move. The second method may work better when there are multiple rescuers. The First Responder at the patient's head must maintain head alignment during the log roll, regardless of the patient's arm positioning. Check with your instructor for the preferred method in your jurisdiction.)

3. The second rescuer should kneel between the patient's shoulders and hips. If other rescuers are available, all of them should kneel along the side of the patient from shoulders to knees.

4. Rescuer(s) should grasp the patient's shoulders, hips, knees, and ankles. If only one rescuer is available to roll the patient, he should grasp the heavy parts of the torso—the shoulders and hips.

5. The rescuer at the patient's head should signal and give directions: "On three, slowly roll: 1 . . . 2 . . . 3 . . . roll together." All rescuers should slowly roll the patient in a coordinated move and carefully keep her spine in a neutral, in-line position until she is supine.

Sometimes the patient is already supine but must be placed on a blanket or spine board. If this is the case, then perform steps 1 through 5 above, maintaining control of the patient when she is rolled onto her side. Without removing your hands, continue with the following (Scan 5-6):

1. The First Responder at the patient's head should continue stabilization of the patient's head and neck until rescuers position a blanket or long spine board (backboard) behind the patient.

2. At a signal from the rescuer at the head, they should slowly roll the patient in a coordinated move onto the blanket or spine board.

3. Finally, they should make sure the patient is positioned on the center of the spine board. If they must adjust the patient's position, they must keep her head and spine in neutral alignment.

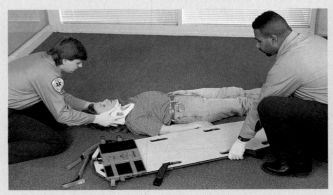

1. Manually stabilize the patient's head and neck as you place the board parallel to the patient. Maintain manual stabilization throughout the log roll.

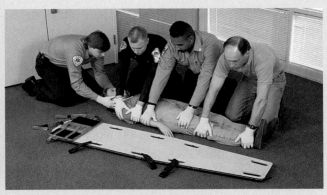

2. Kneel at the patient's side opposite the board at the shoulder, waist, and knees. Reach across the patient and position your hands.

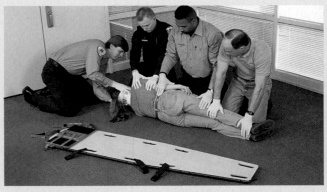

3. On command from the rescuer at the head, roll the patient toward you as a unit. The spine board should be put in place.

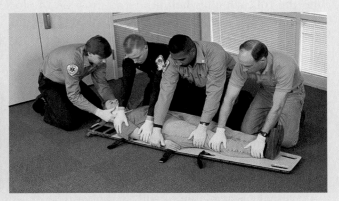

3. Place the patient onto the board, rolling her as a unit.

EQUIPMENT

EMTs and ALS personnel will often ask First Responders to assist with packaging, lifting, moving, and loading patients into the ambulance. In order to help with these tasks, First Responders must be familiar with the various carrying and packaging devices that may be used (Scan 5-7). Many First Responder courses do not include information and practice on immobilization devices. Your instructor will teach you the procedures if First Responders are expected to perform them in your jurisdiction. Do not try to learn the procedures on your own.

When you package a patient on an immobilization device, you must first stabilize the head and neck by selecting and applying the appropriate size cervical collar (Scans 5-8 and 5-9). These collars, also called extrication collars, are rigid supports that rescuers apply to help maintain stability and alignment with the body in patients who have suspected neck and spine injuries (Scans 5-10 and 5-11). Again, do not try to learn the steps of placing a collar on a patient without proper instruction. Your instructor will teach you the steps if First Responders are required to use collars in your jurisdiction. (Refer to Chapter 11 for care of patients with spinal injuries.)

Typical equipment that may be used for packaging and loading the patient includes:

- *Wheeled stretcher*—This device is sometimes called a stretcher, cot, or gurney. It is secured in the back of an ambulance to transport the patient. There are many brands and types of wheeled stretchers. Many ambulance providers use one known as a single-operator stretcher, which has collapsible legs that fold as they are pushed onto the ambulance. With this type of stretcher, rescuers do not have to lift the patient. In addition, the head and the foot ends of many stretchers can be elevated to make the patient comfortable or to assist in caring for certain conditions such as shock.

- *Portable stretcher*—Portable or folding stretchers are often used in multiple-casualty incidents (incidents with many patients). The stretchers may be canvas, aluminum, or heavy plastic, and they usually fold, roll up, or collapse for easy storage. Aluminum and plastic stretchers are now commonly used because it is easy to disinfect them.

- *Stair chair*—The stair chair helps rescuers move patients on stairways and through tight places where a traditional stretcher will not fit. Newer brands are made of canvas on sturdy folding frames and are easy to store. They have wheels that allow rescuers to roll them over flat surfaces like a wheelchair, and some models are designed to maneuver and slide easily down stairways just by tilting them.

- *Scoop (orthopedic) stretcher*—This device is called the scoop stretcher because it splits vertically into two pieces, which can be used to "scoop" the patient up. Newer models are sturdier and more inflexible than older ones and provide support to the spine. However, a scoop stretcher is commonly used for picking up and moving a patient with hip injuries or multiple injuries rather than for spine injuries. It is also used for transferring patients from a bed or the floor to a wheeled stretcher or from the wheeled stretcher to the hospital bed. Follow your local protocols for using this device.

- *Spine board*—There are two types of spine boards, or backboards: long and short. The long spine board is used for patients who are found lying down or standing and must be immobilized. Short spine boards are used primarily for removing patients from vehicles when it is suspected that they have neck or spine injuries. Once secured to the short spine board, the patient can be moved from a sitting position in the vehicle to a supine position on a long spine board.

- *Vest extrication devices and short spine boards*—The extrication vest is used to help immobilize patients found in a seated position and remove them from a vehicle. It wraps around the patient's torso to stabilize the spine and has an extended section above the vest with side flaps for stabilizing the patient's head and neck. Rescuers secure the patient's head, neck, and torso with straps and padding. The vest has handles that aid in lifting the patient onto a long spine board.

  Short spine boards are also used to remove patients in a seated position from vehicles when they have neck or spine injuries. Once secured to the

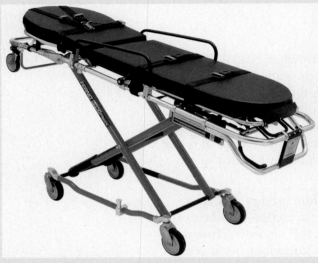

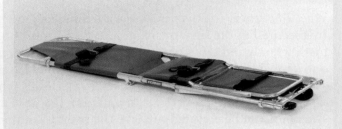

Portable Stretcher. Beneficial in multiple-casualty incidents.

Wheeled Stretcher. Head can be elevated to benefit some patients. (Ferno Corporation)

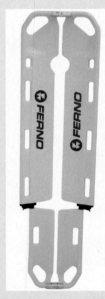

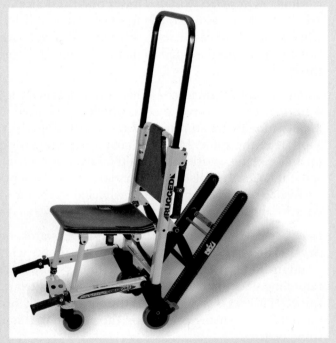

Scoop (Orthopedic) Stretcher. Allows quick immobilization of hip or multiple injuries as well as quick patient transfer. New devices are sturdy enough to support spinal injuries. (Ferno Corporation)

Stair Chair. For use on stairs or tight places. (Stryker EMS)

continued...

Patient Carrying Devices

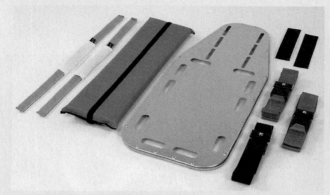

Short Spine Board. Used to remove patients from vehicles.

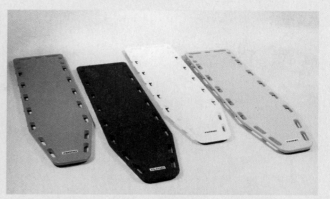

Long Spine Board. Used for patients found lying down or standing.

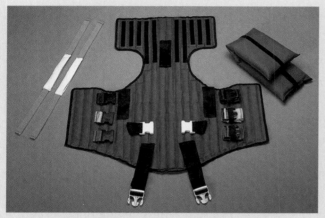

Vest-Type Extrication Device. Wraps help stabilize the patient's head, neck, and spine.

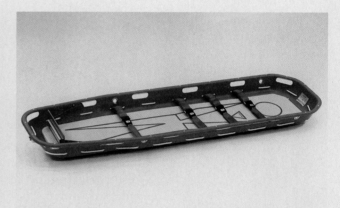

Basket Stretcher. Used to transport over rough terrain.

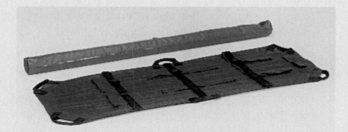

Flexible Stretcher. Used in restricted areas or narrow hallways.

Cervical Spine Immobilization Collars

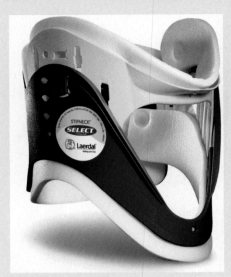

(Laerdal Medical Corporation)

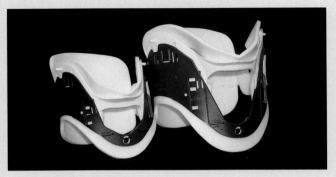

(Philadelphia Collar Corporation)

short spine board, rescuers move the patient from a sitting position in the vehicle to a supine position on a long spine board. EMS personnel often use the vest extrication device instead of the short spine board because it is easy and quick to apply.

- *Full-body spinal immobilization devices*—Different types include body-splinting devices called composite backboards, full-body splints, and full-body vacuum splints. (Some areas may still use wooden boards, but they are not as easy to disinfect if their protective surface is damaged. Composite boards are easy to disinfect.) Full-body spinal immobilization devices are used for patients with multiple injuries or suspected spine injuries.

- *Basket stretcher*—This stretcher is typically used in more rural settings to move a patient from one level to another or over rough terrain.

- *Flexible stretcher*—This stretcher is made of canvas, rubberized, or other flexible material such as heavy plastic, often with wooden slats sewn into pockets. The flexible stretcher usually has three carrying handles on each side. Because of its flexibility, it can be useful in restricted areas or narrow hallways.

- *Pedi-boards*—Special spinal immobilization boards are made to fit infants and children. The back of a child's head is larger than an adult's, so boards have a depression in the head end to fit it. However, it is still necessary to pad the child's body from the shoulders to the heels to ensure his airway is in a neutral position while secured on the board.

Sizing a Cervical Spine Immobilization Collar

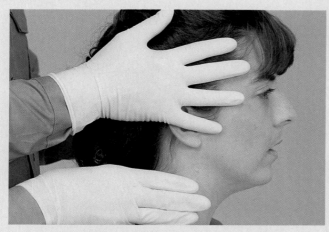

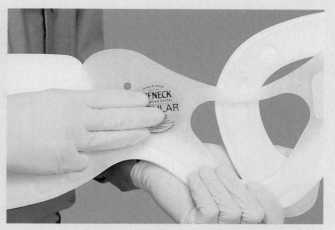

1. To size a cervical spine immobilization collar, first draw an imaginary line across the top of the shoulders and the bottom of the chin. Use your fingers to measure the distance from the shoulder to the chin.

2. Check the collar you select. The distance between the sizing hole (black fastener) and lower edge of the rigid plastic should match that of the number of stacked fingers previously measured against the patient's neck.

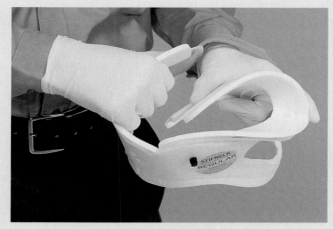

3. Assemble and pre-form the collar.

Applying a Cervical Spine Immobilization Collar to a Sitting Patient

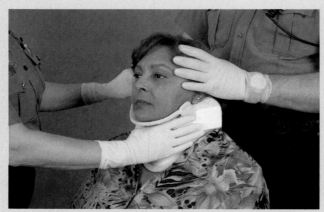

1. After selecting the proper size, slide the cervical spine immobilization collar up the chest wall. The chin must cover the central fastener in the chin piece.

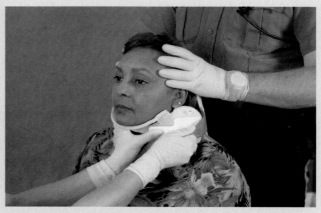

2. Bring the collar around the neck and secure the Velcro. Recheck the position of the patient's head and collar for proper alignment. Make sure the patient's chin covers the central fastener of the chin piece.

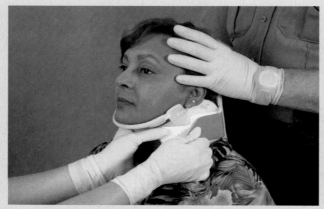

3. If the chin is not covering the fastener of the chin piece, re-adjust the collar by tightening the Velcro until a proper sizing is obtained. If further tightening will cause hyperextension of the patient's head, then select the next smaller size.

NOTE: With the collar alone in place, there can still be movement of the lower cervical region. Manually maintain the patient's head in a neutral position.

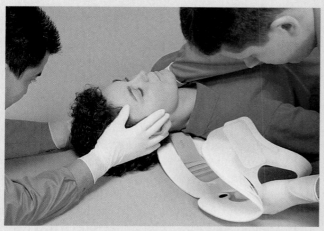

I. Slide the back portion of the cervical spine immobilization collar behind the patient's neck. Fold the loop Velcro inward on the foam padding.

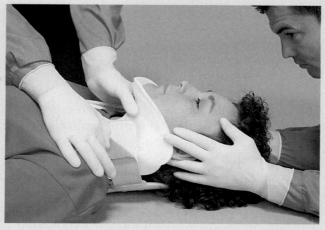

2. Position the collar so that the chin fits properly. Secure the collar by attaching the Velcro.

ALTERNATIVE METHOD

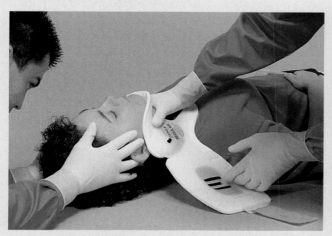

I. An alternative method of applying the collar to a supine patient is to start by positioning the chin piece and then sliding the back portion of the collar behind the patient's neck.

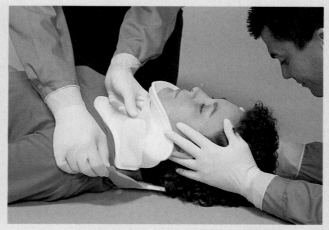

2. Hold the collar in place by grasping the trachea hole. Attach the loop Velcro so it mates with (and is parallel to) the hook Velcro.

Chapter Review

SUMMARY

Whenever possible, you should not move a patient. Only move patients when you must reposition them to care for life-threatening problems. Assess the patient, monitor the patient's condition, keep the patient at rest, and move him only when a dangerous environment presents a life threat or further injury or when your care requires repositioning. Before you move a patient or an object, first plan what you will do and how. Get help rather than risk injury. When you lift, use proper **body mechanics**. That is, position your feet at shoulder's width apart; use your legs, not your back, to lift; never twist as you lift; keep your back as straight as possible; and keep the weight you are lifting close to your body.

Emergency moves are carried out quickly when the scene is hazardous, care of the patient requires repositioning, or you must reach another patient who needs life-saving care. A heavy patient or one who is unresponsive or unable to move alone may be moved by using one of the drag methods. Always drag the patient along the long axis of the body, keeping his head as low as possible. The use of a drag may also be appropriate where there are possible spinal injuries.

Nonemergency moves are the preferred choice when the situation is not urgent, the patient is stable, and you have adequate time and personnel to move him. Most nonemergency moves are NOT appropriate for patients with suspected spine injuries and are carried out after you have completed a thorough patient assessment. It is best to splint any suspected fractures before these moves.

The direct ground lift is a nonemergency move that can be used for patients with no neck or spine injuries. You should have two, three, or more people to help. The patient must be supported at the head, neck, back, and knees. A rescuer should control and support the patient above and below the buttocks. Another rescuer should support the patient's knees and ankles. When moving the patient, you should keep the patient rolled toward your chest.

The extremity lift is a good nonemergency move, but it should not be used if the patient has possible head, neck, or spine injuries, is unresponsive, or has injuries to the upper or lower extremities (including the shoulder and hip). This lift requires two rescuers, with you lifting the patient at the shoulders and your helper lifting the patient at the knees.

Transfer patients from a bed to a stretcher using the direct carry method or the draw sheet method.

Sometimes it is necessary to position patients to ensure they can maintain an airway, breathe, and drain fluids. Use the **recovery position** for unresponsive patients, who are breathing and have no spine injuries. Use a position of comfort or a semi-sitting position for responsive patients who have no spine injuries, such as those with chest pain, nausea, or difficulty breathing.

First Responders may be asked to assist with lifting, moving, and immobilizing patients. Many types of equipment are available, including wheeled, portable, scoop (orthopedic), basket, and flexible stretchers, full-body spinal immobilization devices, the stair chair, and short spinal immobilization devices, such as the extrication vest and short spine boards. There are also special immobilization devices for infants and children called pedi-boards.

Using poor body mechanics is dangerous, not only to you but also to your patient and coworkers.

✔ Learn and practice proper methods of lifting and moving patients until you are able to perform them effortlessly.

Remember that it is also dangerous to push yourself past your physical limits.

✔ Never hesitate to ask for assistance from other EMS providers if a patient or equipment is too heavy for you to lift alone.

Each EMS system has various types of equipment for packaging and carrying patients.

✔ Find out what kinds of patient carrying and immobilization devices are used on the ambulances in your community and become proficient in using them.

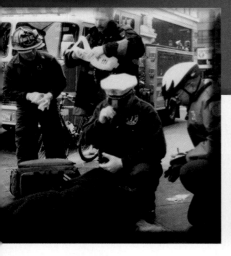
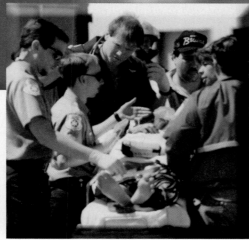
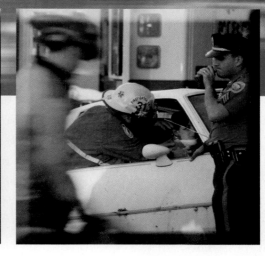

Airway Management

CHAPTER 6

Breathing is life. We take in each life-giving breath through simple passages—our mouth, nose, and windpipe. These few important parts of our bodies form an airway into our lungs. Blood that circulates to the lungs drops off carbon dioxide and picks up oxygen. The heart then pumps the oxygen to the rest of the body. When the blood returns to the heart with waste gases, it is pumped to the lungs to exchange those gases with oxygen. This continuous process is a simple one that we don't usually think about—until we cannot do it. This chapter will briefly explain the process of breathing. It will then list the steps to take for patients who are not breathing or who are having difficulty breathing because of airway obstructions.

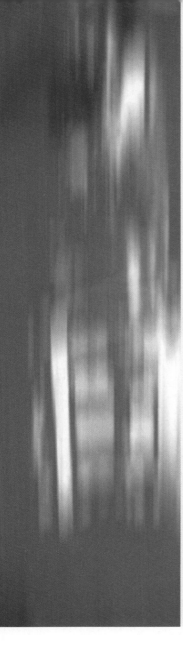

NATIONAL STANDARD OBJECTIVES

This chapter focuses on the objectives of Module 2, Lesson 2–1, of the U.S. DOT's First Responder National Standard Curriculum and serves as an instructional aid to help you meet any specific objectives added to the course by your local EMS system.

By the end of this chapter, you will be able to
(from cognitive or knowledge information):

2–1.1 Name and label the major structures of the respiratory system on a diagram. (pp. 99–100)

2–1.2 List the signs of inadequate breathing. (pp. 100–101)

2–1.3 Describe the steps in the head-tilt, chin-lift. (pp. 101–102)

2–1.4 Relate mechanism of injury to opening the airway. (pp. 101, 111–112)

2–1.5 Describe the steps in the jaw thrust. (pp. 102–103)

2–1.6 State the importance of having a suction unit ready for immediate use when providing emergency medical care. (pp. 112, 129–131)

2–1.7 Describe the techniques of suctioning. (pp. 129–131)

2–1.8 Describe how to ventilate a patient with a (pocket) resuscitation mask or barrier device. (pp. 103–107)

2–1.9 Describe how ventilating an infant or a child is different from an adult. (pp. 108–109)

2–1.10 List the steps in providing mouth-to-mouth and mouth-to-stoma ventilation. (pp. 103, 107, 110–111)

2–1.11 Describe how to measure and insert an oropharyngeal (oral) airway. (pp. 125–128)

2–1.12 Describe how to measure and insert a nasopharyngeal (nasal) airway. (pp. 128–129)

2–1.13 Describe how to clear a foreign body airway obstruction in a responsive adult. (pp. 114–120, 121)

2–1.14 Describe how to clear a foreign body airway obstruction in a responsive child with a complete obstruction or a partial obstruction and poor air exchange. (pp. 114–120, 121–122)

2–1.15 Describe how to clear a foreign body airway obstruction in a responsive infant with a complete obstruction or a partial airway obstruction and poor air exchange. (pp. 114–120, 122–124)

2–1.16 Describe how to clear a foreign body airway obstruction in an unresponsive adult. (pp. 114–120, 122)

2–1.17 Describe how to clear a foreign body airway obstruction in an unresponsive child. (pp. 114–120, 122)

2–1.18 Describe how to clear a foreign body airway obstruction in an unresponsive infant. (pp. 114–120, 122–124)

LEARNING TASKS

Chapter 6 explains the functions of the airway and breathing. As you work through this chapter, you will come to understand better the reasons that airway and breathing are the first and most important steps in patient care. By the end of the chapter, you should be able to:

✔ State three reasons why we must breathe to stay alive.

When patients stop breathing, a First Responder only has a few minutes to assist them in starting the breathing process again. But if the delay is too long, patients will die. The time between breathing and not breathing is critical, and you need to understand what happens in those few minutes. Be able to:

✔ Explain the difference between clinical death and biological death and the approximate times for each before brain cells begin to die if the patient does not receive oxygen.

Feel comfortable enough to
(by changing attitudes, values, and beliefs):

2–1.19 Explain why basic life support ventilation and airway protective skills take priority over most other basic life support skills. (pp. 94, 96–97, 133)

2–1.20 Demonstrate a caring attitude towards patients with airway problems who request emergency medical services. (pp. 109–110)

2–1.21 Place the interests of the patient with airway problems as the foremost consideration when making any and all patient care decisions. (pp. 109–110)

2–1.22 Communicate with empathy to patients with airway problems, as well as with family members and friends of the patient. (pp. 109–110)

Show how to
(through psychomotor skills):

2–1.23 Demonstrate the steps in the head-tilt, chin-lift. (pp. 101–102)

2–1.24 Demonstrate the steps in the jaw thrust. (pp. 102–103)

2–1.25 Demonstrate the techniques of suctioning. (pp. 129–131)

2–1.26 Demonstrate the steps in mouth-to-mouth ventilation with body substance isolation (barrier shields). (pp. 106–107)

2–1.27 Demonstrate how to use a (pocket) resuscitation mask to ventilate a patient. (pp. 103–106)

2–1.28 Demonstrate how to ventilate a patient with a stoma. (pp. 110–111)

2–1.29 Demonstrate how to measure and insert an oropharyngeal (oral) airway. (pp. 125–128)

2–1.30 Demonstrate how to measure and insert a nasopharyngeal (nasal) airway. (pp. 128–129)

2–1.31 Demonstrate how to ventilate infant and child patients. (pp. 108–109)

2–1.32 Demonstrate how to clear a foreign body airway obstruction in a responsive adult. (pp. 114–120, 121)

2–1.33 Demonstrate how to clear a foreign body airway obstruction in a responsive child. (pp. 114–120, 121)

2–1.34 Demonstrate how to clear a foreign body airway obstruction in a responsive infant. (pp. 114–120, 122–124)

2–1.35 Demonstrate how to clear a foreign body airway obstruction in an unresponsive adult. (pp. 114–120, 122)

2–1.36 Demonstrate how to clear a foreign body airway obstruction in an unresponsive child. (pp. 114–120, 122)

2–1.37 Demonstrate how to clear a foreign body airway obstruction in an unresponsive infant. (pp. 114–120, 122–124)

When we breathe, pressure inside the lungs changes so that air flows in and out. Breathing in is an active process that requires muscle contractions, but breathing out is a passive process that works as muscles relax. The lungs function by pressure changes similar to blowing up a balloon and allowing it to deflate. Think about that process and be able to:

✔ Relate, in a very general way, changes in volume and pressure in the lungs to the process of breathing.

When First Responders help a patient to breathe, sometimes they ventilate with too much pressure and too frequently, so that the exhalation phase is not complete. When this happens, the lungs get overfilled and the extra air may go to the stomach. If that happens, you must notice and know what to do about it. So, be able to:

✔ State two things to do when air gets in the patient's stomach (gastric distention) from assisted ventilations.

Sometimes, events or actions cause our airway to become blocked, and it becomes difficult or impossible to breathe. What are the causes? How can you tell if someone is having a problem? What can First Responders do to help? You must be able to:

- ✔ List five factors that may cause airway obstruction.
- ✔ List three signs of partial airway obstruction.
- ✔ State when you should care for a partial airway obstruction as if it were a complete airway obstruction.
- ✔ Describe two things you will commonly notice about a responsive patient with a complete airway obstruction.

In addition, for a patient with injuries, always consider the possibility of an injury to the spine. If there is any reason to suspect one, stabilize the injured patient's head and neck while opening the airway so you do not cause further spinal damage. Be able to explain why and:

- ✔ Demonstrate the techniques used for patients with possible neck or spine injuries.

The Occupational Safety and Health Administration (OSHA) and the Centers for Disease Control and Prevention (CDC) guidelines state that EMS personnel can reduce the risk of contracting infectious diseases by using pocket face masks with one-way valves and high-efficiency particulate air (HEPA) filter inserts when ventilating patients. Always have one on hand. Also wear latex or vinyl gloves during assessment and care of all patients.

BREATHING

WHY WE BREATHE

respiration the act of breathing; the exchange of oxygen and carbon dioxide that takes place in the lungs.

To maintain life, we breathe. The act of breathing is called **respiration**. During the breathing process, oxygen is brought into the body and carbon dioxide is expelled. The body's cells, tissues, and organs need oxygen for life and energy, and all life processes require energy. The body uses oxygen to produce the energy needed to contract muscles, send nerve impulses, digest food, and build new tissues.

In addition to supplying the cells with oxygen, breathing also removes carbon dioxide from cells. As the body uses oxygen to produce energy, carbon dioxide is given off as a waste product. The process of breathing keeps up a constant exchange of carbon dioxide and oxygen. If breathing is not adequate or if it stops, carbon dioxide accumulates in the body's cells and becomes a deadly poison. An increase in carbon dioxide shows up in certain signs and symptoms: the person pants to try to rid the body of the excess carbon dioxide; the person becomes drowsy as brain cells react to excess carbon dioxide; as brain cells start to die, the person may start to hallucinate and lose the ability to make breathing efforts. The individual will become unresponsive and, if someone does not assist ventilations, will go into a coma and die.

By regulating the blood and tissue levels of carbon dioxide, the respiratory system plays a key role in keeping a normal acid-base balance. This is measured using the pH scale. A low pH indicates too much acid and may be caused by a buildup of carbon dioxide, as may be seen in respiratory failure. Cells live and function within a very narrow range of pH. If breathing is not adequate or if it fails, this balancing function stops. If blood pH level goes too far one way or the other on the scale, cells stop functioning and die. The brain is also very sensitive to improper levels of pH balance. Without proper pH, brain functions quickly cease, including those that control breathing.

When breathing stops, the heart will stop shortly after. This is because the heart is made of muscle cells that require a continuous supply of oxygen to contract. The moment when both heartbeat and respirations have stopped is called **clinical death**. Over the next 4 to 6 minutes, oxygen is depleted and cells begin to die. This is the period when it is critical for the patient to receive oxygen and assisted ventilations. If the patient's cells do not receive oxygen within 10 minutes, they quickly die. The organ affected first, and the most critical one, is the brain. **Biological death** occurs during this 6- to 10-minute time frame (Figure 6.1). A patient is biologically dead when the brain cells die. Clinical death can be reversed. Biological death is irreversible.

How We Breathe

Breathing is automatic. Even though you can control depth and rate sometimes, that control is short-term and is soon taken over by involuntary orders from the respiratory centers of the brain. If you try to hold your breath, these centers will urge you to breathe, then take over and force you to breathe. If you try to breathe slow, shallow breaths while running, these brain centers will automatically adjust the rate and depth of breathing to suit the needs of your body. Asleep, or even unresponsive, if there is no damage to these respiratory centers and the heart continues to circulate oxygenated blood to the brain, breathing will be an involuntary, automatic function. The needs of your cells, not your will, are the determining factors in the control of breathing.

The lungs are very elastic and expandable. This expansion is limited by the size of the chest cavity and the pressure within the cavity pushing back on the lungs. To **inspire** (inhale air), the size of the chest cavity must increase and the pressure inside the cavity must decrease. A simple law governs respiration: as volume increases, pressure decreases (Figure 6.2).

If you take the air out of a small balloon and place the same amount of air into a larger balloon, the final pressure inside the large balloon will not be as great as it was in the smaller one. Why? The larger balloon has a greater volume to be filled. The air from the small balloon will produce less pressure inside the large one.

clinical death the moment that breathing and heart actions stop.

biological death when the brain cells die. This is usually within 10 minutes of respiratory arrest.

remember

The process of biological death may be delayed by cold temperatures, especially in cold-water drowning situations. This is because the oxygen-requiring cell functions are profoundly slowed by the cooling of the body. Always perform resuscitation procedures on cold-water drowning victims, even if they have been in the water longer than 10 minutes.

inspire to inhale air. *Opposite* expire.

FIGURE 6.1
Without oxygen, brain cells begin to die within 10 minutes. Cell death may begin in as little as 4 minutes.

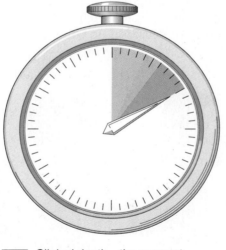

Clinical death—the moment breathing and heartbeat stop

Brain damage—within 4–6 minutes

Biological death—within 10 minutes brain cells begin to die

FIGURE 6.2
An equal amount of air delivered to each balloon will not produce the same pressure. An increase in volume means a decrease in pressure.

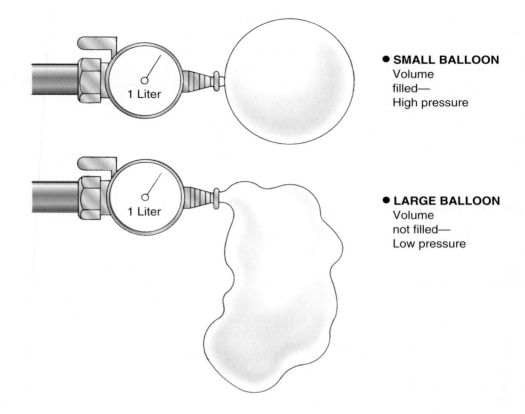

● **SMALL BALLOON**
Volume
filled—
High pressure

● **LARGE BALLOON**
Volume
not filled—
Low pressure

diaphragm the dome-shaped muscle that separates the chest and abdominal cavities. It is the major muscle used in breathing.

inspiration refers to the process of breathing in.

FIRST➤ The volume of the chest cavity is increased by muscle contraction. This may sound backwards because contractions usually make things smaller. However, as the muscles between the ribs contract, they pull the front of the ribs up and out. When the **diaphragm** contracts, it flattens downward. Both actions result in an increase in the size and volume of the chest cavity.

With each **inspiration**, the volume of the chest cavity increases, causing a decrease in the pressure within the lungs. (Figure 6.3 illustrates the breathing process.) When this happens, the lungs expand automatically. As the lungs expand, the volume inside each lung increases. This means that the pressure inside each lung will decrease. As you know, air moves from high pressure to low pressure. (A

INSPIRATIONS AND EXPIRATIONS

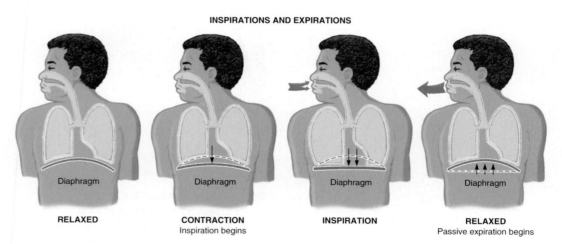

Diaphragm

RELAXED

Diaphragm

CONTRACTION
Inspiration begins

Diaphragm

INSPIRATION

Diaphragm

RELAXED
Passive expiration begins

FIGURE 6.3
Changes in volume and pressure produce inspiration and expiration.

punctured automobile tire demonstrates this fact.) So, when the pressure inside the lungs becomes less than the pressure in the atmosphere, air rushes into the lungs. It moves from high pressure (atmosphere) to low pressure (lungs). It will continue to do so until the pressure in the lungs equals the pressure in the atmosphere.

For **expiration** to occur, the process is reversed. The diaphragm and the muscles between the ribs relax, which reduces the volume in the chest cavity. In the smaller cavity, pressure builds in the lungs until it becomes greater than the pressure in the atmosphere and we must exhale. Air flows from high pressure (full lungs) to low pressure (atmosphere).

Inspiration is an active process. Rib and diaphragm muscles contract, causing expansion of the chest cavity. In contrast, expiration is a passive process. Muscles do not have to work to relax and allow air to leave the lungs and return to the atmosphere. ■

expiration refers to the passive process of breathing out.

Respiratory System Anatomy

FIRST➤ Several important parts of the respiratory system have been discussed: the respiratory centers in the brain and the muscles of respiration, including the diaphragm and those between the ribs. Other major structures of the respiratory system include the upper and lower airways (Figure 6.4):

- *Nose*—the primary path for air to enter and leave the system.
- *Mouth*—the secondary path for air to enter and leave the system.
- *Throat*—an air and food passage, which is also called **pharynx**.
- *Larynx*—an air passage at the top of the windpipe. The **larynx** is also known as the voice box (the anatomic structure that contains the vocal cords).
- *Bronchial tree*—tubes that branch from the windpipe and take air to the lungs. Its two main branches are the primary bronchi, one for each lung. These

pharynx (FAR-inks) the throat.

larynx (LAR-inks) the airway between the throat and the windpipe. It contains the voice box.

FIGURE 6.4
The respiratory system.

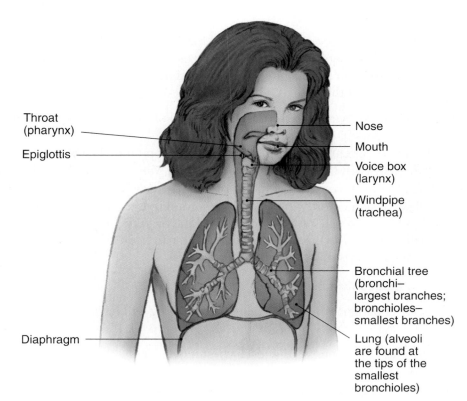

Throat (pharynx)
Epiglottis
Nose
Mouth
Voice box (larynx)
Windpipe (trachea)
Bronchial tree (bronchi– largest branches; bronchioles– smallest branches)
Diaphragm
Lung (alveoli are found at the tips of the smallest bronchioles)

branch into secondary bronchi in the lobes of the lungs. The secondary bronchi then branch into bronchioles, many of which have *alveoli*, the microscopic air sacs where the exchange of gases actually takes place.

- *Lungs*—elastic organs containing the bronchioles, small branching air passages in the lungs, and alveoli. These are the small air sacs at the end of the bronchioles where blood cells replenish their oxygen supply and release their accumulated carbon dioxide. Some of the bronchioles are called terminal bronchioles and do not have these microscopic air sacs. They are blind tubes, coming to an end that is closed off. As air enters these terminal bronchioles, they expand pathways wide enough to allow air to enter deeply into the lungs. This is important since some diseases will harden or close off these terminal bronchioles and reduce the ease of breathing.

- *Trachea*—an air passage to the lungs below the larynx. The **trachea** is also called the windpipe.

- *Epiglottis*—a leaf-shaped structure that covers the larynx when we swallow. The **epiglottis** prevents food and fluids from entering the windpipe. ■

trachea (TRAY-ke-ah) the windpipe.

epiglottis (EP-i-GLOT-is) a flap of cartilage and other tissues that is located above the voice box. It helps to close off the airway when a person swallows.

Respiratory Cycle

When our breathing muscles (the diaphragm and those between the ribs) contract and enlarge the chest cavity, oxygen flows through the mouth and nose, into the throat, past the open epiglottis, and into the trachea. Oxygen then flows into the left and right branches of the bronchi, then through the smaller bronchioles to the clusters of alveoli. The alveoli are surrounded by tiny blood vessels called *capillaries*. Gases—oxygen and carbon dioxide—can easily pass through the thin capillary membranes. Oxygen passes through alveoli to the blood, which delivers it to all body cells. Carbon dioxide passes from the blood cells in the capillaries back to the alveoli and out through the bronchial tree to the mouth or nose.

ASSESSMENT

Signs of Normal Breathing

FIRST➤ As you approach a patient and form a general impression, you can quickly determine if he is comfortable and breathing normally or if he is distressed and having trouble breathing. As you perform an initial assessment of the patient, you will:

- Look for the even and effortless rise and fall of the chest associated with normal breathing.
- Listen for air entering and leaving the nose or mouth. The sounds should be quiet like a soft breeze (no gurgling, gasping, wheezing, or other unusual sounds).
- Feel for air moving into and out of the nose or mouth.
- Observe skin color. While every person's skin is a different color, the skin should not be pale or ashen or tinted blue or gray. Look for these signs especially around the lips and eyes and in the nail beds, where they will be obvious if the patient is not ventilating properly. ■

Signs of Inadequate Breathing

FIRST➤ A patient who has inadequate breathing will have the following signs and symptoms:

- No chest movements, or uneven chest movements.
- No air heard or felt at the nose or mouth.
- Noisy breathing or gasping sounds.

NOTE

The rate and depth of breathing should be in the normal range while sitting quietly (at rest). For the adult—12 to 20 breaths per minute. For the child—15 to 30 breaths per minute. For the infant—25 to 50 breaths per minute.

- Breathing that is irregular, too rapid, or too slow.
- Breathing that is too shallow or deep and labored, or appears to be an effort, especially in infants and children.
- Breathing that uses muscles in the upper chest and around the neck.
- Nostrils that flare when breathing, especially in children.
- Skin that is tinted blue, gray, or ashen. (cianosis)
- Sitting or leaning forward in a tripod position to make breathing easier. ■

PULMONARY RESUSCITATION

Pulmonary refers to the lungs. *Resuscitation* is any effort to revive or to restore normal breathing function. When you perform **pulmonary resuscitation**, you are providing artificial or assisted ventilations to the patient in an attempt to restore the normal delivery of oxygen into the blood and removal of carbon dioxide. This is also referred to as rescue breathing.

Since you provide air that has already been in your lungs to the patient, you might wonder if you are providing enough oxygen. The atmosphere contains about 21% oxygen. The air exhaled from your lungs contains almost 16% oxygen. This is more than enough oxygen to keep most patients biologically alive until they can receive supplemental oxygen and care at a hospital.

pulmonary resuscitation (PUL-mo-ner-e re-SUS-si-TAY-shun) to provide breaths to a patient in an attempt to artificially maintain normal lung function. Also called rescue breathing or artificial ventilation.

OPENING THE AIRWAY

As part of your initial assessment of the patient, make certain that he has an open airway and adequate breathing. In an unresponsive patient, the muscles begin to relax and the tongue, a muscle, will drop into the back of the throat and obstruct the airway. The simple act of opening the airway could relieve this problem. If a patient is responsive and showing signs of obstruction (panicked looks and movements such as hands at the throat), the problem is not likely to be the tongue. Immediately begin the steps to relieve airway obstructions (discussed later in this chapter).

Repositioning the Head

FIRST➤ Simply repositioning the head may be enough to open the airway. If the patient is lying down with his head on several pillows or up against some object with head flexed forward, tilt the head back slightly by removing pillows or repositioning him so that the head is not flexed forward. You may place one flat pillow beneath the patient's shoulders to help maintain the airway. A large fluffy pillow may open the airway too far (that is, it may hyperextend it). Patients under the influence of alcohol or drugs often have trouble holding a head position that will keep the airway open. ■

There are two methods of opening the airway. The first, the head-tilt, chin-lift maneuver, is used for ill or injured patients with no possibility of spinal injury. The second, the jaw-thrust maneuver, is used for patients who have a mechanism of injury that indicates possible spinal injury.

Head-Tilt, Chin-Lift Maneuver

To perform the head-tilt, chin-lift maneuver, place one hand on the patient's forehead and tilt it back slightly. At the same time, place the fingertips of your other hand under the bony parts of the chin. (Be careful not to compress the soft tissues under the jaw.) Lift up the patient's chin so the lower teeth are almost touching the upper teeth (Figure 6.5). This maneuver will move the tongue out of the back of the throat and allow air to flow freely as the patient

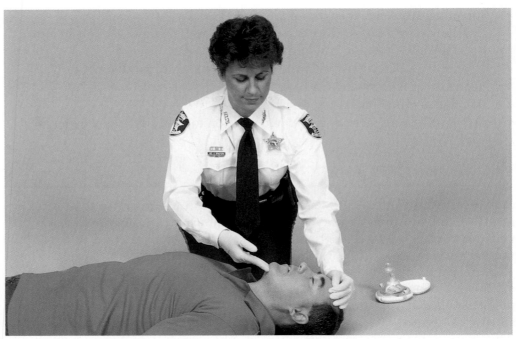

FIGURE 6.5
If there are no spinal injuries, use the head-tilt, chin-lift maneuver to open the airway.

breathes. It will also move the neck, which you do not want to do if the patient has a possible spinal injury. In such cases, use the next maneuver, the jaw-thrust.

Jaw-Thrust Maneuver This maneuver is the only recommended procedure for patients with possible neck or spine injuries (Figure 6.6). Position yourself at the top of the patient's head. Reach forward and place one hand on each side of the chin

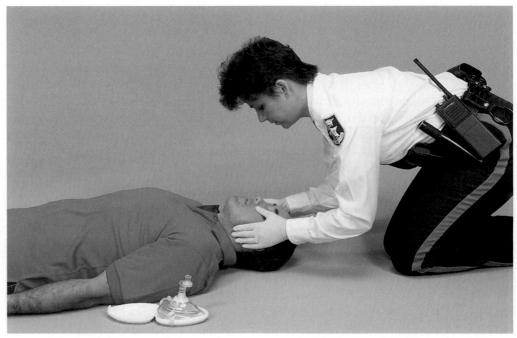

FIGURE 6.6
Use the jaw-thrust maneuver if there are possible neck or spinal injuries.

behind the jaw, just below the ears. You may press your thumbs against the cheek-bones for leverage. Push the jaw forward. Do not tilt or rotate the patient's head.

RESCUE BREATHING

All First Responders should use barrier devices. When First Responders perform rescue breathing, they can come into direct contact with the patient's body fluids, such as respiratory secretions and saliva droplets, blood, or vomitus. Take all steps necessary to ensure protection from infectious diseases. Use personal protective equipment and *barrier devices* (pocket face masks or face shields). Always protect yourself when performing rescue breathing or CPR.

One example of a barrier device is the pocket face mask. It should fit the patient and seal easily to the facial contours of the adult, child, or infant. A face mask should be easy to clean, made of durable plastic, have a replaceable one-way valve and filter, have an available oxygen inlet and, as an option, have a head strap to hold it in place.

Another example of a barrier device is the face shield, which is a durable plastic sheet with a filter. It is small enough to be packaged in a case and attached to a key ring, but it is large enough to cover the patient's lower face and act as a barrier to help prevent direct contact with body fluids.

NOTE: *The mouth-to-mouth and mouth-to-nose procedures are no longer accepted as safe practices. Citizens learn these methods because they do not normally carry barrier devices, and they would usually perform assisted ventilations on family members. EMS personnel would not use these techniques. However, it is common for all rescuers to learn how to deliver mouth-to-mouth and mouth-to-nose techniques, because of the possibility of being in situations where there are no protective devices or where there are more patients than devices at the scene. Those who advocate rescue breathing without protective devices state that it is a decision of the rescuer as to whether or not to provide ventilation without adequate rescuer protection.*

In addition, remember that protective gloves should be worn throughout any patient encounter.

MOUTH-TO-MASK VENTILATION

The mouth-to-mask technique of providing assisted ventilation (rescue breathing) is recommended for rescue personnel. A **pocket face mask** allows you to provide ventilations without direct contact with the patient's mouth and nose. The mask should have a one-way valve in the stem so that you can provide ventilations into one port while the patient exhales through another port. This is meant to prevent the patient's exhaled air and any body fluids from reaching the rescuer. The pocket face mask that you use should also come with a disposable filter called a *high-efficiency particulate air (HEPA) filter* (Figure 6.7). It snaps inside the pocket face mask and traps air droplets and secretions that may contain dangerous pathogens.

remember
You can reduce your risk of contracting infectious diseases by using a pocket face mask with one-way valve and HEPA filter when ventilating patients.

pocket face mask a device used to help provide ventilations. It has a chimney with a one-way valve and HEPA filter. Some have an inlet for supplemental oxygen.

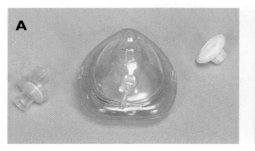
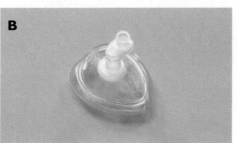

FIGURE 6.7
A. Pocket face mask parts: one-way valve, mask, HEPA filter. **B.** Assembled pocket face mask.

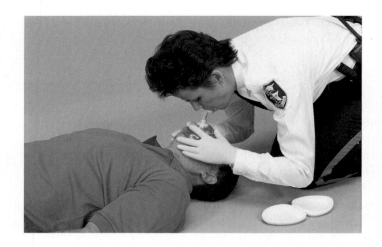

remember

If your patient is an unresponsive infant or child *and you are alone*, provide one minute of artificial ventilation and then call 9-1-1. If you are working with a partner or others are around, have one of them call 9-1-1 while you continue ventilating.

The pocket face mask is made of soft plastic material that can be folded and carried in your pocket. It is available with or without an oxygen inlet. You provide mouth-to-mask ventilations through a chimney on the mask (Figure 6.8). If the mask has a second port for oxygen, you can simultaneously ventilate the patient with air from your own lungs and with additional oxygen from an oxygen source (Figure 6.9).

Another advantage of the pocket face mask is that it allows you to use both hands to maintain a proper head-tilt or jaw-thrust and still hold the mask firmly in place. It is relatively easy to keep a good seal between the face mask and a patient's face with this device. The pocket face mask also can be used with or without an airway adjunct (discussed later in the chapter).

FIRST➤ To provide mouth-to-mask ventilations, make sure you are wearing protective gloves. Then follow these steps (Figure 6.10):

1. Determine if the patient is unresponsive. If so, and your patient is an adult, alert dispatch before starting resuscitation.

2. Properly position the patient and yourself. Then open the airway with the head-tilt, chin-lift maneuver or jaw-thrust maneuver.

3. Check for breathing:

   –**Look** for chest movements. Does the chest rise and fall evenly?

   –**Listen** for air flow from the mouth or nose. Are there unusual sounds (gurgling, crowing, snoring)?

FIGURE 6.9
Providing supplemental oxygen to the patient through the oxygen inlet on the pocket face mask.

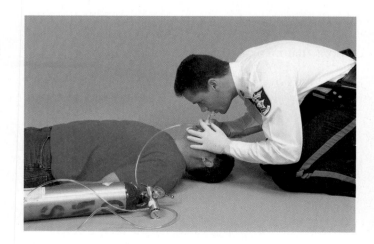

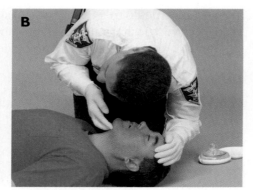

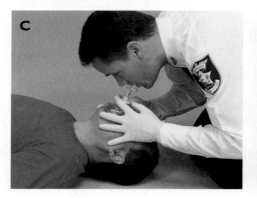

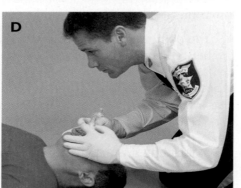

FIGURE 6.10
Mouth-to-mask ventilation.
A. Open the airway. **B.** Look, listen, and feel for air exchange. **C.** Ventilate as you watch for the chest to rise. **D.** Allow passive expiration as you watch for the chest to fall.

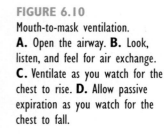

–**Feel** for air exchange against your cheek at the patient's mouth and nose.

–**Observe** skin color, such as a blue or gray tint or a pale or ashen appearance.

Take no more than 10 seconds to determine if the patient is breathing. If not, then attach the one-way valve to the face mask. Position the proper size mask on the patient's face so that the apex (upper tip of the triangle) is over the bridge of the patient's nose and the base is between the lower lip and the projection of the chin.

4. Firmly hold the mask in place while keeping the airway open:

   –Place both thumbs and index fingers on the cone of the mask to form a "C" around both sides. Apply even pressure on both sides of the mask.

   –Place the third, fourth, and fifth fingers of each hand under the jaw to form an "E" on both sides of the patient's jaw. Lift the jaw forward.

5. Take a deep breath and exhale slowly into the port of the one-way valve attachment on the mask chimney (1.5 to 2.0 seconds for adults; 1.0 to 1.5 seconds for infants and children). Air will enter through the airway openings, the patient's slightly open mouth, and the nose. Watch for the patient's chest to rise.

   Remember that there is no need to remove your mouth to allow the patient to exhale. The chimney has a one-way valve and the patient's exhaled air will escape through separate vents.

6. Continue this cycle of providing a breath every 5 seconds for an adult and every 3 seconds for a child or an infant. ■ BIRTH → 8 years old.

If air does not enter on the initial breath, reposition the patient's head, replace the mask, and try again. If air still does not enter, perform the steps for clearing an obstructed airway (explained later).

Dentures can cause an airway obstruction and interfere with your efforts to ventilate a patient. If dentures are secure, leave them in. If they are loose, remove them.

It may be difficult to get a good mask-to-face seal when dentures are removed. Make sure you position the mask properly, and open the airway appropriately.

You will know you are providing adequate ventilations to the patient when you:

- See the chest rise and fall with each ventilation.
- Ventilate 12 times a minute for adults and 20 times a minute for infants and children.

Your efforts are NOT adequate and you must make adjustments when:

- The chest does not rise and fall with each ventilation.
- Your rate is too slow or too fast.
- You do not have an appropriate seal on the mask, which allows air to leak out between the face and the mask.

Mouth-to-Barrier Ventilation

Use a face shield when performing mouth-to-barrier ventilation. Make sure you also are wearing protective gloves. Then follow these steps:

1. Determine if the patient is unresponsive. If so, alert dispatch before starting resuscitation on an adult patient.
2. Properly position the patient and yourself. Then open the airway with the head-tilt, chin-lift maneuver or jaw-thrust maneuver.
3. Check for breathing. Look, listen, and feel for air exchange and observe skin color. Take no more than 10 seconds to determine if the patient is breathing.
4. If the patient is not breathing, properly position a protective face shield between you and the patient and hold it in place with your fingers.
5. Keep the airway open as you pinch the nose closed with the thumb and forefinger of the hand on the patient's forehead. (You can use your thumbs or your cheek to seal the nose when performing the jaw-thrust maneuver.)
6. Open your mouth wide and take a deep breath.
7. Place your mouth over the face shield opening. Make a tight seal by pressing your lips against it.
8. Exhale slowly into the patient's airway until you see the chest rise and feel resistance to the flow of your breath. If this first attempt to provide a breath fails, reposition the patient's head or re-open the airway with the jaw-thrust maneuver and try again.
9. Break contact with the face shield to allow the patient to exhale. Quickly take in another deep breath and ventilate the patient again. You will give two initial ventilations.
10. If the patient does not begin breathing again, check for a pulse. If the patient has a pulse but is not breathing, continue with the following steps:

    –Take a deep breath.

    –With a face shield, ventilate the patient until you see the chest rise.

    –Break contact with the mouth and release the pinch on the nose to let the patient exhale.

    –Turn your head to watch the patient's chest fall.

    –Take a deep breath to begin the cycle again.

For an adult patient, deliver one breath every five seconds or at a rate of 12 breaths per minute. For an infant or child, deliver one breath every three seconds or at a rate of 20 breaths per minute. Every few minutes, stop and check for a pulse. If there is no pulse, begin CPR. If the patient has a pulse, continue pulmonary resuscitation until the patient begins to breathe unaided, until someone trained in pulmonary resuscitation can replace you, or until you are too exhausted to continue.

If you are following the correct procedures, and the patient's airway is not obstructed, you should be able to feel resistance to your ventilations as the patient's lungs expand, see the chest rise and fall, hear air leaving the patient's airway as the chest falls, and feel air leaving the patient's mouth as the lungs deflate. Monitor the patient to determine if he has begun to breathe unassisted.

The most common problems with the mouth-to-barrier technique are:

- Failure to form a tight seal over the face-shield opening and the patient's mouth (often caused by failing to open your mouth wide enough to make an effective seal as well as pushing too hard in an effort to form a tight seal).

- Failure to pinch the nose completely closed.

- Failure to tilt the head back far enough to open the airway.

- Failure to open the patient's mouth wide enough to receive ventilations.

- Failure to deliver enough air during a ventilation.

- Providing breaths too quickly (less than 1.5 to 2.0 seconds per breath for adults and 1.0 to 1.5 seconds for infants and children).

- Failure to clear the airway of obstructions.

Two additional problems, air in the patient's stomach and vomiting, will be covered later in this chapter.

Mouth-to-Nose Ventilation

Patients may have injuries to the mouth and jaw, missing teeth or dentures, and airway obstructions that will make the previous techniques ineffective. For these patients, you will have to use the mouth-to-nose technique. (Depending on the location of the obstruction, mouth-to-nose ventilation may not work if mouth-to-mask or mouth-to-barrier ventilation has failed, but it should be tried.)

Most of this procedure is the same as mouth-to-barrier ventilation. The differences in the mouth-to-nose procedure are that you will:

- Use your thumb to seal the mouth shut. Do not pinch the nose.

- Seal your mouth around the patient's nose.

- Deliver ventilations through the nose and be sure to keep the patient's mouth closed.

- Break contact with the nose and open the mouth slightly to allow the patient to exhale. Keep your hand on the patient's forehead to keep the airway open.

Note that like mouth-to-mouth ventilation, mouth-to-nose ventilation exposes the rescuer to potentially infectious body fluids.

remember

Deliver one breath every five seconds to adults, and one breath every three seconds to infants and children.

NOTE

You may use the jaw-thrust maneuver with the mouth-to-nose technique. Seal the patient's mouth with your cheek.

Special Patients

Among your patients as a First Responder are infants and children, elderly patients, neck breathers, and trauma victims (some with possible neck and spine injuries).

Infants (Birth to 1 Year) and Children (1 to 8 Years) The airways of infants and children have several physical characteristics that are different from adults. In the infant and child, the:

- Mouth and nose are much smaller and more easily obstructed than in an adult.

- Tongue takes up more space in the mouth and throat.

- Windpipe is smaller and more easily obstructed by swelling. It also is softer, more flexible, and easily obstructed by opening the airway too far (hyperextension).

- Chest muscles are not as well developed, causing the infant and child to depend more on the diaphragm for breathing.

- Chest cavity and lung volumes are smaller, so air getting into the stomach (gastric distention) occurs more commonly.

The First Responder must recognize and aggressively care for airway and respiratory problems in infants and children. *Respiratory distress and failure lead to cardiac arrest with little chance of survival.*

FIRST▶ When assisting ventilations for an infant (Figure 6.11) or small child, make sure you are wearing protective gloves. Then:

1. Open the airway and check for breathing. If the patient is not breathing, give two breaths.

   –If air enters, check the pulse. If no pulse, start CPR. If there is a pulse, ventilate for one full minute. Then alert the EMS dispatcher or have someone else call 9-1-1.

FIGURE 6.11
Ventilating an infant.

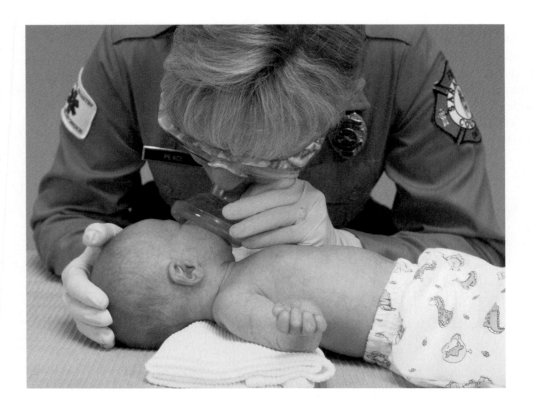

–If air does not enter on the initial breath, reposition the head and try again. If air still does not enter, perform the steps for an obstructed airway (later in this chapter).

2. Lay the patient on a hard surface.

3. Open the airway with a slight head-tilt, chin-lift maneuver and check for breathing. For an infant, keep the airway open by placing the head in a neutral position. For a child, keep the airway open by placing the head in a "sniffing position" (tilted slightly back, as when a person sniffs). Use the jaw-thrust maneuver if you suspect spinal injury.

4. Position a proper size pocket face mask or face shield on the patient.

5. Assist ventilations with gentle but adequate breaths. The volume of breath for the infant or child is determined by ventilating until you see the chest rise. Be aware of resistance to your breaths and watch for the chest to rise.

6. Allow the patient to exhale.

7. Give ventilations at a rate of one breath every 3 seconds for infants and children. Take 1.0 to 1.5 seconds per breath. ■

NOTE: *It is helpful to place a folded towel or similar object under an infant's shoulders to help in maintaining an open airway.*

Terminally Ill Patients   Many terminally ill patients choose to spend their remaining time at home with family and friends. Many others enter a hospice program, which supports and advises the patient and family or makes arrangements with their doctors for advance directives such as DNR orders. For guidelines on how to care for hospice or DNR patients, check your jurisdiction for training programs and follow your local protocols.

Elderly Patients   Elderly patients may require special care because of changes in their bodies that are normal for aging. First, the lungs may have lost some elasticity, and the rib cage may be more rigid and more difficult for you to expand when assisting ventilations. The jaw joints and neck may be arthritic, which can make it difficult to open the airway, but you will be able to get sufficient air in the patient with the usual maneuvers. With the mouth-to-mask technique, air will still enter the nose, even if the mouth will not open, but your ventilations may have to be a little more forceful (Figure 6.12). Patients who have lost their teeth and have not been using dentures have receding chins and sunken cheeks that make it difficult

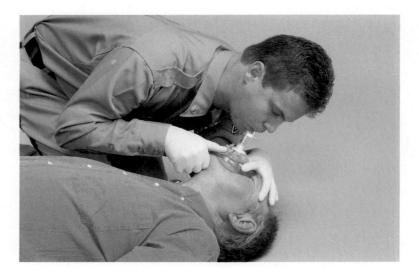

FIGURE 6.12
Ventilating an elderly patient.

to seal a mask to the face. Always be aware of resistance to your ventilations and the rise and fall of the patient's chest.

Second, realize that the elderly patient's bones may be more brittle than the bones of younger patients. If elderly patients have fallen, they are more likely to suffer spinal injury. When such injuries are possible or when you are in doubt, use the jaw-thrust maneuver in place of the head-tilt, chin-lift to open the airway.

Finally, you may be faced with bystanders who say such things as "He's so old. Let him die in peace." It is not their right to make that decision. You are charged with the responsibility to assist all patients who need care, unless direct orders stating otherwise have been given to you by a physician. What bystanders tell you may not be what the patient wants. Any time there is conflict in care priorities, contact medical direction.

laryngectomy (lar-in-JEK-to-me) the total or partial removal of the larynx.

stoma (STO-mah) any permanent opening that has been surgically made. The opening in the neck of a neck breather.

Neck Breathers   Some people have had a surgical procedure called a **laryngectomy** to remove part or all of their larynx (voice box). An opening is made outside the throat to the windpipe (trachea) so there is an adequate airway for breathing. These patients breathe through the opening made in the neck (Figure 6.13). This opening, not the mouth or nose, is now the beginning of their airway.

FIRST►   The opening in the neck is called a **stoma**. Since the patient no longer takes air into the lungs by way of the nose and mouth, you will have to use the mouth-to-mask-to-stoma technique to assist ventilations. Always look to see if there is a stoma. If so, ventilate the patient through the stoma. Currently, there is no specific mask for ventilating these patients, but a pediatric (infant's) mask often fits and works well to establish a seal around the stoma. You may also assist ventilations with a protective face shield or by attaching a bag-valve resuscitator directly to the patient's stoma tube if one is in place in the stoma opening. Follow the protocols of your jurisdiction. Remember, direct contact increases the risk of infection. ■

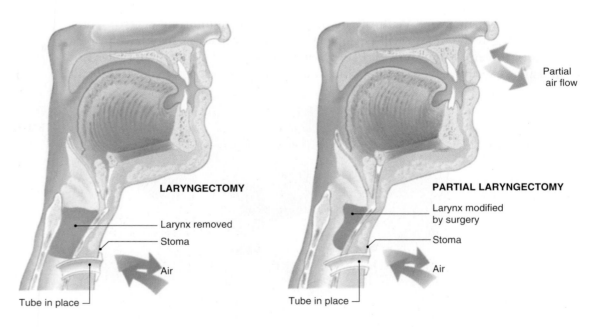

LARYNGECTOMY

Larynx removed
Stoma
Air
Tube in place

PARTIAL LARYNGECTOMY

Partial air flow

Larynx modified by surgery
Stoma
Air
Tube in place

FIGURE 6.13
The neck breather's airway has been changed by surgery.

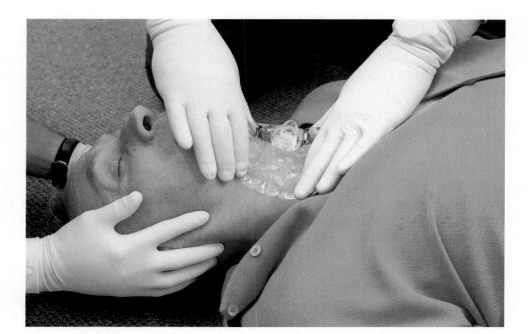

FIGURE 6.14
Using a barrier device to ventilate a stoma patient.

When ventilating a stoma patient (Figure 6.14), you should wear gloves and:

1. Keep the patient's head in a neutral or normal position. Do not tilt the head.

2. Clean away mucus or encrusted matter from around the neck opening or breathing tube. Do not remove the breathing tube.

3. Use the same procedures as you would for mouth-to-mask or mouth-to-barrier resuscitation, EXCEPT:

   –Do not pinch the patient's nose closed.

   –Place the mask or face shield on the neck over the stoma.

If the chest does not rise, the patient may be a partial neck breather. This means that the patient takes in and expels some air through the mouth and nose. In such cases, you will have to pinch the nose closed, seal the mouth with the palm of your hand, and ventilate through the stoma.

Crash Victims Opening the airway and assisting ventilations are easier for you to perform when the patient is lying down. This means that collision victims who are not breathing but who are still in their vehicles must be repositioned. You know that you risk causing further spine injury if you move them, but you must be realistic. If you wait for other EMS personnel to arrive, or if you take time to put on a rigid cervical collar and secure the patient to a spine board, the patient will be biologically dead from lack of oxygen to the brain. Airway and breathing are always the first priorities of patient care.

Without risking your own safety, reach the victim as quickly as possible. Look, listen, and feel for breathing before moving him. If he is breathing, the airway is open and you do not have to move him. If you believe the mechanism of injury may have caused damage to the spine or neck and the patient is not breathing, stabilize the head and open the airway with the jaw-thrust maneuver. Then check again for breathing. If the patient is breathing, keep the airway open while maintaining the head and neck in a neutral position. Monitor breathing until assistance arrives. If the patient is not breathing and he is in a position where you cannot maintain an airway while you assist ventilations, you will have to reposition him.

Your instructor will show you methods to practice so you can reposition a patient with maximum head stabilization and as little spinal movement as possible. If you have help, hold the patient's head and neck in line with the rest of the spine with both of your hands and forearms and work swiftly with your helpers to lay the patient flat.

Air in the Stomach and Vomiting

A common problem with assisted ventilations is that over-inflating the lungs will force air into the patient's stomach. Remember to carefully watch the chest rise as you ventilate. It will only rise so far. Do not keep ventilating when it stops rising. When the chest rises completely, allow the patient to exhale. Forcing more air than the lungs can hold during ventilation can cause or worsen inflation of the stomach. Air in the stomach will cause the abdomen to distend. This condition is called **gastric distention**.

Watch for gastric distention when you ventilate a patient. Excessive distention will force the patient's diaphragm upward into the chest cavity, which will reduce lung capacity. Reduced lung capacity restricts ventilations and reduces oxygen flow to the body. Gastric distention also can cause extra pressure in the stomach, which can result in the patient vomiting.

Do not worry about slight bulging or distention, but you will have to make adjustments if you notice extensive bulging. In cases of air in the stomach where you see a noticeable bulge, reduce the force of your ventilations and:

- Reposition the patient's head to ensure an open airway.

- Be prepared for vomiting. If the patient begins to vomit, turn the patient (not just the head) to one side so the vomitus will flow out of the airway and not back into it. (Vomitus can obstruct the airway and damage the lungs.) Have suction equipment on hand if you carry it on your unit.

- Stabilize the head and move the patient as a unit if you suspect neck or spine injuries. If the patient is an unresponsive medical patient with no indication of injury, place him in the recovery position.

- Do not push on the stomach to release the air. This may cause vomiting, which can block the airway or enter the lungs. Even if the patient is on his side when he vomits, the vomitus will not simply flow out. With your gloved hand, clear his mouth with gauze and finger sweeps or use suctioning equipment.

gastric distention inflation of the stomach.

AIRWAY OBSTRUCTION

CAUSES OF AIRWAY OBSTRUCTION

FIRST▸ Many factors can cause the airway to become partially or fully obstructed, including a foreign object lodging in the airway or excess saliva or respiratory secretions accumulating in the mouth and interfering with breathing.

The following conditions are upper airway obstructions that you may be able to relieve (Figure 6.15):

- *Obstruction by the tongue*—the tongue falls back in the throat to block the airway.
- *Obstruction by the epiglottis*—the patient attempts to force inspirations when he is having difficulty breathing. This effort may create a negative pressure that can force the epiglottis and tongue to block the airway.

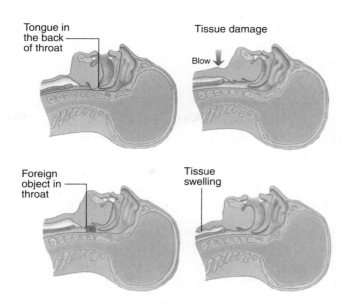

Tongue in
the back
of throat

Tissue damage

Blow ↓

Foreign
object in
throat

Tissue
swelling

FIGURE 6.15
Possible causes of airway obstruction.

- *Foreign objects (also called mechanical obstructions)*—objects and other matter, such as pieces of food, ice, toys, dentures, vomitus, and liquids pooling in the back of the throat can block the airway.

  The following obstructions may be impossible for you to relieve, but you must still attempt to assist ventilations:

- *Tissue damage*—tissue damage can be caused by punctures to the neck, crush wounds to the neck and face, upper-airway burns from breathing hot air (as in fires), poisons, and severe blows to the neck. The tissues of the throat and windpipe become swollen and make it difficult for air to flow through the airway.
- *Infections*—pharyngeal and epiglottic (ep-i-GLOT-ik) infections can produce airway obstruction. ■

Signs of Partial Airway Obstruction

A patient who is having difficulty breathing may have only a partial obstruction and may still be able to move some air.

FIRST➤ The signs of partial airway obstruction include the following:

- Unusual breathing sounds, such as:
  - *Snoring*—usually caused by the tongue partially or intermittently obstructing the back of the throat.
  - *Gurgling*—usually caused by fluids or blood in the airway or by a foreign object in the windpipe, which stimulates excess fluids.
  - *Crowing*—usually caused by spasms of the larynx (voice box).
  - *Wheezing*—usually due to swelling or spasms along the lower airway, but it does not always mean there is an airway problem. Wheezing may sound serious but is not usually associated with airway obstruction. It is more common during exhalation.
  - *Stridor*—a high-pitched harsh sound usually caused by a blockage in the throat or larynx (voice box) and typically heard when the patient inhales.
- Breathing is present, but skin is blue, gray, or ashen at the lips, earlobes, fingernail beds, or tongue. The usual presentation in a responsive patient is fear,

panic, or agitation. Nothing invokes terror in a person like a threatened airway or the inability to breathe.

● Breathing keeps changing from normal to labored. ■

If a responsive patient has some air exchange with a partial airway obstruction, encourage him to cough. A forceful cough indicates that he has enough air exchange. Encourage him to continue coughing so that any foreign materials may be dislodged and expelled. Do not interfere with the patient's efforts to clear the airway.

If the patient has poor air exchange and cannot cough or can only cough weakly, begin care as if there is a complete airway obstruction. (Care steps will follow later in the chapter.) Do the same if he has poor air exchange at first assessment or when good air exchange becomes poor air exchange.

Signs of Complete Airway Obstruction

When the airway is completely obstructed, the responsive patient will try to speak and cough but will not be able to. The patient often will grasp her neck and open her mouth, which is the universal sign of an inability to breathe (Figure 6.16). The unresponsive patient will not have any of the typical chest movements or the other signs of good air exchange.

CORRECTING UPPER AIRWAY OBSTRUCTION—FOREIGN BODY

When a patient shows the universal sign of airway obstruction, move swiftly to clear the airway. When the patient is unresponsive, act quickly to determine if there is an airway obstruction and clear the airway. Since so many cases of airway obstruction are caused by relaxation of the tongue, always make certain that the airway is open using a manual maneuver. Once this has been done, move on to the recommended techniques for clearing obstructions from the airway. Perform the following steps for the patients listed.

Back Blows for Infants

Back blows create pressure in the chest that helps to dislodge an obstruction. Use back blows only on infants.

FIRST▶ For an infant with a complete airway obstruction, you will:

FIGURE 6.16
Universal sign of choking.

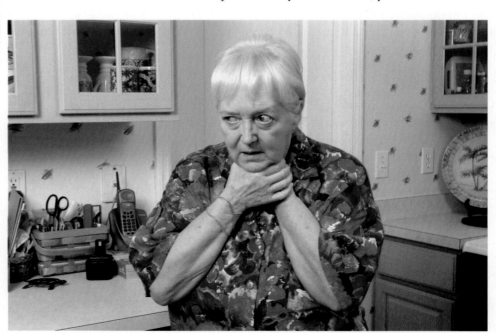

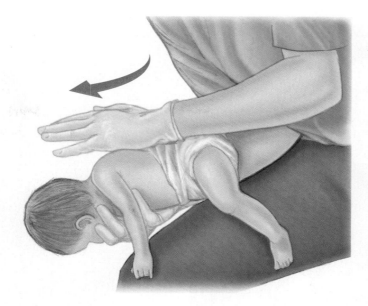

1. Support the infant, face down, on your forearm (Figure 6.17). Use your hand to support the infant's jaw and chest. You can assure better patient support if you are seated or kneeling and resting your forearm on your thighs. Keep the infant's head lower than the chest.

2. Use the heel of your other hand to deliver five sharp and rapid blows to the midline of the infant's back between the shoulder blades. ■

Do not place the infant or very small child into this head-down position if he has a partial airway obstruction and you observe that he is breathing adequately or coughing to clear the airway.

Abdominal Thrusts for Adults and Children

To perform abdominal thrusts, press into the abdomen just below the rib cage with your fists. This forceful thrust will create a pressure that causes an artificial cough. The cough pushes trapped air in the lungs upward through the airway, which can dislodge an obstruction.

If the patient with an airway obstruction is responsive and is standing or sitting:

1. Position yourself behind the patient.

2. Slide your arms under the patient's armpits and wrap them around the patient's waist (Figure 6.18).

3. Make a fist and place the thumb side against the midline of the abdomen, just above the navel. Keep your fist below the rib cage and avoid the area just below the breastbone (sternum) at the level of the xiphoid process.

4. Grasp your fist with your free hand and apply pressure as an inward and upward thrust. Deliver separate rapid inward and upward thrusts. Repeat them until the airway is cleared or the patient becomes unresponsive.

5. Reevaluate the responsive patient after 5 thrusts.

If the patient with an airway obstruction is unresponsive (Scan 6-1) or becomes unresponsive, you will:

1. Call 9–1–1.

2. Place the patient on his back.

warning

Do not practice abdominal thrusts on your classmates or any other person. While this procedure must be practiced so you learn to perform the important steps, it can be dangerous when performed on a responsive, healthy person. Practice only on the manikins that are provided by your instructor.

NOTE

If the patient is very large or if you are small, you can deliver effective thrusts if you straddle one leg of the patient. For the child patient (between 1 and 8 years of age), you may kneel at the child's feet or place the child on a table and stand at his feet.

warning

Do not use abdominal thrusts on infants or children under one year of age.

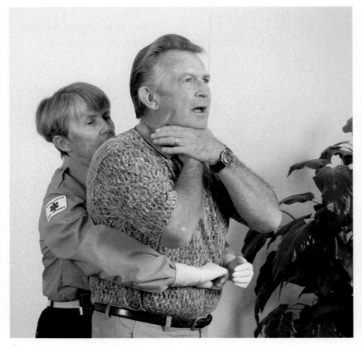
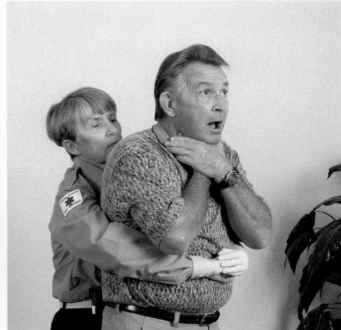

A **B**

FIGURE 6.18
Correct positioning is important for delivering abdominal thrusts.

3. Attempt to ventilate.

4. Kneel and straddle the patient's hips. This position helps you deliver effective, abdominal thrusts.

5. Place the heel of one hand on the abdomen at the midline between the navel and the rib cage. Your fingers should point toward the patient's chest. Keep your hand below the patient's rib cage and avoid the area just below the breastbone.

6. Place your free hand over the positioned hand.

7. Press your hands inward and upward toward the diaphragm.

8. Deliver five rapid abdominal thrusts.

Because abdominal thrusts can damage internal organs, do not use them on infants up to one year of age. This technique may rupture or lacerate the liver, lungs, and heart, or internally damage the heart. It may also break ribs. The American Heart Association (AHA) does not recommend abdominal thrusts for infants.

Chest Thrusts for Special Patients

Chest thrusts create pressure in the chest or an artificial cough that can dislodge an obstruction. Use them in place of abdominal thrusts when the patient is under one year of age or when the patient is pregnant. You may also use it on patients who are so large that you cannot wrap your arms around the waist.

To use the chest-thrust technique on an adult patient or a pregnant patient who is standing or seated (Figure 6.19), you will:

1. Position yourself behind the patient and slide your arms under the armpits so that you can encircle the chest with your arms.

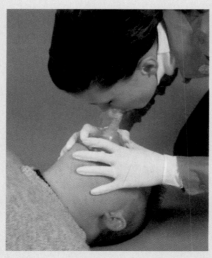

1. Open the airway. Look, listen, and feel for breathing. Attempt to ventilate.

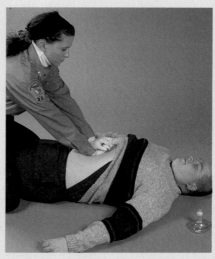

2. If ventilations are unsuccessful, reposition the head and attempt to ventilate again. If there is an obstruction, deliver abdominal thrusts.

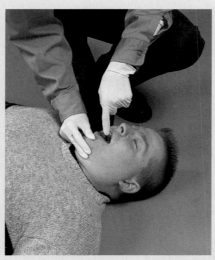

3. Open the mouth and look for foreign bodies. If you see an object, use a finger sweep to clear the mouth.

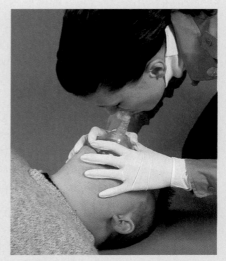

4. Attempt ventilations again and, if necessary, repeat the sequence of abdominal thrusts, finger sweeps, and ventilations.

2. Form a fist with one hand and place the thumb side on the breastbone about two or three finger-widths above the lower tip.

3. Grasp your fist with your free hand and deliver distinct thrusts directly backward until the object is expelled or the patient loses responsiveness. Do not deliver thrusts in an upward or downward direction or off to one side.

FIGURE 6.19
Chest thrust to a pregnant patient.

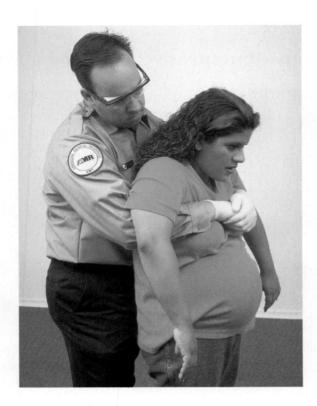

FIRST> If you must perform chest thrusts on a very large adult or a pregnant patient who is lying down (Figure 6.20) and you cannot straddle the hips or one leg, you should:

1. Kneel beside the patient's chest.
2. Place the heel of one hand on the midline of the breastbone, two to three finger-widths from the lower tip. Lift and spread your fingers so that they will not apply pressure on the ribs.
3. Place your free hand on top of this hand.
4. Lean forward until your shoulders are directly over the midline of the patient's chest.
5. Deliver distinct thrusts in a downward direction, applying enough force to compress the chest cavity. Continue until the object is expelled or the patient loses responsiveness. ■

If you perform chest thrusts on an infant (Figure 6.21), you will:

1. Support the infant on your forearm. The infant should be face down with head lower than body.
2. Deliver five back blows.
3. Sandwich the infant between your arms and then turn him over to a face-up position on your thigh. Support his head as you turn him. Keep the head lower than the trunk. Apply five *quick, distinct chest thrusts*, using the tips of two or three fingers. Press along the midline of the breastbone (sternum), one finger-width below an imaginary line drawn directly between the nipples.

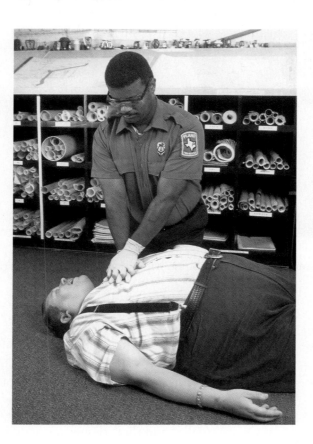

FIGURE 6.20
Chest thrust to a supine obese patient.

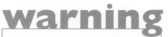

Do not use the finger sweep technique on responsive patients or on unresponsive patients who have a gag reflex.

NOTE

Finger sweeps can dislodge dentures. If this happens, remove them from the patient's mouth. Do not attempt to replace them.

Finger Sweeps

The finger sweep is the next step in clearing the airway. You will only perform finger sweeps if you can see the object in the mouth and it is dislodged or partially dislodged (Figure 6.22). Be sure you do not force the object back down the patient's throat.

To perform a finger sweep, make certain that you are wearing protective gloves and then follow these steps:

1. Place the patient on his back.
2. Use one hand to steady the forehead and tilt it back slightly. This should open the mouth just far enough for you to place the thumb of the other hand against the patient's lower teeth and your index finger against the upper teeth.

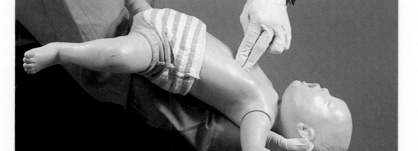

FIGURE 6.21
Chest thrust to an infant.

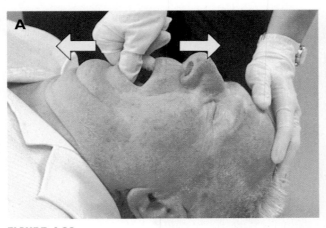
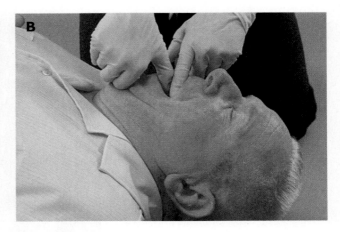

FIGURE 6.22
A. Open the mouth with the crossed-finger technique. **B.** Then use a finger sweep to remove foreign objects.

3. Open the patient's mouth by crossing your thumb and index finger (crossed-finger technique).

4. Once the mouth is open, grasp the lower jaw and tongue and lift slightly. This is known as the tongue-jaw lift (Figure 6.23).

5. Look into the mouth. If you see the object there, use your finger to sweep it out. You may have to turn the patient's head to one side to help. *When you use this technique on infants and children, use your little finger.* Remember, their airways are smaller and their tissues more delicate. Do not attempt to sweep the mouth if you do not see an object. Sweeping without first looking is called "blind" finger sweeps. If you do not see an object, there is nothing to sweep.

A responsive person has a gag reflex. Probing the mouth with your finger may cause vomiting. The patient may vomit and inhale this vomitus into the lungs. *Use a finger sweep only on unresponsive patients.*

CORRECTING AIRWAY OBSTRUCTIONS—COMBINED PROCEDURES

The American Heart Association (AHA) has researched the proper techniques to be used in cases of partial and complete airway obstruction. As part of their Basic Cardiac Life Support Program, the AHA has shown that a specific sequence of actions will provide the rescuer with the greatest chance of clearing a patient's airway. Most EMS systems use the procedures set by the AHA.

FIGURE 6.23
Tongue-jaw lift.

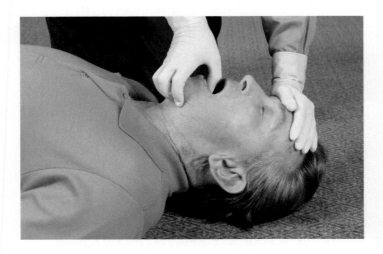

Procedures used to clear the airway are considered effective if any of the following occurs:

- Patient shows good air exchange or spontaneous breathing.
- Patient regains responsiveness.
- Skin color improves.
- Foreign object is expelled from the mouth.
- Foreign object is expelled into the mouth where it is visible to the rescuer and can be removed.

Adult or Child—Responsive

FIRST➤

1. Determine that there is complete obstruction or a partial obstruction with poor air exchange. Ask, "Are you choking?" or "Can you speak?" Look and listen for signs of complete obstruction or poor air exchange. Tell the patient you will help.
2. Position yourself to give up to five abdominal thrusts in rapid succession (or chest thrusts for a pregnant or obese patient.
3. If the patient's airway remains obstructed, repeat the thrusts until the airway is cleared or until the patient loses responsiveness. ■

Adult or Child—Loses Responsiveness

FIRST➤

1. Help the patient to the ground to prevent injury from a fall. Position him on his back. Make sure your gloves are on.
2. Quickly alert EMS dispatch at once if the patient is an adult. If the patient is an infant or child, alert dispatch after giving one minute of ventilation if the obstruction is cleared quickly; or call if the obstruction is not cleared and attempts to ventilate are not successful.
3. Use the tongue-jaw lift to open the mouth. Look for the object and perform finger sweeps only if you see the object.
4. Open the patient's airway by using the head-tilt, chin-lift maneuver for the adult. Use a slight head-tilt with chin-lift for the child.
5. Give two ventilations. If your attempt to ventilate fails, reposition the head and attempt to ventilate again. If this fails . . .
6. Perform five abdominal thrusts in rapid succession.
7. Check the mouth for foreign bodies and perform a finger sweep. If you cannot find and remove the obstruction . . .
8. Open the airway and repeat your attempt to ventilate the patient. If this fails. . . .
9. Repeat the sequence of:

   –Repositioning and attempting ventilations.

   –Providing abdominal thrusts.

   –Looking for objects and performing finger sweeps.

   –Attempting to ventilate. ■

Continue these efforts until the obstruction is cleared. Even if you can do no more than partially dislodge the obstruction, you will be able to provide some air exchange. Then when the obstruction is cleared, proceed with two breaths and check for signs of circulation.

Adult or Child—Unresponsive

FIRST➤

1. Check to see if the patient is unresponsive. Make sure your gloves are on. Alert EMS dispatch at once for an adult patient. If the patient is a child, alert EMS after giving one minute of ventilation if the obstruction is cleared quickly; or call if the obstruction is not cleared and attempts to ventilate are not successful.

2. Open the airway.

3. Attempt to give the patient two adequate ventilations. If you are not successful . . .

4. Reposition the patient's head and repeat your attempt to ventilate the patient. If you are not successful . . .

5. Deliver five abdominal thrusts, then check the mouth for the object. Finger sweep if you see the object. If these procedures fail . . .

6. Attempt to ventilate and repeat the sequence: reposition and attempt ventilations, provide abdominal thrusts, perform finger sweeps, and attempt to ventilate until successful. Once the obstruction is cleared, proceed with two breaths and then check the pulse. ■

Chest thrusts must be used for infants, obese patients, and women in the later stages of pregnancy.

Infant—Responsive

FIRST➤

1. Assess breathing to make sure the problem is due to an airway obstruction. If you are working alone, call out for help.

2. Support the infant's head as you place the infant face down on your forearm. Use your thigh to support your forearm. Remember to keep the infant's head lower than the trunk.

3. Rapidly deliver five back blows. If this fails . . .

4. Support the infant's head, and sandwich him between your arms. Turn the infant over onto his back and keep the head lower than the trunk. Use your thigh to support your forearm.

5. Locate the compression site and deliver five chest thrusts with the tips of two or three fingers along the midline of the breastbone.

6. Continue with the sequence of back blows and chest thrusts until the object is expelled or the infant loses responsiveness. ■

Infant—Loses Responsiveness

FIRST➤

1. Make sure your gloves are on. Give one minute of ventilations if the obstruction is quickly cleared. Then alert dispatch if the obstruction is not cleared quickly and attempts to ventilate are not successful.

2. Place the infant on his back and open the mouth with the tongue-jaw lift. Look in the mouth. If you see the object, use your little finger to sweep the mouth.

remember

Chest thrusts must be used for infants, obese patients, and women in the later stages of pregnancy.

3. Open the airway and attempt to ventilate. If this fails, reposition the head and attempt to ventilate again. If unsuccessful . . .

4. Deliver five back blows. If this fails . . .

5. Deliver five chest thrusts.

6. Use the tongue-jaw lift. Look for and remove any visible foreign objects.

7. Reattempt to ventilate. If this fails . . .

8. Continue the sequence of back blows, chest thrusts, finger sweep of visible foreign object, and attempts to ventilate; reposition and attempt to ventilate again until you are successful. Once the obstruction is cleared, proceed with two breaths and then check the pulse. ■

Infant—Unresponsive

FIRST▶ See Scan 6-2.

1. Establish unresponsiveness by tapping or shaking the infant's foot. Make sure your gloves are on. When working alone, give one minute of ventilation, then alert dispatch.

2. Position the infant on his back on a flat surface or on your forearm. Be sure to support the infant's head.

3. Open the airway. Assess breathing. If the infant is not breathing . . .

4. Attempt to ventilate. If this fails . . .

5. Reposition the infant's head and attempt to ventilate again. If this fails . . .

6. Support the infant's head and place him face down on your forearm. Support your forearm with your thigh and keep the infant's head lower than his trunk. Deliver five back blows. If this fails . . .

7. Sandwich the patient between your arms, and place him in a face-up position on your thigh. Deliver five chest thrusts. If this fails . . .

8. Use the tongue-jaw lift and remove any visible foreign objects.

9. Open the airway and attempt to ventilate. If this fails, reposition the head and attempt to ventilate again. If this fails . . .

10. Repeat the sequence of:

    –Five back blows.

    –Five chest thrusts.

    –Looking for and removing visible foreign objects and . . .

    –Attempt to ventilate, reposition, and attempt to ventilate again until you are successful. ■

If the infant is in respiratory arrest and you have cleared the airway enough to provide adequate ventilations, deliver two breaths and check for heart action to see if CPR must be started (see Chapter 8).

AIDS TO RESUSCITATION

NOTE: *Some jurisdictions and agencies do not require First Responders to use special equipment for breathing and circulation. This part of the chapter is provided for those who must learn such skills to meet the requirements of their EMS agency. These skills must be learned and practiced on manikins under your instructor's supervision. The pocket face mask with*

Clearing the Airway—Unresponsive Infant

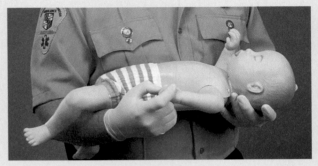

1. Determine unresponsiveness. Position the patient.

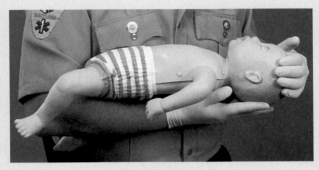

2. Open the airway. Establish breathlessness.

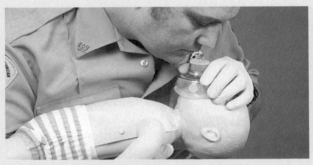

3. Attempt to ventilate. If this fails, reposition the patient's head and try again.

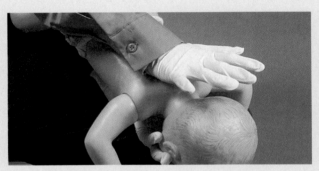

4. Deliver five back blows.

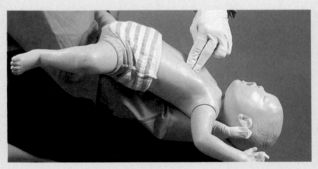

5. Deliver five chest thrusts.

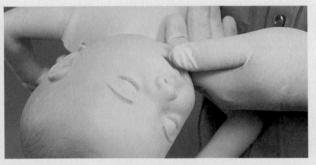

6. Look for and remove visible objects with a finger sweep.

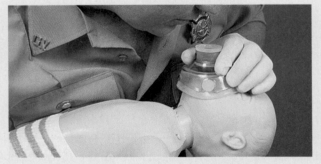

7. Attempt to ventilate again and, if necessary, repeat the sequence of back blows, abdominal thrusts, removing visible objects, and ventilations.

one-way valve and HEPA filter were covered earlier in this chapter. Students who are training to use the bag-valve-mask ventilator and provide oxygen therapy should refer to Appendix 2.

The use of rather simple but special adjunct equipment can help First Responders provide more effective resuscitation. The EMS system uses a variety of respiratory and circulatory support equipment, much of which is considered to be part of advanced life support and is beyond the scope of First Responder training courses. But three pieces of adjunct equipment are commonly taught in First Responder programs. These devices are the two types of airways—the **oropharyngeal airway (OPA)** and the **nasopharyngeal airway (NPA)**—and the pocket face mask discussed earlier in this chapter.

The advantages of using these pieces of adjunct equipment include:

● Oropharyngeal and nasopharyngeal airways help the rescuer maintain an open airway for the patient, allowing him to deliver more effective ventilations.

● Pocket face mask is an important piece of personal protective equipment that acts as a barrier device for infection control.

One disadvantage of all adjunct equipment is that it can delay the beginning of resuscitation if it is not readily available. Your pocket face mask, even adjunct airways, should always be as handy as your latex or vinyl gloves. Never delay the start of ventilations or CPR while you try to find, retrieve, or set up adjunct airway equipment. Another disadvantage of some adjunct equipment is that it must be maintained, cleaned, and kept in working order. Unless cared for properly, adjunct devices can fail to function. Always dispose of non-reusable patient care items or thoroughly disinfect all reusable adjunct equipment after each use.

OROPHARYNGEAL AIRWAYS

Oro refers to the mouth. *Pharyngeo* refers to the throat. An oropharyngeal airway is a device, usually made of plastic, that can be inserted into a patient's mouth and into the back of the throat. It helps to maintain an open airway for breathing or resuscitation.

Once a patient's airway is open, an oropharyngeal airway can be inserted to help keep it open. The device has a flange that fits against the patient's lips. The rest of the airway holds down the patient's tongue and curves back into the throat.

Use oropharyngeal airways only on *unresponsive* patients who do not have a gag reflex. These devices can stimulate the gag reflex and cause vomiting in responsive patients. If the patient vomits, he can aspirate or breathe the vomitus back into the lungs, a serious complication. If the patient is responsive, even if disoriented or confused, do not insert an oropharyngeal airway. Do not continue to insert or leave the airway in the patient's mouth if you meet any resistance or if the patient begins to gag as you insert it.

If you carry a suction unit and are trained to use it, have it ready for any patient who is unresponsive and may need an airway. Follow your local guidelines for using airways.

Rules for Using the Oropharyngeal Airway

● Open the patient's airway first. Inserting an oropharyngeal airway does not replace this step.

● Use only in unresponsive patients with no gag reflex. If the patient gags, do not use the airway.

oropharyngeal (or-o-fah-RIN-je-al) **airway (OPA)** a curved breathing tube inserted into the patient's mouth. It will hold the base of the tongue forward. Also called oral airway.

nasopharyngeal (na-zo-fah-RIN-je-al) **airway (NPA)** a flexible plastic tube that is lubricated and then inserted into a patient's nose to the level of the nasopharynx (back of the throat) to provide an open airway. Supplemental oxygen may be delivered through this tube. Also called nasal airway.

- When inserting the airway, take care not to push the patient's tongue back into the throat.

- While inserting the airway, listen for gagging. Remove the device immediately if the patient begins to gag.

- Once the device is in place, continue to monitor the patient's airway. If the patient regains responsiveness, he may attempt to remove, displace, or cough up the airway. You must be ready to assist or remove it. Continue to monitor respiration.

Measuring the Oropharyngeal Airway

There are numerous standardized sizes of oropharyngeal airways designed to fit infants, children, and adults (Figure 6.24). To use this device effectively, you must be able to select the correct size for the patient. Before using an airway, hold the device against the patient's face and measure to see if it extends from the center of the mouth to the angle of the lower jaw. The airway also may be sized by holding it at the corner of the patient's mouth and seeing if it will extend to the tip of the earlobe on the same side of the face. If the airway is not the correct size, do not use it on the patient; select another airway and re-measure to check correct size before inserting.

Sometimes it is difficult to find the correct size oropharyngeal airway for a patient. If the airway is too long, it might become displaced by muscular action and block the airway. If the device is too short, it will curve into the tongue instead of into the back of the throat, and it may also block the airway. The device must be the correct size to be used.

Inserting the Oropharyngeal Airway

To insert an oropharyngeal airway, you should (Scan 6-3):

1. Have a pocket face mask or face shield ready. Don latex or vinyl gloves.
2. Remove dentures or partial plates only if they are loose.
3. Place the patient on his back. Measure an airway.
4. Cross your thumb and forefinger. Then scissor open the patient's mouth at the corner, or pull down on the chin with your thumb.
5. Position the airway so that its tip is pointing toward the roof of the patient's mouth.
6. Insert the airway and slide it along the roof of the mouth, past the uvula (the soft tissue hanging down at the back of the mouth). Be certain not to push the tongue back into the throat.

FIGURE 6.24
Various sizes of oropharyngeal airways.

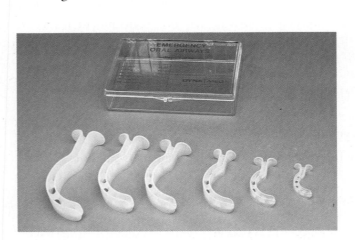

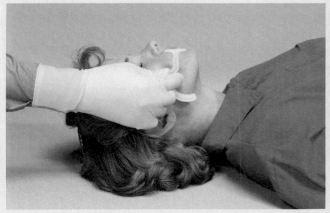

1. Select an oropharyngeal airway. One way to measure is from the center of the mouth to the angle of the lower jaw.

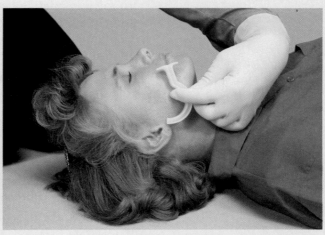

2. Another way to measure is from the corner of the mouth to the tip of the earlobe.

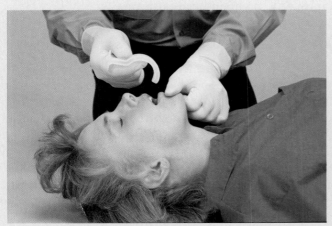

3. Insert the airway, with the tip pointing to the roof of the patient's mouth.

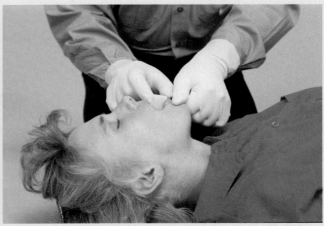

4. Rotate the airway into position.

NOTE: Never practice the use of airways on anyone. Manikins should be used for developing airway skills.

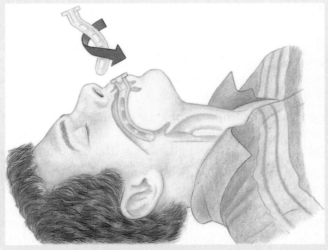

5. When the airway is positioned properly, the flange rests against the patient's lips.

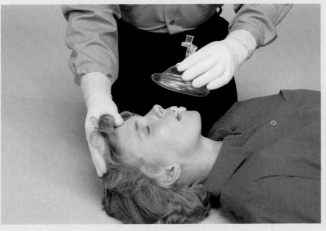

6. The patient is ready for ventilation.

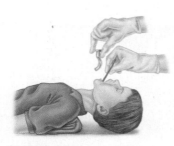

7. Rotate the airway 180 degrees (one-half turn) until the tip is pointing down the patient's throat.

8. Open the airway, using the head-tilt, chin-lift or jaw-thrust maneuver. Keep the airway open. Check to see that the flange of the airway is against the patient's lips. If the airway is too long, it will keep slipping out of the mouth and the flange will not rest on the lips. If the airway is too short, the patient's mouth may remain slightly open in an awkward position. Remove a too-long or too-short airway, and replace it with one of the correct size.

9. Ventilate the patient with the mouth-to-mask technique.

To minimize injury to the mouth of the infant or child while inserting an oropharyngeal airway, the following alternative method is recommended (Figure 6.25):

1. Use a tongue blade to gently place downward pressure on the tongue.

2. Insert the oropharyngeal airway with the tip pointing toward the tongue and throat, in the same position it will be in after insertion, rather than upside down.

The oropharyngeal airway is inserted in this way because the mouth is smaller than an adult's and the upper portion of the oral cavity is more easily injured. Rotating the airway can damage the soft palate or the uvula.

The oropharyngeal airway is an adjunct. It does not maintain the head in an open-airway position. You must still maintain head position.

NASOPHARYNGEAL AIRWAYS

The nasopharyngeal airway is being used more frequently because it is easy to insert, it does not stimulate a gag reflex, it does not have to be removed if the patient regains responsiveness or starts breathing, and it is more comfortable for the patient. It is a soft, flexible tube that is inserted through the nose rather than in the mouth. It is easy to insert because you do not have to reposition the patient's head and pry open the mouth. If there is any injury to the mouth, teeth, or oral cavity, the nasopharyngeal device will still allow you to provide an open airway for the patient. The only precaution is for patients with possible skull or facial fracture. If there is any indication of head or mid-face (including nasal) injury or the mechanism of injury suggests either or both, do not insert the nasopharyngeal airway.

Inserting the Nasopharyngeal Airway

To insert a nasopharyngeal airway, you should (Figure 6.26):

1. Don gloves and have a face mask ready.

2. Select the largest diameter nasopharyngeal airway that will fit into the patient's nostril without force. The size can be compared to the patient's little finger. Length is also critical since too long an airway can stimulate the gag reflex. The nasopharyngeal airway should be at least as long as the distance between the patient's earlobe and the tip of his nose. It can be longer.

3. Use a water-based lubricant on the outside of the tube before you insert it. Do not use petroleum jelly or any other non-water-based lubricant. These will damage the nasal cavity and pharynx (throat) and will increase the risk of infection.

4. Keep the patient's head in a neutral position, while you gently push the tip of the nose upward. Insert the airway through the nostril straight back, not angled upward toward the eye. If the airway has a beveled (angled) edge, it should point toward the septum (the divider between the two nostrils). Gently advance the airway until the flange rests firmly against the patient's nostril.

warning

Do not attempt to insert a nasopharyngeal airway if there are indications of nasal injury or if you see clear fluid flowing from the nose.

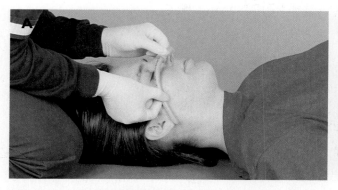
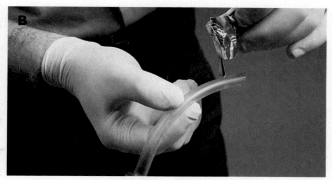
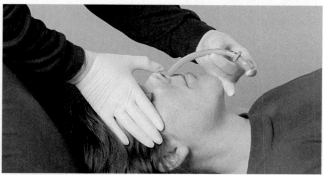

FIGURE 6.26
Inserting a nasopharyngeal airway.
A. Measuring. **B.** Lubricating. **C.** Preparing to insert.

Never force the airway. If the airway will not advance into the nostril easily, remove it, re-lubricate it if necessary, rotate it 180 degrees so the beveled edge points toward the septum, and try it in the other nostril. (It does not matter if the natural curve of the airway is arcing in the other direction. It will adjust as you insert it.) If the airway will not advance into the other nostril, make another attempt with an airway that is slightly smaller in diameter.

5. Ventilate with a pocket face mask or with a face shield.

warning

If you continue to meet resistance while inserting the nasopharyngeal airway, do not continue your attempts.

SUCTION SYSTEMS

Typically, a First Responder will reposition the patient on his side (recovery position) or use finger sweeps appropriately to clear blood, mucus, and other body fluids from the airway. However, a suction device can assist in keeping a patient's airway clear. More and more First Responder units are carrying suction devices, and training programs are including suctioning techniques.

There are several types of portable suction units that range from the hand-operated devices to the mechanically powered ones. They may be manually powered, oxygen- or air-powered, or electrically powered units (Figure 6.27). The vacuum pressure and flow must be adequate for mouth, throat (pharyngeal), and stoma suctioning. All units must have thick-walled, non-kinking, wide-bore tubing; a non-breakable collection container (bottle); and sterile, disposable semi-rigid but flexible tubes and/or rigid suction tips. The longer flexible simi-rigid suction tips are usually called *catheters;* the rigid suction tips are sometimes referred to as *tonsil suction tips* (for example, the Yankauer suction tip).

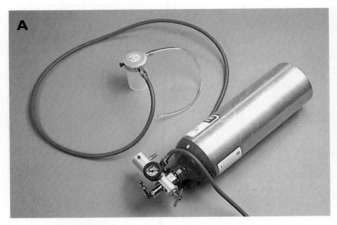

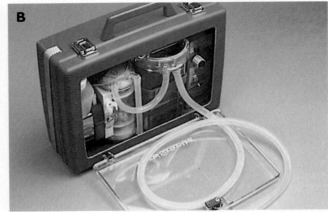

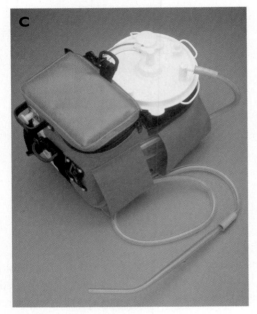

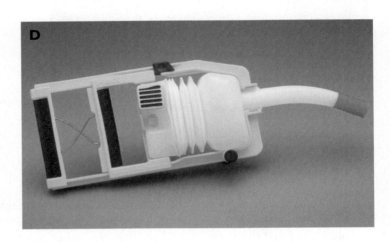

FIGURE 6.27
A. Oxygen-powered suction unit. **B.** Electrically powered suction unit. **C.** Portable electrical suction unit. **D.** Portable hand-operated suction unit.

NOTE

A manually powered suction unit may have a rubber bulb or a hand- or foot-operated device to produce the vacuum. Follow manufacturer and local EMS system guidelines for generating the vacuum.

SUCTIONING TECHNIQUES

USE PERSONAL PROTECTIVE EQUIPMENT. Because of droplets in the air, a face mask and eye protection are essential. Remember, any patient may be a source of infection.

There are many variations to the techniques used to suction the mouth, throat, or stoma. One example of a long-standing procedure is given below. You MUST follow the guidelines established by your local EMS system's Medical Director. They may include:

- Follow all infection control guidelines. Use personal protective equipment.

- Never suction for longer than 15 seconds at a time. Some guidelines require a maximum of 10 seconds for the breathing patient and 5 seconds for the non-breathing patient before attempting to ventilate.

- Measure the tip of the catheter before inserting it in the patient's mouth. Measure from the patient's earlobe to the corner of the mouth and place your fingers at that point. Insert the tip or catheter no farther than that point where you have your fingers placed.

- Never suction as you are inserting the catheter. Place the suction tip or catheter in the patient's mouth BEFORE starting suction.
- Suction only as you remove the tip or catheter. Twist and turn the tip or catheter as you are removing it from the mouth, throat, or stoma.

General guidelines for suctioning a patient's mouth, throat, or stoma include the following:

1. Attach the catheter and test for suction.
2. Position yourself at the patient's head, and turn him to the side. If practical, turn the entire patient, not just the head. Follow guidelines for spinal protection.
3. Measure the flexible catheter or rigid tip between the earlobe and the corner of the mouth, or from the center of the mouth to the angle of the jaw (just like the oropharyngeal airway). Hold the tip or catheter in your fingers at the point where it reaches the mouth. You will insert the tip or catheter only that far into the patient's mouth.
4. Open the patient's mouth and clear obvious matter and fluid from the oral cavity by turning the patient and draining the mouth or by using finger sweeps.
5. Insert the tip or catheter to your finger position. Usually, the tip is inserted to the base of the tongue (Figure 6.28). If you are using a rigid pharyngeal tip, place the convex (curved-out) side against the roof of the mouth, with the tip at the base of the tongue.
6. Apply suction ONLY when the tip or catheter is in place at the back of the mouth or base of the tongue and as you begin to withdraw it. Twist and turn it from side to side and sweep the mouth. This twisting action prevents the end of the tip or catheter from grabbing mouth tissue. Follow all the rules stated above. REMAIN ALERT FOR THE PATIENT'S GAG REFLEX AND FOR SIGNS OF VOMITING.

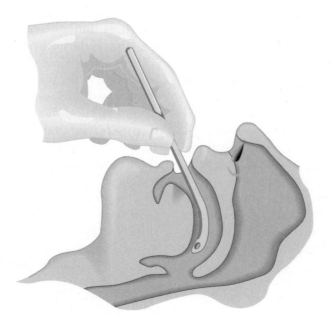

FIGURE 6.28
Positioning a rigid pharyngeal (throat) tip. Do not push it down the throat or into the larynx.

Chapter Review

We breathe to bring in oxygen, remove carbon dioxide, and help regulate the pH level of our blood, a process called **respiration.** The major muscle of breathing, the **diaphragm,** and the muscles between our ribs contract to increase the volume of the chest cavity. Increased volume decreases the pressure in the chest cavity and allows the lungs to expand. As the lungs expand, the pressure inside decreases and allows air to fill the lungs. When we exhale, changes in chest size and pressure cause air in the lungs to flow out. All this is an involuntary, automatic process, which is mainly controlled by the respiratory centers of the brain.

Clinical death occurs when an individual stops breathing and the heart stops beating. **Biological death** occurs when the brain cells start to die. Without oxygen, lethal changes take place in the brain cells within 4 to 6 minutes. Brain death may start within 10 minutes.

In addition to the respiratory centers in the brain, the diaphragm, and the muscles between the ribs, the respiratory system includes the nose and mouth, the **pharynx** (throat), **larynx** (voice box), the **epiglottis,** the **trache**a (windpipe), the bronchial tree, and the lungs.

To assess normal breathing, **look** for chest movements, **listen** and **feel** for air movement, and observe skin color for blue, gray, white (pallor or paleness), or ashen tints. Suspect problems when you note changes in breathing rate and depth, skin color, and breathing effort.

Opening the airway is the first important step in patient care. Simply repositioning the patient's head may solve breathing problems. The **head-tilt, chin-lift maneuver** is used to open the airway of patients with no neck or spine injuries. The **jaw-thrust maneuver** is used when there are possible neck or spine injuries. Only a slight head-tilt with chin-lift, or **sniffing position,** is used for children. The infant's head is kept in the neutral position to maintain the airway.

Mouth-to-mask ventilation is the recommended procedure for performing assisted ventilations. Use a pocket face mask with one-way valve and HEPA filter. Some jurisdictions train First Responders to use the bag-valve mask (see Appendix 2).

Mouth-to-barrier ventilation is another procedure that helps to provide protection from infectious disease.

Mask-to-stoma ventilation is used for neck breathers. Methods that do not use a mask or some other barrier increase the risk of infectious disease transmission.

Watch for **gastric distention** when you perform assisted ventilations. Reposition the head and adjust your ventilations to correct gastric distention. Be on guard for vomiting.

When caring for car-crash victims, stabilize the patient's head and use the jaw-thrust maneuver to open the airway. If you must reposition the patient in order to assist ventilations, open the airway and ventilate while stabilizing his head in the best way you can.

When you begin artificial ventilation, start with two adequate breaths. Assist ventilations for the non-breathing adult at a rate of one breath every five seconds. This rate can also be expressed as 12 breaths per minute. For infants and children, the rate is one breath every three seconds or 20 breaths per minute.

A variety of problems can cause **partial or complete airway obstruction.** These include the tongue, the epiglottis, foreign objects, tissue damage, tissue swelling, and disease.

In addition to the signs of inadequate breathing, listen for snoring, gurgling, crowing, wheezing, and stridor sounds. For complete obstruction, there will be no chest movements, no sounds of respiration, and no air exchange felt at the nose and mouth.

Encourage patients with partial obstructions to cough. If they cannot cough, if their coughing is very weak, or if there is poor air exchange, provide care as if there is a complete airway obstruction.

To clear an obstructed airway, deliver abdominal thrusts to adults and to children (older than one year of age) in rapid succession. Deliver slow, distinct chest thrusts for infants (less than one year of age), obese adults, and pregnant patients.

Responsive patients with airway obstructions will look distressed and will often grasp their necks trying to communicate. Ask patients, "Can you speak?" or "Can you cough?" or "Are you choking?" If they can respond, the obstruction is partial.

Relieve airway obstructions with the combined procedures of attempting to ventilate, manual thrusts (back blows for infants only), finger sweeps (do not perform blind finger sweeps), and opening the airway and attempting ventilations again.

Airway adjuncts, such as the **oropharyngeal airway** and the **nasopharyngeal airway,** help the First Responder maintain the patient's airway while providing ventilations. Measure the oral airway by one of two methods: from the center of the mouth to the angle of the jaw, or from the corner of the mouth to the earlobe. Begin inserting the oropharyngeal airway upside down in adults and turn it to the correct position to seat it properly in the oral cavity. For infants and children, insert the oropharyngeal airway in the right-side-up position. Turning the airway in pediatric patients may damage the oral cavity. The nasal airway should be slightly smaller in diameter than the patient's nostril and at least as long as the distance between the tip of the nose and the earlobe. Lubricate the nasopharyngeal airway with a water-soluble gel before inserting it. Reassess the patient's airway after inserting any airway adjunct.

REMEMBER AND CONSIDER

Making sure that a patient has an open airway and knowing how to maintain and manage it is the most important care you can provide. All other patient care activities are secondary, because if people cannot breathe, they die. The steps for opening an airway are simple and easy to perform. The skills required to maintain and manage an airway take practice. Practicing airway maintenance and management skills helps you develop an ability and proficiency that will help you act quickly in a stress-filled emergency.

✔ Do you remember and can you perform the different ways to open an airway?

✔ Why is it important to know when to use one technique rather than the other?

You will practice measuring and inserting nasopharyngeal and oropharyngeal airways on manikins in class. You will also practice using pocket face masks and possibly bag-valve masks, too. Go back to your station and check the response units and aid kits for airways and masks.

✔ What kinds and sizes of airways do you have? Where are they located? Are they kept in several places that are easy to get to?

✔ What kinds of pocket face masks do you have? Which one is easiest for you to use? Have you tried using one on a person or just a manikin? Ask a member of your family, a friend, or other EMS company member if you can position one on his or her face so you can get used to the placement and grip. Ask the person to breathe in and exhale normally. Check your seal. Does air leak out around the cheeks, or does it exit through the one-way valve only? If you feel you have to press hard to get a seal, then you may not have the mask in the correct position. Reposition it until you get a good seal. Be sure to thoroughly wash and dry the mask after practice.

Remember the signs of an obstructed airway and how to manage the patient in all three situations: responsive, becomes unresponsive, is unresponsive when you arrive.

✔ What do you do if you cannot get air into the unresponsive patient with your first or second breath? What if you are doing obstructed airway procedures on a responsive patient who is showing signs of obstructed airway and the patient becomes unresponsive? Have you ever had to perform obstructed airway procedures on anyone? Ask care providers in your company to tell you their experiences. Ask people you know who are different sizes (tall and short) and various girths (slender and stout) if you can practice your positions on them. Where do you place yourself or the patient when he or she is much taller or shorter than you, when his or her girth is larger than your arms can reach? Is it more difficult to find the correct position on the abdomen when someone is obese?

WARNING: *Even though obstructed airway procedures do not require extremely forceful thrusts, they can cause discomfort or injury. Therefore, while you can practice positioning on people of different sizes, perform the complete maneuver only on manikins.*

How does your company's suctioning unit work?

Is the suction unit a portable battery-operated one, or a hand-operated unit, or do you have both kinds? Do you know how to assemble and disassemble them? Where are the replacement parts and tubing kept? Where do you dispose of the contents? Do you have labels for the collection containers in case the hospital wants the contents? What would you put on a label?

Will you be able to manage a patient with a stoma?

Do you know anyone with a stoma? Where can you get information on stoma patients? Check the Internet for web pages and local directories for phone numbers of the American Heart Association, the American Lung Association, or your local health department. These resources will give you additional information. Local agencies will probably have speakers willing to give a presentation or show a film at your department on how to manage patients with stomas.

How often do you practice your assisted ventilation skills?

Do you know that motor skills will rapidly deteriorate if you do not use them? Practice makes perfect and in order to be able to assist ventilations quickly and accurately, you must practice them frequently. There are many steps to perform when you assist ventilations, but once you are familiar with them and develop an automatic response, they flow in a very logical sequence. But that automatic response only comes with practice. Check with your company and find out how often they hold drills. Do you have manikins at your station? Find out if you can get them out and practice on them when you are on duty. Even without the actual manikins, you can review the pictures in the text and mentally picture yourself performing each step. Go through the motions even without the manikin.

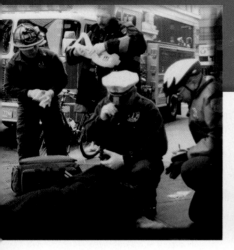
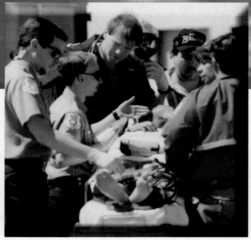
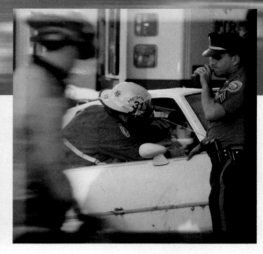

Assessment of the Patient

CHAPTER
7

A First Responder may be active in a small part of the initial care of one patient or have responsibilities that involve all aspects of emergency care for another. Whatever your role, it is always true that your patient assessment skills are the foundation for all the care that you will provide.

Patients cannot receive the care they need until their problems are identified. You must assess each patient in order to detect possible illness or injury and determine the direction of the emergency care needed. Such assessment must be done in a specific and orderly fashion to minimize the chance of overlooking an important sign or symptom.

Remember that patient assessment performed well generally leads to appropriate patient care. Performed poorly, it can lead to dire consequences for the patient.

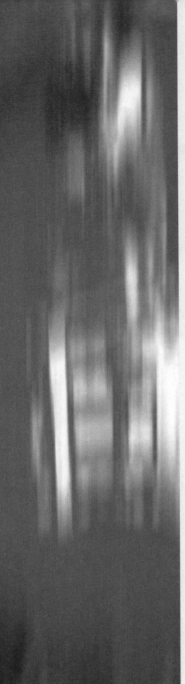

NATIONAL STANDARD OBJECTIVES

This chapter focuses on the objectives of Module 3, Lesson 3–1, of the U.S. DOT's First Responder National Standard Curriculum and serves as an instructional aid to help you meet any specific objectives added to the course by your local EMS system.

By the end of this chapter, you will be able to
(from cognitive or knowledge information):

3–1.1 Discuss the components of scene size-up. (pp. 145–149)

3–1.2 Describe common hazards found at the scene of a trauma and a medical patient. (pp. 146–148)

3–1.3 Determine if the scene is safe to enter. (pp. 146–148)

3–1.4 Discuss common mechanisms of injury/nature of illness. (pp. 147–148)

3–1.5 Discuss the reason for identifying the total number of patients at the scene. (p. 148)

3–1.6 Explain the reason for identifying the need for additional help or assistance. (p. 148)

3–1.7 Summarize the reasons for forming a general impression of the patient. (p. 153)

3–1.8 Discuss methods of assessing mental status. (p. 154)

3–1.9 Differentiate between assessing mental status in the adult, child, and infant patient. (pp. 154, 157–158)

3–1.10 Describe methods used for assessing if a patient is breathing. (p. 156)

3–1.11 Differentiate between a patient with adequate and inadequate breathing. (p. 156; see also Chapter 6)

3–1.12 Describe the methods used to assess circulation. (pp. 156–157)

3–1.13 Differentiate between obtaining a pulse in the adult, child, and infant patient. (pp. 157–158, 167–168)

3–1.14 Discuss the need for assessing the patient for external bleeding. (pp. 156–157)

3–1.15 Explain the reason for prioritizing a patient for care and transport. (p. 157)

3–1.16 Discuss the components of the physical exam. (pp. 158–162)

3–1.17 State the areas of the body that are evaluated during the physical exam. (pp. 171–178)

3–1.18 Explain what additional questions may be asked during the physical exam. (pp. 163–166)

3–1.19 Explain the components of the SAMPLE history. (p. 165)

3–1.20 Discuss the components of the ongoing assessment. (p. 178)

3–1.21 Describe the information included in the First Responder hand-off report. (p. 178)

Feel comfortable enough to
(by changing attitudes, values, and beliefs):

3–1.22 Explain the rationale for crew members to evaluate scene safety prior to entering. (pp. 145–149)

LEARNING TASKS

In addition to the objectives listed in the previous section, you should be able to:

✔ State the three things you must say to a responsive patient upon your arrival at the scene.

✔ Describe the personal protective equipment you should wear during the assessment of a patient.

✔ Describe how to ensure an open airway.

✔ Differentiate between a sign and a symptom.

✔ Define and describe how to take vital signs, and indicate what you are looking for in terms of rate, character, and what is considered normal.

✔ Define baseline vital signs and explain why they are important when obtaining additional sets of vital signs.

3–1.23 Serve as a model for others by explaining how patient situations affect your evaluation of the mechanism of injury or nature of illness. (pp. 147–148)

3–1.24 Explain the importance of forming a general impression of the patient. (p. 153)

3–1.25 Explain the value of an initial assessment. (pp. 149–158)

3–1.26 Explain the value of questioning the patient and family. (pp. 147–148, 163–166)

3–1.27 Explain the value of the physical exam. (pp. 171–178)

3–1.28 Explain the value of an ongoing assessment. (p. 178)

3–1.29 Explain the rationale for the feelings that these patients might be experiencing. (pp. 148–149, 165–166)

3–1.30 Demonstrate a caring attitude when performing patient assessments. (pp. 148–149, 165–166)

3–1.31 Place the interests of the patient as the foremost consideration when making any and all patient-care decisions during patient assessment. (pp. 163–166)

3–1.32 Communicate with empathy during patient assessment to patients as well as with family members and friends of the patient. (pp. 163–166)

Show how to
(through psychomotor skills):

3–1.33 Demonstrate the ability to differentiate various scenarios and identify potential hazards. (pp. 145–149)

3–1.34 Demonstrate the techniques for assessing mental status. (p. 154)

3–1.35 Demonstrate the techniques for assessing the airway. (p. 156)

3–1.36 Demonstrate the techniques for assessing if the patient is breathing. (p. 156; see also Chapter 6)

3–1.37 Demonstrate the techniques for assessing if the patient has a pulse. (pp. 156–157, 167–168)

3–1.38 Demonstrate the techniques for assessing the patient for external bleeding. (pp. 156–157)

3–1.39 Demonstrate the techniques for assessing the patient's skin color, temperature, condition, and capillary refill (infants and children only). (pp. 156–157, 170)

3–1.40 Demonstrate questioning a patient to obtain a SAMPLE history. (p. 165)

3–1.41 Demonstrate the skills involved in performing the physical exam. (pp. 163–166)

3–1.42 Demonstrate the ongoing assessment. (p. 178)

✔ Distinguish between a stable and an unstable patient.

✔ List examples of significant mechanisms of injury.

✔ List, in correct order, the steps of the focused history and physical exam for a trauma patient with no significant mechanism of injury.

✔ List, in correct order, the steps of the rapid trauma assessment for a trauma patient with a significant mechanism of injury.

✔ List, in correct order, the steps of the focused history and physical exam for a responsive medical patient.

✔ List, in correct order, the steps of the rapid physical exam for an unresponsive medical patient.

✔ List 10 First Responder rules that apply to patient assessment.

✔ Define the detailed physical exam and the ongoing assessment.

WARNING: *Patient assessment procedures can bring you into contact with a patient's blood and body fluids. Take body substance isolation (BSI) precautions whenever you care for a patient. It is important. Latex, vinyl, or other synthetic gloves should always be worn during assessment and emergency care. Eye protection may also be required depending on the type of emergency and patient condition. Wear any other items of personal protection required for your safety and that of your patients. Follow OSHA, CDC, and local guidelines to help prevent the spread of infectious diseases. Review the personal safety and protection information in Chapter 3.*

OVERVIEW OF PATIENT ASSESSMENT

patient assessment the gathering of information to determine a possible illness or injury. It includes interviews and physical examination.

Many EMS systems use an assessment-based approach to providing care to patients. This is to say that First Responders and EMTs are trained to identify, prioritize, and care for major signs and symptoms. What they will not do is try to diagnose a patient's specific problems. For example, a First Responder will do what he can to make sure a patient with difficulty breathing has an open airway and supplemental oxygen. What he will *not* do is waste critical time attempting to figure out the underlying cause of the patient's difficulty. Once all life threats have been cared for, the First Responder will complete a more thorough assessment of the patient, try to identify any less obvious signs and symptoms, and gather a pertinent patient history.

STABLE VS. UNSTABLE

stable a term used in reference to the scene or a patient when conditions have a steady quality; remaining steady or the same.

unstable a term used in reference to the scene or a patient when conditions do not have a steady quality; unsteady or not remaining the same.

The components of patient assessment and the order in which they are performed may vary from patient to patient based on the patient's problem. But before you study those components, you must know two terms that apply to both the scene and the patient: **stable** and **unstable**.

A stable scene is a safe scene. The conditions at a *stable scene* allow for rescuers to safely access and provide care to patients. An *unstable scene* is one that is not safe or has the potential of becoming unsafe. An example may be a motor-vehicle crash site. It is not unusual to find vehicles or objects that can move or shift position (an overturned car or a broken, leaning utility pole, for instance). In addition, fire could break out or fuel and other fluids could leak and increase the danger, causing the scene to become even more unstable.

Patients also may be classified as *stable* or *unstable*. In this sense, stable means that there is a steady quality to the patient's vital signs and clinical condition. Whether slow or rapid, changes to this steady state indicate an unstable patient. Note: a patient who appears to be stable can become unstable without warning.

ASSESSMENT COMPONENTS

For most patients, a First Responder's assessment should begin as follows:

1. Perform a scene size-up so that you can ensure your own safety and the safety of your patient.

2. Perform an initial assessment so that you can identify and care for any immediate life threats.

medical patient one who has or describes symptoms of an illness; a patient with no injuries.

trauma patient one who has a physical injury caused by an external force.

The initial assessment is a set of procedures meant to detect and correct life-threatening problems. The remaining components of patient assessment change slightly with each of the four types of patient: **medical patients**—responsive and unresponsive; and **trauma patients**—those who have a significant mechanism of injury and those who do not.

Patient Assessment—Responsive Medical Patient

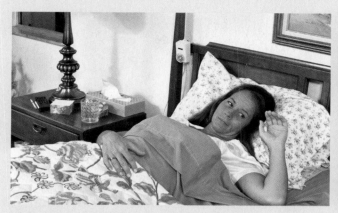

1. Size up the scene. Enter only if it is safe to do so.

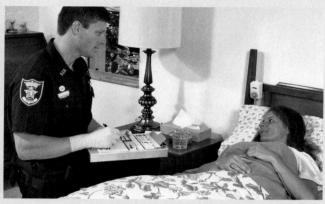

2. Perform an initial assessment. Care for immediate life threats first.

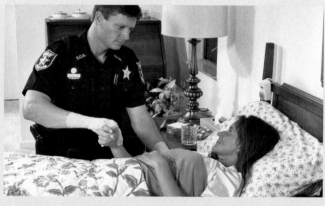

3. Perform a focused history and physical exam based on the patient's chief complaint. Take vital signs.

4. Perform an ongoing assessment.

Note that, at times, the type of patient you are caring for is not so clearly defined. For example, a patient experiencing a medical problem may fall and injure himself. Or a medical problem may have actually caused a motor-vehicle collision. Your patient assessment will need to include elements for both medical and trauma emergencies. What should guide your assessment should be the more serious of the patient's problems.

Medical Patients

Responsive Medical Patient   For a responsive medical patient, you will (Scan 7-1):

- Perform a scene size-up and an initial assessment.

- Perform a focused history and physical exam based on the patient's chief complaint.

- Obtain vital signs, including pulse, respirations, and skin signs. Blood pressure and pupil assessment may be included for some First Responders.

- Perform an ongoing assessment, including a reassessment of the patient's vital signs in order to identify any changes in the patient's condition.

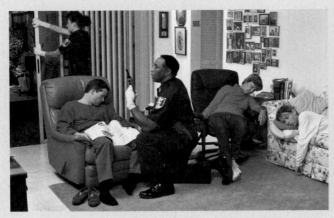

1. Size up the scene. Enter only if it is safe. If it is not, contact dispatch for assistance. Ventilate closed spaces or remove yourself and the patients from the area quickly.

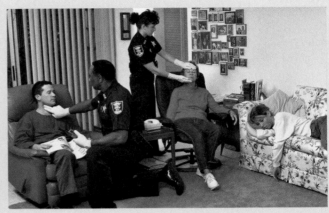

2. Perform an initial assessment. Care for immediate life threats first.

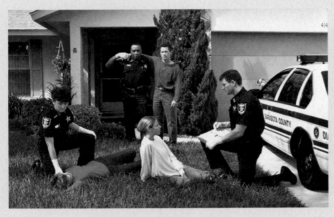

3. Perform a rapid physical exam to look for signs of illness. Take vital signs.

4. Perform an ongoing assessment.

Unresponsive Medical Patient For an unresponsive medical patient, you will (Scan 7-2):

- Perform a scene size-up and an initial assessment. Care for any major problems as you detect them.

- Perform a rapid physical exam to look for signs of illness.

- Take the patient's vital signs.

- Attempt to interview the patient's family or bystanders to determine the patient's chief complaint and **nature of illness (NOI)**.

- Perform an ongoing assessment, including a reassessment of vital signs in order to identify any changes in the patient's condition.

nature of illness (NOI)
what is medically wrong with the patient; a complaint not related to an injury.

Patient Assessment—Responsive Trauma Patient
(No Significant Mechanism of Injury)

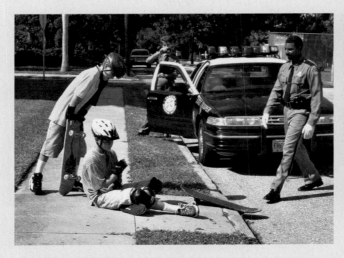

1. Size up the scene. Determine the mechanism of injury. Enter only if it is safe to do so.

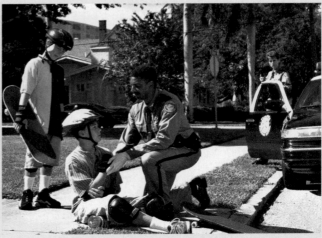

2. Perform an initial assessment. Simultaneously, as you check for an open airway, adequate breathing, and serious bleeding, gather a patient history.

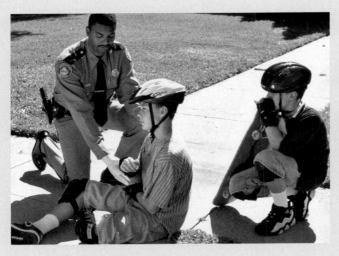

3. Examine the patient based on his complaints. Take baseline vital signs. Perform a detailed physical exam as needed.

4. Perform an ongoing assessment

Trauma Patients

No Significant Mechanism of Injury   For a trauma patient with no significant mechanism of injury, you will (Scan 7-3):

- Perform a scene size-up and an initial assessment. Include a scan of the scene to determine the cause of the patient's injuries. That cause should be referred to as the **mechanism of injury (MOI)**.

- Interview the patient while checking for adequate breathing and serious bleeding.

mechanism of injury (MOI) the force or forces that may have caused injury.

Patient Assessment—Unresponsive Trauma Patient
(Significant Mechanism of Injury)

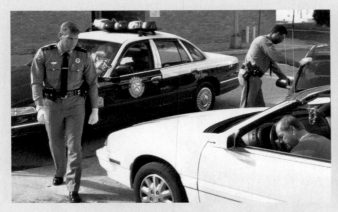

1. Size up the scene. Determine the mechanism of injury. Enter only if it is safe to do so.

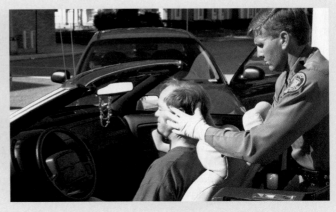

2. Perform an initial assessment. Manually stabilize the patient's head and neck. Simultaneously, as you check for an open airway, adequate breathing, and serious bleeding, gather a patient history.

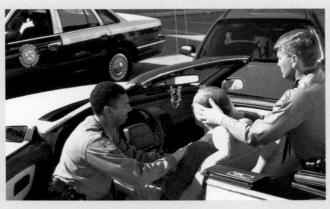

3. Perform a rapid trauma assessment to detect any serious injuries. Take baseline vital signs. Perform a detailed physical exam.

4. Perform an ongoing assessment.

• Conduct a physical exam of the patient based on the patient's chief complaint.

• Determine vital signs.

• Perform a detailed physical exam as needed.

• Perform an ongoing assessment, including a reassessment of vital signs in order to identify any changes in the patient's condition.

Significant Mechanism of Injury For a trauma patient with a significant mechanism of injury, you will (Scan 7-4):

• Perform a scene size-up. Include a scan of the scene and note the mechanism of injury.

- Perform an initial assessment. Manually stabilize the patient's head and neck. Check for an open airway, adequate breathing, and a pulse. Also, check for serious bleeding. Care for any life threats as you detect them.

- Perform a rapid trauma assessment to look for serious injuries. Simultaneously, begin to question family and bystanders about the incident.

- Take vital signs if the patient appears to be unstable.

- Perform a detailed physical exam if time allows.

- Perform an ongoing assessment, including a reassessment of vital signs in order to identify any changes in the patient's condition.

FIRST RESPONDER ASSESSMENT-BASED CARE

FIRST➤ A typical patient assessment contains seven major components. While only some portions of them apply to the First Responder, you should be familiar with all of them in order to communicate with other EMS responders properly. These components include (Figure 7.1):

- *Scene size-up*—Note if the scene is safe or has been made safe.
- *Initial assessment*—Detect and correct any life-threatening problems. Remember, a patient may become unstable and require care for life-threatening problems that develop. Such a change may occur during any step of the patient assessment or emergency care.
- *Focused history and physical exam*
  -*Trauma patient.* For the injured patient, perform a physical exam based on information obtained from the patient, the mechanism of injury. Take vital signs and, if possible, obtain a patient history from the patient, family, or bystanders. Note if the patient has changed since the initial assessment and provide appropriate care.
  -*Medical patient.* For the patient who is ill, obtain a history, perform any required physical exam, and take vital signs. As with all patients, remain alert for changes, making certain that you maintain airway, breathing, and circulation.
- *Detailed physical exam*—When time permits, perform a more detailed head-to-toe physical exam. This exam is called for in all cases involving trauma patients with a significant mechanism of injury.
- *Ongoing assessment*—Monitor the patient to detect any changes. Repeat the initial assessment (usually done en route to the hospital), correct any additional life-threatening problems, repeat vital signs, and evaluate and adjust as needed any **interventions** performed, such as dressing and bandaging. You will find that the condition of your patient will improve, stay the same, or get worse.
- *Communications*—Communicate patient information to the higher-level providers who will be taking over patient care.
- *Documentation*—Accurately and completely fill out all required written reports and forms. ■

interventions actions taken to correct or stabilize a patient's illness or injury.

FIRST➤ The typical First Responder program stresses five major parts of patient assessment. They include:

- Scene size-up.
- Initial assessment.
- Focused assessment (trauma and medical), including a history and physical exam.
- Detailed assessment (head-to-toe exam).
- Ongoing assessment. ■

Patient Assessment

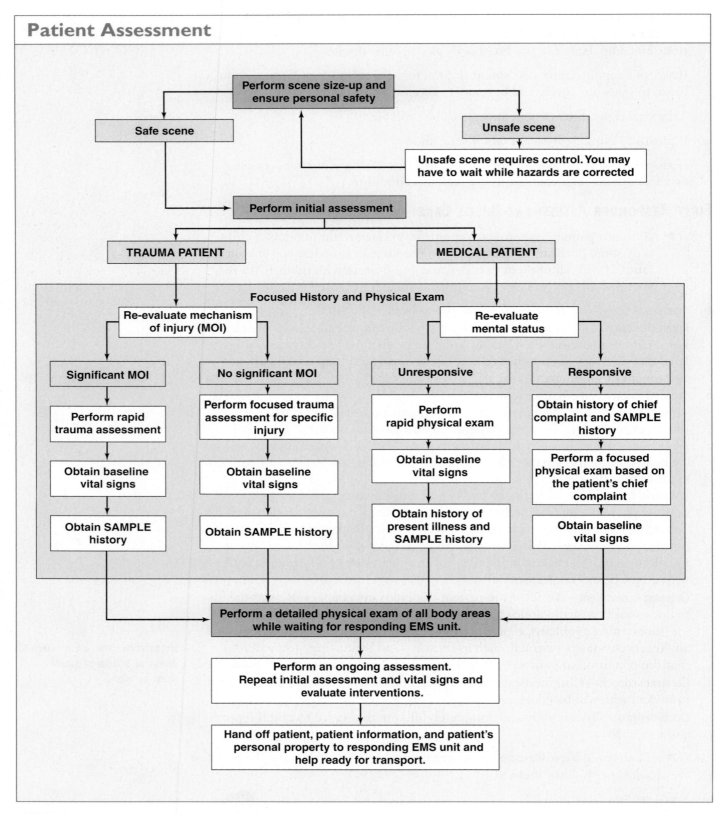

FIGURE 7.1

While the responsibilities of the First Responder may differ from one EMS system to another, most use an assessment-based approach to patient care. After ensuring one's own personal safety, a First Responder's first concern is to safely detect and begin to correct life-threatening problems in his patient. The second concern is to safely identify and provide care for problems that are serious or may become serious. The third concern is to safely monitor the patient to quickly detect any changes in his condition.

SCENE SIZE-UP

Safety is a primary goal of the **scene size-up**. Scene size-up actually begins with the information you receive from your dispatcher, before you arrive at the emergency scene. While en route to the scene, bring to mind the dispatcher's description of the emergency. Think about the types of injuries or hazards you may find at that particular scene, or the signs and symptoms you may see in a patient with that particular emergency.

FIRST➤ When you arrive on scene, take appropriate BSI precautions and make sure the scene is safe to enter. Note whether it is *stable* or *unstable*. When the scene is safe to enter, remain cautious. Continue to evaluate scene safety throughout the call. Next, look for the mechanism of injury at calls involving a trauma patient (Figure 7.2). Identify the nature of illness at medical emergencies (Figure 7.3). Note the number of patients, and anticipate any additional resources that may be needed.

To recap, every patient assessment begins with scene size-up, which includes (Scan 7-5):

● Take BSI precautions.
● Determine if the scene is safe for you, other responders, the patient, and by-standers.

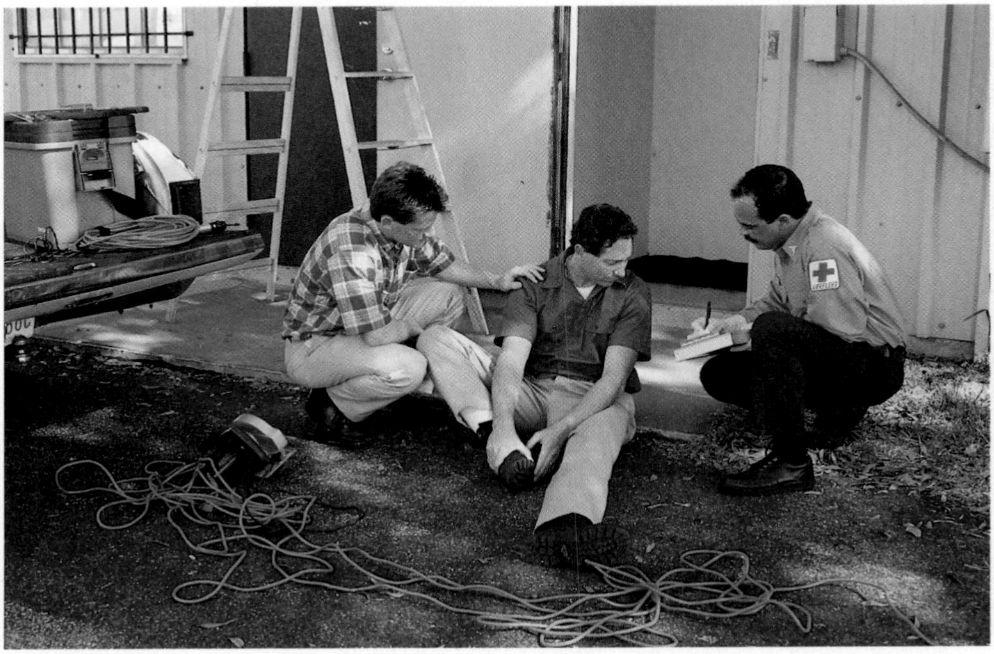

scene size-up steps taken when approaching the scene of an emergency, which consist of taking BSI precautions, determining the safety of the scene, identifying the mechanism of injury or nature of illness, determining the number of patients, and identifying additional resources.

FIGURE 7.2
Clues to the trauma patient's injuries may be gathered upon arrival at the scene.

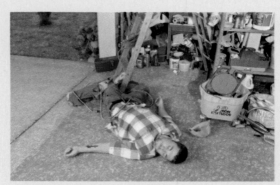

TRAUMA PATIENT

As you approach the trauma patient:

- Take the appropriate BSI precautions.
- Determine if the scene is safe for yourself, the patient, and bystanders.
- Identify the mechanism of injury.
- Determine the number of patients.
- Decide if additional resources are needed (EMTs, ALS providers, Medevac helicopter, fire service, law enforcement)
- Report to EMS dispatch.
- Consider the need for spinal immobilization.

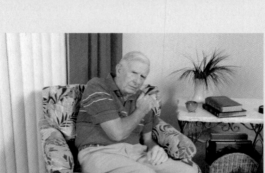

MEDICAL PATIENT

As you approach the medical patient:

- Take the appropriate BSI precautions.
- Determine if the scene is safe for yourself, the patient, and bystanders.
- Identify the nature of illness.
- Determine the number of patients.
- Decide if additional resources are needed (EMTs, ALS providers, Medevac helicopter, fire service, law enforcement)
- Report to EMS dispatch.

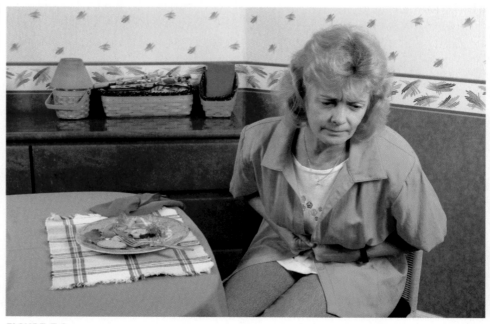

FIGURE 7.3

The medical patient's chief complaint may be apparent as you approach.

- Identify the mechanism of injury or nature of illness.
- Determine the number of patients.
- Identify any additional resources needed. ■

TAKE BSI PRECAUTIONS

(You may wish to review Chapter 3 on personal safety and protection at this time.) Always wear latex or vinyl gloves when caring for any patient. Wear eye protection, and take other BSI precautions as needed, depending on the patient's problem. Remember, BSI precautions are meant to protect you and your patient. So apply personal protective equipment as you approach the patient.

ENSURE SCENE SAFETY

A dangerous and sometimes fatal mistake that responders make is entering an unsafe or hazardous scene. *Never assume that any scene is safe.* First of all, did the scene size-up have you conclude that the scene was stable? A scene is stable or unstable. You may not bypass this evaluation. If the scene is unstable it *must* be considered unsafe. Many factors that are found during the size-up and ongoing scene assessment will force you to classify the scene as unsafe. For example, if a scene has the potential for violence, and you are not a law enforcement officer, do not enter it until law enforcement indicates it is safe for you to do so. If there is a potential for a hazardous materials release, remain a safe distance away. You may never actually enter the scene. Often, appropriately trained and equipped hazardous materials team members will bring properly decontaminated patients to you.

Other examples of hazardous or unsafe scenes include crash/rescue scenes, the release of toxic substances, violent or crime scenes, scenes involving any weapon, and unstable surfaces. Also look for signs of domestic disturbances, electrical hazards, potential for fire or explosions, and guard dogs and vicious, wild, or unusual animals. Be especially careful if the emergency is a result of gang activity. Use all your senses to detect unsafe scenes.

Establish a *danger zone* to keep yourself and others away from harm. An important rule to remember is: *Do not take more victims to the scene.* Every year many rescuers are injured and some are killed by being struck by a vehicle while on scene. In some cases, rescuers are not visible or are too close to traffic. In order to ensure safety at a mishap or unsafe scene, use adequate emergency lights and properly position emergency vehicles. Also remember that weather conditions, such as icy roads, should be of concern to rescuers. Learn to *always* relate scene assessment findings to scene safety. The better your scene size-up, the better your ability to recognize and deal with unsafe scenes.

IDENTIFY THE MECHANISM OF INJURY OR NATURE OF ILLNESS

During the scene size-up, identify the mechanism of injury (MOI) for a trauma patient and the nature of illness (NOI) for a medical patient. Information may be obtained from the patient, if responsive and oriented, from family members or bystanders, and by carefully looking at the scene for clues.

The mechanism of injury (MOI), simply defined, is the combined forces that caused the injury. Did this patient fall? Is there a penetrating wound? Was he involved in a motor-vehicle collision? A damaged steering wheel of a vehicle, for example, should lead you to consider the possibility of a chest injury. A cracked windshield could be an indication of a head injury. Consider spine injuries in a patient who experienced a fall. Recalling your reading in anatomy will help you consider what internal structures may be injured beneath an obvious injury to the body's surface.

Identifying the nature of illness is similar to identifying a mechanism of injury. Look at the patient and the area in which he is found for clues to his problem. Does the patient look as if he is in distress? Does his position suggest where there might be pain or discomfort? Are there medications or is there home oxygen equipment in view? Do you detect any odors, such as vomit or urine? While diagnosing why the patient is having a particular medical problem is not necessary, the nature of illness will guide you in the appropriate direction for care.

Both the mechanism of injury for trauma patients and the nature of illness for medical patients will allow you to consider what serious complications to watch for that may have not yet developed. For example, if the patient is complaining of chest pain, you should consider the possibility of a heart problem and the potential for cardiac arrest. Be prepared.

DETERMINE THE NUMBER OF PATIENTS AND ADDITIONAL RESOURCES

The final part of the scene size-up is to determine the number of patients and whether or not you have sufficient resources to handle the call. It is important to account for all patients involved. How many people were in the vehicle? Did someone walk away from a crash scene? Did a patient get thrown from the vehicle?

Once you are certain of the number of patients involved in the emergency, you must determine if additional resources are needed. More than one EMT unit may be required to handle several patients. In fact, you may require additional resources even on calls with only one patient. You may need additional lifting help if a heavy patient must be carried down stairs. You may require a fire department response to help with extrication (to disentangle and free patients from entrapment) or to make a motor-vehicle collision scene safe. Or the patient may require air transport to a specialty medical facility such as a regional trauma center.

An important part of scene size-up is recognizing when additional resources are needed—and calling for them early. If you put off calling for assistance, you may become so involved in patient care that you forget to call for the additional help until it is too late.

ARRIVING AT THE PATIENT'S SIDE

Upon arrival at the patient's side, you should begin by identifying yourself, even when you believe the patient to be unresponsive. A patient who initially appears to be unresponsive may actually be alert. If you wear a uniform, such as that of a law enforcement officer or firefighter, most bystanders and patients will respond to your uniform and allow you to take charge of the scene without question. If you do not wear a uniform, identifying yourself is critical in allowing you to go about your duties. Simply state your name and then the following: "I am a First Responder, and I've been trained in providing emergency care." While many people may not know what a First Responder is, the statement should allow you access to the patient and the cooperation of bystanders.

Your next statement should be to the patient: "May I help you?" As noted in Chapter 2, by answering "yes" to this question, the patient is giving you *expressed consent* to begin assessment and care. The patient may not answer "yes" to your question, but instead may tell you what he believes is wrong and what you must do to help. Even though you may need to perform more steps in the assessment before you can begin specific care and it may be obvious that the care the patient wants is incorrect, the fact that the patient has asked you to begin care implies you have his consent.

Do not ignore a patient's requests. Stop the assessment for a moment and then ask him a specific question about what is wrong. A few seconds to respond to a request such as asking you to look at an injured limb may relax him and indicate that he still has some control. Now, you are in a better position to receive a cooperative response while you explain politely that you are required to gather more information before you can start care.

It is possible for the patient to become upset when you ask additional questions rather than provide the specific care requested. However, most patients will begin to work with you if you state that you must have more information and believe the patient is your best source. Let him know that you must have his cooperation so you will do what is needed to provide proper care.

Sometimes a patient's fear may be so great that he is confused, and will answer, "no" or "just leave me alone." Gaining the patient's confidence by talking with him is usually easy. If the patient is unresponsive or unable to give expressed consent, *implied consent* allows you to care for the patient. This means that if the patient were able to do so, it is assumed that he would give you expressed consent to care for him. (Review Chapter 2 for a more detailed discussion of consent.)

Remember, upon arrival and after conducting a scene size-up, you must:

1. State your name.
2. Identify yourself as a trained First Responder, explaining what this means if necessary. Let the patient and bystanders know that you are with the Emergency Medical Services system. (Do not say "EMS" system. The patient may have no idea what that means.)
3. Ask the patient if you may help.

While you are doing this, remember to look for any obvious life threats such as serious bleeding or breathing problems.

If someone is already providing care to the patient when you arrive, identify yourself as a First Responder. If the person's training is equal to or at a higher level than your own, ask if you may assist. You should still identify yourself to the patient and ask if he wishes you to help. Expressed and implied consent laws still apply.

If you have more training than the person who has begun care, respectfully ask to take over responsibility for the patient. Compliment him on what he has done so far and ask him to assist you. Do not criticize or argue with anyone who may have initiated care. Unless you are a law enforcement officer or there are specific emergency care laws in your state, you cannot order the first provider to relinquish care of the patient to you. Check your local laws and protocols.

INITIAL ASSESSMENT

The **initial assessment** of a patient is designed to detect and correct life-threatening problems that primarily involve the patient's airway, breathing, and circulation. Each problem is corrected as it is found. These problems are serious enough that, if they are not immediately corrected, the patient may die. The initial assessment is begun as soon as you reach the patient. Life-saving procedures must be done as soon as you discover they are needed.

initial assessment the part of a patient assessment that is used to detect and immediately correct life-threatening problems involving the patient's airway, breathing, and circulation.

FIRST> The initial assessment has six components (Scans 7-6, 7-7, and 7-8).

Initial Assessment—Responsive Trauma Patient
(No Significant Mechanism of Injury)

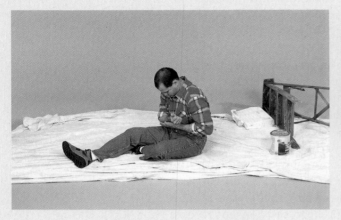

1. Form a general impression of the patient.

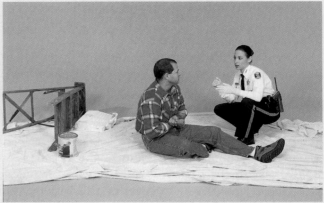

2. Assess the patient's mental status. Initially, this may be to determine if the patient is responsive or unresponsive.

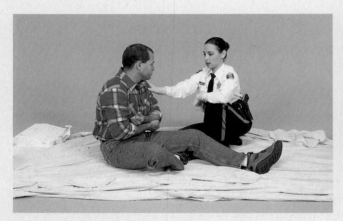

3. Assess the patient's airway and breathing.

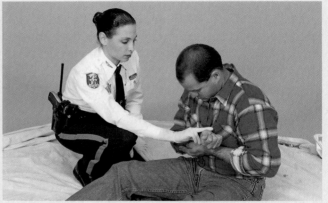

4. Assess the patient's circulation (pulse and major bleeding).

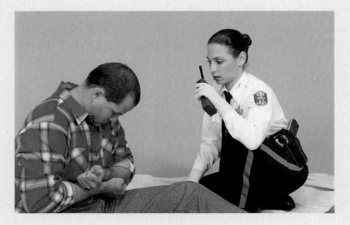

5. Make a decision on the priority or urgency of the patient for transport.

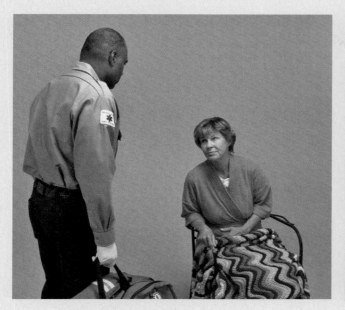

1. Form a general impression of the patient.

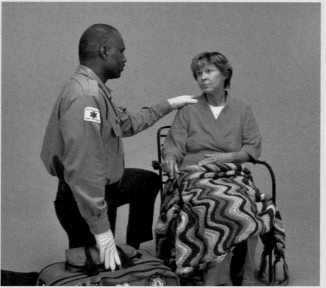

2. Assess the patient's mental status. Initially, this may be to determine if the patient is responsive or unresponsive.

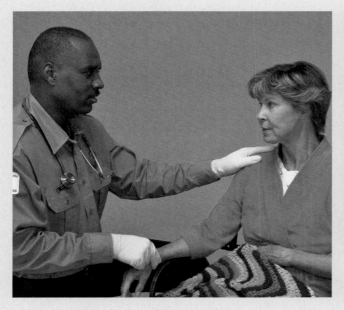

3. Assess the patient's airway, breathing, and circulation.

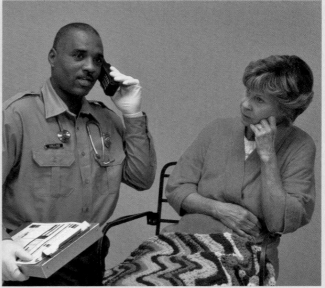

4. Make a decision on the priority or urgency of the patient for transport.

Initial Assessment—Unresponsive Patient
(Medical or Trauma)

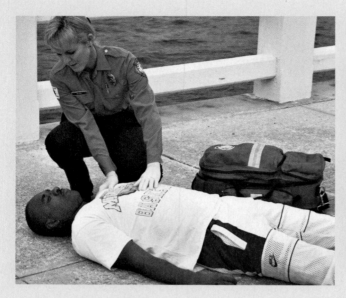

1. As soon as you approach the patient, establish unresponsiveness.

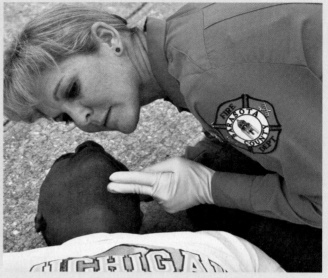

2. Ensure an open airway. Then LOOK, LISTEN, and FEEL for breathing.

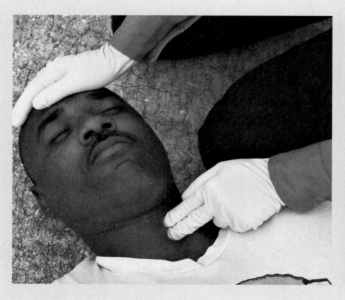

3. Check for a carotid pulse.

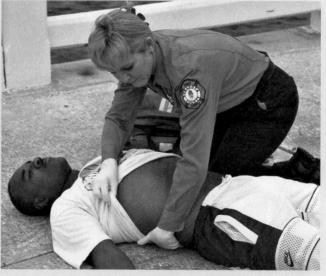

4. Look for and control all major bleeding. Then make a decision on the priority or urgency of the patient for transport.

- Form a general impression of the patient.
- Assess the patient's mental status. Initially, this may be to determine if the patient is responsive or unresponsive.
- Assess the patient's airway.
- Assess the patient's breathing.
- Assess the patient's circulation (pulse and bleeding).
- Make a decision on the priority or urgency of the patient for transport. ■

FIRST➤ While conducting the initial assessment, you will look for life-threatening problems in three major areas. These are:

- *Airway*—Is the patient's airway open?
- *Breathing*—Is the patient breathing adequately?
- *Circulation*—Does the patient have an adequate pulse to circulate blood? Is there serious bleeding? Did the patient lose a large quantity of blood prior to your arrival? Is the patient developing shock? ■

This assessment and the actions taken are known as the **ABCs of emergency care**, which stand for:

A — Airway
B — Breathing
C — Circulation

During patient assessment, if a life-threatening problem is detected, it may be necessary to start *simultaneous actions* focused on the ABCs of emergency care. For example, a trauma patient may require manual stabilization of his head and neck at the same time you are opening his airway, providing ventilations, and controlling bleeding. A medical patient may require you to assess his mental status at the same time you are taking a pulse and assessing his breathing. Simultaneous actions may prove to be very challenging. It is essential that you know how to assess a patient's ABCs, as well as how to provide the care related life-threatening problems require.

FORM A GENERAL IMPRESSION

To begin your initial assessment, form a general impression of the patient and the patient's environment. You may also be given information by the patient or bystanders at this time, such as the reason why EMS was called. The term for the reason why EMS was called, in the patient's own words, is the **chief complaint**.

First Responders have always formed a general impression when they first see a patient, even if they are not immediately aware of doing so. With experience, you may form one on intuition alone. You may notice if the patient looks very ill, pale, or cyanotic (blue coloring to the skin). You may notice unusual details such as odors, temperature, and living conditions. You may immediately see serious injuries, or see that the patient looks quite stable. This impression forms an early opinion of how seriously ill or injured the patient is.

Your decision to request immediate transport or to continue assessing the patient may be based solely on your general impression.

ABCs of emergency care refers to the patient's airway, breathing, and circulation as they relate to the initial assessment.

chief complaint the reason EMS was called, usually in the patient's own words.

ASSESS MENTAL STATUS

Your actual assessment of a patient begins with the patient's mental status, or level of responsiveness. If you do not suspect trauma, especially spinal injury, check for responsiveness by gently squeezing the patient's shoulder and shouting, "Are you okay?" Speak loudly enough to wake the patient if he is merely sleeping.

Classify the patient's mental status by using the letters **AVPU**, which stand for *alert, verbal, painful,* and *unresponsive.*

- *Alert*—The alert patient will be awake, responsive, oriented, and talking with you.

- *Verbal*—The patient who is verbal may appear to be unresponsive at first, but will respond to a loud stimulus.

- *Painful*—If the patient does not respond to verbal stimuli, he may respond to painful stimuli, such as a sternal (breastbone) rub or a gentle pinch to the shoulder. Be careful not to injure the patient when applying painful stimuli. Never forcefully pinch the skin. Never stick the patient with a sharp object.

- *Unresponsive*—If the patient does not respond to either verbal or painful stimuli, he is unresponsive.

Note that the term *verbal* does not mean the patient is answering your questions or initiating a conversation. In assessing mental status the term is a simple measure of responsiveness. The patient may speak or he may grunt or groan, and may even say "huh." It is possible that the patient may have a medical condition such as a stroke or a problem associated with trauma such as a head injury. Either of these examples may cause the patient to loose the ability to speak. In rare cases, a pre-existing condition may have rendered the patient unable to speak prior to the emergency. Often, when such a condition is present the patient will have a medical identification device, such as a card, bracelet, or necklace (Figure 7.4). Check with bystanders. They may know the patient and alert you to the problem.

Try to assess mental status without moving the patient. But if the patient is unresponsive, you may need to reposition him to check for breathing, pulse, and serious bleeding, or to perform CPR. Follow the procedures shown in Scan 7-9.

Always suspect the presence of neck or spine injuries in the unresponsive trauma patient. Moving this type of patient may cause additional serious injuries, but it may be necessary to check for life-threatening problems. (Moving a patient safely was covered in Chapter 5.)

AVPU a memory aid for the classifications of mental status, or levels of responsiveness. The letters stand for *alert, verbal, painful,* and *unresponsive.*

FIGURE 7.4
Example of a medical identification bracelet.

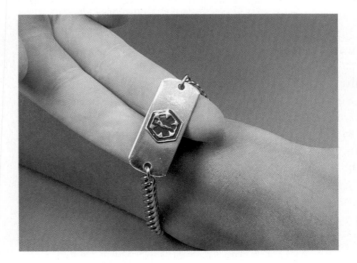

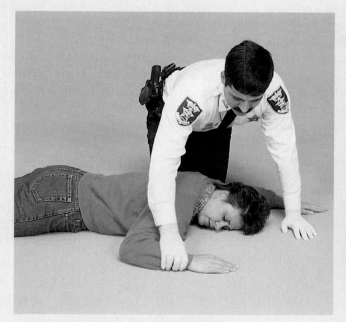

1. Straighten the legs and reposition arms.

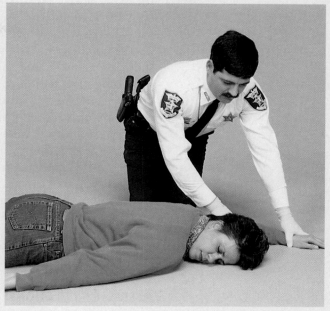

2. Place the arms close to the patient's side. They will help splint the torso as you roll the patient.

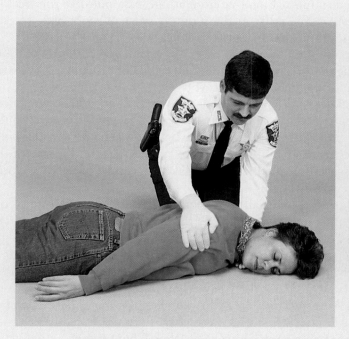

3. Cradle the head and neck, and then grasp the distant shoulder. Move the patient as a unit onto her side.

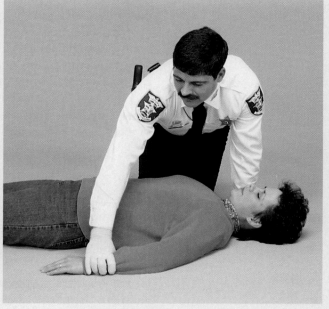

4. Move the patient onto her back.

WARNING: This maneuver is used to initiate basic life support when you must act alone. For all other situations, use a log roll.

ASSESS AIRWAY AND BREATHING

If the patient is unresponsive, stabilize the head and neck and use the jaw-thrust maneuver to ensure an open airway. If you do *not* suspect a spinal injury, position the patient flat on his back and position yourself by his side. Use the head-tilt, chin-lift maneuver to open the airway of a patient with no spine injury. Remember, for patients with suspected spinal injury, use the jaw-thrust.

Then check for adequate breathing. With the airway open, place your ear over the patient's nose and mouth, and watch the chest for movement. If the patient is breathing, you will hear and feel the exhaled air on your ear, and you will see the chest rise and fall with each respiration. Listen to the quality of the breaths. Are there any noises that indicate a possible obstruction?

Determining breathing status should take no more than 10 seconds. The patient is not breathing if there is no chest movement, even if you hear noises coming from the patient's mouth. Sporadic respirations are called *agonal respirations*. They typically occur just prior to death.

If the patient is breathing, there will be a pulse. At this point, you can go on and check for serious bleeding. If the patient is not breathing, or if there is an airway obstruction, you must take immediate action to correct the problem. (The procedures to follow were covered in Chapter 6.)

ASSESS CIRCULATION

Check for a Pulse

carotid pulse the pulse that can be felt on either side of the neck.

If the patient is not breathing, check for a **carotid pulse** at the neck (see Scan 7-8.3). You do this to determine if blood is circulating. The pulse at the neck is considered more reliable than the pulse at the wrist. A pulse at the wrist—the radial pulse—may not be present if the patient is in shock.

To assess the carotid pulse, first locate the patient's Adam's apple. Place the tip of your index and middle fingers directly over the midline of this structure. Now, slide your fingertips to the side of the neck closest to you. Do not slide your fingertips to the opposite side of the patient's neck, as this may apply improper pressure and close the airway. Do not attempt to take a carotid pulse on both sides of the neck at the same time. This may interfere with circulation to the brain. You should detect a pulse in the groove between the trachea (windpipe) and the large muscle on the side of the neck. Only moderate pressure is needed to feel it. Take the carotid pulse for 5 to 10 seconds. Frequent practice will make this skill easy to master.

It is not important during the initial assessment to count the exact rate of the pulse. You only want to confirm the presence of a pulse. If the pulse is very rapid or weak, the patient may be in shock. If there is no pulse, alert dispatch and begin CPR. If there is a pulse, but no breathing, begin artificial ventilations using a pocket face mask or other barrier device.

If the patient is not breathing but does have a pulse, the patient may have an airway obstruction or be in respiratory arrest. You must take immediate action to ventilate the patient before the heart stops. If the chest does not rise during ventilations, the patient may have an airway obstruction. (See Chapter 6.)

Check for Serious Bleeding

The next step in the initial assessment is checking for serious bleeding. While any uncontrolled bleeding may eventually become life-threatening, you will only be concerned with profuse bleeding during the initial assessment. Blood that is bright red and spurting may be coming from an *artery*. Because blood in arteries is under a great deal of pressure, large amounts of blood may be lost in a short period of time. Flowing blood that is darker in color is most likely coming from a *vein*. Even if the bleeding is slow, it may be life-threatening if the patient has been bleeding for a long period of time. Look at the amount of blood that has been lost on the ground, in clothing, and in the hair. Your concern is for the total amount of blood that has been lost, not just how fast or slow the bleeding is. (Methods of controlling serious bleeding are covered in Chapter 10.)

In some EMS systems, First Responders also check skin color, relative skin temperature, and skin moisture, as well as a radial pulse at this time. An abnormal finding such as pale, cool, clammy skin could indicate a serious circulation problem, such as shock or heart problems.

Assessment of circulation may be altered slightly when you immediately see profuse, spurting, or rapidly flowing bleeding. In this case, attempt to slow the bleeding at the same time you are evaluating the patient's breathing. Do what you can to control the bleeding, but never neglect the patient's airway and breathing status.

DETERMINE PATIENT PRIORITY

Information you give to dispatch will help determine the priority of the patient for transport. A *high-priority patient* should be transported immediately, with little time spent on the scene. High-priority conditions include a poor general impression, unresponsiveness, breathing difficulties, severe bleeding or shock, complicated childbirth, chest pain, and any severe pain.

SPECIAL CONSIDERATIONS FOR INFANTS AND CHILDREN

Your assessment of an infant or a child will differ from that of an adult in a few ways. It is important for you to realize that children are not little adults. They react to illness and injury differently. For example:

- Infants and children are often shy and distrustful of strangers. When checking the mental status of an unresponsive infant, talk to him and flick the bottom of his feet. An infant or a child who pays no attention to you or what you are doing may be seriously ill.

- Opening the airway of an infant involves moving the head into a neutral position, not tilting it back as with an adult.

- Opening the airway of a child requires only slight extension.

- Breathing and pulse rates are faster in infants and children than in adults. The pulse to check in an infant or a small child is the **brachial pulse**. It is taken at the brachial artery in the upper arm, not at the neck or wrist.

brachial pulse the pulse that can be felt in the medial side of the upper arm between the elbow and shoulder.

An additional part of checking an infant's or a child's circulation is **capillary refill**. When the end of a child's fingernail is gently pressed, it turns white because blood flow is restricted. When the pressure is released, the nail bed turns pink again, usually in less than 2 seconds. This is a good way to evaluate the circulation of blood in an infant or a child. If it takes longer than 2 seconds for the nail bed to become pink again or if it does not return to pink at all, there may be a problem with circulation, such as shock or blood loss. If the infant's nail beds are too small, you may perform the same test on the top of his foot or back of his hand. To judge the amount of time it takes for the blood to flow back, count, "one-one thousand, two-one thousand," or simply say "capillary refill."

capillary refill the return (refill) of blood into the capillaries after it has been forced out by fingertip pressure to the patient's nail bed. Normal refill time is two seconds or less.

Usually, when adult patients have a serious problem, they become worse gradually. The downward trend often can be spotted in time to take appropriate action.

However, an infant's or child's body can compensate so well for a problem such as blood loss that he may appear stable for some time, and then suddenly become much worse. Children can actually maintain a near-normal blood pressure up to the time when almost half of their total blood volume is gone. That is why blood pressure is not a reliable assessment of a child's circulation. Checking capillary refill time is more reliable.

It is vital for the First Responder to recognize the seriousness of a child's illness or injury early, before it is too late. You will learn about other considerations in approaching and assessing infants and children in Chapter 13.

ALERT DISPATCH

There is a natural tendency for First Responders to contact EMS dispatch as soon as they arrive on the scene of an emergency. If you find an unresponsive adult, you should notify dispatch immediately, even before beginning CPR. Many EMS providers now carry defibrillators. The earlier the defibrillation of a cardiac-arrest patient can be initiated, the greater the chance of that patient's survival. In other cases, it is best to gather some information, such as the type of emergency and number of patients, before you call dispatch.

The information you give EMS dispatch can determine the type and level of response sent. Many EMS dispatch centers are now using an emergency medical dispatch system, or *priority dispatching*. This system determines if basic life support (BLS) or advanced life support (ALS) is needed, or a combination of both. It also determines the response mode used, such as "cold" (Code 2) with no lights or siren or "hot" (Code 3) with lights and siren.

If you have notified dispatch once, but then obtain additional information, you may contact them again to update the responding units. Update the responding EMS units with a brief report by radio including the patient's mental status, age and sex, chief complaint, airway and breathing status, circulation status, and interventions and their results.

FOCUSED HISTORY AND PHYSICAL EXAM

focused history and physical exam the step of patient assessment that follows the initial assessment and includes the patient history, physical exam, and vital signs.

A **focused history and physical exam** should be performed after the initial assessment. It assumes that life-threatening problems have been found and corrected. If you have a patient with a life-threatening problem that you must continually care for (performing CPR on a cardiac-arrest patient, for example), you may not get to this assessment component.

The main purpose of the focused history and physical exam is to discover and care for the patient's specific injuries or medical problems. It is a very systematic approach to patient assessment. It also may assure the patient, family, and bystanders that there is concern for the patient and that something is being done for the patient immediately.

The focused history and physical exam includes a physical exam that hones in on a specific injury or medical complaint, or it may be a rapid exam of the entire body. It also includes obtaining a patient history and taking vital signs. The order in which these steps are accomplished is based on the patient's type of emergency (Table 7-1).

FIRST➤ Some important terms associated with the focused history and physical exam are introduced below. There is more about each one later in the chapter. The terms include:

TABLE 7-1 FOCUSED HISTORY AND PHYSICAL EXAM

TRAUMA PATIENT	MEDICAL PATIENT
Significant Mechanism of Injury	**Unresponsive Medical Patient**
• Perform a rapid trauma assessment. • Take vital signs. • Gather SAMPLE history.	Perform a rapid physical exam. Take vital signs. Gather SAMPLE history.
No Significant Mechanism of Injury	**Responsive Medical Patient**
• Perform a focused trauma assessment. • Take vital signs. • Gather SAMPLE history.	Gather SAMPLE history. Perform focused physical exam. Take vital signs.

- *Patient history*—Gathering information by asking questions and listening. Whenever possible, the patient is your primary source for information. Family and bystanders are also sources of information.
- *Rapid physical exam*—This is a quick, less detailed head-to-toe assessment of the most critical patients.
- *Focused physical exam*—This is an exam conducted on stable patients. It focuses on a specific injury or medical complaint.
- *Vital signs*—These include pulse, respirations, skin signs, and pupils. In some areas, First Responders also include assessment of blood pressure. The first set of vital signs taken on any patient is referred to as the *baseline vital signs*. All subsequent vital signs should be compared to the baseline set to identify developing trends.
- *Symptoms*—These are felt and reported by the patient. **Symptoms** include chest pain, dizziness, and nausea. Symptoms are also called *subjective findings*.
- *Signs*—These are what you see, feel, hear, and smell as you examine the patient. **Signs** include cool, clammy skin or abnormal vital sign measurements. Another term for signs is *objective findings*. ■

Objective findings can be seen, felt, or in some way measured scientifically. Subjective findings are influenced by the person, who in this case is the patient reporting the symptoms. The objective portion of patient assessment is considered part of the science of medicine; the subjective portion as part of the art of medicine.

Many of the signs and symptoms you will find during the physical exam are the result of the body's compensating mechanisms. For example, to compensate for blood loss, the body will increase pulse and breathing rates and close down, or constrict, blood vessels in the extremities, all of which results in cool, clammy, pale skin. These actions are attempts to circulate an adequate amount of oxygenated blood to the more important parts of the body. Adequate flow of oxygenated blood to all cells of the body is called **perfusion**. Inadequate blood flow can lead to *shock*.

Any abnormal findings during your exam indicate a problem that should not be ignored. Note, however, that when most people see something wrong, they want to take care of it or fix it immediately. Remember, this is correct during the initial assessment where you are finding and correcting life threats. But you should not interrupt a focused history and physical exam to care for a problem that is not likely to get worse. You can stop bleeding from getting worse, but there is little you

symptoms subjective indications of illness or injury that cannot be observed by another person but are felt and reported by the patient.

signs objective indications of illness or injury that can be seen, heard, felt, and smelled by another person.

perfusion the adequate flow of oxygenated blood to all cells of the body.

can do to stop a broken leg from getting worse. It is important to complete your examination. *By stopping to care for an injury that is not life-threatening, you may delay or forget the remainder of the exam and miss a more important problem.*

FOCUSED HISTORY AND PHYSICAL EXAM—TRAUMA PATIENT

A *trauma patient* is one who has received a physical injury of some type. Your assessment of a trauma patient will consist of a physical exam, vital signs, and patient history. The type of physical exam you perform and the order in which you do the various steps will be based on your initial assessment, what the patient and bystanders tell you, and the mechanism of injury.

The trauma patient is classified as either having no significant mechanism of injury (probably not causing a serious injury) or having a significant mechanism of injury (probably causing a serious injury). The assessment is different for each type of patient.

To assess a trauma patient with *no significant mechanism of injury*, perform a *focused trauma assessment* on the area that the patient tells you is injured (Scan 7-10). Obtain vital signs and gather a patient history. Provide continued care during the ongoing assessment. (There is usually no need to perform a detailed physical exam on a patient with no significant mechanism of injury.)

To detect and care for serious injuries in a patient with a *significant mechanism of injury*, perform a *rapid assessment* of the entire body (Scan 7-11). Obtain vital signs and gather a patient history. Then, if time permits, perform a *detailed physical exam.* Provide continued care during the ongoing assessment.

Significant mechanisms of injury include:

- Ejection from a vehicle.

- Death of one or more passengers in a motor-vehicle crash.

- Falls greater than 15 feet.

- Rollover vehicle collision.

- High-speed vehicle collision.

- Vehicle-pedestrian collision.

- Motorcycle crash.

- Unresponsiveness or altered mental status.

- Penetrations of the head, neck, chest, or abdomen.

Significant mechanisms of injury for a child include:

- Falls of more than 10 feet.

- Bicycle collision.

- Medium-speed vehicle collision.

NOTE: *Many years of careful medical studies have demonstrated that people are more likely to be seriously injured in falls that are three times the patient's height. Injuries may be serious in shorter falls, often depending on the nature of the surface on which the patient lands and how the patient strikes the surface. Based on research, First Responders should consider all falls as potentially serious. Assess the patient without bias.*

Focused History and Physical Exam—Trauma Patient
(No Significant MOI)

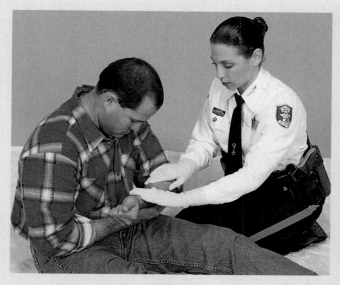

1. Examine the area that the patient tells you is injured.

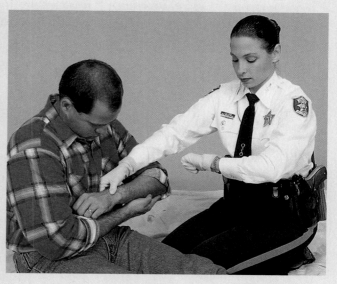

2. Take vital signs and gather a patient history.

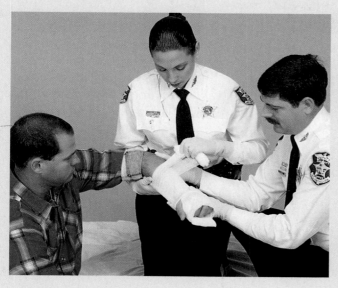

3. Provide appropriate care for the injury.

FOCUSED HISTORY AND PHYSICAL EXAM—MEDICAL PATIENT

The focused history and physical exams for a medical patient and a trauma patient are similar, but the order and emphasis are different. For a medical patient, you are more concerned with the medical history of the patient.

For the *unresponsive medical patient,* perform a *rapid physical exam* to determine if there are any obvious signs of illness. Take vital signs. Gather a patient history, if possible. Provide care as needed.

Focused History and Physical Exam—Rapid Assessment
(Significant MOI or Unresponsive Medical Patient)

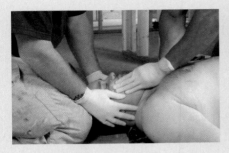

1. First, have your partner stabilize the patient's head and neck. Then check the head (scalp and face).

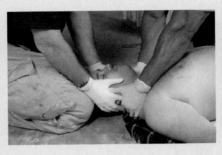

2. Check the patient's neck. Apply a cervical collar, if you are trained to do so.

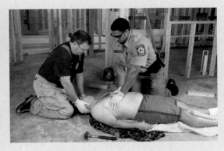

3. Check the chest.

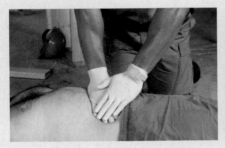

4. Check each quadrant of the abdomen.

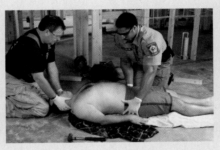

5. Check the pelvis, pressing gently down and inward.

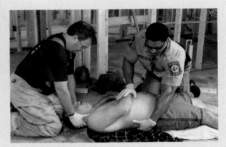

6. Check the back and buttocks by sliding your hands under the patient. (If you have to reposition the arms to check the back, first make sure that there are no injuries to the arms.)

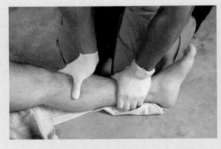

7. Check the extremities, legs first and then the arms.

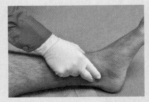 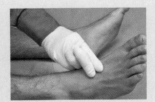

8. Check for circulation, sensation, and motor function.

For the *responsive medical patient* (Scan 7-12), gather a patient history, observing patient signs and asking about the history of the illness and symptoms. The patient's chief complaint helps direct the questioning. Perform a *focused physical exam* based on the patient's problem areas. Take vital signs. Provide care as needed. Provide continued care during the ongoing assessment.

Medical patients rarely require a detailed physical exam and if one is necessary, there is usually a significant mechanism of injury or the rescuer believes there is a potential for injuries, such as when a medical patient has fallen.

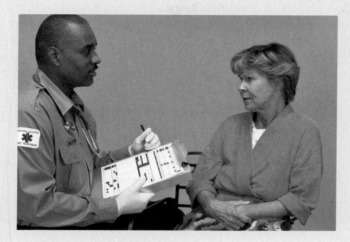

1. Gather a SAMPLE history.

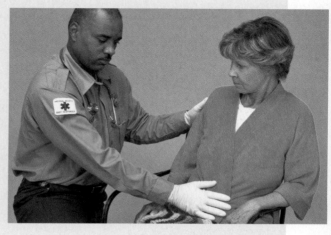

2. Perform a focused physical exam based on the patient's problem areas.

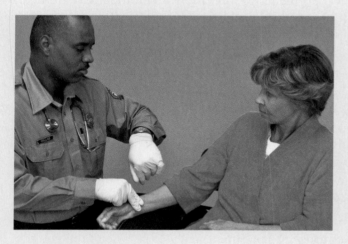

3. Take vital signs.

PATIENT HISTORY

Patient Interview

An alert patient is your best source of information. Direct your questions to him. Ask questions clearly at a normal rate and in a normal tone of voice. Avoid leading questions. Do not falsely reassure the patient. Do not say things such as "Everything will be fine" or "Take it easy, everything's okay." The patient knows this is not true and will lose confidence in you if you attempt to provide false reassurance. Phrases such as "I'm here to help you" or "I'm doing everything I can to help you" are more appropriate.

FIRST➤ When interviewing a patient who is alert, ask the following questions:

1. *What is your name?* This is an essential piece of information. It shows your patient that you are concerned for him as a person. Remember his name and use it often. Also, if your patient's mental status decreases, you can call him by name to elicit a response.

2. *How old are you?* As a First Responder, you do not need to know more than the general age of your adult patient. But the age of a child is important, as it may determine what type of care is provided. Ask all children their age. It may be appropriate to ask an adolescent his age in order to be certain that he is a minor. Also ask minors: *How can I contact your parents?* Children may already be upset at being hurt or ill without a parent being there to help them. Always re-assure them that someone will contact their parents.

3. *What is wrong?* This will usually be the patient's chief complaint. No matter what is wrong, ask if there is any pain. When an extremity is involved, ask if there is numbness, tingling, or a burning sensation in the limb. Any of these could indicate possible nerve or spinal injury. As you learn more about various illnesses and injuries, you will also learn additional questions to ask.

4. *How did it happen?* When caring for trauma patients, knowing how the patient was injured will help direct you to problems that may not be noticeable or obvious to you or the patient. If your patient is lying down, determine if he got into that position himself or was knocked down, fell, or was thrown. Do this for patients with medical problems, as well. Remember, the injury to the patient may be the result of a medical problem. This information may indicate the possibility of a spinal injury or internal bleeding.

5. *How long have you felt this way?* You want to know if the patient's problem occurred suddenly or if it has been developing for the past few days or over a period of time.

6. *Has this happened before?* It is especially important to ask this question of medical patients. You want to know if this is the first time or if it is a recurring, or chronic, problem. This question is not usually asked of trauma patients, unless you suspect a recurring problem. If your patient has been hit by a car, it is not necessary to ask him if this has happened before.

7. *Are there any current medical problems?* Has the patient been feeling ill lately, seen a doctor, or is he being treated by a doctor for any problems?

8. *Are any medications being taken?* Your patient may not be able to tell you the exact name of a medication he is taking, especially if he is taking several. He may be able to tell you just general medication categories, such as "heart pills" or "water pills." Ask not only about prescription medications but over-the-counter medications as well. Routine use of simple medications such as aspirin may alter the treatment the patient receives at the hospital.

   Do not use the terms *drugs* or *recreational drugs* in general. They imply mis-use or abuse. Some patients may think that you are trying to gather evidence and become uneasy. Instead, ask the patient if he can think of anything else that he might be taking. If you still feel that the patient has not given all the in-formation needed, explain your feelings to the EMTs who take over patient care. Be certain that your concern is stated in both your patient assessment notes and the patient assessment record used by the EMTs. Law enforcement officers who are First Responders should follow Standard Operating Proce-dures, keeping in mind that the assessment and care of the patient may require the issue of illegal drug use to be set aside for the moment. Do as you have been trained and required to do as a law enforcement officer.

9. *Do you have any allergies?* Allergic reactions can vary from simple hives or itch-ing to life-threatening airway problems and shock. Knowing that the patient is allergic to a substance will enable you to keep it away from him. Be sure to ask

specifically about allergies to medications, adhesive tape, and latex (as used in gloves), since the patient may come in contact with any of these during care.

10. *When did you last eat?* This is an important question if your patient is a candidate for surgery. It also is important information when dealing with a patient who is having a diabetic emergency. ■

When obtaining a patient history, EMS systems use the acronym **SAMPLE** as a memory aid for questions to be asked. Each letter of the word SAMPLE represents a specific question or series of questions:

S — Signs/symptoms?
A — Allergies?
M — Medications?
P — Pertinent past medical history?
L — Last oral intake?
E — Events leading to the illness or injury?

SAMPLE history a system of information gathering that allows the rescuer to ask questions about past or present medical or injury problems. Letters stand for *signs/symptoms, allergies, medications, pertinent past medical history, last oral intake,* and *events leading to the illness or injury.*

When taking a history, maintain patient eye contact. This will improve personal communication and build the patient's confidence in you. If you look away while asking questions or while listening to answers, it may indicate to your patient that you are not as concerned as you should be or not giving the patient your full attention. A simple touch can also improve communications. You touch the patient's forehead to note relative skin temperature and moisture. But by touching the patient, you are also showing caring and concern. However, respect a patient's wish not to be touched. Patients are often fearful and anxious. Your calm, caring, and professional attitude often can do as much for the patient as any medical care you provide.

Bystander Interview

You may encounter a patient who is unresponsive or unable to answer your questions regarding his history. If this is the case, you must depend on family or bystanders for information. Ask specific, directed questions to shorten the time required to obtain the information. Questions to bystanders include:

1. *What is the patient's name?* If the patient is a minor, ask if the parents are there or if they have been contacted.

2. *What happened?* You can receive valuable information when asking this question. If the patient fell from a ladder, did he appear to faint or pass out first? Was he hit on the head by something? Clues from the answers to this question are limitless.

3. *Did you see anything else?* For example, was the patient holding his chest before he fell? This gives the bystander a chance to think again and add anything he remembers.

4. *Did the patient complain of anything before this happened?* You may learn of chest pain, nausea, shortness of breath, a funny odor where the patient was working, and other clues.

5. *Did the patient have any known illness or problems?* Family or friends who know the patient may know his medical history, such as heart problems, diabetes, allergies, or other problems that may cause a change in his condition.

6. *Does the patient take any medication?* Again, family or friends who know the patient may be aware of the medications he takes. When talking with the patient, family, friends, or bystanders, remember to use the word *medication* or *medicine* instead of *drugs.* Medicines or medications are considered prescriptions for le-

gitimate medical purposes. The public views drugs as illegal substances. Remember to ask the patient if he is taking over-the-counter medications.

The patient history and physical exam can be done simultaneously. There is no need to wait to take vital signs until the SAMPLE history has been completed. You may obtain the SAMPLE history while performing the physical exam of the patient or while controlling bleeding from a wound. You can do both at the same time.

Most of the questions listed above are questions you would normally ask about someone who is hurt or ill. You would usually introduce yourself and ask for a name, just as you would ask what was wrong and how it happened. Much of your First Responder training is simply formalized common sense.

Medical Identification Devices

Medical identification devices can provide important information if the patient is unresponsive and a history cannot be obtained from family or bystanders. A common one is the Medic Alert device worn on a necklace or a wrist or ankle bracelet. One side of the device has a Star-of-Life emblem. Information on the patient's medical problem is engraved on the reverse side, along with a phone number for additional information. If you must move the patient or any of his extremities, take care to check for a medical identification device. Be sure to alert the EMTs who take over care that the patient is wearing one, and tell them what is on it, such as diabetes, heart condition, or penicillin allergy.

VITAL SIGNS

FIRST➤ Vital signs can alert you to problems that require immediate attention. Taken at regular intervals, they can help you determine if the patient's condition is getting better, worse, or staying the same. For most First Responders, **vital signs** include pulse, respirations, and skin signs. Some First Responders include pupils and determining blood pressure. (Taking blood pressure is described in Appendix 1.) ■

vital signs objective signs that include assessment of the patient's pulse, respirations, skin, blood pressure, and pupils.

baseline vital signs the first determination of vital signs; used to compare with all repeated readings of vital signs in order to identify trends.

The first set of vital signs is called **baseline vital signs**. Compare all other vital sign readings to the baseline vital signs. This comparison helps determine if the patient is stable or unstable, improving or growing worse, and benefiting or not benefiting from care procedures. For example, comparing baseline vital signs before and after administering oxygen to the patient can tell the EMTs who take over patient care objective information about how that intervention may be affecting the patient.

Certain combinations of vital signs point to possible serious medical or traumatic conditions. For example, cool, clammy skin, a rapid, weak pulse, and increased breathing rate can indicate possible shock in the presence of a significant mechanism of injury. Hot, dry skin with a rapid pulse may indicate a serious heat-related emergency. You can determine which patients are a high priority for immediate transport by taking vital signs.

For an adult, a continuous pulse rate of less than 60 beats per minute or above 100 beats per minute is considered abnormal. Likewise, a respiratory rate above 28 breaths per minute or below 8 breaths per minute is considered to be serious. You should be concerned about these vital signs because they indicate unstable situations that could become life-threatening, and the patient could worsen quickly. Stay alert and monitor the patient closely. Keeping the patient quiet, at rest, caring for shock, and reassuring the responsive patient can make a difference in the outcome.

Pulse

When taking a patient's pulse, you must assess for three characteristics: *rate*, *strength*, and *rhythm* (Figure 7.5). Rate is a count of the number of heartbeats per minute and is used to determine if the patient's pulse is normal, rapid, or slow. Strength is the force of the pulse. It will be either *strong* or *weak*. Rhythm is the steadiness of the pulse, which will be either *regular* or *irregular*.

During the initial assessment, you checked the carotid pulse in the patient's neck. During the focused history and physical exam, the **radial pulse** is measured. The term *radial pulse* refers to the radial artery found in the lateral portion of the forearm, on the thumb side of the wrist. If for any reason you are unable to feel the radial pulse, assess the carotid pulse. The absence of a radial pulse when there is a carotid pulse indicates possible shock. A radial pulse may not be detectable if the patient's blood pressure is too low or if there is an extremity injury that is interrupting blood flow to the distal arm. Do not start CPR based only on the absence of a radial pulse.

radial pulse the pulse that can be felt on the thumb side of the wrist.

FIRST▶ To measure a radial pulse rate:

1. Use the three middle fingers of your gloved hand. Do not use your thumb, since it has its own pulse, which could be mistaken for the patient's.

2. Place your fingertips on the anterior side of the patient's wrist, just above the crease between hand and wrist. Slide your fingers from this position toward the thumb side of the wrist (lateral side). Keeping the fingertip of the middle finger on the crease between wrist and hand will ensure you are placing the fingertip over the site of the radial pulse.

3. Apply moderate pressure to feel the pulse beats. If the pulse is weak, you may have to apply more pressure. Too much pressure can cause pain to the patient or slow blood flow. By having all three fingers in contact with the patient's wrist and hand, you should be able to judge how much pressure you are applying.

4. Once you feel the pulse, make a quick judgment as to the rate. Does the pulse feel normal, rapid, or slow?

5. Count the beats for 30 seconds.

6. While counting, assess strength and rhythm.

7. Multiply your 30-second count by 2 to determine the number of beats per minute. ■

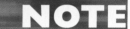

NOTE

If the patient's pulse is irregular, count the pulse rate for a full minute.

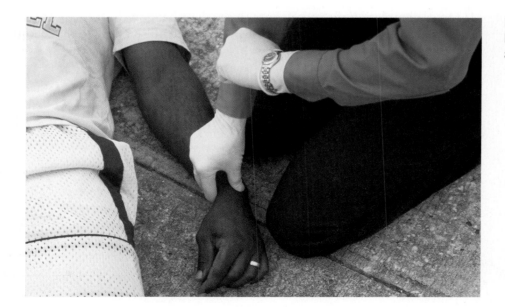

FIGURE 7.5
Rate, strength, and rhythm are characteristics of a pulse.

The normal pulse rate for adults at rest is between 60 and 100 beats per minute. Any rate above 100 is considered rapid (tachycardia), and any rate below 60 is considered slow (bradycardia). In emergency situations, because of anxiety or excitement, it is not unusual for the pulse to be about 100 beats per minute. You should consider a pulse rate over 100 or under 60 to be an indication of a serious problem. One exception to this is a well-conditioned athlete whose normal resting pulse may be about 50 beats per minute or less.

Newborn infants can have pulse rates around 120 to 160 beats per minute. Children up to 5 years old will show ranges from 80 to 140 beats per minute, depending on their age. The normal range of the pulse of children from 5 to 12 years of age is 70 to 110 beats per minute. Adolescents typically have a pulse rate ranging from 60 to 105 beats per minute.

Measuring pulse rates efficiently takes experience. Practice taking both "at rest" rates and rates after mild exercise of both males and females, adults and children. Practice often. It will help you develop an ability to judge normal and rapid rates quickly and accurately.

See Table 7-2 for the relationship between pulse and certain emergency problems you may see as a First Responder.

Respirations

As with pulse rates, you should determine both *rate* and *character* of the patient's respirations (breathing) (Figure 7.6). The respiratory rate is a count of the patient's breaths and is classified as *normal*, *rapid*, or *slow*. The character includes *rhythm*, *depth*, *sound*, and *ease* of breathing. A single respiration is one entire cycle of breathing in and out.

While you are counting respirations, note if the rhythm is *regular* or *irregular*. At the same time, decide if the depth of breathing is *normal*, *shallow*, or *deep*. Listen for any abnormal sounds during breathing, such as snoring, gurgling, gasping, wheezing, or crowing. Notice if the breathing is easy or whether it appears *labored*, *difficult*, or *painful*. If the patient is responsive, ask if he is having any problems or pain while he breathes. A patient who has to work at breathing is in serious condition.

Table 7-3 shows some of the problems that are associated with variations in respirations.

FIRST➤ To measure respiratory rate and character, follow these steps:

1. After completing the pulse count, leave your hand in the same position at the patient's wrist, as if you were still counting the pulse rate. Do this because many patients will unknowingly alter their respiratory rate when someone is watching them breathe.

2. Observe the patient's chest move and listen for sounds.

TABLE 7-2 ASSESSMENT SIGN—PULSE

OBSERVATION	POSSIBLE PROBLEM
Rapid, strong pulse	Internal bleeding (early stages), fear, heat emergency, overexertion, high blood pressure, fever
Rapid, weak pulse	Shock, blood loss, heat emergency, diabetic emergency, failing circulatory system
Slow, strong pulse	Stroke, skull fracture, brain injury
No pulse	Cardiac arrest

3. Count the number of breaths the patient takes in 30 seconds. (One breath = one inspiration plus one expiration.) Multiply the number of breaths by 2 to obtain the respiratory rate.

4. While counting respirations, note rhythm, depth, sound, and ease of breathing. ■

If you cannot visually count the patient's respiratory rate from watching chest movement, gently place your hand on the patient's chest near the xiphoid process. Let the patient know you are going to touch his chest and why. This will allow you to feel each inspiration and expiration. However, do not do this procedure if there are obvious injuries to the chest or abdomen.

TABLE 7-3 ASSESSMENT SIGN—RESPIRATIONS

OBSERVATION	POSSIBLE PROBLEM
Rapid, shallow breaths	Shock, heart problems, heat emergency, diabetic emergency, heart failure, pneumonia
Deep, gasping, labored breaths	Airway obstruction, heart failure, heart attack, lung disease, chest injury, diabetic emergency
Slowed breathing	Head injury, stroke, chest injury, certain drugs
Snoring	Stroke, fractured skull, drug or alcohol abuse, partial airway obstruction
Crowing	Airway obstruction, airway injury due to heat
Gurgling	Airway obstruction, lung disease, lung injury due to heat
Wheezing	Asthma, emphysema, airway obstruction, heart failure
Coughing blood	Chest wound, chest infection, fractured rib, punctured lung, internal injuries

Normal respiratory rates for adults at rest are from 12 to 20 breaths per minute. Older adults breathe more slowly than younger adults. For adults, a respiratory rate of over 28 or below 8 breaths per minute is serious. Infants breathe from 25 to 50 times per minute. If the patient is a child between one and five years of age, a rate over 30 or below 20 breaths per minute is serious. A rate over 30 or below 15 breaths per minute is serious for children six to ten years old.

Skin Color, Temperature, and Moisture

FIRST ➤ Skin color, relative skin temperature, and skin moisture are assessed at the patient's forehead (Figure 7.7), unless this is not possible. The patient's abdomen may also be used as a site for this assessment. Some jurisdictions may have you check the extremities. Use the back of your hand to determine if the skin is *normal, hot,* or *cool.* At the same time, notice if the skin is *dry* or *moist.* Look for goose bumps, which are associated with chills. Observe skin color. Does it appear normal, or is the color abnormal in any way? ■

Tables 7-4 and 7-5 list some of the problems associated with skin color, relative skin temperature, and moisture.

Blood Pressure

While patient assessment is more reliable when the patient's blood pressure is taken and monitored, some First Responders do not carry the necessary equipment to measure this vital sign (Figure 7.8). If your EMS system requires that you determine blood pressure, see Appendix 1.

Pupils

Many EMS systems have the First Responder assess the patient's pupils as part of taking vital signs. The technique used and information gathered are given on page 173 as part of the head-to-toe examination. Table 7-6 provides observations you may make when assessing a patient's pupils and lists possible causes.

FIGURE 7.7
Color, temperature, and moisture are characteristics of the skin.

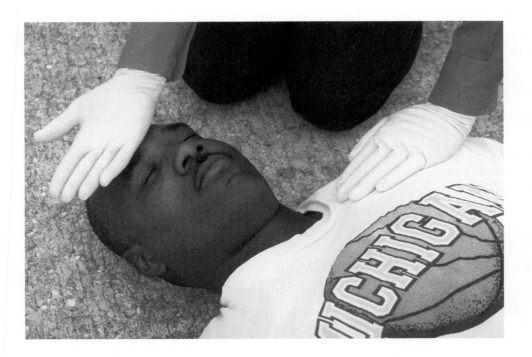

TABLE 7-4 ASSESSMENT SIGN—SKIN COLOR

OBSERVATION	SIGNIFICANCE/POSSIBLE CAUSES
Pink	Normal in light-skinned patients; normal in inner eyelids, lips, and nail beds of dark-skinned patients
Pale	Constricted blood vessels possibly resulting from blood loss, shock, decreased blood pressure, emotional distress
Blue (cyanotic)	Lack of oxygen in blood cells and tissues resulting from inadequate breathing or heart function
Red (flushed)	Heat exposure, high blood pressure, emotional excitement; cherry red indicates late stages of carbon monoxide poisoning
Yellow (jaundiced)	Liver abnormalities
Blotchiness (mottling)	Occasionally in patients in shock

PHYSICAL EXAM

If your trauma patient has no significant mechanism of injury and appears to have an isolated minor injury (supported by the mechanism of injury and what the patient tells you), perform a *focused trauma assessment* on the injury site and the area close to it. If the patient has a significant mechanism of injury, a serious injury, or is unresponsive, perform a *rapid trauma assessment* of the entire body.

The physical exam of a medical patient may be brief. If the patient is responsive, perform a *focused physical exam* based on the patient's chief complaint. If the patient is unresponsive, conduct a *rapid physical exam* of the entire body.

Use the memory aid **DCAP-BTLS** to help you remember what to look for during any physical exam. The letters stand for *deformities, contusions, abrasions, punctures and penetrations, burns, tenderness, lacerations,* and *swelling.* Each part of the body is examined for these injuries, as well as some others specific to each body part.

Rapid Trauma Assessment—Trauma Patient with Significant MOI

The **rapid trauma assessment** is a head-to-toe physical exam of the patient that should take no more than two to three minutes. It is performed on patients who have a significant mechanism of injury (MOI), as described previously. These patients will most likely have a high priority for transport. Remember, no matter what other injuries a patient has or does not have, a patient who is unresponsive or

DCAP-BTLS a memory aid used to recall what to look for in a physical exam. The letters stand for *deformities, contusions, abrasions, punctures/penetrations, burns, tenderness, lacerations,* and *swelling.*

rapid trauma assessment a quick, safe head-to-toe exam of the trauma patient.

TABLE 7-5 ASSESSMENT SIGN—SKIN SIGNS

SKIN SIGNS	SIGNIFICANCE/POSSIBLE CAUSES
Cool, clammy	Shock, heart attack, anxiety
Cold, moist	Body is losing heat
Cold, dry	Exposure to cold
Hot, dry	High fever, heat emergency, spinal injury
Hot, moist	High fever, heat emergency
Goose bumps accompanied by shivering, chattering teeth, blue lips, and pale skin	Chills, communicable disease, exposure to cold, pain, or fear

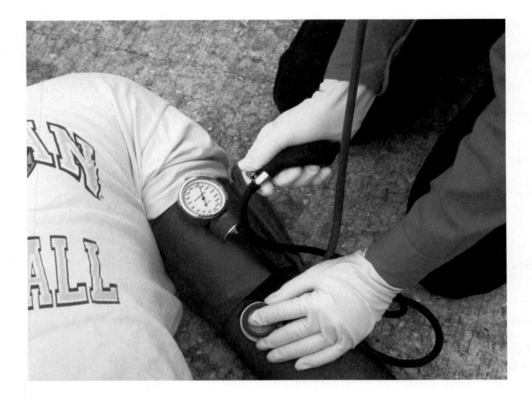

has an altered mental status is a high priority for immediate transport. Take great care not to move the patient. Neck and spine injuries may be present. If available, another First Responder can take vital signs while you perform the exam to save time.

It is usually not necessary for the First Responder to remove the patient's clothing during a head-to-toe exam. Of course, you may remove or readjust clothing that interferes with your ability to examine the patient. Cut away, lift, slide, or unbutton clothing covering a suspected injury site, especially the chest, back, and abdomen, so you can fully inspect the area. If you suspect an injury to the upper leg, you may need to cut away the clothing covering it. Also, check the patient's clothing for evidence of bleeding.

Suspect internal injuries if your responsive patient indicates pain in the area or pain when you touch the area during your exam. If the patient is unresponsive, you may wish to remove or rearrange clothing covering the chest, abdomen, and back to examine those areas of the body completely. If you must remove or rearrange the clothing of a responsive patient, tell him what you are doing and why. Take

TABLE 7-6 ASSESSMENT SIGN—PUPILS

OBSERVATION	POSSIBLE PROBLEM
Dilated, nonreactive pupils	Unresponsiveness, shock, cardiac arrest, bleeding, certain medications, head injury
Constricted, nonreactive pupils	Central nervous system damage, certain medications
Unequal pupils	Stroke, head injury

great care to respect the modesty of the patient. Also protect him from harsh weather conditions and temperatures.

Many EMS systems recommend or require having another woman present when a male First Responder examines a female patient. However, do not delay examining any patient. As a trained First Responder in an emergency situation, your intentions should be respected.

While performing a rapid trauma assessment, avoid contaminating your patient's wounds and aggravating his injuries. Be sure to take the appropriate BSI precautions. Remember, each area of the body is checked for DCAP-BTLS, plus other problems specific to that area. *If you are dealing with an unresponsive trauma patient, you should suspect that the patient has a neck and spine injury. Do what you can to manually stabilize the head and neck before continuing with your assessment.*

FIRST ➤ To perform your assessment:

1. *Check the scalp for cuts and bruises* (Figure 7.9). Take care not to move the patient's head. Run your fingers through the patient's hair, looking for blood. Gently feel for cuts, swelling, or any other injuries. Do not part the hair over a suspected scalp injury. This could restart bleeding. Gently slide your gloved fingers under the back of the patient's neck and upward to the back of the head. Check your gloved fingers for blood.

2. *Check the skull for deformities and depressions and check the face* (Figure 7.10). Note any depressions or bony projections that would indicate an injury to the skull. Check the facial bones for any signs or symptoms of a possible fracture or crushing, swelling, heavy discoloration, or depressions of the bones.

3. *Examine the patient's eyes* (Figure 7.11). Note any cuts, impaled objects, or signs of chemical burns. Have the patient open his eyes, or gently open the eyes of an unresponsive patient. Look for cuts, foreign objects, or burns. Check the pupils for size, equality, and reaction to light. A penlight would be helpful for this. If outside in bright sunlight, cover the patient's eye with your hand. Remove your hand quickly and watch for reaction of the pupil to the light. Pupils that are *dilated* or *constricted* may indicate possible drug usage, shock, or cardiac arrest. *Unequal pupils* may indicate a brain or spine injury. Pupils that react sluggishly may indicate shock.

4. *Look at the inner surface of the eyelids (conjunctiva).* A pale color may indicate major blood loss. During the rest of the exam, be alert for external bleeding or signs of internal bleeding.

5. *Inspect the ears and nose for blood, clear fluid, or bloody fluid* (Figure 7.12). Use a penlight or other light source for this. Blood in the nose may be caused by a simple nasal tissue injury. But it could also mean a skull fracture. Blood in the ears or clear or bloody fluids in the ears or nose are strong indications of a skull fracture.

6. *Inspect the mouth for possible airway obstructions, bleeding, and tissue damage* (Figure 7.13). If your patient is unresponsive, you will have to open his mouth. Consider all unresponsive trauma patients to have neck and spine injuries, so open the mouth gently, without moving the head. Look for broken teeth, bridges, dentures, and crowns. Check for chewing gum, food, vomitus, and foreign objects. In children, take extra care in looking for toys, balls, and other objects in the mouth and the back of the throat. If you find any objects, follow

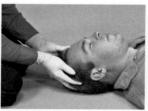
FIGURE 7.9
Examine the scalp. (Step 1)

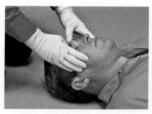
FIGURE 7.10
Check the skull and face. (Step 2)

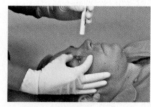
FIGURE 7.11
Examine the eyelids, eyes, and pupils. (Steps 3 and 4)

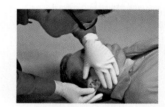
FIGURE 7.12
Check the ears and nose for blood and fluids. (Step 5)

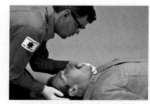
FIGURE 7.13
Examine the mouth for obstructions, bleeding, and tissue damage. (Step 6)

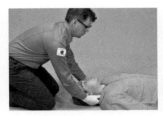

FIGURE 7.14
Check the cervical spine for point tenderness and deformity. (Step 7)

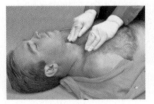

FIGURE 7.15
Check the front of the neck for injuries and openings. Also look for a medical identification device. (Step 8)

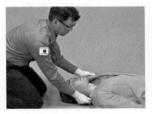

FIGURE 7.16
Inspect the chest for injuries. (Step 9)

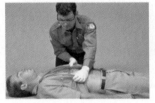

FIGURE 7.17
Check the collarbones for tenderness and deformity. (Step 10)

the directions given in Chapter 6. Inspect the mouth for blood and note any odd breath odors.

7. *Check the cervical spine for point tenderness and deformity* (Figure 7.14). Any *point tenderness* (pain to gentle finger pressure) or deformity should be considered an indication of a possible spinal injury. If you have already immobilized the patient's head and neck, continue with the exam. If not, stop the exam and immobilize the head and neck now, before continuing. Next, gently check the patient's chin for point tenderness and deformity, steadying the patient's chin with one hand. Look for any medical identification device. If one is found, make note of what it says but do not remove it.

8. *Check the front of the neck for injury and deformity* (Figure 7.15). Also notice if the patient has a stoma, a surgical opening in the front or side of his neck. (See Chapter 6 for details about such patients.)

9. *Inspect the chest for cuts, bruises, penetrations, and impaled objects* (Figure 7.16). If necessary, bare the chest and upper abdomen. Leave impaled objects in place. Do not remove them. Also check for medical identification devices.

10. *Examine the chest for possible collarbone or breastbone fracture* (Figures 7.17 and 7.18). Feel the collarbones (clavicles) and the breastbone (sternum) for tenderness and deformity.

11. *Examine for rib fracture* (Figure 7.19). Gently apply pressure to the sides of the chest with your hands. Warn the patient of possible pain. Pain here indicates possible rib fractures.

12. *Observe and feel for equal expansion of both sides of the chest* (Figure 7.20). Note any portion that appears to be floating or moving in opposite directions to the rest of the chest. This could indicate an injury called a *flail chest* in which several ribs are fractured in two places, causing them to float in the chest. When baring the chest of female patients, provide them with as much privacy as possible.

13. *Inspect the abdomen for cuts, bruises, penetrations, distention, and impaled objects.*

14. *Feel the abdomen for tenderness* (Figure 7.21). Prepare the patient for the possibility of pain. If the patient tells you his abdomen already hurts, leave the area alone, but ask him to describe the pain and where exactly it is located. Gently press on the abdomen with the palm side of the fingers, noting any areas that are rigid, swollen, or painful. As you press on the area, ask the patient if it hurts. Note if the pain is *local* (just one spot) or *general* (spread over a wide area). Check each abdominal quadrant and note any problems in that specific quadrant.

15. *Feel the lower back for point tenderness and look for deformity* (Figure 7.22). Take care not to move the patient. Gently slide your gloved hands into the area of the lower back that is formed by the curve of the spine. Check your gloves for blood.

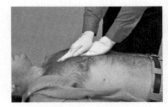

FIGURE 7.18
Check the sternum for tenderness and deformity. (Step 10)

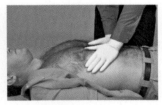

FIGURE 7.19
Gently apply pressure to the sides of the chest to check for rib fractures. (Step 11)

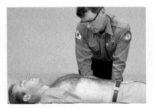

FIGURE 7.20
Check for the equal expansion of the chest. (Step 12)

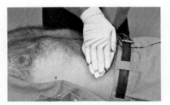

FIGURE 7.21
Inspect the abdomen for injuries. (Steps 13 and 14)

16. *Feel the pelvis for injuries and possible fractures* (Figure 7.23). After checking the lower back, gently slide your hands from the small of the back to the lateral wings of the pelvis. Warn the patient of possible pain and *gently* compress the pelvis. Press in and down at the same time, noting any pain or deformity.

17. *Note any obvious injury to the genital (groin) region.* Look for bleeding and impaled objects. Do not expose the area unless you feel there is an injury. In male patients, check for *priapism*, the persistent erection of the penis caused by spinal injury. If there is any reason to suspect spinal injury and clothing prevents you from noting the presence of an erect penis, gently brush the genital region with the back of your hand. Priapism (PRI-ah-pizm) is an important indication of spinal injury and should be noted as a serious consideration during the head-to-toe exam.

18. *Examine the legs and feet* (Figure 7.24). Examine each leg and foot individually. Compare one limb to the other in terms of length, shape, and any apparent swelling or deformity. Do not move or lift the legs. Do not change the position of the legs or feet. Note any discoloration, bleeding, bone protrusions, and obvious fractures. If you think there is a fracture, warn the patient about possible pain and apply light fingertip pressure to the site. Note any point tenderness. *Do not touch possible fracture (painful, swollen, or deformed) sites if the skin is broken.*

19. *Check for distal pulse* (Figure 7.25). Confirm the circulation of blood through the leg and foot by feeling for a distal pulse. The most useful is the *posterior tibial* (TIB-e-al) *pulse,* felt behind the medial ankle. If the patient is wearing boots, do not remove them if the patient has indications of crush injury to the leg or foot, objects impaled in the leg or foot, severe leg or foot fractures, or any indications or possibilities of spinal injury, unless you must to stop obvious bleeding.

    Another distal pulse is the *dorsalis pedis* (dor-SAL-is PEED-is) *pulse,* which is located lateral to the large tendon of the big toe. This pulse can be important in assessment because some patients do not have a posterior tibial pulse. Some EMS systems do not have First Responders use the dorsalis pedis pulse in the exam because they would have to unlace or remove the patient's shoe to feel this pulse.

    What you can do about a problem of circulation is minimal. Do not cause additional injury to the patient for the sake of taking a distal pulse. When possible, check both legs for a distal pulse. You may also check capillary refill in *pediatric patients* (infants and children) at this time.

20. *Check the lower extremities for motor function and sensation* (Figures 7.26 and 7.27). Do not do this on patients with possible fractures or dislocations of the lower limbs. Do not aggravate possible injuries by removing shoes. If you cannot rule out paralysis, assume the patient has spinal injury.

    Touch each toe and have the patient tell you if he can feel it. You may grasp the toes through the patient's shoe if you believe there are no injuries to the toes. Have the patient gently press the sole of each foot against the palm of your hand and, with your hand on the top of his foot, have him pull up, or flex

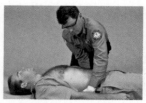

FIGURE 7.22
Check the lower back for point tenderness and deformity. (Step 15)

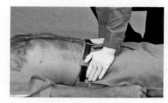

FIGURE 7.23
Gently apply pressure to check for pelvic injuries. Then inspect the genital region. (Steps 16 and 17)

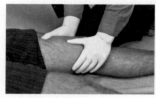

FIGURE 7.24
Examine the legs and feet. DO NOT lift or move them. (Step 18)

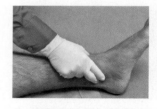
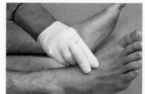

FIGURE 7.25
When possible without risk to the patient, check for distal pulse. (Step 19)

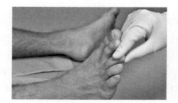

FIGURE 7.26
Check for motor function and sensation. (Step 20)

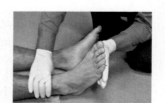

FIGURE 7.27
Can the patient push his foot against the palm of your hand? (Step 20)

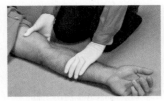

FIGURE 7.28
Check the arms and hands for injuries. (Step 21)

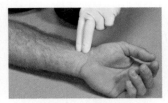

FIGURE 7.29
Take a radial pulse. Remember, you did this for one arm when finding vital signs. (Step 21)

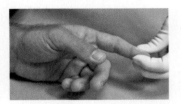

FIGURE 7.30
Can the patient tell you which finger was touched? (Step 21)

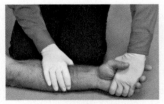

FIGURE 7.31
Can the patient grip your hand? (Step 21)

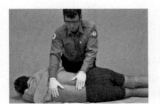

FIGURE 7.32
If there are no injuries to the head, neck, spine, or extremities, inspect the back surface. (Step 22)

his foot, lifting your hand. Then pinch the top of the foot. Do these tests on both feet. If the patient does not respond to any one of these tests, assume spinal injury.

21. *Examine the upper extremities from the shoulders to the fingertips* (Figures 7.28 through 7.31). Examine each limb separately. The procedures are similar to those of the lower extremities.

–Note any cuts, bruises, impaled objects, bleeding, deformities, swelling, discoloration, protruding bones, or obvious fractures. Check for point tenderness at any suspected site of fracture. Do not touch open fracture sites.

–Confirm a radial (wrist) pulse in both arms. Do not measure pulse rate. Simply confirm circulation. You may also check capillary refill in pediatric patients.

–Check for motor function and sensation. If alert, have the patient identify the finger you touch and grip your hand. When checking grip, test both hands at once to determine equality of strength. Have the patient grip your index finger and middle finger together; having the patient squeeze your whole hand may be painful for you. If the patient is unresponsive, pinch the back of his hand.

–Look for a medical identification device.

WARNING *You must suspect that your patient has a spinal injury if he fails to respond properly on any test of the leg or arm. Also, an alert patient who cannot move his hands or arms may suddenly stop breathing due to a spinal injury. The patient may also show signs and symptoms of shock. Continually monitor the patient.*

22. *Inspect the back surfaces of the patient for bleeding and obvious injury* (Figure 7.32). Do not lift or roll the patient if there is any indication of skull, neck, spine, or serious extremity injury. Consider any unresponsive trauma patient as having a neck injury. ■

Focused Trauma Assessment—Trauma Patient with No Significant MOI

When your trauma patient has no significant mechanism of injury, the steps of the **focused trauma assessment** are appropriately simplified. Instead of examining the patient from head to toe, you focus your assessment on just the areas that the patient tells you are painful or that you suspect may be injured because of the mechanism of injury. The assessment includes a physical exam, vital signs, and a SAMPLE history.

Your decision on which areas of the patient's body to assess will depend partly on what you see and partly on the patient's chief complaint (why EMS was called in the patient's own words). Be sure to consider potential injuries based on the mechanism of injury. For example, if the patient's chief complaint is pain in his leg after falling down several stairs, you may also consider possible back or neck injuries, and care for the patient accordingly. Use the memory aid DCAP-BTLS to help you properly perform your assessment.

Rapid Physical Exam—Unresponsive Medical Patient

The **rapid physical exam** of an unresponsive medical patient is almost the same as the rapid trauma assessment of a trauma patient with a significant mechanism of injury (MOI). You will rapidly assess the patient's head, neck, chest, abdomen, pelvis, extremities, and posterior. As you assess each area of the body, look for signs of illness. Be sure to assess for:

● *Neck*—neck vein distention and a medical identification device.

● *Chest*—presence and equality of breath sounds.

- *Abdomen*—distention, firmness, or rigidity.
- *Pelvis*—incontinence of urine or feces.
- *Extremities*—circulation, sensation, motor function, and medical identification devices.

Focused Physical Exam—Responsive Medical Patient

The **focused physical exam** of a responsive medical patient is usually brief. The most important assessment information will be obtained through the SAMPLE history and the taking of vital signs. Focus the exam on the body part that the patient has a complaint about. For example, if the patient complains of abdominal pain, focus your exam on that area of the body. As with the trauma patient, use DCAP-BTLS as a memory aid for what to look for, as well as problems specific to each body part.

Completing the Exam

Upon completing the physical exam of the patient, you must consider all the signs and symptoms found that could indicate an illness or injury. Certain combinations of signs and symptoms can point to one specific problem. A finding as simple as pain in a certain region of the body may be significant. The lack of certain findings may also lead you to a conclusion. For example, if a patient has an obvious injury but feels no pain at the site, you must consider problems such as spinal injury, brain damage, shock, or drug abuse.

During your assessment of the patient, and throughout the time you are caring for him, remember the first rule of emergency care: *Do no further harm.* Be sure to do only what you have been trained to do. Avoid adding injury and aggravating existing injuries and problems. (See a summary of Rules for Patient Examination in Table 7-7.) Later in your training you will learn what you can do to help the patient based on the findings in your physical exam.

focused trauma assessment an examination of the area the patient tells you is injured.

rapid physical exam a quick, safe head-to-toe exam of the medical patient.

focused physical exam an examination of the medical patient's problem areas.

TABLE 7-7 RULES FOR PATIENT EXAMINATION

1.	Do no further harm.
2.	If anything about the patient's awareness or behavior does not seem "right," consider that something is seriously wrong.
3.	Patients who appear stable may worsen rapidly. You must be alert to all changes in a patient's condition.
4.	Watch the patient's skin for color changes.
5.	Look over the entire patient and note anything that appears to be wrong.
6.	Unless you are certain that the patient is free of spinal injury, assume every trauma patient has a spinal injury.
7.	Tell the patient that you are going to examine him, what you will be doing, and why you are doing it. Stress the importance of the exam.
8.	Take vital signs.
9.	Conduct a head-to-toe exam. If anything looks, sounds, feels, smells, or "seems" wrong to you or the patient, assume that there is something seriously wrong with the patient.
10.	Failure of the patient to respond properly on any test for sensation or motor function in the leg or arm must be considered a sign of spinal injury.

DETAILED PHYSICAL EXAM

detailed physical exam a complete head-to-toe exam.

Usually, a full **detailed physical exam** is performed on the patient while en route to the hospital or medical facility. If the response time of the EMTs is lengthy, the First Responder may perform this exam if time permits. Sometimes, the First Responder is a part of the crew or may accompany the ambulance crew to assist in continuing care of the patient. During that time, a detailed physical exam is done by repeating the rapid trauma assessment in *much more detail and by taking more time*. Detailed physical exams are performed on trauma patients with a significant mechanism of injury. First Responders also may perform a detailed physical exam on responsive medical patients, but may be too involved in necessary patient care to do one on unresponsive medical patients.

ONGOING ASSESSMENT

ongoing assessment last step in patient assessment, used to detect changes in a patient's condition; includes repeating initial assessment, reassessing and recording vital signs, and checking interventions.

When performing the **ongoing assessment** either at the scene or en route to the hospital, repeat the initial assessment, reassess vital signs, and check any interventions to ensure they are still effective. Reassess the patient, watching closely for any changes in his condition. Repeating assessments and noting any changes in patient condition are ways of *trending* a patient's condition. Remember that patients will get better, get worse, or stay the same. Seriously ill or injured patients should be reassessed every 5 minutes. A good rule to follow is that by the time you finish the ongoing assessment from start to finish, it is time to start over with the beginning of the next ongoing assessment. Patients who are not seriously ill or injured should be reassessed every 15 minutes.

HAND-OFF TO EMTS

When additional EMS providers arrive at the scene, it is important to communicate with them well. Give the responding EMTs a verbal report including:

- Patient's mental status.
- Age and sex.
- Chief complaint.
- Airway, breathing, and circulatory status.
- Physical findings.
- SAMPLE history.
- Interventions applied and the patient's response to them.

Some EMS systems also require the First Responder to provide a written report to the EMT crew. It usually includes the same information as the verbal report. The First Responder's written report and the information in it will become part of the EMT crew's patient care report.

Accuracy is vital in any verbal or written report because care given by the responding EMTs and the hospital emergency department staff may be based, in part, on your evaluation of the patient.

Chapter Review

Patient assessment is one of the most important skills you will learn as a First Responder. Even though it may seem time-consuming, it is necessary to properly and completely examine the patient if you are to determine what care the patient requires. You must detect life-threatening problems and correct them as quickly as possible. Then you must detect problems that may become life-threatening if they go unnoticed. Always keep the following in mind:

- *Arrival*—Perform a scene size-up. Make sure the scene is safe to enter. Gain information quickly from the scene, the patient, and bystanders. If possible, determine the patient's nature of illness or mechanism of injury.

- *Initial Assessment*—Determine if the patient is responsive. If you suspect a spine injury, maintain manual stabilization of the head and neck. Make certain that the patient has an open airway, adequate breathing, and a pulse. Control all serious bleeding.

- *Focused History and Physical Exam*—Look over the scene, and look over the patient. Look for medical identification devices. Begin gathering information by asking questions and listening. The more organized your interview and physical exam are, the better your chances of gaining the needed information.

As part of your examination of the patient, take vital signs. Remember that baseline vital signs—plus repeated **vital signs** over time—are valuable to the personnel who take over patient care. Determine the pulse and respiratory rate and character. Determine skin color, relative skin temperature, and moisture. In some areas, First Responders also assess pupils and measure blood pressure.

The physical exam of a patient varies somewhat depending on whether the patient is a medical or trauma patient.

A head-to-toe exam consists of the following:

- *Head*—Check the scalp for cuts, bruises, swellings, and the skull and facial bones for deformities, depressions, and other signs of injury. Inspect the eyelids and the eyes for injury and check pupil size, equality, and reactions to light. Note the color of the inner surface of the eyelids. Look for blood, clear fluids, or bloody fluids in the nose and ears. Examine the mouth for airway obstructions, blood, and any odd odors.

- *Neck*—Examine the cervical spine for point tenderness and deformity. Recheck to see if the patient has a stoma. Note obvious injuries and look for medical identification devices.

- *Chest*—Examine the chest for cuts, bruises, penetrations, and impaled objects. Check for possible bone fractures. Look for equal expansion and note chest movements.

- *Abdomen*—Examine the abdomen for cuts, bruises, penetrations, and impaled objects. Check for local and general pain as you examine the abdomen for tenderness.

- *Lower back*—Feel for point tenderness, deformity, and other signs of injury. Check the rest of the back last and only if it is safe to roll the patient (no suspected back injuries).

- *Pelvis*—Press in and down to check for possible fractures and note any signs of injuries.

- *Genital region*—Note any obvious injuries. Look for priapism when examining male patients.

- *Extremities*—Examine for deformities, swelling, bleeding, discoloration, bone protrusions, and obvious fractures. Check for point tenderness on all suspected closed fracture sites. Check for distal pulse. In pediatric patients, check for capillary refill. Determine motor function and sensation as appropriate. Remember to look for medical identification devices.

While EMTs usually complete the **detailed physical exam** en route to the hospital, in some systems First Responders may assist by repeating the initial assessment and vital signs. If you also assist with the **ongoing assessment,** note any changes in patient condition or the need for additional interventions.

It is extremely important that you constantly review the systematic approach to patient assessment.

✔ Take time now to review the rules for patient exam in Table 7-7. You might consider copying each of these rules on a 3 × 5 card and keeping them as quick reminders.

Consider the importance of vital signs and what they can tell you about a patient's condition. Keep in mind:

✔ In an adult, a pulse rate of less than 60 beats per minute or above 100 beats per minute is considered serious.

✔ In an adult, a respiratory rate above 28 breaths per minute or below 8 breaths per minute is considered serious.

✔ Skin signs can signal serious problems such as shock, heart attack, decreased blood pressure, and heat and cold emergencies.

✔ Also remember the memory aids DCAP-BTLS and SAMPLE. Work with a partner and practice using them in various scenarios.

INVESTIGATE...

Additional vital signs that some First Responders may be required to take include determining blood pressure and examining the patient's pupils.

✔ Find out if your service requires you to know how to take a patient's blood pressure. If so, review Appendix 1. Does your service require examination of the patient's pupils? If so, review Table 7-6.

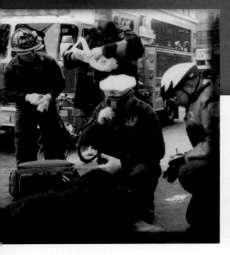
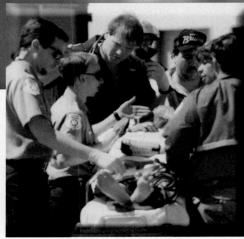
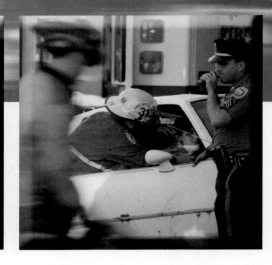

CPR and Automated External Defibrillators (AEDs)

CHAPTER 8

Research and statistics show that there are nearly one million deaths each year from cardiovascular disease. About a quarter of those people die suddenly from cardiac arrest. Over the years, researchers studied and refined CPR so that emergency care providers can learn it easily and provide it effectively when a patient needs it. First Responders are often the closest and quickest sources of assistance for those experiencing cardiac arrest. So make a point of practicing often, keeping your skills up to date with the best research findings, and getting recertified as often as recommended in your area.

This chapter outlines one- and two-rescuer CPR as well as automated external defibrillation, skills that can help save lives.

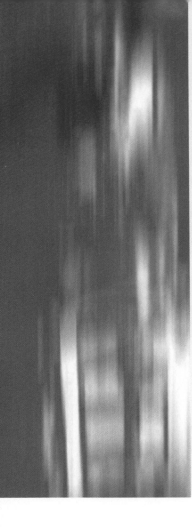

NATIONAL STANDARD OBJECTIVES

This chapter focuses on the objectives of Module 4, Lesson 4-1, of the U.S. DOT's First Responder National Standard Curriculum and serves as an instructional aid to help you meet any specific objectives added to the course by your local EMS system.

By the end of this chapter, you will be able to (from cognitive or knowledge information):

4–1.1 List the reasons for the heart to stop beating. (p. 185)

4–1.2 Define the components of cardiopulmonary resuscitation. (pp. 186–193)

4–1.3 Describe each link in the chain of survival and how it relates to the EMS system. (p. 184)

4–1.4 List the steps of one-rescuer adult CPR. (pp. 193–197)

4–1.5 Describe the technique of external chest compressions on an adult patient. (pp. 190–191)

4–1.6 Describe the technique of external chest compressions on an infant. (p. 214)

4–1.7 Describe the technique of external chest compressions on a child. (pp. 213–214)

4–1.8 Explain when a First Responder is able to stop CPR. (pp. 221–222)

4–1.9 List the steps of two-rescuer adult CPR. (pp. 197–200)

4–1.10 List the steps of infant CPR. (pp. 215–218)

4–1.11 List the steps of child CPR. (pp. 213–216)

Feel comfortable enough to (by changing attitudes, values, and beliefs):

4–1.12 Respond to the feelings that the family of a patient may be having during a cardiac event. (pp. 211–218, 221)

LEARNING TASKS

This chapter explains the functions of the heart and lungs as they work together to circulate life-giving, oxygen-filled blood to the brain and other vital organs. It also will help you apply that knowledge during your study of CPR. As you work through this chapter, you will be able to:

✔ Recognize the signs of cardiac arrest.
✔ Explain how CPR works to keep the brain and other vital organs supplied with oxygen rich blood.

It is important that you learn the very specific steps of performing CPR so you may perform them in an emergency without hesitation. One way you can develop proficiency is to work with your classmates and coach one another as you use manikins to:

✔ Locate the proper compression site on an adult, child, infant, and newborn.
✔ Describe adult and pediatric CPR.
✔ Practice performing CPR on adult and pediatric manikins.

It can be difficult and tiring to maintain one-rescuer CPR for any length of time. Two-rescuer CPR has some distinct advantages, but it takes a little more training and practice. After this chapter, you will be able to:

✔ State the advantages of two-rescuer CPR over one-rescuer CPR.

4–1.13 Demonstrate a caring attitude towards patients with cardiac events who request emergency medical services. (pp. 221–222)

4–1.14 Place the interests of the patient with a cardiac event as the foremost consideration when making any and all patient-care decisions. (pp. 184, 210–211, 218–220, 221)

4–1.15 Communicate with empathy with family members and friends of the patient with a cardiac event. (p. 221)

Show how to
(through psychomotor skills):

4–1.16 Demonstrate the proper technique of chest compressions on an adult manikin. (pp. 190–191)

4–1.17 Demonstrate the proper technique of chest compressions on a child manikin. (pp. 213–214)

4–1.18 Demonstrate the proper technique of chest compressions on an infant manikin. (p. 214)

4–1.19 Demonstrate the steps of adult one-rescuer CPR on a manikin. (pp. 193–197)

4–1.20 Demonstrate the steps of adult two-rescuer CPR. (pp. 197–200)

4–1.21 Demonstrate child CPR on a manikin. (pp. 213–216)

4–1.22 Demonstrate infant CPR on a manikin. (pp. 215–218)

When you become tired during two-rescuer CPR, you may switch or change positions with your partner. This switch takes practice so that CPR remains effective. With practice, you should be able to:

✔ List, step by step, the sequence of procedures for changing positions during two-rescuer CPR.

✔ State how long compressions may be interrupted when checking for breathing and a carotid pulse.

When you apply new knowledge, you must be able to determine if you are applying it correctly. Watch one another as you practice and be able to:

✔ List the proper compression/ventilation ratios used during adult and pediatric CPR.

✔ State how you can determine that CPR is being performed correctly.

✔ Discuss some of the complications that can occur while performing CPR.

A heart attack is only one of the many causes of cardiac arrest. You must be able to:

✔ List other causes of cardiac arrest.

✔ Discuss some of the unique considerations when performing CPR on victims of trauma and drowning.

When you approach any emergency scene, be sure to perform all the patient assessment steps. Remember and be able to:

✔ Demonstrate the steps of the initial assessment to determine if a patient is in cardiac arrest.

Your jurisdiction may allow First Responders to use an automated external defibrillator (AED) and have them ready for use on your unit or where you work. You must complete appropriate training before using an AED, and in your training you will:

✔ List the criteria for the use of an AED.
✔ Demonstrate the proper use of an AED for a patient in cardiac arrest.

CARDIOPULMONARY RESUSCITATION (CPR)

CHAIN OF SURVIVAL

Chapter 1 described the chain of human resources and services in the EMS system. If each link in the chain works quickly and efficiently, the EMS system can provide effective prehospital emergency care. The "chain of survival" is another linked system of patient-care events. For a patient to have the best chance of survival following a **cardiac arrest**, each link in this chain must be strong. The links in the chain of survival include early access to EMS, early CPR, early defibrillation, and early advanced life support (ALS):

cardiac arrest when the heart stops beating. Also, the ineffective circulation caused by erratic muscle activity in the lower chambers of the heart (ventricular fibrillation).

- *Early access.* Early access refers to recognizing a possible cardiac emergency and having a quick way to call for the help the patient needs. It usually begins with a family member or bystander calling 9-1-1 (or the emergency phone number for the area). The dispatcher can then activate an appropriate EMS response.

- *Early CPR.* The sooner that CPR can be initiated, the sooner circulation can be restored to the patient's brain and vital organs. Pre-arrival instructions provided by an Emergency Medical Dispatcher to the 9-1-1 caller can help sustain life until more advanced assistance arrives on scene.

- *Early defibrillation.* Defibrillation is the application of an electric shock to a patient's heart in an attempt to convert a lethal rhythm to a normal one. The time from cardiac arrest to defibrillation is an essential factor in the survival rate of out-of-hospital cardiac-arrest patients. The less time, the better.

- *Early advanced life support (ALS).* ALS is the care provided by more highly trained personnel such as EMT-Intermediates and EMT-Paramedics. ALS providers have many hours of training in the recognition and care of emergencies. In addition to defibrillators, they provide other early interventions, such as oxygen to support ventilation, intravenous access to fluids, and medications that control heart rate and rhythm, relieve pain, and help to stabilize the patient.

Each link in the chain is essential to improving patient survival. However, research has shown that of all the links, early defibrillation has the most effect on positive patient outcomes. In recent years, defibrillator technology has improved to the point that an automated external defibrillator (AED) can be operated with minimal training. Today, AEDs may even be found in many public areas such as airports, shopping malls, stadiums, and other public gathering places.

If First Responders in your jurisdiction are permitted to use AEDs, your instructor or medical director will provide the appropriate training. Do not attempt to use one without training.

CIRCULATION AND CPR

When everything is working properly, the human circulatory system keeps well-oxygenated blood moving to all parts of the body. At the center of the circulatory system is the heart. When the heart beats, it acts as a pump. Blood from the body flows into the heart and is sent to the lungs. In the lungs, the blood gives up carbon dioxide gathered while circulating through the body and exchanges it for oxygen. This oxygen-rich blood is then sent back to the heart, where it is pumped back out to the body.

As blood flows through the body, it picks up nutrients from the small intestines as well as secretions from special glands that are carried to the organs and tissues. Blood gives up wastes to the kidneys and picks up carbon dioxide from the tissues in exchange for oxygen it picked up in the lungs. This constant exchange of nutrients for wastes and oxygen for carbon dioxide is important for life and body function. One vital organ that needs a constant flow of oxygen is the brain.

There is a strong relationship between the brain and the activities of circulation and breathing (Figure 8.1). That relationship includes the following:

- When breathing stops, blood circulating to the brain will contain little or no oxygen.

- Without enough oxygen, the brain cannot direct the work of all other body functions. The heartbeat becomes irregular, then slows, and finally stops beating altogether.

- When the heart stops beating, the oxygen supply in the brain is then used up in about four to six minutes.

FIRST➤ When the heart stops beating, a person is said to be in **cardiac arrest**. The signs of cardiac arrest are (in the order in which you would check them during your initial assessment):

- Patient is unresponsive.
- Patient is not breathing.
- Patient has no pulse or other signs of circulation, such as breathing, coughing, or movement. ■

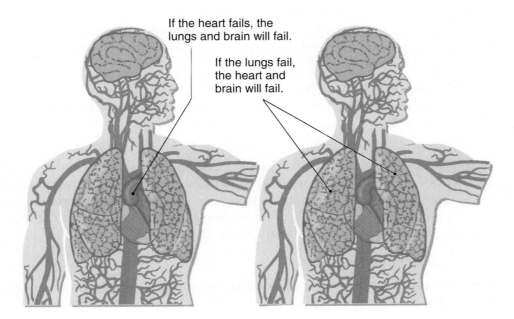

If the heart fails, the lungs and brain will fail.

If the lungs fail, the heart and brain will fail.

FIGURE 8.1
The activities of the heart, lungs, and brain are interdependent.

CPR—What It Is

Cardiopulmonary resuscitation, or CPR, is an emergency procedure that involves the application of both external chest compressions and ventilations when heart and lung actions stop. (*Cardio-* refers to the heart, and *pulmonary* refers to the lungs. *Resuscitation* means to revive.) You studied pulmonary resuscitation in Chapter 6. When performing CPR, you will perform that skill. In addition, you will compress the chest to circulate blood to the brain, lungs, and the rest of the patient's body.

First➤ During CPR you must:

- Maintain an open airway.
- Ventilate or breathe for the patient.
- Perform chest compressions to circulate the patient's blood. ■

CPR—How It Works

Clinical death occurs the instant a patient's breathing and pulse stop. *Biological death* occurs approximately 4 to 6 minutes following clinical death. During this 4-to-6-minute period, irreversible brain damage begins. Approximately 10 minutes after breathing and pulse have stopped, it is unlikely the patient will ever regain responsiveness.

By performing CPR early, you can circulate oxygenated blood to brain and help to delay the onset of biological death and irreversible brain damage. However, the time frame for beginning CPR is not always within 10 minutes after the onset of cardiac arrest. In a cold-water near-drowning, for example, people have been successfully resuscitated after being submerged 20 minutes or more. Usually, you will not know exactly when a patient's breathing and pulse actually stopped, even if a bystander reported the person to be unresponsive for what seemed to them a long time. Such estimates are generally unreliable. So, in general, you will almost always start CPR in cases of cardiac arrest.

CPR is a series of specific steps that must be performed in a certain manner. (Note, however, that for adults, children, and infants the steps vary slightly to accommodate size and anatomical differences.) Generally, CPR begins with the patient lying on his back on a firm surface. You will compress the patient's chest straight down along its midline at a point over the lower half of the breastbone (sternum). This increases pressure in the chest (thoracic) cavity, which forces blood out of the heart and into the arteries to circulate to all parts of the body. When compression is relaxed and pressure is released, blood flows into the veins and back to the heart. One-way valves in the patient's heart and veins keep the blood moving in the proper direction.

First➤ During CPR, your breaths provide oxygen to the patient's blood, which is then circulated to the brain and other vital organs with each compression. ■

There may be times when no appropriate barrier device is available and the rescuer does not want to take the risk of being exposed to the patient's bodily fluids. According to the American Heart Association, providing compressions only is significantly better than providing no assistance at all, and it minimizes the risk of the rescuer coming in contact with bodily fluids. Studies have shown that there is some air movement in and out of the lungs with each chest compression.

When to Begin CPR

First➤ As a First Responder, always perform an initial assessment on your patient. Your actions leading to CPR should include the following:

1. *Form a general impression of the patient.* As you approach, note what the patient looks like. Form an immediate opinion and react based on that opinion. Does the patient look sick, appear to be having trouble breathing, or seem unresponsive? Also note the sex, general age, and level of distress of the patient.

2. *Assess responsiveness.* Is the patient alert, responsive to verbal or painful stimuli, or unresponsive? Start with a gentle shake or squeeze on the shoulder and shout, "Are you okay?" If there is no response, rub the sternum or pinch the shoulder. If the adult patient is unresponsive, this is a serious emergency and you must make sure that an ambulance has been requested.

3. *Assess the airway.* Open the airway using the head-tilt, chin-lift or jaw-thrust maneuver, as appropriate. Quickly inspect the anterior neck looking for a possible stoma.

4. *Assess breathing.* Look, listen, and feel for breathing for no more than 10 seconds. If the patient is not breathing, deliver two slow initial breaths. If you do not see the chest rise, the airway may be obstructed, perform the steps to clear the airway and, when it is clear, provide two ventilations.

5. *Assess circulation.* Take no more than 10 seconds to assess for a pulse and any other signs of circulation, such as breathing, coughing, and movement. If there are no signs of circulation, proceed to step 6.

    To assess for a pulse:

    –*Adult or child* (1–8 years old)—check the carotid pulse in the neck (Figure 8.2).

    –*Infant* (one month to 1 year old)—check the **brachial pulse** in the upper arm (Figure 8.3).

    –*Neonate* (birth to one month old)—check the **apical pulse** by listening over the left side of the rib cage just below the nipple with your ear or a stethoscope (Figure 8.4).

    –*Newborn* (just delivered)—check for pulsations by placing your fingertips at the base of the umbilical cord.

6. *Position the patient.* Place the patient on his back and on a firm surface and begin CPR. Advanced life support (ALS) personnel with defibrillators and EMTs

brachial (BRAY-key-al) **pulse** the pulse located on the inside (medial) aspect of the upper arm; used to evaluate circulation of an infant.

apical (AP-i-kal) **pulse** the pulse felt or heard over the apex or lower part of the heart.

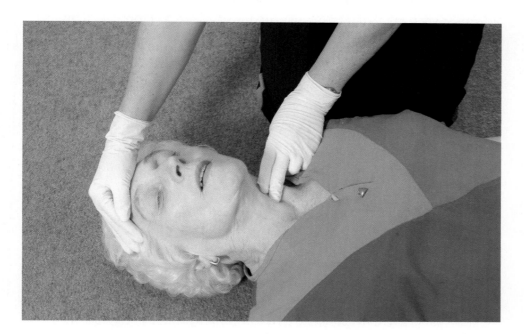

FIGURE 8.2
Use the carotid (neck) pulse for an adult and a child.

FIGURE 8.3
Feel for a brachial (medial upper arm) pulse for an infant.

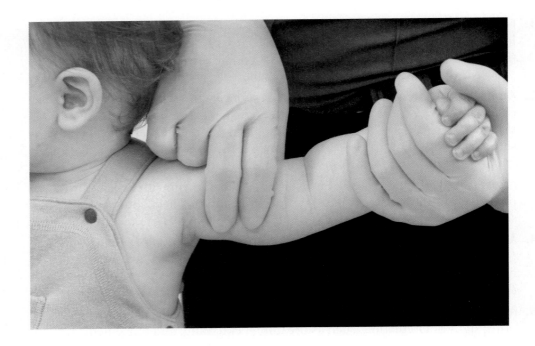

with oxygen and ventilation devices can be dispatched to the scene while you begin CPR. If you are alone and the patient is a child or an infant, begin CPR immediately and continue for one minute. Then, if not already done, call 9-1-1. ■

NOTE: *From here on, discussion centers on adult CPR, unless noted otherwise. Pediatric CPR is discussed in detail later in this chapter.*

Locating the CPR Compression Site

External chest compressions are not effective unless they are delivered to a specific site on the patient's chest (Scan 8-1). If you apply compressions to the wrong site, you may injure the patient or provide ineffective CPR. Steps for locating the compression site on an adult patient are listed below.

FIRST➤ After determining that the adult patient needs CPR, you will:

1. Place the patient face up on a firm surface such as the ground or floor. This is necessary for CPR to be effective. If the patient is in bed, move him to the floor or place a board under his back. Do not delay CPR to find a board.

FIGURE 8.4
Check the apical (over the chest) pulse for a neonate.

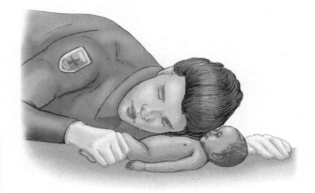

Locating the CPR Compression Site

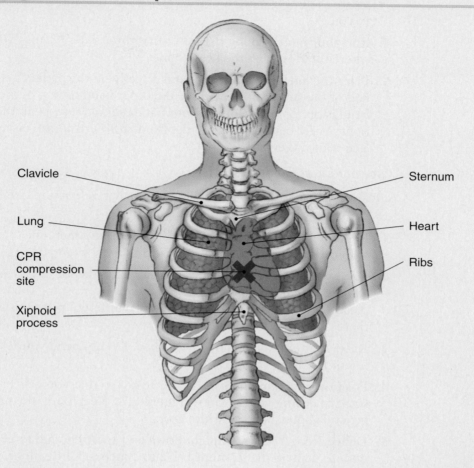

Clavicle

Lung

CPR compression site

Xiphoid process

Sternum

Heart

Ribs

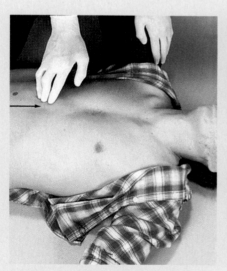

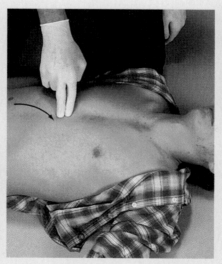

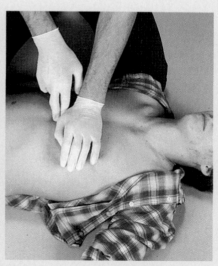

1. Use the index and middle fingers to locate the lower margin of the rib cage.

2. Move your fingers along the margin of the ribs to the notch where the ribs meet the sternum.

3. Place the heel of one hand on the lower half of the sternum and your other hand on top of the first.

2. Kneel at the patient's side between his lower ribs and shoulder.

3. Use your index and middle fingers of the hand closest to the patient's waist to locate the lower margin of the rib cage on the side of the patient's chest closest to you.

4. Run your fingers along the lower margin of the ribs until you find the notch where the ribs meet the breastbone.

5. Place the heel of your other hand directly on the patient's chest over the lower half of the sternum. Now place the other hand on top of the first, so that one hand is on top of the other. Your hands should now be in the center of the patient's chest between the nipples (Figure 8.5). You may either extend or interlace your fingers. ■

External Chest Compressions

FIRST➤ The correct technique for external chest compressions on an adult patient includes the following:

1. Keep the heels of both hands parallel to each other, one on top of the other, with the fingers of both hands pointing away from you.

2. Keep your fingers off the chest, either extended or interlaced (Figure 8.6). For some it may be easier to do compressions by grasping the wrist of the hand placed at the compression site. Practice different positions until you find one that is comfortable for you.

3. Keep your elbows straight and locked. Do not bend your elbows when delivering or releasing compressions.

4. Position your shoulders over your hands so that you deliver compressions straight down over the chest (Figure 8.7). Keep both of your knees on the ground about shoulder width apart.

5. Deliver compressions straight down and apply enough force to the adult patient to depress the sternum 1-1/2 to 2 inches. CPR will be effective for the patient and less tiring for you if you bend from the hips in a smooth up-and-down motion. Perform chest compressions at a rate of approximately 100 per minute.

FIGURE 8.5
During CPR, pressure in the chest cavity increases with compression, which forces blood into circulation.

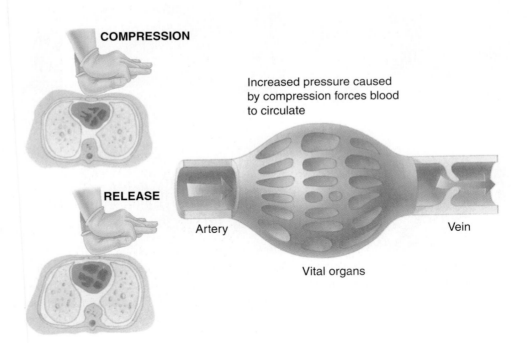

COMPRESSION

Increased pressure caused by compression forces blood to circulate

RELEASE

Artery

Vein

Vital organs

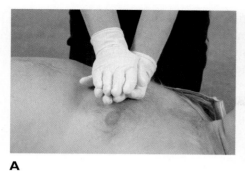
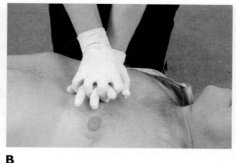
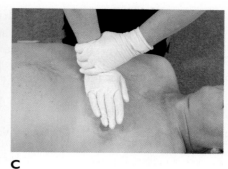

A   B   C

FIGURE 8.6
Positioning the hands at the CPR compression site.

6. Release pressure on the chest completely to allow the patient's heart to refill. Do not bend your elbows in order to release pressure. Do not lift your hands off the patient's chest. Lift up from your hips to return your shoulders to their original position. The release of pressure should take the same amount of time as compression (50% compression and 50% release). ■

Providing Ventilations During CPR

Along with chest compressions (artificial circulation), you must provide artificial ventilation when performing CPR. Breaths are provided between each set of compressions, using a pocket face mask, face shield, or bag-valve mask. Open the patient's airway using the head-tilt, chin-lift or, if you suspect spinal injury, use the jaw-thrust maneuver. Place and seal the mask or barrier device over the patient's face and ventilate until you see the chest rise and fall.

There are four special factors to consider when providing ventilations during one-rescuer adult CPR:

- Deliver each breath slowly over 1.5 to 2.0 seconds.

- Provide two slow back-to-back breaths after every 15 compressions.

- Do not over-ventilate the patient. If you force too much air into the patient's lungs, the excess air will begin to fill the stomach and may eventually cause gastric distention. To prevent this, feel for resistance as you ventilate and watch for the patient's chest to rise.

- Establish a regular pattern of breathing for yourself. Do not try to breathe or hold your breath with each compression.

warning

Do not practice artificial ventilations on a healthy person. Only practice on manikins.

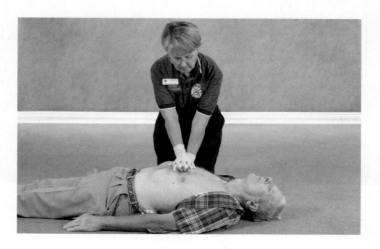

FIGURE 8.7
Position your shoulders directly over the compression site.

To provide effective mouth-to-mask ventilations, you may position yourself either at the top of the patient's head (cephalic) or laterally at the patient's side (Figure 8.8). The cephalic (sef-FAL-ik) position is preferred for patients with a pulse but no respirations and for two-rescuer CPR. The lateral position is preferred for one-rescuer CPR. Practice both on manikins. Determine which one enables you to provide the most effective CPR to a patient. Remember that good CPR delays the onset of biological death and increases the patient's chances for survival.

Rates and Ratios of Compressions and Ventilations

FIRST➤ Effective CPR depends on the correct rate and ratio of compressions and ventilations. For adult CPR, you must:

- Deliver compressions at a rate of approximately 100 per minute.
- Provide ventilations at a ratio of two breaths for every 15 compressions. Deliver each breath slowly over 1.5 to 2.0 seconds.
- Once you have begun CPR, avoid interruptions that are longer than 10 seconds. Interrupt CPR only for pulse and breathing checks and to move the patient for transport or from a dangerous area. After the first minute of CPR and every few minutes thereafter, stop CPR to check for a return of spontaneous breathing and signs of circulation. Take no more than 10 seconds to check for the spontaneous return of pulse and breathing. ■

The rate for chest compressions should be approximately 100 per minute. Note that the rate refers to the speed rather than the number of compressions the rescuer delivers in one minute. Because a single rescuer must interrupt chest compressions to deliver breaths and check pulse periodically, the actual number of compressions will be less than 100 per minute. Practicing CPR becomes more important when the actual number of compressions the rescuer delivers depends on the accuracy and consistency of the compressions and the time it takes for the rescuer to open the airway and deliver breaths.

To be sure that you provide compressions at the proper rate of 100 per minute, count out loud as you deliver compressions: "One—and, two—and, three—and, four—and . . ." until you reach 15. Then, deliver two slow ventilations over 1.5 to 2.0 seconds each, quickly relocate the CPR compression site, and continue the next set of compressions.

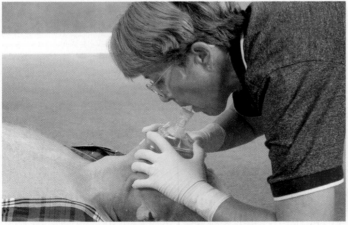
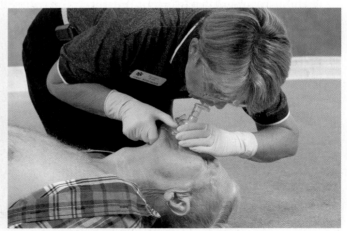

A   **B**

FIGURE 8.8
Deliver ventilations using (A) the cephalic position or (B) the lateral position.

Effective CPR

FIRST➤ You can be certain that you are performing adult CPR correctly if:

- Another trained person feels for the carotid pulse as you compress the patient's sternum. Do not try to deliver compressions with one hand while you check for a pulse at the carotid artery with the other.
- You see the chest rise and fall during ventilations. ■

If you are performing CPR correctly, you may notice the patient's skin color improve, but this does not always occur. Sometimes the patient may try to swallow, gasp, or move his limbs. These actions do not necessarily mean that the patient is recovering; however, they are signs of life and do mean that you should stop CPR and check for the return of breathing and pulse.

FIRST➤ Check for the return of breathing and signs of circulation after performing CPR for one minute (four cycles of two breaths and 15 compressions). If the patient has a pulse but is not breathing, stop compressions and continue with ventilations only. If there is no pulse, continue CPR and check for signs of circulation every few minutes. Most patients will not regain a heartbeat and breathing with CPR alone. Patients will usually require defibrillation and possibly other special medical procedures before they regain heart function. CPR delays the onset of biological death until special medical procedures can be provided. ■

> **remember**
> Oxygen must reach the air-exchange levels of the patient's lungs if CPR is to be effective.

ADULT CPR

The following offers step-by-step outlines for performing one-rescuer adult CPR and two-rescuer CPR. These procedures follow the American Heart Association (AHA) recommendations. Your instructor will tell you if the AHA has made any recent changes. Otherwise, learn the procedures as they are presented. Do not create your own methods or shortcuts. The extensive research done by the AHA has found these procedures to be most efficient in saving the lives of patients in cardiac arrest. Also, remember that the following steps are a part of the initial assessment. (See Table 8-1 for a summary of CPR techniques.)

ONE-RESCUER CPR—ADULT

FIRST➤ To perform one-rescuer CPR on an adult (Scan 8-2):

1. *Check for responsiveness.* Gently shake or squeeze the patient's shoulder and ask, "Are you okay?" If the patient is not responsive, call out for help. If you are alone with an unresponsive adult patient, call 9-1-1 immediately to get ALS with a defibrillator en route (Figures 8.9 and 8.10).

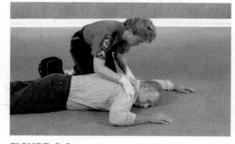

FIGURE 8.9
Determine unresponsiveness.

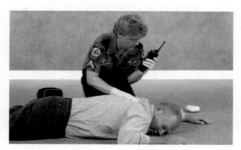

FIGURE 8.10
Activate EMS immediately if the patient is unresponsive.

TABLE 8-1 SUMMARY OF ONE-RESCUER CPR TECHNIQUES

PROCEDURE	ADULT	CHILD	INFANT	NEWBORN
Compressions				
Method	Heels of two hands	Heel of one hand	2 or 3 fingers	2 thumbs with hands encircling chest (preferable) or 2 fingers
Depth	1½" to 2"	1" to 1½"	½" to 1"	⅓ the depth of the chest
Rate	100/minute	100/minute	At least 100/minute	120/minute
Ventilations				
Method	Mouth-to-barrier device			
Ratio of Compressions to Breaths				
	15:2	5:1	5:1	3:1
Counts				
	1 and 2 and 3 and 4 and 5 … 15 and breathe, breathe	1, 2, 3, 4, 5, breathe	1, 2, 3, 4, 5, breathe	1, 2, 3, breathe

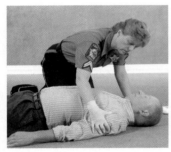

FIGURE 8.11
Properly position the patient and yourself.

2. *Position the patient* face up on a hard surface. Kneel beside the patient's chest (Figure 8.11).

3. *Open the airway* by using the head-tilt, chin-lift maneuver or, if you suspect a spinal injury, by using the jaw-thrust maneuver (Figure 8.12). Look at the anterior neck to see if the patient has a stoma.

4. *Check for breathing.* Place your ear next to the patient's nose and mouth and look, listen, and feel for air exchange. Assess for no more than 10 seconds (Figure 8.13).

5. *Provide two slow breaths,* back-to-back. Watch for chest rise and feel for resistance (Figure 8.14). Follow the steps for mouth-to-mask or mouth-to-face shield ventilation or for using a bag-valve mask (see Appendix 2).

6. *Clear the airway,* if necessary. Use the techniques of abdominal thrusts, finger sweeps, and ventilations.

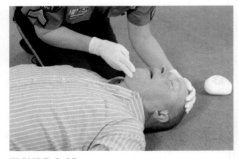

FIGURE 8.12
Open the airway.

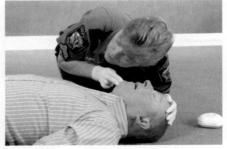

FIGURE 8.13
Check for breathing.

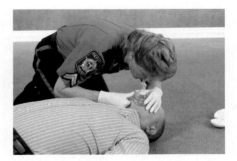

FIGURE 8.14
Use a barrier device to provide two slow breaths.

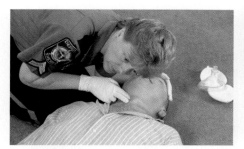

FIGURE 8.15
Check for signs of circulation.

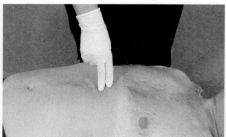

FIGURE 8.16
Locate the CPR compression site.

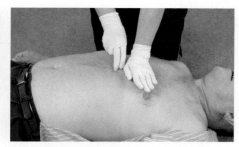

FIGURE 8.17
Position your hands on the lower half of the sternum and between the nipples.

7. *Check for a pulse* and other signs of circulation, such as breathing, coughing, or movement (Figure 8.15). This should take no more than 10 seconds. If the patient has a carotid pulse, but no respirations, provide one breath every five seconds. If there is no pulse . . .

8. *Locate the CPR compression site* (Figure 8.16). Place the heels of your hands on the lower half of the sternum (Figure 8.17). Keep your fingers off the patient's chest and deliver 15 compressions.

9. *Provide chest compressions* (Figure 8.18). Keep your arms straight, elbows locked, and shoulders directly over the compression site. Bend at the hips to use your upper body weight when performing compressions.

    —Deliver compressions directly over the CPR compression site.

    —Compress the patient's breastbone 1-1/2 to 2 inches.

    —Deliver compressions at a rate of 100 per minute, counting "One—and, two—and, three—and . . ." until you reach 15.

    —Release pressure completely to allow the heart to refill. Each release should take the same amount of time as a compression. Do not take your hands off the patient's chest while doing chest compressions.

    —Deliver 15 compressions, then . . .

10. *Provide two slow breaths,* back-to-back. Use a barrier device and provide ventilations at a rate of two breaths after every 15 compressions and watch for chest rise (Figure 8.19).

11. *Continue CPR.* Deliver 15 compressions at the rate of 100 per minute followed by two ventilations for one minute, which is four sets of compressions and ventilations.

12. *Recheck for signs of circulation* after one minute or four cycles of CPR (Figure 8.20). Do not interrupt CPR for any longer than is absolutely necessary. If the

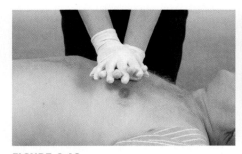

FIGURE 8.18
Keep your fingers off the patient's chest and deliver 15 compressions.

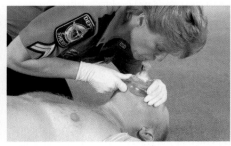

FIGURE 8.19
Use a barrier device to provide two slow breaths.

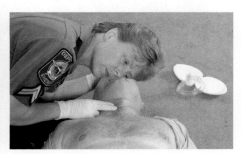

FIGURE 8.20
Reassess for signs of circulation after one minute or four cycles of CPR.

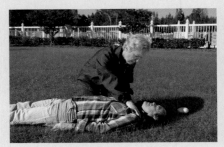

1. Establish unresponsiveness and activate EMS. Position the patient and yourself.

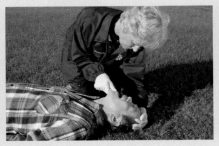

2. Open the airway.

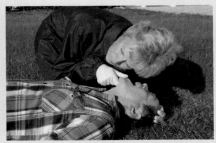

3. Look, listen, and feel for breathing for no more than 10 seconds.

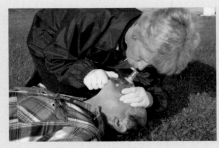

4. Give two slow breaths over 1.5 to 2.0 seconds each.

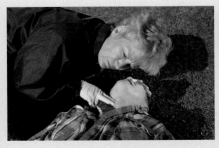

5. Check for signs of circulation for no more than 10 seconds.

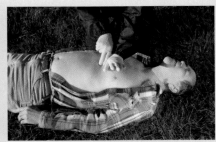

6. Locate the compression site.

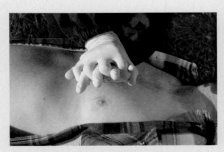

7. Position your hands.

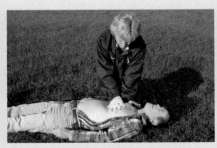

8. Begin compressions. Compression rate is 100 per minute.

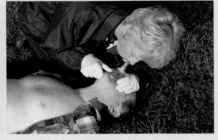

9. Give two ventilations. One cycle = two ventilations every 15 compressions.

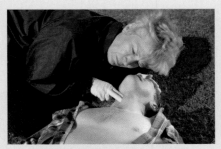

10. Recheck pulse after the first minute and every few minutes thereafter.

patient regains a pulse and/or breathing, stop CPR. If there is a pulse but no breathing, continue ventilations at the rate of one breath every five seconds. If there is no pulse . . .

13. *Continue CPR.* Check for signs of circulation every few minutes. Provide CPR until another trained person can take over, the patient regains a pulse and breathing, or you are too tired to continue. ■

Note that health-care providers, such as First Responders, who have a duty to perform CPR, should also be trained, equipped, and authorized to use an automated external defibrillator (AED).

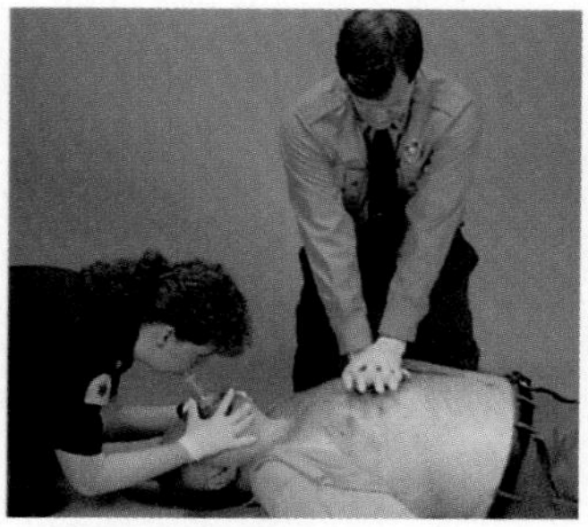

TWO-RESCUER CPR

All EMS personnel should learn and remain proficient in both one-and two-rescuer CPR techniques. CPR that is performed by two rescuers who have trained together and are familiar with the techniques is more efficient and less tiring for both rescuers (Figure 8.21). Two-rescuer CPR minimizes the transition time between ventilations and compressions and, therefore, maximizes the effectiveness of both.

Use of an AED is also more efficient with two rescuers. One rescuer can begin to set up the AED and attach the electrodes to the patient, while the other rescuer begins an initial assessment of the patient. If you arrive on scene and find that an AED is being used, ensure that the individuals are performing the steps properly and taking the necessary safety precautions. Offer to assist them and support their actions. You may also need to relieve or guide someone who is unsure of the procedures.

Changing from One- to Two-Rescuer CPR

When you assess an adult who has collapsed, your first action is to assess for unresponsiveness. Tap or gently shake the patient and shout "Are you okay?" If there is no response, remember: *phone first.* Direct someone to activate the EMS system (or phone the emergency number provided by your job or industry's first-aid department, if that is the policy). If you are alone, leave the patient long enough to call for help. Then return and continue your assessment.

In many situations a bystander may start one-rescuer CPR before First Responders arrive. Upon arrival, assess the patient's breathing and pulse before taking over and performing two-rescuer CPR with your partner.

If you arrive as a lone First Responder and determine that the bystander's CPR techniques are inadequate or incorrect, take over one-rescuer CPR. If the bystander is CPR-trained but has no barrier device and is reluctant to ventilate a stranger, perform the ventilations yourself with your own pocket face mask. Have the bystander take over chest compressions and monitor his effectiveness.

FIRST➤ If a First Responder member of the EMS system is performing CPR when you arrive, begin two-rescuer CPR. To help you make a smooth transition from one-rescuer to two-rescuer CPR, follow these steps:

1. The first rescuer is performing CPR when another rescuer arrives and identifies herself. The first rescuer continues CPR while the second rescuer activates the EMS System, if not already done.

2. While the first rescuer continues the cycle of 15 compressions and two breaths, the second rescuer checks for a pulse in the carotid artery, which is generated with each compression.

FIGURE 8.21
First Responder positions for two-rescuer CPR.

remember

Each rescuer should use his own barrier device with one-way valve and HEPA filter insert in order to perform two-rescuer CPR safely.

3. At the end of a cycle, following the two slow breaths, the first rescuer stops and assesses for signs of circulation for no more than 10 seconds. If there are no signs of circulation, the second rescuer, moves to the chest on the opposite side from the first rescuer and resumes chest compressions. The first rescuer, now the ventilator, resumes ventilations, providing two ventilations after every 15 compressions.

4. The second rescuer, now the compressor, provides compressions at the rate of 100 per minute with a pause after every 15 compressions to allow for two ventilations.

5. If the rescuer performing compressions becomes tired, both rescuers can change positions. ■

If the First Responder who arrives on scene to see CPR being performed is equipped with an AED, he will immediately set it up, turn it on, and attach electrodes in preparation for early defibrillation.

Compressions and Ventilations

During two-rescuer CPR, deliver 15 compressions at a rate of 100 compressions per minute. After every 15 compressions, deliver two ventilations.

The rescuer providing compressions will count aloud so that both rescuers will be able to establish and maintain the correct rate. By hearing the count, the rescuer providing ventilations will be prepared to provide a breath after every 15 compressions (while the first rescuer pauses to allow for adequate ventilation).

NOTE: *ALS providers who insert an endotracheal tube (considered a "protected airway") will perform two-rescuer CPR at a ratio of five compressions to one ventilation and will not pause their compressions to provide ventilations. First Responders and EMT-Basics who cannot "protect" the airway will always perform one- or two-rescuer CPR at the 15 compressions to two ventilations ratio and will pause after 15 compressions to allow the ventilator to provide breaths.*

CPR Procedure

FIRST➤ Scan 8-3 outlines the complete sequence for two-rescuer CPR for an adult. Note that one rescuer is called the *ventilator*, and the other rescuer is called the *compressor*. Both rescuers are shown on the same side of the patient for teaching purposes. In actual two-rescuer CPR, rescuers normally place themselves on opposite sides of the patient because they will not be in each other's way. If the ventilator uses a pocket face mask or a bag-valve mask and supplemental oxygen (see Appendix 2), his position is usually at the top of the patient's head (cephalic position), though it may be at the patient's side (lateral position). For either position, the ventilator must ensure a proper mask-to-face seal to provide the most effective ventilations. Your instructor will demonstrate how to ventilate a patient in both positions, using the barrier devices and oxygen delivery equipment that your jurisdiction requires First Responders to use. ■

The ventilator will check frequently for a carotid pulse, which should be felt with each compression. If a carotid pulse cannot be found, the ventilator will have the compressor recheck hand position, body position (arms straight, shoulders over sternum, bend at hips), and depth of compressions.

After the first minute of CPR, and every few minutes thereafter, both rescuers will stop CPR and the ventilator will assess for signs of circulation for no more

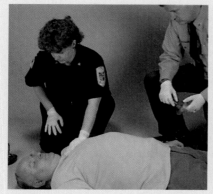

1. Determine unresponsiveness. Activate EMS. Position the patient.

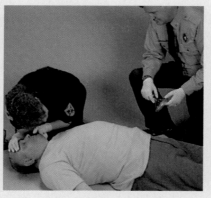

2. Open the airway. Look, listen and feel for breathing for no more than 10 seconds.

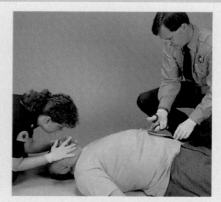

3. Give two slow breaths over 1.5 to 2.0 seconds each.

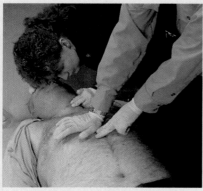

4. Assess for signs of circulation. Locate the CPR compression site.

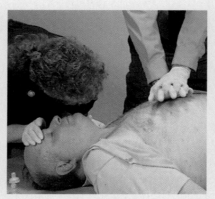

5. Say "No pulse." Begin compressions. Deliver 15 compressions at a rate of 100 per minute.

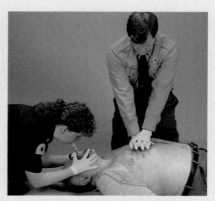

6. Provide two slow breaths after each set of 15 compressions.

7. Continue with two ventilations every 15 compressions.

NOTE: Assess for spontaneous breathing and pulse for no more than 10 seconds at the end of the first minute (about seven cycles of 15 compressions and two breaths), and then every few minutes thereafter.

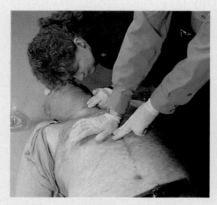

8. Check compression effectiveness. Deliver 15 compressions at rate of 100 per minute.

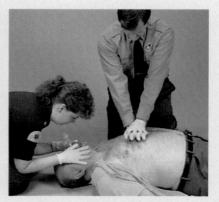

9. Reassess breathing and pulse after one minute. No pulse—say "Continue CPR." Pulse—say "Stop CPR." Monitor the patient's breathing and pulse.

than 10 seconds. The ventilator will determine if there is breathing and a pulse and take the appropriate action:

- *Pulse, no breathing*—say "There is a pulse." Continue rescue breathing only.

- *No pulse, no breathing*—say, "No pulse, continue CPR."

- *Pulse and breathing*—say, "Stop CPR." Monitor the patient.

If CPR is continued, the ventilator will check for the return of spontaneous breathing and pulse every few minutes. This interruption of CPR compressions should last for no more than 10 seconds.

Changing Positions

FIRST▶ Either rescuer may request a change in position if he becomes tired. However, it is usually the compressor who needs the break. Unless the ventilator finds that the compressor cannot generate a pulse during compression, the compressor will decide when to change positions. At the beginning of a cycle, the compressor will give a clear signal to the ventilator to switch places, but will complete a set of 15 compressions before any moves are made. At the end of 15 compressions, the ventilator will provide two ventilations. Then the rescuers will quickly change positions (Scan 8-4). Your instructor will teach you the preferred switching signals to use. ■

Following the position change, the ventilator will assess for signs of circulation for no more than 10 seconds and direct the compressor depending on the findings of the assessment. See Scan 8-5 for a summary of one- and two-rescuer adult CPR.

Potential Problems

After 15 compressions, the ventilator must provide two slow breaths over 1.5 to 2.0 seconds. Resistance from the patient's airway, rescuer fatigue, and many other factors can cause the ventilator to miss providing the breath to the patient at the appropriate time. If you should miss a breath, do not wait another 15 compressions. Provide a ventilation after any compression as soon as possible during the next set of compressions. Resume your normal ventilations after the 15th compression.

In addition, changing positions or adding a second rescuer while one-rescuer CPR is being performed has its challenges. Each person performs the change a little differently than the next. For this reason, practice two-rescuer CPR with several different partners.

AUTOMATED EXTERNAL DEFIBRILLATION

American Heart Association guidelines state that health-care providers should be trained and equipped to provide defibrillation at the earliest possible moment for victims of sudden cardiac arrest. Almost all jurisdictions have approved and adopted the use of automated external defibrillators (AEDs). Your organization or department may have purchased one or more AEDs and may include AED training in emergency care programs. AEDs assist emergency-care providers in assessing the patient's heart rhythm and in restoring the normal heart beat when certain kinds of abnormal heartbeats, called *arrhythmias*, are present.

The fact that most sudden cardiac deaths occur away from hospitals is the reason why there are CPR programs for EMS personnel and for laypeople. Two early problems with recognizing and caring for cardiac-arrest patients are being resolved. The first problem—delay in starting CPR—has been dramatically reduced

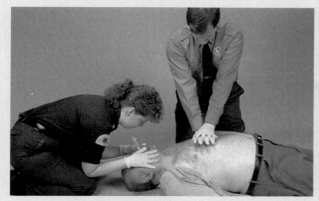

1. When fatigued, the compressor calls for a switch and then gives a clear signal to change.

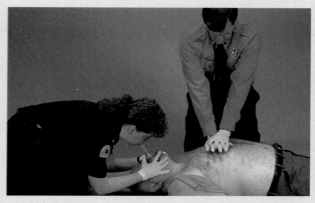

2. Compressor completes 15 compressions. Ventilator provides two ventilations.

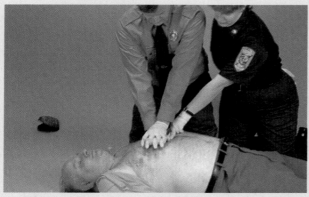

3. Ventilator moves to chest and locates compression site.

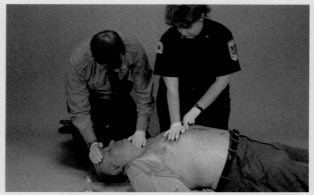

4. New ventilator checks for signs of circulation (10 seconds) and says "No pulse, continue CPR." (Note: Additional breaths are not given.)

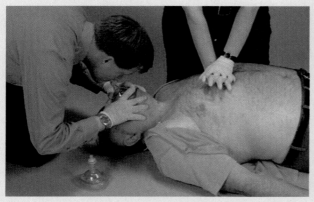

5. New compressor begins compressions and new ventilator breathes after 15 compressions.

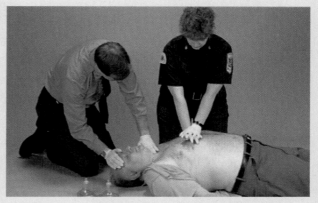

6. New ventilator and new compressor continue until compressor is fatigued and calls for a change.

CPR Summary—Adult Patient

ONE RESCUER	FUNCTIONS	TWO RESCUERS
	• Establish unresponsiveness • If no response, call 911 • Position patient • Open airway • Look, listen, and feel (no more than 10 seconds)	
	• Deliver two breaths (1½–2 sec each). If unsuccessful, reposition head and try again. Clear airway if necessary.	
	• Check carotid pulse . . . (5–10 seconds) If no pulse . . . • Begin chest compressions	
	DELIVER COMPRESSIONS	
	1½–2 inches 100/min | 1½–2 inches 100/min	
	DELIVER VENTILATIONS **10–12 breaths/min**	
	15:2 • Pause to allow ventilations	
	• Do four cycles • Ventilator checks pulse for effective CPR	
	CONTINUE PERIODIC ASSESSMENT	

Changing Positions

• Compressor—signal to change; finsh compression cycle • Ventilator—two ventilations	New ventilator checks pulse. If no pulse, says "No pulse, continue."	Continue CPR sequence

NOTE: Wear latex or vinyl gloves. Rescuers should have their own pocket face masks with one-way valves and HEPA filter inserts.

through the training of more citizens who can administer CPR before EMS personnel arrive. The second problem stems from the fact that many heart attacks are fatal no matter how soon CPR is started. These deaths are often caused by lethal heart rhythms that must be corrected as soon as possible if the patients are to survive.

In response, First Responders, EMTs, and citizens are now being trained in the use of an amazing device called an automated external defibrillator, or simply, an AED. AEDs assess a heart's rhythm, determine if defibrillation is necessary, and can deliver an electrical shock to the patient's heart in an attempt to convert a lethal (deadly) rhythm to a normal one.

The U.S. Senate has passed the Cardiac Arrest Survival Act, which does two things. First, it instructs the secretary of Health and Human Services to make recommendations to promote public access to defibrillation programs in federal buildings and other public buildings across the country. This step helps to ensure the health and safety of everyone by encouraging ready access to the tools needed to improve cardiac arrest survival rates. Second, the act extends Good Samaritan protection to AED users and to those who acquire AEDs in those states that do not currently have AED Good Samaritan legislation. This Good Samaritan legislation will enable and encourage more placement and use of AEDs in public places and encourage laypeople to respond in a cardiac emergency and use an AED.

The Cardiac Arrest Survival Act is a critical step toward increasing cardiac-arrest survival rates, but just as critical is the training of those who will use AEDs. Training will provide the information needed to understand the heart's electrical system functions and dysfunctions and the procedures for assessing and providing initial care to a person with chest pain or cardiac arrest. Training will also provide instruction for operating an AED and emphasize all necessary precautions.

EXTERNAL DEFIBRILLATION

Defibrillators are designed to deliver an electrical shock that will stimulate the heart to begin beating normally. The shock does not start a heart that is stopped, or in arrest, but it will convert certain lethal rhythms and give the heart a chance to spontaneously re-establish an effective rhythm on its own. The entire process is called *defibrillation*.

Manual defibrillators carried by most ALS providers are different from the AEDs mentioned in this chapter. Manual defibrillators require that the rescuer be able to interpret the patient's heart rhythm and deliver an appropriate shock depending on that interpretation. Interpreting heart rhythms requires significant training beyond the level of most First Responders and EMT-Basics.

NOTE: *Some patients with specific heart conditions may have a small automated defibrillator surgically implanted inside their chest or abdomen. These devices are very much like external AEDs only much smaller. You might not know that this was in place unless the patient or a family member tells you it is there. Your care of a patient in cardiac arrest will not change with the presence of an internal defibrillator.*

There are many AEDs on the market (Figure 8.22). Among these are two basic types: fully automated and semi-automated. The fully automated AED assesses the patient's heart rhythm, advises that a shock is necessary, and delivers the shock without any input from the rescuer. Semi-automated defibrillators analyze the patient's rhythm and simply advise the rescuer if a shock is needed. It is then up to the rescuer to push the shock button and deliver the shock.

AEDs are capable of recognizing two very specific abnormal heart rhythms and either delivering a shock or alerting the rescuer that a shock is advised. They

FIGURE 8.22
Examples of AEDs.

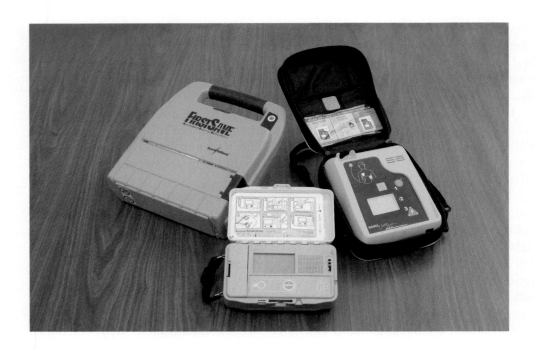

are *fibrillation* (fib-ri-LAY-shun) and *ventricular tachycardia* (ven-TRIK-u-ler tak-e-KAR-de-ah).

Fibrillation is a disorganized electrical activity within the heart that renders the heart incapable of pumping blood. The most common cause of fibrillation is a heart attack. Fibrillation results in a disorganized quivering of the heart muscle much like a spasm or seizure (Figure 8.23). The most common type of fibrillation affects the lower half (ventricles) of the heart and is called *ventricular fibrillation* (ven-TRIK-u-ler fib-ri-LAY-shun), or *VF* for short. When a person's heart goes into VF, the brain and other vital organs no longer receive an adequate supply of oxygenated blood and the person becomes unresponsive. VF does not produce a pulse, so the patient will be found unresponsive with no pulse and no breathing. It is believed that 50% to 60% of all adult cardiac-arrest patients are in ventricular fibrillation (VF) in the first few minutes following cardiac arrest. The sooner that VF can be defibrillated, the better the patient's chances are for survival.

AEDs also can recognize *ventricular tachycardia*, or *V-tach* for short. V-tach is a rapid rhythm that originates in the ventricles. It does not pump blood very efficiently. Less than 10% of the prehospital cardiac-arrest cases have this problem. Defibrillation may help some of these patients.

In situations where there is no electrical activity within the heart, AEDs will not be effective. This rhythm is called *asystole* (ah-SIS-to-le), or sometimes referred to as "flat line."

EMS AND DEFIBRILLATION

Time is one of the most critical elements in the effort to save the life of a victim of cardiac arrest. Minimizing the times between collapse and the initiation of CPR, between CPR and the delivery of the first shock, and between defibrillation and the arrival of more advanced care is the goal of a strong chain of survival. The time between the moment a person collapses until defibrillation can be divided into four segments:

1. *EMS access time*—the time from patient collapse until the EMS system is alerted.

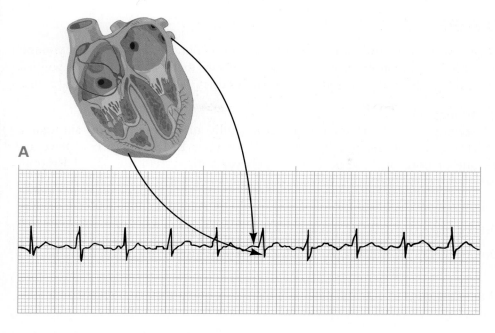

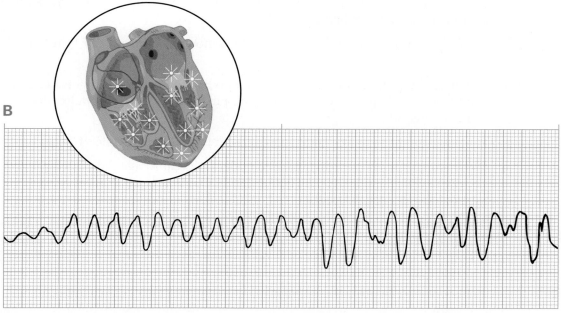

FIGURE 8.23

(A) Normal heart rhythm, or normal sinus rhythm, and (B) ventricular fibrillation.

2. *Dispatch time*—the time from the call to EMS dispatcher until the alert of the personnel who will respond and defibrillate.

3. *Response time*—the time it takes for the person or crew to reach the patient.

4. *Shock time*—the time it takes from reaching the patient until the first shock is delivered.

The goal of every EMS system is to reduce the time of each of these four segments. In particular, having rescuers with defibrillators available 24 hours a day is shortening the time from dispatch to the arrival of the defibrillator. If the patient can receive the first shock within 3 to 5 minutes of collapse, survival is more likely.

USING AEDS

A defibrillator must be ready for use at any given moment. Make certain that you follow your EMS and manufacturer guidelines to ensure that the defibrillators you use are in working order and prepared for use. Always carry fully charged spare batteries.

Basic Warnings

First Responders may be trained to use either fully automated or semi-automated defibrillators. The physician advisory board for your EMS system may have approved one or both of these devices. Whichever your system uses, First Responders are responsible for noting certain warnings when working with AEDs:

- Follow the same precautions that you would for operating any electrical device.

- Do not place the AED on a patient who is not in cardiac arrest.

- Do not place defibrillator patches over a patient's medication patch or implanted pacemaker.

- Do not attempt to defibrillate a patient who is in physical contact with rescuers, bystanders, or other patients.

- Do not attempt to assess or shock a patient who is moving or when the defibrillator or its leads are being moved.

- Do not attempt to defibrillate a patient in a moving ambulance or other moving vehicle.

- Do not attempt to defibrillate a patient who has an obstructed airway. The patient who is in respiratory arrest but not in cardiac arrest (assess pulse) does not need defibrillation.

- Do not attempt to defibrillate a patient who is lying in a puddle of water.

- Do not attempt to defibrillate a child under one year of age. Your medical director may have guidelines for defibrillating children from 12 months to 8 years old with a special pediatric AED. Check your local protocols.

Defibrillating patients on metal surfaces has been an issue and training courses have emphasized that doing so would transfer the shock to other persons. American Heart Association guidelines indicate that metal surfaces pose no shock hazard to either the patient or the rescuer.

Protocols for the use of AEDs for trauma patients vary by state and jurisdiction. Follow your EMS system's protocols and carefully assess the patient and mechanism of injury or the nature of the illness. If you are not certain as to what you are to do, phone or radio the emergency department physician or EMS medical direction.

First Responder Care

The use of a defibrillator must follow specific procedures of care and assessment. You must determine if the patient is indeed a candidate for the placement of an AED. Before you may place an AED on the patient, the patient must:

- Be unresponsive.

- Be over the age of one year.

- Have no carotid pulse.

- Have no respirations.

- Have a clear airway.

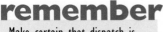

remember

Make certain that dispatch is informed of the emergency.

NOTE

On the basis of the published evidence to date, the Pediatric Advanced Life Support Task Force of the International Liaison Committee on Resuscitation (ILCOR) has made the following recommendation as of July 2003: "AEDs may be used for children one to eight years of age who have no signs of circulation. Ideally, the device should deliver a pediatric dose."

All of these criteria must be met before you can place an AED on a patient in suspected cardiac arrest.

Perform an initial assessment to confirm that the patient is indeed in cardiac arrest and that he has a clear airway. If you are first on the scene and have confirmed the patient meets all of the criteria, place the AED immediately. If you do not have an AED, start CPR.

If you arrive on scene with a defibrillator and someone else is providing CPR, your job will be to prepare and attach the defibrillator. Make certain that both of you are clear of the patient before delivering a shock.

Attaching the Defibrillator

The procedure for attaching the defibrillator to a patient is the same for both semi-automated and fully automated devices. While the first rescuer performs CPR, the rescuer operating the defibrillator should perform the following steps:

remember
Always follow the manufacturer's manual and your EMS system's guidelines for the defibrillator you will be using.

1. Bare the patient's chest. If the patient's chest is wet, quickly wipe it dry. If the ground beneath the patient is wet, move the patient to a dry surface.

2. Next, place electrodes on the patient's bare, dry chest one at a time. It may be necessary to shave the chest, as hair may prevent the electrodes from sticking properly. Place one pad on the patient's upper right chest below the collarbone (clavicle) and next to the breastbone (sternum). Place the second pad on the patient's left side well below the armpit. Most pads and devices have illustrations on them showing the correct placement of the pads (Figure 8.24).

3. Finally, ensure that the electrodes are firmly plugged into the device. Some electrodes come pre-connected and others need to be plugged in after the pads have been placed. Follow the specific directions for your device.

AEDs will not function properly unless the pads fully adhere to the patient's chest and the cables are tightly inserted into the device. If either of these problems exist, the "no contact" or "check electrodes" prompt will sound or appear on the AED.

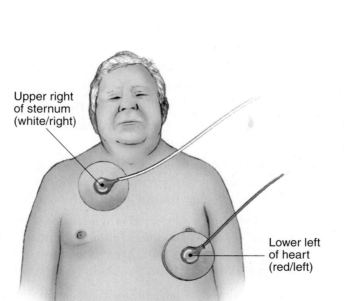

Upper right
of sternum
(white/right)

Lower left
of heart
(red/left)

FIGURE 8.24
Correct placement of defibrillator pads.

Automated External Defibrillation

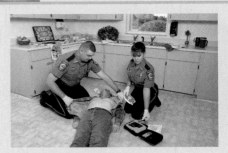

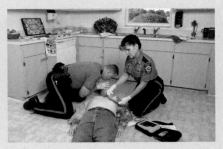

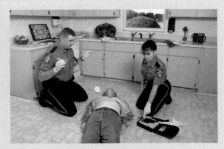

1. Turn on the AED and bare the patient's chest.

2. Place the pads and connect cable to device (if not pre-connected).

3. Press the "analyze" button to begin analyzing the patient's rhythm and follow the prompts.

Operating the Fully Automated Defibrillator

The following describes the operational procedures for a typical fully automated defibrillator. There are many defibrillator models available. You must be familiar with the one that you will use. Follow the manufacturer's operating manual for the specific AED you will be using.

Once turned on and attached to the patient, the latest models of fully automated defibrillators will assess the patient's heart rhythm, determine if a shock is indicated, charge to the pre-set energy level, and deliver the shock to the patient, all without further input from the rescuer. Many of these defibrillators have voice and text prompts that advise the rescuer with messages such as, "Shock advised. Do not touch the patient," "Charging. Stand clear," "Stop CPR. Check breathing and pulse." Should this voice system fail, the rescuer is expected to know what to do and how to ensure personal safety.

To operate a fully automated external defibrillator, you should (Scan 8-6):

1. Assess the patient to confirm that he is in cardiac arrest and that he has a clear airway.

2. Have your partner or someone trained in basic life support begin CPR while you set up the AED. If you are alone, do not start CPR. Instead make sure that EMS has been called and immediately attach the AED.

3. Turn on the AED and attach the electrodes. Once the electrodes are in place, the AED will begin to analyze the patient's rhythm.

4. Depending on the patient's rhythm, the AED will deliver up to three consecutive or "stacked" shocks.

5. Following the third shock, the AED will advise you to assess the patient. If there are no signs of circulation, provide one minute of CPR. (AEDs are programmed to pause for one minute after each stack of three shocks.)

6. After one minute, the AED will advise you to stop CPR. It will then re-analyze the heart rhythm and, if indicated, deliver up to three more stacked shocks. This sequence of three shocks and one minute of CPR will continue until a maximum of nine shocks have been delivered.

If at any time the patient goes into a rhythm that is not shockable, the AED will advise you to assess for a pulse and, if there is no pulse, to begin CPR. If the patient does have a pulse, leave the defibrillator attached to monitor the patient.

Maintain an open airway and continue life support procedures until more advanced care arrives and takes over. The patient would benefit from oxygen therapy and, if necessary, assisted ventilations.

The AED sequence presented here is a typical protocol that is pre-programmed into many AEDs from the factory. Each EMS system has its own protocols for the use of AEDs and may differ from what is presented here. Some jurisdictions may require First Responders to give a different number of shocks before transporting or continuing CPR, while others may require rescuers to perform CPR for one full minute or perform some other step before preparing and attaching the defibrillator. Always know and follow local protocols before attempting to use an AED.

Operating the Semi-Automated Defibrillator

The following is an example of the operational procedures for a semi-automated defibrillator. There are several semi-automated models currently available. Follow the instructions given in the manufacturer's manual for your specific model and always follow your EMS system's protocols for the defibrillator that you will be using.

Semi-automated defibrillators are also called *shock advisory defibrillators*. Once turned on and applied to the patient, they will analyze the rhythm and advise if a shock is necessary. Some models require the rescuer to push a button to begin the analyze sequence. In either case, the AED will automatically charge to a pre-set energy level. At this point it is necessary for the rescuer to push the shock button to deliver the shock (Figure 8.25).

The same assessment and safety procedures that apply to the fully automated defibrillator also apply to the operation of the semi-automated defibrillator. Some older models may not have a voice synthesizer. Regardless of the model, they all require the rescuer to push a button to deliver the shock.

To operate a semi-automated defibrillator, you should:

1. Assess the patient to confirm that he is in cardiac arrest and that he has a clear airway.

2. Have your partner or someone trained in basic life support begin CPR while you set up the AED. If you are alone, do not begin CPR. Instead make sure that EMS has been called and immediately attach the AED.

3. Turn on the AED and attach the electrodes. Once the electrodes are in place, the AED will begin to analyze the patient's rhythm. If necessary, push the analyze button.

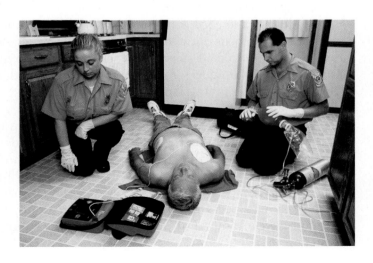

FIGURE 8.25
Operating a semi-automated defibrillator. Do not apply shock until everyone, including you, is clear of the patient.

4. If a shockable rhythm is detected, the AED will advise so and charge to the appropriate energy level. When appropriate, the AED will prompt you to push the shock button to deliver a shock.

5. Depending on the patient's rhythm, the AED will deliver up to three consecutive or "stacked" shocks. Deliver each shock by pushing the shock button.

6. Following the third shock, the AED will advise you to assess the patient. If there are no signs of circulation, provide one minute of CPR. (AEDs are programmed to pause for one minute after each stack of three shocks.)

7. After one minute, the AED will advise you to stop CPR. It will then re-analyze the heart rhythm and, if indicated, advise the rescuer to deliver up to three more stacked shocks. This sequence of three shocks and one minute of CPR will continue until a maximum of nine shocks have been delivered.

The maximum number of shocks that any AED will deliver is typically pre-set at the factory, as is the energy level of each shock, and follows local protocols. If you are in doubt as to what to do, contact medical direction.

Potential Problems

Most of the problems with defibrillator operations can easily be corrected. Most problems involve the poor attachment of the pads and/or cables. Making certain that the pads are in full contact with the patient's chest and that the cables are tightly connected to the device will be all that is needed to correct these problems.

Make sure the patient's chest is dry and free of anything that can prevent the pad from adhering well, such as hair or medication patches that occupy the pad placement sites. With gloved hands, remove any medication patches and wipe off any medication remaining on the patient's chest. If you have to shave the pad placement areas of the patient's chest, use a disposable safety razor provided in the AED kit for this purpose.

Most AEDs are pre-programmed to run self-diagnostic checks every 24 hours. Should one of these self-checks detect a failure of any of the AED's internal systems, an error message and/or audible alarm will sound alerting the rescuer of the failure. It is important to know the specific error messages that can be displayed by your specific device. Some errors are only advisory in nature and allow continued use of the device, while others indicate a failure of a major system, rendering the AED inoperable. Be sure to read the manufacturer's operating manual for the device you use and become familiar with all error messages and alarms.

Assessment and Quality Assurance

To be effective, a prehospital defibrillation program requires ongoing evaluation in order to identify and correct any problems. This process of assessment and quality assurance should focus on specific situations that involve standard operating procedures, physician-directed standing orders, care delivered by the rescuers, performance of the equipment, routine maintenance, and effectiveness of training programs. Changes in any aspect of the program must be the result of physician evaluation and orders.

Some AEDs have a voice-recording device built in that will provide an audible record of the resuscitation and defibrillation incident. All AEDs have an internal recording device that can capture a digital recording of the patient's heart rhythm, including when shocks are delivered. This information can be downloaded onto a computer so that a physician can evaluate the event to determine how the various aspects of the defibrillation program performed. Evaluation is an important part of any AED program and serves to improve and ensure quality patient care.

Be certain to carefully document all incidents involving the use of an AED. Your notes should include the time you arrived on scene, your assessment findings, how many shocks you delivered, and when they were delivered.

Part of your equipment inspection and assessment should include the operation of your defibrillator recording devices. Follow the manufacturer's manual and your EMS system's recommendations to correct any problems before the unit is put into service. In addition, it is important to ensure that the AED kit includes the necessary supplies at all times, such as an extra battery, an extra set of electrode pads, razors, and towels. You may find it helpful to carry duplicate supplies with the unit.

PEDIATRIC CPR

Throughout this chapter and for purposes of field resuscitation, all pediatric patients under the age of one year are referred to as infants. However, pediatric patients are commonly referred to as one of the following based on age:

- *Child*—1 to 8 years of age.

- *Infant*—includes the neonate period through 1 year of age.

- *Neonate*—the infant during the first 28 days of life.

- *Newborn*—the infant in the first minutes to hours after birth.

In general, you should use adult CPR techniques on a child over eight years old. However, because children develop at different rates, you may find that many infants and children are large for their age. Some adolescents are small enough to be mistaken for children. So, the above age categories are guidelines, not absolutes. It is more important to begin CPR and check for effective ventilations and compressions than to spend time determining a patient's exact age. For example, if you think the patient is under the age of one year and find that you cannot adequately compress the chest with just two fingers, then begin one-handed compressions as you would if the patient was older than one year.

PREPARING FOR CPR

Positioning the Patient

Just as you do for adults, place pediatric patients face up on a hard, flat surface. Be aware that when a child is on his back, his large head may cause the neck to flex forward, potentially closing the airway. To help ensure an open airway, maintain the head in a neutral position. It may be necessary to provide support under the shoulders with a folded blanket or towel (Figure 8.26).

Opening the Airway

FIRST➤ For the infant and child with no spinal injury, use the head-tilt, chin-lift maneuver. Tilt the head gently back to a neutral or slightly extended position with one hand. A slight head-tilt is often all that is needed. Place your fingers under the bony part of the chin and lift to finish the technique of opening the airway. Be careful not to compress the soft tissues of the neck, as this may obstruct the airway. In cases of suspected spinal injury, use the jaw-thrust maneuver. Airway obstructions should be cared for as described in Chapter 6. ■

FIGURE 8.26

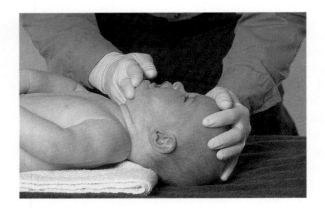

To help keep the head and neck in a neutral position, place a folded blanket or towel under the shoulders fill the void.

Assessing Breathing

To assess for breathing, place your ear next to the patient's nose and mouth. Then look, listen, and feel for air exchange for no more than 10 seconds. Look for the rise and fall of the chest and abdomen. Listen and feel for exhaled air. If there is breathing, maintain an open airway. Place the patient in the recovery position, if you do not suspect spinal injury. If there is no breathing, use an appropriate barrier device and give two slow breaths over 1.0 to 1.5 seconds while watching for the chest to rise.

Checking for Signs of Circulation

FIRST➤ Follow these steps when assessing for signs of circulation in a pediatric patient:

1. With your ear next to the patient's nose and mouth, look, listen, and feel for breathing.

2. Feel for a pulse and other signs of circulation, such as breathing, coughing, or movement, for no more than 10 seconds.

   —**Child** (1–8 years old)—use two fingers of one hand to assess the carotid pulse in the neck. Locate the Adam's apple and slide your fingers into the groove at the side of the neck closest to you.

   —**Infant** (one month to 1 year old)—locate the brachial pulse on the medial side of the arm between the elbow and armpit (Figure 8-27).

   —**Neonate** (birth to one month old)—check for an apical pulse, the sound of the heartbeat over the left side of the chest just below the nipple. Listen with your ear to the chest wall or through a stethoscope.

   —**Newborn** (just delivered)—feel for a pulse at the base of the umbilical cord. ■

FIGURE 8.27
For infants, feel for a brachial pulse.

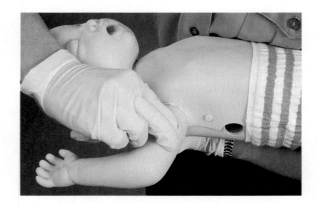

PEDIATRIC CPR TECHNIQUES

Ventilations

If your assessment finds that the patient has a good pulse, but is not breathing adequately or not at all, you will need to provide rescue breaths (ventilations). With the airway open and using an appropriate barrier device, provide slow rescue breaths at a ratio of one breath every three seconds for children and infants. The pediatric airway may be highly resistant to airflow, and you may have to blow hard to deliver an adequate volume of air. The correct volume for each ventilation is the volume that causes the chest to rise. Be careful not to overinflate the lungs, as this may cause air to enter the stomach (gastric distention) and, eventually, vomiting.

NOTE: *The following ventilation steps are optional if barrier devices are not available. It is unusual for infants and children to have contagious diseases and it is generally considered comparatively safer to give mouth-to-nose or mouth-to-mouth ventilations to pediatric patients than to adults.*

If the patient is an infant or a very small child, you may find it easier to seal your mouth over the patient's mouth and nose. If the patient is a child or a very large infant, seal your mouth over the patient's mouth and pinch the nostrils closed. If you do not see chest rise after repositioning the airway, follow the steps for clearing a foreign body airway obstruction.

FIRST➤ Provide one breath every three seconds using an appropriate barrier device or mouth-to-mouth or mouth-to-nose technique if a barrier device is not available. Watch carefully for the rise and fall of the patient's chest. ■

External Chest Compressions

External chest compressions and artificial ventilation can easily be performed by a single rescuer or shared between two trained rescuers depending on available resources. Compressions are necessary whenever a patient shows no signs of circulation. Chest compressions squeeze the heart between the breastbone (sternum) and backbone (spine). The squeezing of the heart combined with the increased pressure developed with each compression is what helps circulate blood to the brain and other vital organs.

FIRST➤ *Child*—After finding the compression site, use the heel of one hand to apply compressions (Figure 8.28). Depress the child's sternum 1 to 1-1/2 inches with each compression at a rate of 100 per minute.

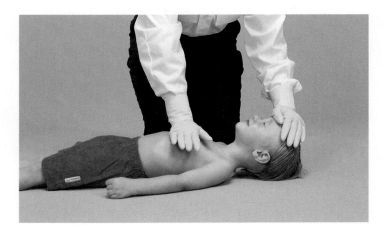

FIGURE 8.28
For child chest compression, use the heel of one hand.

FIGURE 8.29
For infant chest compression, use
the tips of two fingers.

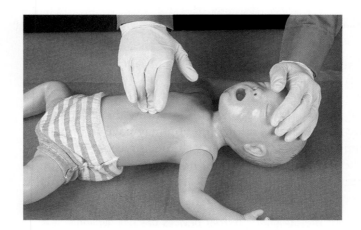

Maintain an open airway with one hand while compressing the chest with the heel of the other hand. Compress at a rate of approximately 100 per minute. After each set of five compressions, pause just long enough to provide a breath. Watch carefully for the rise and fall of the child's chest. ■

FIRST ➤ *Infant* —Apply compressions to the lower half of the breastbone (sternum). Place two fingers on the sternum, one finger-width below the imaginary nipple line (Figure 8.29). Compress the infant's sternum 1/2 to 1 inch, which is equal to about 1/3 to 1/2 the depth of the chest, at a rate of at least 100 per minute.

Maintain an open airway with one hand while compressing the chest with two fingers of the other hand. Provide a rescue breath after each set of five compressions. Watch carefully for the rise and fall of the infant's chest. ■

When there are two rescuers, the preferred method for chest compressions for the infant is the two-thumbs encircling-hands technique. One rescuer (the compressor) places both thumbs side-by-side over the lower half of the infant's sternum or about one finger's width below the nipple line (Figure 8-30). For very small infants or newborns, you may place one thumb on top of the other (Figure 8-31). The other rescuer provides ventilations.

FIGURE 8.30
For the infant, place two thumbs side by side on the middle third of the sternum just below an imaginary line drawn across the nipples.

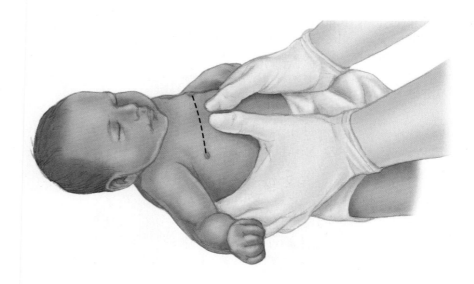

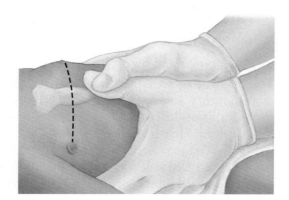

FIGURE 8.31
For newborns, place one thumb on top of the other.

CPR Rates and Ratios

FIRST➤ *Infant* —Deliver compressions at the rate of at least 100 per minute. Perform compressions and ventilations at a ratio of 5:1. To assure the correct compression rate, count aloud: "One, two, three, four, five," and provide one breath. ■

FIRST➤ *Child* —Deliver compressions at the rate of 100 per minute. Perform compressions and ventilations at a ratio of 5:1. To assure the correct compression rate, count aloud: "One, two, three, four, five," and provide one breath. ■

The following steps outline key points for infant or child CPR:

1. Determine unresponsiveness by gently tapping the child on the shoulder or the bottom of the infant's feet and shout, "Are you all right?" If no response . . .

2. Direct someone to call EMS. If you are alone, provide one minute of CPR before calling EMS. (There are exceptions to this rule such as in the case of near drowning, congenital heart disease, or respiratory failure.)

3. Position the patient. Place the child supine (face up) on a flat, hard surface. You may support small infants on your forearm.

4. Open the airway. Use the head tilt—chin lift maneuver or, if you suspect spinal injury, use the jaw-thrust maneuver.

5. Check for breathing. Place your ear next to the patient's nose and mouth and look, listen, and feel for breathing. If the patient is not breathing, maintain the airway and . . .

6. Using an appropriate barrier device, provide two slow breaths, each being 1.0 to 1.5 seconds in duration, while watching for adequate chest rise. Look for and clear any airway obstruction as necessary using the tongue-jaw lift. Use your gloved finger to sweep the mouth only if you see the obstruction.

7. Check for signs of circulation. Determine the presence of a carotid pulse in a child or a brachial or apical pulse in an infant. If there is a pulse but no respirations, provide ventilations at a rate of one breath every three seconds. If there are no signs of circulation, or it is an infant with a heart rate of less than 60 per minute . . .

8. Provide chest compressions. Place two fingers in the center of the chest, one finger width below the nipple line. Compress at a rate of at least 100 per

minute and provide ventilations at a 5:1 ratio for children and infants and a 3:1 ratio for neonates.

Activating the EMS System

The majority of pediatric cardiac arrests result from some type of respiratory failure or respiratory arrest. For this reason, most pediatric patients who need CPR are treated a little differently than adults. With pediatric patients, it is recommended that the lone First Responder provide one minute of rescue support before activating EMS. You may be able to carry the child or infant and continue emergency care while calling EMS. If the patient begins to breathe and regains a pulse, place him on his side in the recovery position (Figure 8-32). Do not place anyone in the recovery position if you suspect a spinal injury. Monitor the breathing patient or continue CPR on the pulseless, nonbreathing patient until help arrives.

RESUSCITATING THE NEWBORN INFANT

About 6% of all newborns need life support, and for newborns with very low birth weights, the percentage rises. While it may be rare for the First Responder to deliver an infant in the field, it is even rarer for that infant to require basic life support. However, you must have the knowledge and skill to recognize and manage a newborn in distress. The following information will discuss the issues unique to newborns and their resuscitation.

Rapid Assessment and Initial Stabilization

Call for ALS support immediately for any out-of-hospital childbirth. This precaution is to ensure that any newly born infant has all possible life support if it should be needed. Resuscitating a newly born infant requires at least two rescuers, one of whom will manage the airway and perform ventilations and the other of whom will monitor the heart rate and perform compressions. An additional team per infant is required if there are multiple births.

Suctioning and Stimulation   During delivery, suction the mouth and nose immediately after the head delivers. Use a bulb syringe or other appropriate device to suc-

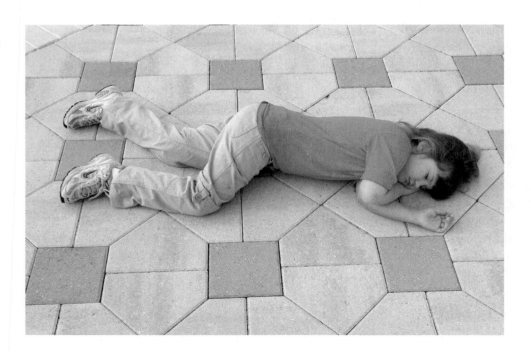

FIGURE 8.32
If the patient begins to breathe and regains a pulse, place her in the recovery position.

tion the mouth first and then the nose. Suctioning will usually stimulate the newborn to breathe if he is not already breathing. If suctioning does not stimulate breathing, first try rubbing his back or flicking the soles of his feet.

Warmth It is important to keep the infant warm and dry. A cool environment causes the infant to become chilled. Low temperatures reduce the drive to breathe. Always keep newborns warm throughout all procedures.

Airway If the newborn has a lot of oral secretions, turn him onto his side to allow drainage. Support him in this position by placing another towel behind his back. Suction the mouth and back of the throat (pharynx) if necessary.

Positioning Place the newborn on his back or side with the head in a neutral or slightly extended position. If needed, place a small folded towel under the newborn's shoulders to help maintain an open airway.

Evaluation Assess and support the ABCs by evaluating respiratory effort, heart rate, and color as described in the following sections. Also assess and support body temperature; the newborn should be kept warm and dry.

Oxygen and Ventilations

A newly born infant who is crying vigorously and is flushed from the effort has good respiratory effort. One who is listless, gasping, and pale or bluish in color has poor respiratory effort and needs oxygen. If available, deliver oxygen at no less than 10 liters per minute using the blow-by method through a face mask or through a makeshift funnel made from a paper cup attached to oxygen tubing. Hold the oxygen source close to the side of the newborn's face to maximize the inhaled concentration. (Blowing oxygen directly into the face can cause periods of **apnea**.)

apnea (AP-ne-ah) the temporary cessation of breathing.

If you must assist breathing, use an appropriate size bag-valve device attached to 100% oxygen. It is also critical to use an appropriate size mask to assure a good seal and proper oxygen delivery to the newborn. Provide assisted ventilations at a rate of 40 to 60 breaths per minute.

If you are also providing compressions, ventilate once every five compressions or approximately 30 times per minute. Watch carefully for the chest to rise with each breath. If the chest does not rise, reposition the newborn's head and mask and try to ventilate again. Suction again if needed. By now, ALS should be on the way. After providing ventilations for 30 seconds, check heart rate by listening for the apical pulse (over the left chest) with your ear or with a stethoscope. In a newborn, you can feel the base of the umbilical cord for a pulse, which will continue to pulsate for several minutes after birth.

If the heart rate is at least 100 beats per minute and spontaneous respirations are now present, gradually discontinue assisted ventilations and provide gentle stimulation by rubbing the skin. If respirations are inadequate or the heart rate is below 100 beats per minute, continue with assisted ventilations.

(For information on oxygen delivery, see Appendix 2. Follow local protocols and medical direction and only deliver oxygen if First Responders are allowed to do so in your jurisdiction.)

Chest Compressions

Because the normal pulse rate for a newborn is so high (120 to 160 beats per minute), a pulse rate below 60 is not sufficient to support life. If the heart rate of a newborn is less than 60 beats per minute you must begin chest compressions. For newborns whose heart rate is between 60 and 80 beats per minute and rising, it is recommended that you assist ventilations and carefully monitor the heart rate. First Responders should concentrate on providing effective ventilations until the heart rate is less than 60 beats per minute, at which time it becomes necessary to support circulation by providing compressions along with ventilations.

Just as with the infant patient, there are two techniques for performing chest compressions on newborns: the two-finger technique and the two-thumbs encircling-hands technique. The two-finger technique is the preferred method for the single rescuer. The two-thumbs encircling-hands technique is preferred when two rescuers are available for CPR.

Depress the sternum approximately 1/3 the depth of the chest using a smooth compression and relaxation technique. Do not lift your thumbs (or fingers) from the chest during the relaxation phase.

Check the pulse rate periodically and discontinue compressions when the newborn's own heart rate reaches 80 beats per minute or greater. Always provide assisted ventilations with 100% oxygen while you are performing chest compressions. The compression-to-ventilation ratio in newborns is 3:1. Deliver three compressions followed by one slow breath. (Check protocols in your jurisdiction to see if the ratio is smaller. Some medical directors require a 1:1 ratio.) Compress at a rate of 120 per minute.

It takes practice to provide effective CPR on newborns. Take every opportunity in class and at your station to practice the procedures on infant manikins. Remember, these cases are rare and you will not get a lot of real-life practice, but you must be ready to provide the skill when needed.

Ensuring Effective CPR for All Patients

Unless the proper techniques are carried out, CPR will not be effective and the patient will die. To assure effective CPR for all patients, be sure to remember these important points:

- Place the patient face up (supine) on a hard surface.

- Maintain an open airway using the most appropriate technique.

- Use an appropriate barrier device, place it securely over the face, and ensure a good seal.

- During ventilations watch the chest for adequate rise and fall.

- Compress smoothly and to the proper depth and relax pressure completely between compressions to allow the heart to refill.

- Use the correct rates and ratios.

- Limit necessary interruptions such as pulse and breathing checks to no more second 10 seconds and 15-to-30 seconds for patient moves.

FIRST➤ First Responders must be aware of complications that may be caused by using improper CPR techniques. Certain complications occur because the rescuer places his hands improperly during compressions (Figure 8.33).

- If you place your hands too high on the patient's chest, you can cause damage to the collarbones (clavicles) and not provide adequate compression of the heart.
- If your hands are too low, there is a risk of damaging internal organs.
- If you place your hands too far to either side, you may fracture the ribs and possibly damage an internal organ.

Lungs
Heart
Spleen
Liver
Stomach

Too far right:
May fracture ribs and cause lacerations to lung and liver

Too far left:
May fracture ribs and cause lacerations to lung and heart

Too high:
May fracture collar bone

Too low:
May depress xiphoid process into liver

You must carefully locate the CPR compression site and properly position your hands to avoid these problems. In some cases, rib fractures occur even when you are properly performing CPR. In adult patients, whose chests are not as pliable and whose bones are more brittle, the ribs may actually break during correct compressions. Children's chests are very pliable; their ribs are not likely to break. On any patient, you may hear a cracking sound while performing compressions, which may be a separation of the cartilage that connects the ribs to the sternum. This separation occurs when you compress the sternum to the depth required for appropriate CPR and circulation. If you think you have heard ribs crack, do not stop CPR. Check the position of your hands, reposition them properly, and resume CPR. A fractured rib will heal; stopping CPR will result in death.

Another problem occurs if you attempt to force too much air into the patient's lungs. The excess air overflows out of the lungs and enters the stomach by way of the esophagus. When too much air enters the stomach, it can result in gastric distention. Do not try to force this air out of the stomach. To do so might cause the patient to vomit, which could lead to an airway obstruction. In some cases, the patient may inhale (aspirate) stomach contents and, if you try to provide breaths, you will force the vomitus into the lungs.

To avoid or reduce the amount of air forced into the stomach, always look for the patient's chest to rise as you deliver ventilations. Adjust the size of your breaths so that you see the chest rise, and then allow the patient to passively exhale. If you see the stomach begin to bulge, reposition the patient's head and adjust your ventilations. Remember: The key to minimizing the air that enters the stomach is to provide slow ventilations and only enough to see appropriate chest rise.

If the patient vomits, stop CPR. Take time to clear the patient's airway as best you can by repositioning the patient for drainage and by using your gloved fingers to sweep the mouth. After clearing the airway, resume CPR. ■

SPECIAL CPR SITUATIONS

MOVING THE PATIENT

Usually, there are only two reasons for a First Responder to move a patient who is receiving CPR: transport and immediate danger at the scene. Most of the time, the patient is moved after the EMTs assume responsibility for care. In the majority of moves, you may be asked to help lift and carry the patient. You may assist EMTs in ventilating patients if you have been trained to use oxygen and oxygen delivery equipment. You may also be asked to continue compressions as part of two-rescuer CPR.

TRAUMA

Many factors complicate CPR when dealing with a victim of trauma. Severe injuries to the patient's face may interfere with your attempts to provide ventilations. Crushing injuries to the patient's chest may lessen the effectiveness of chest compressions. Head, neck, and spine injuries may require that you handle the patient in a special manner.

Many rescuers are unsure about starting CPR on trauma patients. When rescuers find obvious indications of spinal injuries, they may feel it is more important to immobilize the spine before they start CPR. If rescuers find a patient with a crushed chest, they may be afraid of causing internal injuries if they perform chest compressions. Patient injuries should not prevent you from starting CPR. If you delay or do not start CPR, the patient will die.

Moving the trauma patient into proper position is a major problem. One concern is spinal injury, but CPR is not effective if the patient is in a seated position. Nor is CPR likely to be effective if the patient is on a soft surface, such as a car seat. Patients must be moved to hard surfaces and placed on their backs. While doing so, take into account the possibility of neck and spine injury and use your hands and arms to initially control and stabilize the head and neck whenever you have to move a patient.

When moving an adult, cradle the head and shoulders in your forearms and attempt to move the patient so that his head stays in line with his body. When moving an infant or a child, always use one hand to support the head and neck of the patient. Again, for CPR to be effective, the patient must be lying face up on a hard surface.

If you must move the patient after starting CPR because of the dangers at the scene, then do so. Try not to interrupt CPR for more than 15 to 30 seconds during a move. The total move may have to be done in several stages if conditions allow. Even if your patient has possible neck and spine injuries, start CPR as soon as possible. Do not delay CPR in order to fully stabilize the neck and spine with a collar and immobilization devices. Use the jaw-thrust maneuver for ventilations in order to reduce the chances of causing greater injury to the patient.

NEAR DROWNING

Rescuer safety and emergency care procedures at the scene of a drowning or near-drowning incident require special training in water rescue (see Appendix 4). If CPR is needed, begin as soon as possible, but remember your personal safety comes first. You may begin ventilations while the patient is still in the water. Be aware that mouth-to-mask methods may be difficult to perform under these conditions. In a diving incident, suspect neck injury and use the jaw-thrust maneuver to open the airway. Very little water is ever aspirated and any water in the lungs will be absorbed into the circulation as you ventilate the patient. Chest compressions are not effective when the patient is in the water. Attempts to begin compressions while the patient is in the water will delay removing the patient from the water and starting effective CPR.

ELECTRIC SHOCK

Some of the special problems of emergencies involving electricity will be covered in Chapter 10. Your first priority is to avoid placing yourself in danger. Assess the patient and start artificial ventilation as soon as possible after you are sure the power is turned off. CPR, when needed, is performed in the same way for a victim of electric shock as it is for any other patient in cardiac arrest.

CPR—RESPONSIBILITIES OF THE FIRST RESPONDER

When caring for someone in cardiac arrest, your duties are to have someone activate EMS and to start CPR immediately. Only a physician at the scene who has accepted responsibility for the patient may order you not to begin CPR. Bystanders and members of the patient's family may tell you that the patient would not want to be resuscitated. You are not to obey such requests. Even though the patient may have a terminal illness or may be very old, you will still need to provide CPR unless there is an advanced directive such as an official do not resuscitate (DNR) order. Quickly let the family know that you understand their feelings, but your duty as a First Responder is to begin CPR. Suggest that they try to contact the patient's doctor to get further directions. If the family does not have an advance directive from the patient and doctor, you must begin CPR. Without an advance directive such as a DNR, you have no way of knowing that this is what the patient would have you do. (Be sure you are familiar with prehospital DNR orders in your region.) If in doubt, contact medical direction for assistance, and when EMTs arrive, you or one of them should talk with the family to comfort and reassure them. Offer to call friends or other family members for them, and make sure they know where their family member is being transported.

The longer a patient is in cardiac arrest before CPR is started, the less likely CPR will be effective. However, there are documented cases of adults in cardiac arrest for over 10 minutes who have been resuscitated with no major brain damage. Children and infants usually can survive longer periods of time in cardiac arrest than adults. Do not refuse to begin CPR because someone has been in cardiac arrest for 10 minutes, though in most cases, CPR will probably not be effective. However, the moment the patient was seen to collapse and the moment of cardiac arrest are usually not the same. A patient may be unresponsive with minimum lung and heart function for quite some time before cardiac arrest occurs. Always start CPR immediately.

Cold-water drowning victims can be successfully resuscitated after long periods of submersion. There are documented cases of arrest that have lasted over 45 minutes before successful resuscitation. The same is true of people whose body temperatures are lowered by cold (hypothermia). You must provide resuscitation. The emergency department staff will continue resuscitation while they rewarm the patient's body. They will not declare biological death until the patient is rewarmed adequately and all efforts to revive him have failed.

First➤ Once you have started, continue to provide CPR until:

- Spontaneous circulation begins. Then provide ventilations only.
- Spontaneous circulation and breathing begin.
- Equally or more highly trained members of the EMS system or someone certified in CPR can continue in your place.
- You turn over responsibility for patient care to a physician.
- You are exhausted and no longer able to continue. ■

Rescuers are often concerned that they may have to stop CPR when they become exhausted, but you must be realistic. If you reach that point, realize that you have done all you could. CPR has its physical limitations on the rescuer. It also has its physical limitations on the patient. If you are becoming exhausted and know that you will not be able to continue, look for help from bystanders. Even if they are not trained in CPR, you may be able to tell them what they should do.

If you wish to reduce the chances that you will have to stop CPR because of fatigue, then you should:

- Keep yourself in good physical condition. Exercise to improve your heart and lung functions.

- Become a CPR or basic cardiac life support instructor. Help the American Heart Association (AHA), American Red Cross, National Safety Counsel, American Safety and Health Institute, or similar agencies in their efforts to train all citizens in basic cardiac life support. Your efforts to train others will help increase the number of bystanders who are able to assist you in providing CPR.

- Support your local EMS system so that they may have the personnel and equipment needed to reach all victims in your area.

- Practice what you have learned about CPR. Your instructor can tell you how to review CPR, keep yourself up to date, and have access to manikins for practice.

Chapter Review

SUMMARY

Like the chain of EMS resources, the chain of survival is also a linked system of patient-care events. These events include early access, early CPR, early defibrillation, and early advanced life support (ALS). Remember that the chain of survival is different for adults and children.

There is a strong relationship between the brain and the activities of breathing and circulation. When the heart stops beating, a patient is in cardiac arrest and cannot circulate oxygenated blood to the brain. The major signs of cardiac arrest are unresponsiveness, no breathing, and no pulse.

Check for breathing by placing your ear next to the patient's nose and mouth and looking, listening, and feeling for air exchange. Check for a pulse and other signs of circulation, such as breathing, coughing, and moving. Check the carotid pulse on an adult and a child (1 to 8 years); a brachial pulse on an infant (under 1 year of age); and listen for an apical pulse over the chest of a newborn (birth to 28 days) or check for a pulse at the base of the umbilical cord of a newly born infant.

If a patient is unresponsive, check airway, breathing, and circulation (ABCs). After determining that the adult patient is unresponsive, alert the EMS system. If you are alone and caring for a pediatric patient, provide one minute of CPR before activating EMS. To provide proper CPR, you will:

1. Position the patient supine on a hard surface and open the airway. Be careful not to overextend the neck of an infant or child.

2. Check for breathing for no more than 10 seconds. If the patient is not breathing . . .

3. Provide two *slow* breaths. (Clear the airway if necessary.)

4. Check for signs of circulation including a pulse. If there are none . . .

5. Find the appropriate compression site:

   —*Adult and child*—on the center of the chest between the nipples, well above the notch where the ribs come together (xiphoid process).

   —*Infant and newborn*—on the center of the chest, one finger width below an imaginary line drawn between the nipples.

6. Position your hands for compressions:

   —*Adult*—Place your two hands together, one on top of the other, then place the heel of the lower hand on the sternum. You may extend or interlace the fingers. Keep your fingers off the patient's chest.

   —*Child* (age 1 to 8 years)—Place the heel of one hand over the lower half of the sternum being sure to keep the fingers off the chest.

   —*Infant* (age 1 month to 1 year)—Place two fingers on the sternum one finger width below the nipple line.

7. Provide external chest compressions:

   —*Adult* (over 8 years old)—at a rate of 100 per minute and a depth of 1 1/2 to 2 inches.

   —*Child* (age 1 to 8 years)—at a rate of 100 per minute and a depth of 1/3 to 1/2 the depth of the chest.

   —*Infant* (age 1 month to 1 year)—at a rate of at least 100 per minute and a depth 1/3 to 1/2 the depth of the infant's chest.

   —*Newborn* (birth to hours old)—at a rate of at least 120 per minute and a depth of 1/3 of chest.

8. Compression/ventilation ratios:

   —*Adult*—two breaths every 15 compressions.

   —*Child*—one breath every 5 compressions.

   —*Infant*—one breath every 5 compressions.

   —*Newborn*—one breath every 3 compressions.

9. Check for pulse and other signs of circulation after one minute of CPR and every few minutes thereafter.

   —*Adult*—check carotid pulse.

   —*Child*—check carotid pulse.

   —*Infant*—brachial or apical pulse.

   —*Newborn*—umbilical pulse.

10. If the circulation check shows:

    —*No pulse, no breathing*—continue CPR, checking for a pulse every few minutes.

    —*Pulse, but no breathing*—stop compressions and provide artificial ventilations. Continue to monitor pulse every few minutes.

    —Heart rate less than 60 for a newborn, start CPR. If the heart rate is above 60 beats per minute, continue to assist ventilations and monitor the heart rate to ensure that it increases.

If during CPR you miss a ventilation, do not wait until the end of the next compression cycle to ventilate. Instead, provide breaths after any compression in the next cycle. Check for breathing and pulse after the first minute of CPR and then every few minutes. Do not stop CPR for more than 10 seconds other than to move the patient because of danger on the scene. If you have to move the patient, do not stop CPR for more than 15 to 30 seconds. Continue CPR until the patient regains a pulse and/or breathing, or until you are relieved by an equally or more highly trained person, care for the patient is accepted by a physician, or until you can no longer continue because of exhaustion.

Start CPR immediately on a patient in cardiac arrest, even if you may worsen existing injuries. Without CPR, the patient will go from clinical death to biological death within 10 minutes. If the patient has a do not resuscitate (DNR) order, do not start resuscitation. Check with your jurisdiction about advance directives.

First Responders use AEDs in many jurisdictions. These life-saving units are placed in many public areas, and First Responders should be able to assist the public in using them and in performing CPR. AEDs can convert certain lethal heart rhythms to a normal cardiac rhythm. AEDs are electrical devices and must be used with caution and according to specific protocols. The general steps for the use of a typical AED are:

- Confirm that the patient is unresponsive, has no breathing or pulse, and has a clear airway.
- Turn on the AED and expose the patient's chest and securely attach the pads. Wipe dry or shave hair if necessary.
- Follow the AED's prompts to defibrillate, check breathing and pulse.
- Follow AED prompts for a pulse or start CPR if no pulse.

As long as the heart pumps, the blood circulates. If the heart stops pumping, the blood stops circulating and the First Responder must perform CPR to restart and maintain circulation. You will practice CPR in class and may have done so already. Think about what you have read in the text and what you will do during practice.

✔ What equipment do you need to perform CPR?

✔ How many people do you need to perform CPR?

Were the answers easy? Or did you say, "It depends"? Does it depend on the age or size of the patient? Does it depend on the number of rescuers there to help? On whether you have a barrier device, gloves, or oxygen? Can you do CPR without these things? Is it safe to do so? What are your obligations for performing CPR on someone in cardiac arrest? Do you think you need to carry your own barrier device and gloves with you at all times? What if you do not have a barrier device and someone in a restaurant has a heart attack and goes into cardiac arrest before the ambulance gets there? Is there anything handy that you can use as an impromptu barrier device?

✔ If you start CPR on a cardiac-arrest patient in a public place, how do you work with someone who wants to help but is doing CPR incorrectly?

Do you feel that you could coach someone or give directions while you are performing CPR? Would you ventilate and tell the person how to do chest compressions, or would you do chest compressions and tell the person how to ventilate? Would it be better to send the person for help or to ask him or her to control the crowd while you perform one-rescuer CPR?

Practice chest compressions while you coach a classmate or station member on artificial ventilation. Switch your position and practice ventilations while you coach someone on chest compressions. Do you think this is effective? Can it work? Or do you think it is easier to just do it yourself? How long can you last? Have someone time you while you do CPR until you get tired. How long were you able to perform CPR before you felt you were no longer effective?

Whether you are on duty or off when you are in a public place, you may need to assist in the care of a patient before an ambulance arrives. Plan ahead.

✔ Which public places and stores in your area keep emergency care supplies handy for public use? When you go to the library, the grocery store, the mall, the theater, or restaurants, do you see signs that tell you they have first-aid kits with barrier devices or AEDs available? If you do not see signs, ask if these items are kept for public use in the event of an emergency. Can they be retrieved quickly? Or are they locked away causing someone to wait while the key is found? Many malls are beginning to keep emergency care supplies at special locations or at a first-aid center. Do the security guards know where these supplies are kept? Do they have access to these supplies? How hard is it to locate and retrieve these supplies? What supplies are kept? Are there barrier devices and gloves, different sizes of airways and bag-valve masks, an AED? What training do mall, airport, or other large public-place personnel have for using these items?

Part of the learning experience—and an effective quality assurance step—is wanting to know if your emergency care delivery was appropriate and effective.

✔ How do you find out if the CPR that you performed on a patient was effective? Does your department get follow-up information on patients that you cared for in the prehospital setting? Are you able to check the records for patient outcomes? If the new patient privacy laws will not let you, how can you find out what you must do to get that information from the hospital?

You may find that your procedures were performed correctly, but the patient could not be resuscitated because of other medical or trauma conditions or circumstances. Knowing that you performed correctly is a positive reinforcement for your efforts. Finding out what you need to do to correct your performance is a learning experience.

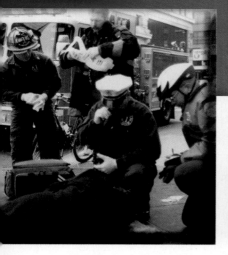
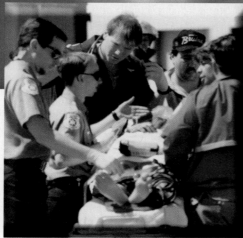
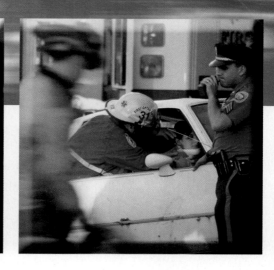

Medical Emergencies

Illnesses and conditions that can affect the body are known as medical emergencies. You must be prepared to provide appropriate emergency care to the various medical patients you may encounter. While some situations require you to intervene with specific skills, others will be referred to as common medical complaints. This chapter provides an overview of medical emergencies and outlines emergency care for specific complaints, including chest pain, congestive heart failure, respiratory emergencies, altered mental status and stroke, seizures, diabetes, and abdominal pain. It also provides emergency care information on poisonings, bites, and stings, heat and cold emergencies, behavioral emergencies, and alcohol and drug abuse.

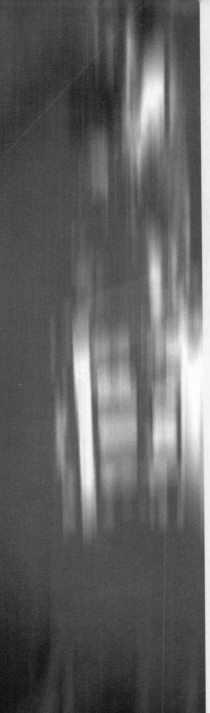

NATIONAL STANDARD OBJECTIVES

This chapter focuses on the objectives of Module 5, Lesson 5–1, of the U.S. DOT's First Responder National Standard Curriculum and serves as an instructional aid to help you meet any specific objectives added to the course by your local EMS system.

By the end of this chapter, you will be able to
(from cognitive or knowledge information):

5–1.1 Identify the patient who presents with a general medical complaint. (pp. 230–231)

5–1.2 Explain the steps in providing emergency medical care to a patient with a general medical complaint. (pp. 230–231)

5–1.3 Identify the patient who presents with a specific medical complaint of altered mental status. (pp. 243–250)

5–1.4 Explain the steps in providing emergency medical care to a patient with an altered mental status. (pp. 243–250)

5–1.5 Identify the patient who presents with a specific medical complaint of seizures. (pp. 246–247)

5–1.6 Explain the steps in providing emergency medical care to a patient with seizures. (pp. 246–247)

5–1.7 Identify the patient who presents with a specific medical complaint of exposure to cold. (pp. 266–269)

5–1.8 Explain the steps in providing emergency medical care to a patient with an exposure to cold. (pp. 266–269)

5–1.9 Identify the patient who presents with a specific medical complaint of exposure to heat. (pp. 262–266)

5–1.10 Explain the steps in providing emergency medical care to a patient with an exposure to heat. (pp. 262–266)

5–1.11 Identify the patient who presents with a specific medical complaint of behavioral change. (pp. 270–273)

5–1.12 Explain the steps in providing emergency medical care to a patient with a behavioral change. (pp. 270–273)

5–1.13 Identify the patient who presents with a specific medical complaint of psychological crisis. (pp. 270–273)

5–1.14 Explain the steps in providing emergency medical care to a patient with a psychological crisis. (pp. 270–273)

Feel comfortable enough to
(by changing attitudes, values, and beliefs):

5–1.15 Attend to the feelings of the patient and/or family when dealing with the patient with a general medical complaint. (pp. 230–231)

5–1.16 Attend to the feelings of the patient and/or family when dealing with the patient with a specific medical complaint. (pp. 231, 234, 235, 239, 241, 243, 244, 247, 265, 266)

5–1.17 Explain the rationale for modifying your behavior toward the patient with a behavioral emergency. (pp. 270–274, 277)

LEARNING TASKS

In addition to the National Standard Objectives, you will need to understand the importance of performing an initial assessment on these patients and identifying any life-threatening conditions. As you work through this chapter, you will also need to know:

✔ Signs and symptoms of a heart attack and the emergency care for patients with chest pain, including those with congestive heart failure.

5–1.18 Demonstrate a caring attitude towards patients with a general medical complaint who request emergency medical services. (pp. 230–231)

5–1.19 Place the interests of the patient with a general medical complaint as the foremost consideration when making any and all patient-care decisions. (pp. 230–231)

5–1.20 Communicate with empathy to patients with a general medical complaint, as well as with family members and friends of the patient. (pp. 230–231)

5–1.21 Demonstrate a caring attitude towards patients with a specific medical complaint who request emergency medical services. (pp. 231, 234, 236, 239, 241, 243, 244, 246, 247, 265, 266)

5–1.22 Place the interests of the patient with a specific medical complaint as the foremost consideration when making any and all patient-care decisions. (pp. 231, 233, 236, 246)

5–1.23 Communicate with empathy to patients with a specific medical complaint, as well as with family members and friends of the patient. (pp. 231, 234, 236, 239, 241, 243, 244, 246, 247, 265, 266)

5–1.24 Demonstrate a caring attitude towards patients with a behavior problem who request emergency medical services. (pp. 270–273)

5–1.25 Place the interests of the patient with a behavioral problem as the foremost consideration when making any and all patient-care decisions. (pp. 270–273)

5–1.26 Communicate with empathy to patients with a behavioral problem, as well as with family members and friends of the patient. (pp. 270–273)

Show how to
(through psychomotor skills):

5–1.27 Demonstrate the steps in providing emergency medical care to a patient with a general medical complaint. (pp. 230–231)

5–1.28 Demonstrate the steps in providing emergency medical care to a patient with an altered mental status. (pp. 243–250)

5–1.29 Demonstrate the steps in providing emergency medical care to a patient with seizures. (pp. 246–247)

5–1.30 Demonstrate the steps in providing emergency medical care to a patient with an exposure to cold. (pp. 266–269)

5–1.31 Demonstrate the steps in providing emergency medical care to a patient with an exposure to heat. (pp. 262–266)

5–1.32 Demonstrate the steps in providing emergency medical care to a patient with a behavioral change. (pp. 270–273)

5–1.33 Demonstrate the steps in providing emergency medical care to a patient with a psychological crisis. (pp. 270–273)

✔ Signs and symptoms of respiratory difficulty and the care for those patients, including patients who appear to be hyperventilating.

✔ Conditions associated with abdominal pain, including signs and symptoms, causes, and emergency care.

✔ Signs and symptoms of poisonings, bites, and stings, including types and emergency care.

✔ Signs and symptoms and emergency care of alcohol and drug-abuse patients.

MEDICAL EMERGENCIES

remember

Part of the patient assessment is to look for medical identification devices.

remember

A systolic pressure greater than 140 mmHg or a diastolic pressure above 90 mmHg may be an indication of high blood pressure. If you detect a low or a falling blood pressure, consider the patient may be developing shock.

Patients may request EMS for a variety of medical complaints. Medical emergencies may be caused by infections, poisons, or the failure of one or more of the body's organs and systems. You must assess each patient and determine the chief complaint as well as any signs and symptoms that might be present. The patient or a bystander may be able to tell you of an existing disease or condition. However, in most cases, what you observe and what the patient describes will be your only clues to the patient's problems.

Note that a patient's medical emergency may be hidden because of an injury. For example, a diabetic patient may collapse because of very low blood sugar or have a car wreck and be injured by the trauma. As a First Responder, you will have to provide care for the patient's injuries. The medical problem, however, should not go unnoticed. During your assessment of a trauma patient, keep in mind there may also be underlying medical problems.

SIGNS AND SYMPTOMS

To detect a medical emergency, you will have to be aware of common signs and symptoms, such as:

- Altered mental status.
- Abnormal pulse rate and character.
- Abnormal breathing rate and character.
- Abnormal skin signs.
- Abnormal pupil size and/or response.
- Unusual breath odors.
- Tenderness or rigidity in the abdomen.
- Muscular activity such as spasms and paralysis.
- Bleeding or discharges from the body.

A patient may complain of some of the following symptoms:

- Pain.
- Fever, or chills.
- Upset stomach and/or vomiting.
- Dizziness or feeling faint.
- Shortness of breath.
- Chest or abdominal pain.
- Unusual bowel or bladder activity.
- Thirst, hunger, or odd tastes in the mouth.
- Burning sensations.

ASSESSMENT

Remember that emergency care for medical emergencies is based on the patient's signs and symptoms. That is why it is so important to complete an appropriate patient assessment. For general medical complaints, you should:

1. Complete a scene size-up before initiating emergency medical care.

2. Complete an initial assessment.

3. Complete a physical exam as needed.

4. Complete ongoing assessments, as appropriate.

5. Comfort and reassure the patient while awaiting additional EMS resources.

FIRST➤ Consider all patient complaints to be valid. When assessing the patient, remember:

- If the patient appears or feels unusual in any way, assume that there is a medical emergency.

- If the patient has abnormal vital signs, conclude that there is a medical emergency. ■

Patient assessment and care for medical emergencies are summarized in Figure 9.1.

SPECIFIC MEDICAL EMERGENCIES

CHEST PAIN AND POSSIBLE HEART ATTACKS

Chest pain is a common medical complaint. There are many conditions that cause chest pain and give the appearance of being a heart attack. Indigestion, stress, and anxiety are among them. As a First Responder, you will not be able to tell the difference. Instead, if a patient is having chest pain, you must conclude that he or she is having, or is about to have, a heart attack (Figure 9.2). Provide care accordingly.

Heart attacks and other problems with the heart are often described using many technical terms, such as angina pectoris, coronary occlusion, acute myocardial infarction (AMI), and acute coronary syndrome (ACS). There are many other terms in common use in medical terminology. Being able to tell one condition from another requires advanced medical training. Simply realize that the heart is a muscle with its own blood vessels. Any damage to the muscle or to the vessels can prevent the heart from getting enough oxygen, which can lead to a heart attack. This is a serious condition. You, as a First Responder, must provide care for all chest pain as a possible heart attack.

FIRST➤ Whenever you suspect that a patient is having, or is about to have, a heart attack, activate EMS. Report the signs and symptoms. It may be possible for dispatch to send an ALS unit. ■

Signs and Symptoms

The following are common signs and symptoms of a heart attack (Scan 9-1):

- Early symptoms generally include chest or upper abdominal sensations of pressure or burning and are often mistaken for indigestion.

- As an attack worsens, pain may localize behind the sternum and radiate to either of the arms or shoulders (usually the left). In some cases, the pain may extend to the hand, neck, jaw, and teeth; back; or upper abdomen.

  The pain may not originate under the sternum. For example, some patients have pain only in the jaw, neck, or arm.

FIRST➤ Many times, the chest pain is associated with other signs and symptoms that are also suggestive of a heart attack in progress. They include:

warning

Always consider chest pain an emergency. Even the patient with a history of heartburn, indigestion, or other stomach or esophageal problems can be having a heart attack.

heart attack a general term used to indicate a failure of circulation to the heart muscle that damages or destroys a portion of the heart.

Care of Medical Emergencies

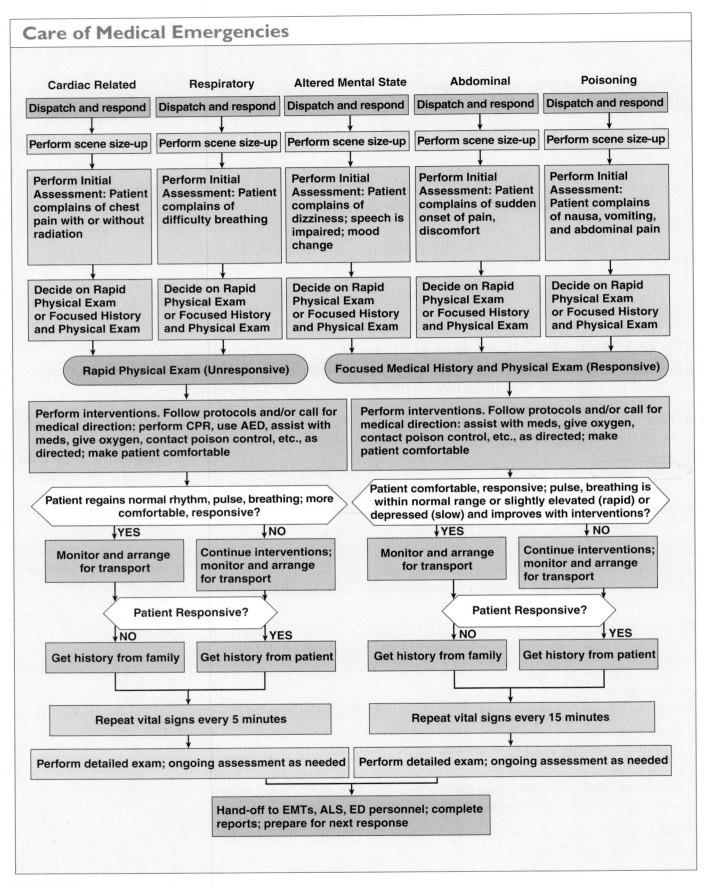

FIGURE 9.1

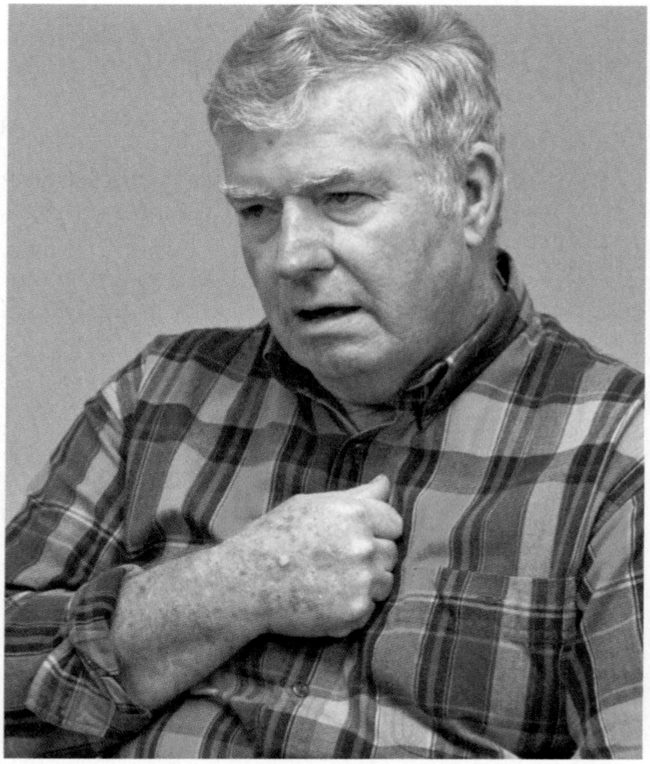

FIGURE 9.2
Chest pain is the primary symptom of a heart attack.

- Shortness of breath.
- Nausea.
- Sweating.
- Weakness. ■

The pain of a heart attack may diminish when physical exertion or emotional stress ends or when the patient takes a prescription medication called nitroglycerin. Additional signs may include an increased pulse rate and an irregular pulse. Patients who have taken repeated doses of nitroglycerin may have low blood pressure as a result of blood vessel dilation.

Sometimes patients who are having a heart attack will deny that they are having one. They will frequently appear frightened and anxious. If there are other signs of a heart attack, or if bystanders report that the patient complained of pain or other discomfort in the areas described above, provide care for a heart attack.

Emergency Care

If the patient is in cardiac arrest (no pulse and not breathing), have someone activate EMS, and then begin CPR. Otherwise, complete the assessment as required, carefully noting the patient's vital signs (Figure 9.3). If the patient is unresponsive when you arrive, gain what information you can from bystanders. If no one saw the patient prior to the loss of responsiveness, suspect that the patient may have had a heart attack.

FIRST➤ Upon gathering signs and symptoms indicating a heart attack or the possibility of a heart attack, you should (Figure 9.4):

1. Perform a scene size-up, including taking BSI precautions.

2. Make certain that the EMS system has been alerted. Stay with the patient and monitor his condition. Make certain that if an AED is available it is kept nearby.

NOTE

If you are trained to administer oxygen, follow your EMS system's protocol for chest-pain patients. Sometimes the patient's pain will decrease when oxygen is administered. If this occurs, it does not mean that the patient's problem has become any less serious.

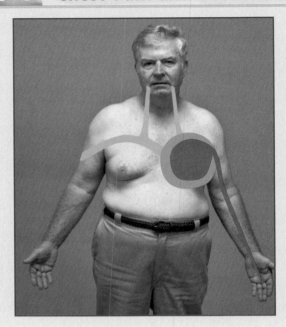

SIGNS AND SYMPTOMS

- Early symptoms generally include chest or upper abdominal sensation of pressure or burning, and are often mistaken for indigestion.
- As an attack worsens, pain may localize behind sternum and radiate to either arm or shoulder (usually the left). Pain may extend to:
  - — Hand.
  - — Neck, jaw, and teeth.
  - — Upper back.
  - — Upper, middle abdomen.
  Some patients have pain only in the jaw, neck, or arm.
- Chest pain may be accompanied by other symptoms that suggest a heart attack, including:
  - — Shortness of breath.
  - — Nausea.
  - — Sweating.
  - — Weakness.
  Pain may diminish when physical exertion or emotional stress ends or when the patient takes nitroglycerin. BP may be high or low.
- Additional signs may include:
  - — Increased pulse rate; irregular pulse.
  - — Low blood pressure (usually a result of repeated doses of nitroglycerin, which dilates blood vessels).

EMERGENCY CARE

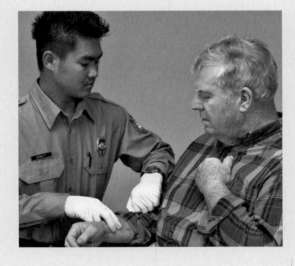

- Make certain EMS has been activated.
- Provide emotional support; reassure and calm the patient.
- Keep the patient at rest. Do not allow the patient to move himself.
- Place the patient in a comfortable position.
- Ensure an open airway and adequate breathing.
- Cover to conserve body heat, but do not overheat.
- Ask if patient took nitroglycerin, when, how much, and over what period of time (see Appendix 3).
- Contact medical facility and let them know:
  - — You have a patient with chest pain.
  - — Patient's history.
  - — If and when the patient took nitroglycerin.
- If local protocols permit, assist patient with prescribed dose of medication. Consult medical direction.
- Provide oxygen as to local protocols
- Do not leave the patient unattended.
- Monitor vital signs.

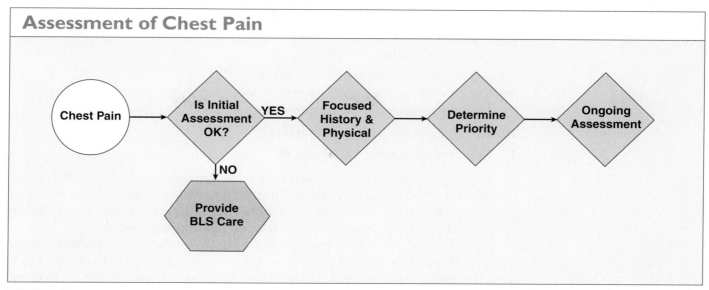

Assessment of Chest Pain

Chest Pain → Is Initial Assessment OK? —YES→ Focused History & Physical → Determine Priority → Ongoing Assessment

Is Initial Assessment OK? —NO→ Provide BLS Care

FIGURE 9.3

3. If possible, provide oxygen per local protocols.

4. Keep the patient at rest. Provide emotional support and reassure the patient.

5. Place the patient into a comfortable position. You should do all the work for the patient. This position should be one that allows for easiest breathing. Many patients with the signs and symptoms of a heart attack are most comfortable in a semi-sitting position. Ensure an open airway and adequate breathing. If the patient has sustained any kind of trauma or injury, do not cause additional problems through incorrect or inappropriate repositioning.

6. Loosen any restrictive clothing as needed for taking vital signs.

7. Cover the patient to prevent chill, but do not overheat the patient.

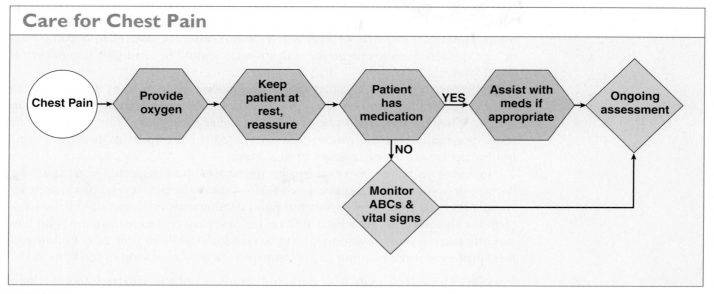

Care for Chest Pain

Chest Pain → Provide oxygen → Keep patient at rest, reassure → Patient has medication —YES→ Assist with meds if appropriate → Ongoing assessment

Patient has medication —NO→ Monitor ABCs & vital signs → Ongoing assessment

FIGURE 9.4

8. Contact medical facility staff and let them know:

—You have a patient with chest pain.

—Patient's history.

—If and when nitroglycerin was taken.

9. Assist the patient with the prescribed dose of medication (nitroglycerin), if your protocols permit. Consult medical direction.

10. Do not leave the patient unattended.

11. Continue to monitor vital signs. ■

Remember, conducting yourself in a calm, professional manner when caring for any type of patient is very important. It is of particular importance in caring for patients with chest pain who can be anxious, restless, or in denial. Their chances for survival may be increased if they can be calmed and kept rested.

A patient may ask if he is having a heart attack. It is best to respond by saying, "Your pain could be a lot of things, but let's not take chances." Do all you can to keep the patient calm and still. Do not argue with patients and do not try to physically restrain them. The stress caused by such efforts could be very harmful. Remain calm and talk to your patient, keeping eye contact whenever possible. Let the patient know that resting is an important part of his care.

Continue to comfort the patient as long as you provide care. Reassure the patient that more highly trained help is on the way. Tell the patient that you are a trained First Responder and that you will be there until further help arrives.

Medications

Normally, First Responders do not administer medications. However, some patients with a history of heart problems have been prescribed medications by their physicians to take when having chest pain. Always ask if a physician has given the patient any medications for the current problem. If medications have been prescribed, then assist the patient in taking them if your local protocols allow (see Appendix 3).

angina pectoris (an-JI-nah PEK-to-ris) chest pain often caused by an insufficient blood supply to the heart muscle.

Patients who suffer from **angina pectoris** will usually have nitroglycerin tablets or spray to take when having chest pain. This chest pain may indicate that the heart muscle needs more oxygen. Placing a nitroglycerin tablet or giving one spray under the patient's tongue will allow the drug to rapidly enter the bloodstream. Nitroglycerin dilates (enlarges) blood vessels, allowing an increase in blood flow to the heart muscle. It also reduces the workload of the heart. In doing so, the patient's blood pressure may be lowered. This can cause the patient to become dizzy or lightheaded. Patients receiving nitroglycerin should be sitting or lying down to avoid fainting.

Nitroglycerin patches, called *transdermal patches*, are named as such to indicate that the medication can pass through the skin and be picked up by the circulatory system. They are too slow to be of use in a cardiac emergency. The manufacturers state specifically that the patches are prescribed for use to help "prevent angina, not for the treatment of an acute angina attack."

In recent years, the use of aspirin for the treatment of suspected heart attack has become commonplace in hospitals and EMS systems. In fact, several pharmaceutical companies have created television and radio commercials encouraging the use of aspirin for this purpose. As a First Responder, you may encounter patients who have recently taken aspirin or who may want to take some while in your care. Follow your local protocols when assisting any patient with the administration of medication.

FIRST➤ Help all patients with signs and symptoms of a heart attack to take their own medications if they have been prescribed by a physician and you are allowed to do so (unless they have taken the prescribed limit prior to your arrival). Continue to monitor the patient and provide care, even if the pain stops. Do not cancel your request for an EMT or more advanced EMS response. ■

CONGESTIVE HEART FAILURE (CHF)

A medical emergency you might encounter that affects both the lungs and the heart is known as **congestive heart failure**. While often confused with a heart attack, it is actually a condition in which the heart cannot pump blood properly. This may be because of problems primarily affecting the lungs or the heart. In either case, fluid builds up in the lungs, leading to respiratory difficulty. In addition to the lungs, fluid can also build up in the feet, ankles, legs, and abdomen. Patients will complain of swelling associated with this fluid build up.

congestive heart failure
the condition in which the heart cannot properly circulate the blood. This causes a backup of fluids in the lungs and other organs.

Signs and Symptoms

FIRST➤ The signs and symptoms of congestive heart failure include (Figure 9.5):

- Shortness of breath. Breathing will be labored, often rapid and shallow. The rate of breathing can be greater than 30 breaths per minute. This is a serious emergency. Patients in this degree of congestive heart failure are frequently very anxious, sweaty, and their blood pressure tends to be very high. These patients may sit upright in a tripod position (sitting forward and leaning on hands or elbows).

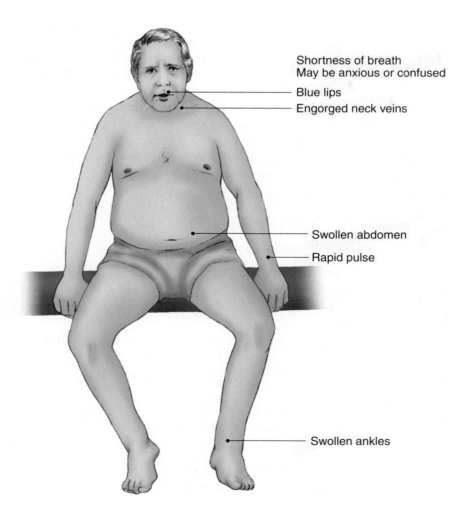

Shortness of breath
May be anxious or confused
Blue lips
Engorged neck veins

Swollen abdomen
Rapid pulse

Swollen ankles

FIGURE 9.5
Signs of congestive heart failure. Note that these signs may be the same for a patient with respiratory difficulty.

- Rapid pulse rate. The rate may be greater than 120 beats per minute.
- Swelling of the feet, ankles, legs, and/or abdomen. (By themselves, these symptoms are seldom an emergency.)
- Neck veins may appear distended or engorged.
- Skin, lips, and nail beds may turn blue (cyanotic).
- Patients may act confused if they are not getting enough oxygen. ■

Emergency Care

FIRST➤ The emergency care for a patient in congestive heart failure is the same as for most patients with a respiratory emergency (see next section). That is, maintain an open airway. Make certain that someone activates the EMS system and requests ALS services if available. Position the patient to provide the greatest ease when breathing, which is usually an upright position. This should be encouraged. If the patient is alert, he should be assisted into a sitting position. Administer high-flow oxygen by nonrebreather mask, if allowed to do so (refer to Appendix 2). Keep the patient covered to conserve body heat, but do not overheat. Reassure the patient and calm him if possible. ■

RESPIRATORY EMERGENCIES

Many conditions cause people to experience difficulty in breathing, or shortness of breath (Scan 9-2). A patient may be unable to stop breathing too rapidly (hyperventilation). Muscle spasms may cause narrowing of the airways (asthma). Or there may be a disease or condition such as emphysema, bronchitis, or pneumonia. Difficulty in breathing may stem from being exposed to a poison or something to which the patient is allergic. Regardless of the cause, a patient's breathing can be considered adequate or inadequate.

Adequate breathing is breathing that is sufficient to support life. It is easy and effortless. Patients should not have to work hard to breathe. Patients should be able to speak full sentences without having to catch their breath. Adequate breathing is characterized by a normal respiratory rate, rhythm, and quality.

Respiratory rate is the number of breaths per minute.

- Normal adult respiratory rate is 12 to 20.
- Normal child respiratory rate is 15 to 30.
- Normal infant respiratory rate is 25 to 50.

The rhythm of breathing is the pattern of the respirations. Respiratory rhythm should be regular. Breaths should be taken at regular intervals and last the same amount of time. Exhaling (breathing out) should take about twice as long as inhaling (breathing in).

The quality of breathing is how well the patient is breathing. Both sides of the chest should rise and fall equally. The depth of respirations should be adequate, and the breathing should be quiet without added sounds (for example, wheezing or stridor).

Inadequate breathing is breathing that is not sufficient to support life. Left untreated, such a condition will eventually result in death. In these patients, you may see the following:

- Rate that is faster or slower than the normal respiratory rate.
- Irregular breathing rhythm or pattern.

RESPIRATORY DIFFICULTY

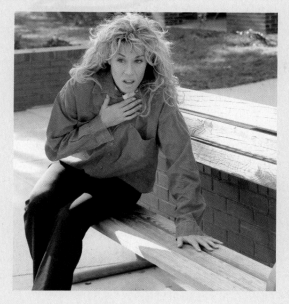

CHRONIC OBSTRUCTIVE PULMONARY DISEASE (COPD)

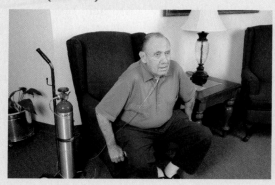

Signs and Symptoms

Usually the patient will have emphysema or chronic bronchitis.

- History of respiratory problems or allergies.
- Cough.
- Shortness of breath.
- Tightness in chest.
- Swelling in lower extremities (advanced cases).
- Rapid pulse (some cases).
- Barrel chest (some cases).
- Dizziness (some cases).
- Blue discoloration (cyanosis).
- Desire to sit upright at all times.

Emergency Care

Provide the same care as you would for respiratory distress. Be certain not to overheat the patient. Do what you can to reduce stress. If appropriate, encourage coughing.

NOTE: If you are allowed to provide oxygen, follow local guidelines for the COPD patient.

Signs and Symptoms

- Difficulty breathing.
- Shortness of breath.
- Temporary cessation of breathing.
- Rapid deep breathing.
- Noisy breathing.
- Dizziness, faintness, or unresponsiveness.
- Restlessness, anxiety, or confusion.
- Strained muscles: face, neck, chest, abdomen.
- Pursed lips or mouth open wide to aid breathing.
- Blue skin color (cyanosis).
- Stabbing chest pains.
- Numbness or tingling in limbs (hands or feet).
- Spasm of the fingers and toes (hyperventilation).

Emergency Care

1. Stay with the patient. Have someone call EMS dispatch.
2. Ensure an open airway. Check for an airway obstruction.
3. Check to see if the patient is allergic to anything at the scene. (Remove substance or move patient.)
4. Keep patient at rest.
5. Cover to conserve body heat.
6. Monitor patient and provide emotional support.
7. Administer oxygen per local protocols.
8. Assist with inhaler per local protocols and medical direction (see Appendix 3).

- Decreased quality of respirations, such as diminished volume of air taken in and exhaled with each breath, or abnormal breath sounds, such as wheezing.

Respiratory difficulty may be caused by a variety of conditions ranging from ongoing medical problems, such as asthma, to sudden illnesses, such as pulmonary embolism. Always listen to what a patient tells you about how he perceives the problem before attempting to make a determination of a patient's condition. The patient may have special medication, which is inhaled and helps certain respiratory conditions. A patient who has an inhaler will want to take the medication but may be too upset or frightened to use it properly. Some jurisdictions allow First Responders to help patients use this kind of medication. Check local protocols and always call for medical direction before assisting a patient with medications.

Signs and Symptoms

respiratory distress any difficulty in breathing.

FIRST➤ For most cases of respiratory difficulty or **respiratory distress**, any or all of the following signs and symptoms may be noticed (Figure 9.6):

- Labored or difficult breathing; a feeling of suffocation.
- Audible breathing sounds.
- Rapid or slowed rate of breathing.
- Unusual pulse rate and character.
- Changes in skin color, particularly of the lips and nail beds. Usually, the color will change to blue or gray.
- Confusion, hallucinations.

FIGURE 9.6
Signs and symptoms of respiratory distress.

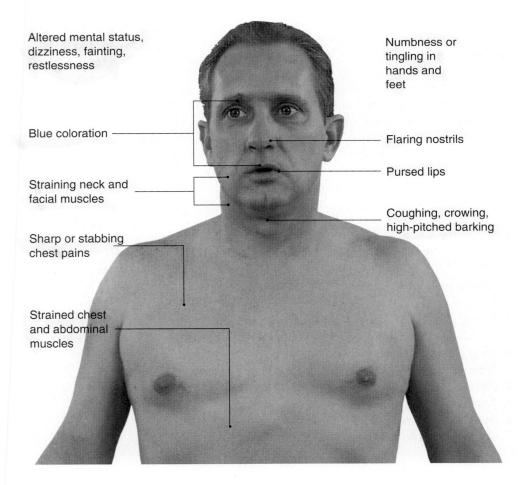

Altered mental status, dizziness, fainting, restlessness

Numbness or tingling in hands and feet

Blue coloration

Flaring nostrils

Pursed lips

Straining neck and facial muscles

Coughing, crowing, high-pitched barking

Sharp or stabbing chest pains

Strained chest and abdominal muscles

There are cases in which the patient may not have any signs and only reports symptoms. You should provide care as described below, being certain to maintain an open airway. Provide oxygen, if allowed to do so. ■

Emergency Care

FIRST➤ When caring for most cases of respiratory difficulty (Figure 9.7):

1. Perform scene size-up, including taking BSI precautions.

2. Have someone activate the EMS system. Arrange for ALS response if available. Never leave the patient alone, since respiratory arrest might develop.

3. Maintain an open airway. Administer oxygen as per local protocols.

4. Make certain that the problem is not caused by an airway obstruction.

5. Make certain that the patient is not allergic to substances at the scene. If this is the case, move the substance or move the patient.

6. Keep the patient at rest.

7. Place the responsive patient in a sitting position. Allow for drainage from the mouth. It often helps if the patient can support himself by the forearms when sitting. This eases the patient's efforts in expanding the chest.

8. Assist with prescribed medication per local protocols and medical direction (see Appendix 3). Obtain vital signs.

9. Cover the patient to conserve body heat, but do not allow the patient to overheat.

10. Continue to monitor the patient, and provide emotional support. ■

Hyperventilation

Breathing that is too rapid and too deep is known as **hyperventilation**. Most of the time, it stems from fear or stress, which may cause the patient to appear anxious and frightened. Patients experiencing hyperventilation are receiving too much oxygen and are not retaining enough carbon dioxide. This could lead to numbness and tingling of the lips, arms, and fingers.

hyperventilation
uncontrolled, rapid, deep breathing that is usually self-correcting; may occur by itself or as a sign of a more serious problem.

FIRST➤ Since most cases of hyperventilation are related to conditions of anxiety, your priority in your care of these patients is to reduce anxiety by reas-

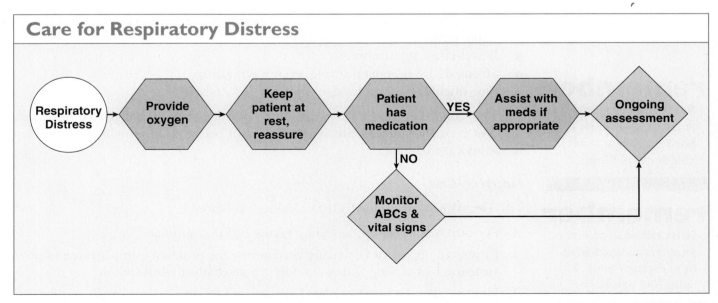

Care for Respiratory Distress

Respiratory Distress → Provide oxygen → Keep patient at rest, reassure → Patient has medication —YES→ Assist with meds if appropriate → Ongoing assessment

Patient has medication —NO→ Monitor ABCs & vital signs → Ongoing assessment

FIGURE 9.7

suring and comforting them. Encourage patients to take slow, deep breaths to slow down their breathing rate. Check with medical direction. ∎

WARNING: *Hyperventilation can be a sign of possible respiratory distress, impending heart attack, or a more serious medical condition. It will be difficult to determine if the condition is related merely to anxiety. Activate the EMS system and provide care for respiratory distress. Be alert for cyanosis (blue discoloration of the skin, lips, and nail beds) or other signs and symptoms of inadequate breathing. Monitor vital signs and be prepared in case the patient has a heart attack or respiratory arrest.*

Stay alert for changes in vital signs, which may indicate medical problems that are more serious than simple hyperventilation. Suspect that there is impending heart attack, poisoning, or other serious medical problems.

Chronic Obstructive Pulmonary Disease

A variety of respiratory conditions can be classified as a **chronic obstructive pulmonary disease (COPD)**. These include emphysema and chronic bronchitis. Other conditions, such as black lung disease, have signs and symptoms similar to emphysema and chronic bronchitis. Usually the patient is middle-aged or older, but COPD can also occur in children and teenagers.

Signs and Symptoms

FIRST▶ The signs and symptoms of COPD may include:

- History of heavy cigarette smoking, respiratory problems, or allergies.
- Persistent cough.
- Shortness of breath. Sometimes the patient breathes through pursed lips and tries to ease breathing effort by sitting forward and leaning on hands or elbows (tripod position).
- Weakness or fatigue.
- Tightness in the chest.
- Periods of dizziness (in a few cases).
- Wheezing.

In advanced cases, there may be:

- Irritability and agitation or lethargy and sleepiness.
- Rapid pulse, sometimes irregular.
- Barrel-chest appearance.
- Strong desire to remain sitting, even when asleep.
- Blue discoloration of the skin, lips, and nail beds. ∎

This condition can be very difficult to distinguish from congestive heart failure. For First Responders, this is less important because care provided by the First Responder is the same.

Emergency Care

FIRST▶ When caring for COPD patients, you should:

1. Perform scene size-up, including taking BSI precautions.
2. Ensure an open airway, making certain that the problem is not because of obstruction by the tongue or some form of mechanical obstruction.
3. Have someone activate the EMS system and report the problem as respiratory difficulty with a history of COPD.

chronic obstructive pulmonary disease (COPD) a variety of lung problems related to diseases of the airway passages or exchange levels, including emphysema complicated by chronic bronchitis.

remember

Monitor COPD patients carefully. The amount of oxygen you administer may have to be adjusted by medical direction.

remember

Do not withhold oxygen from a patient with inadequate breathing or respiratory distress, including COPD patients.

4. Help the patient into a position of comfort, and provide emotional support.

5. Administer oxygen as per local protocols.

6. Monitor vital signs.

7. Assist with medications if permitted to do so.

8. Loosen any clothing to allow monitoring of vital signs.

9. Cover the patient to conserve body heat, but do not overheat the patient. ■

ALTERED MENTAL STATUS

Several conditions may cause a patient to experience an altered mental status, or altered level of responsiveness. This would be characterized by the patient's alertness and responsiveness to his surroundings. Signs and symptoms such as dizziness or hearing loss may not always indicate altered mental status. An altered mental status may be caused by seizures, strokes, diabetic emergencies, poisonings, breathing problems, and cardiac events (Figure 9.8).

Regardless of the underlying cause, you will need to determine the appropriate care procedures by observing and questioning. To start this process, you will need to know and understand the patient's normal mental status. As you may recall from Chapter 7, the AVPU scale (alert, verbal, painful, unresponsive) is used to categorize a patient's mental status (Table 9-1).

Stroke

One potentially serious cause of altered mental status is a **stroke**, or cerebrovascular accident (CVA). Such a condition occurs when blood to the brain is obstructed or when a vessel ruptures. During a stroke, a portion of the brain does not receive

stroke the blocking or bursting of a vessel that supplies blood to the brain. A portion of the brain is damaged or destroyed by this event. Also known as cerebrovascular (SER-e-bro-VAS-cu-ler) accident (CVA).

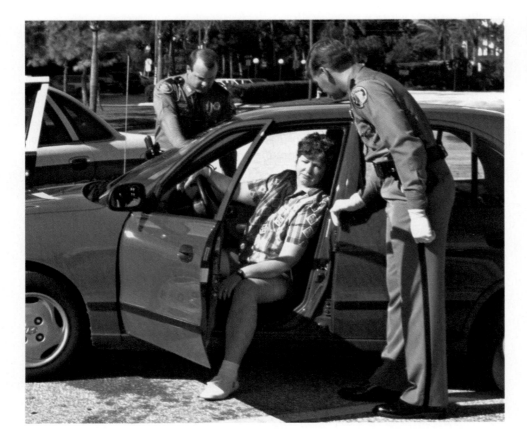

FIGURE 9.8
An altered mental status in a patient may be related to many conditions including low blood sugar.

TABLE 9-1 THE AVPU SCALE

A — Alert	Patient is awake and aware of his surroundings. Often, it is stated that a patient is alert and oriented times four (A & O $\times$ 4), which means the patient is alert and oriented . . . $\times$ 1 to person. He can tell you his name. $\times$ 2 to place. He also can tell you where he is. $\times$ 3 to time. He also can tell you exactly or approximately what time it is. $\times$ 4 to event. He also can tell you the event.
V — Verbal	Patient responds only to verbal stimuli (yelling or raised voice).
P — Painful	Patient responds only to painful stimuli (sternal rub).
U — Unresponsive	Patient is not responsive to any stimuli.

an inadequate supply of oxygenated blood and damage occurs. In some cases, this damage is so great that it may lead to death (Scan 9-3).

Signs and Symptoms

FIRST➤ There are many signs and symptoms for stroke, including:

- Headache. This may be the only symptom at first.
- Collapse or fainting (syncope, SIN-ko-pe).
- Altered mental status.
- Numbness or paralysis, usually to the extremities and/or to the face.
- Difficulty with speech or vision.
- Confusion, dizziness.
- Seizures.
- Altered breathing patterns.
- Unequal pupils.
- Loss of strength, typically to one side of the body.
- Loss of bowel and bladder control.
- Hypertension (patient may report history of high blood pressure). ■

RULE: *If a patient has any of the signs or symptoms of a stroke, including nothing more than a headache, you must conclude that the patient may be having, or is about to have, a stroke. Remember, the risk of having a stroke increases with age.*

Emergency Care

FIRST➤ When caring for a possible stroke patient, you should:

1. Perform scene size-up, including taking BSI precautions.
2. Maintain an open airway. Be prepared to provide ventilations or CPR if needed.
3. Administer oxygen as per local protocols.
4. Make sure someone activates the EMS system.
5. Keep the patient at rest, and protect all paralyzed parts.
6. Provide emotional support. Be certain to make an effort to understand everything that the patient says. Remember, the speech centers of the brain may be affected.

Altered Mental Status—Stroke: Cerebrovascular Accident

CAUSES OF CEREBROVASCULAR ACCIDENTS: STROKE

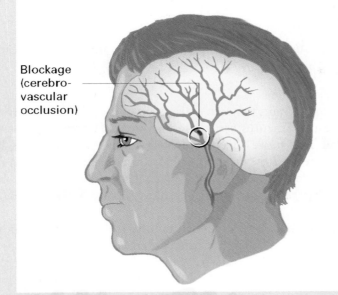

Blockage (cerebro-vascular occlusion)

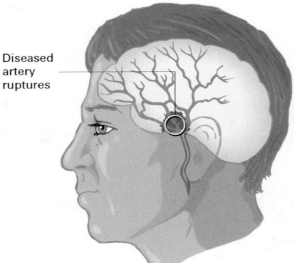

Diseased artery ruptures

CEREBRAL THROMBOSIS (CLOT)

Blockage in arteries supplying oxygenated blood will result in damage to affected parts of the brain.

CEREBRAL HEMORRHAGE (RUPTURE)

An aneurysm or other weakened area of an artery ruptures. This has two effects:

- Area of the brain is deprived of oxygenated blood.
- Pooling blood puts increased pressure on the brain, displacing tissue and interfering with function. Cerebral hemorrhage is often associated with *arteriosclerosis* and *hypertension*.

SIGNS AND SYMPTOMS OF STROKE

- Headache.
- Confusion and/or dizziness.
- Loss of function or paralysis of extremities (usually on one side of the body).
- Numbness (usually limited to one side of the body).
- Collapse.
- Facial paralysis and loss of expression (often to one side of the face).
- Impaired speech.
- Unequal pupil size.
- Impaired vision.

- Rapid or slow pulse.
- Irregular respiration, snoring.
- Nausea, vomiting.
- Convulsions.
- Coma.
- Loss of bladder and bowel control.
- High blood pressure (may have history of hypertension).

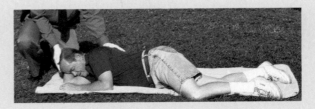

EMERGENCY CARE OF STROKE PATIENTS

- Ensure an open airway.
- Keep the patient calm.
- Monitor vital signs.
- Give nothing by mouth.
- Provide care for shock.
- Place the patient into the recovery position on affected side to protect extremities.
- Administer oxygen per local protocols.

7. Position the patient to allow for drainage from the mouth. This is best done by placing him into the recovery position. Positioning him on the affected side provides more protection for the affected limbs. Do not place a possible stroke patient in a head-down position.

8. Do not allow the patient to become overheated.

9. Do not administer anything by mouth.

10. Continue to monitor the patient. Shock, respiratory arrest, and cardiac arrest are possible. ■

Seizures

seizure irregular electrical activity in the brain that can cause a sudden change in behavior or movement.

Irregular electrical activity in the brain that can cause a sudden change in behavior or movement is called a **seizure**. Seizures can cause uncontrolled muscular movements known as *convulsions*. The more severe convulsions are called *generalized seizures*. Other seizures characterized by a temporary loss of concentration with no dramatic body movements are known as *partial complex seizures*. Older terms, still in use but becoming rare, are *grand mal* for the generalized seizure and *petit mal* for the partial complex seizure.

Seizures can be very frightening for a patient's family, friends, and others to witness. Even though most seizures do not last longer than a minute, it can seem like a much longer period to bystanders. Talk to witnesses to determine what the patient was doing prior to the seizure and if this has happened in the past. While some people have seizures on a regular basis, the patient should still be evaluated by someone with advanced medical training.

A seizure is not a disease, but a sign of an underlying condition. Some of the causes of seizures are:

- Ingestion of drugs, alcohol, or poisons.
- Brain tumors.
- Infections, high fever.
- Diabetic problems.
- Trauma.
- Stroke.
- Heat stroke.
- Epilepsy.
- Unknown.

Signs and Symptoms

FIRST➤ In cases of generalized seizure, any or all of the following may be present:

- Sudden loss of responsiveness, with the patient falling to the ground.
- Patient may report a bright light, bright colors, or the sensation of a strong odor prior to losing responsiveness.
- Patient's body will stiffen.
- Sometimes the patient will temporarily stop breathing and lose bladder and bowel control. This is called *incontinence* or an incontinent bowel or bladder.
- Patient may experience convulsions, jerking all parts of the body. Breathing will be labored, and there may be frothing at the mouth.
- After the seizure, the patient's body completely relaxes.

NOTE

Generalized seizures, or grand mal, usually last only a few minutes and consist of dramatic body movements. Partial complex seizures, or petit mal, last only 10-30 seconds with no dramatic body movements.

- Patient becomes responsive, but he is very tired and confused.
- Patient may complain of a headache. ■

Emergency Care

FIRST▶ Basic care for convulsions includes:

1. Perform scene size-up, including taking BSI precautions.
2. Place the patient on the floor or the ground. Do not force anything into the patient's mouth.
3. Loosen restrictive clothing.
4. Do not try to hold the patient still during convulsions. Your primary job as a First Responder is to protect the patient from injury (Figure 9.9). Keep the patient from striking any nearby objects.
5. After convulsions have stopped, keep the patient at rest, with the head positioned to allow for drainage in case of vomiting (recovery position).
6. Administer oxygen as per local protocols.
7. Protect the patient from embarrassment by asking onlookers to give the patient some privacy. ■

If the patient says that this is the first attack, activate the EMS system. If the patient has a history of seizures and has had other episodes, ask if you may phone the patient's doctor. It is possible that the doctor may wish to see the patient, change medications, or have the patient transported to a medical facility. Remember, the patient has the option to refuse additional care.

After a seizure, the patient will generally feel tired and weak and may not be fully alert. Do not let him wander away. It is best to keep him at rest. Provide emotional support to the patient and family members until additional medical help arrives.

Diabetes

Glucose, a form of simple sugar, is the main source of energy for the body's cells. It is carried to the cells by way of the bloodstream. However, to enter the cells, **insulin**, which is a hormone secreted by the pancreas, must be present. Insulin al-

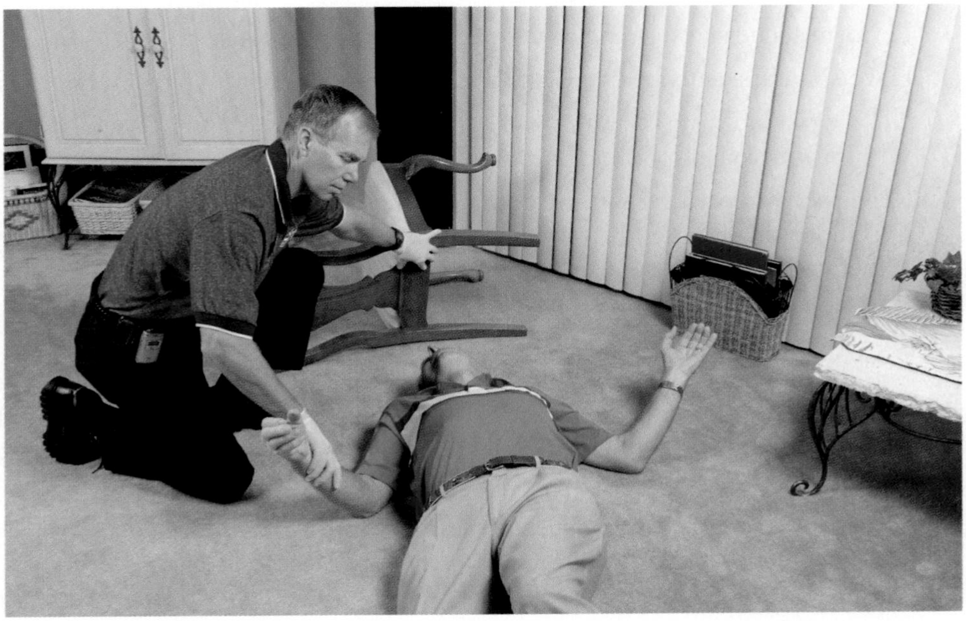

warning
Do not place any object between the teeth of a convulsing patient. Many objects, such as a pencil, can break and obstruct the patient's airway.

glucose (GLU-kohs) a simple sugar that is the primary source of energy for the body's tissues.

insulin (IN-su-lin) a hormone produced in the pancreas that is needed to move sugar (glucose) from the blood into the cells.

FIGURE 9.9
During a seizure, protect the patient from injury.

lows sugar to enter the blood cells so it can be used effectively. In normal, healthy adults this process works well to balance the glucose levels within the body.

Diabetes is a disease that prevents individuals from producing enough insulin or using insulin effectively. While some cases of diabetes can be managed by diet, others require the patient to take doses of insulin or oral hypoglycemic agents. These patients are susceptible to fluctuations in their glucose levels. (See Scan 9-4.)

diabetes usually refers to *diabetes mellitus,* a disease that prevents individuals from producing enough insulin or from using insulin effectively.

hyperglycemia a condition in which the sugar (glucose) level increases in the blood and decreases in the tissue cells. The problem can be serious enough to produce a coma.

Hyperglycemia (High Blood Sugar) **Hyperglycemia** is usually a gradual event, taking several days to develop. Should the individual not take enough insulin, or eat too much for the amount of insulin being taken, or if the diabetes has not been diagnosed, hyperglycemia may occur. It is very important that diabetics keep track of the carbohydrates they consume and relate this amount to the exercise they get and, if on insulin, the amount of insulin they take. Carbohydrates include sucrose (table sugar), as well as starches such as those found in breads, pastas, rice, potatoes, and dairy products. Through the body's manufacture and use of various enzymes, the majority of carbohydrates are broken down into glucose to provide energy to the body and to become part of many of the body's own structural carbohydrates.

NOTE

Some patients who are hyperglycemic may appear to be drunk at first. Do not conclude someone is drunk unless there is obvious alcohol abuse and you have ruled out hyperglycemia. Keep in mind that an alcoholic may also be diabetic.

FIRST➤ The signs and symptoms of severe hyperglycemia are:

- Difficult or abnormal breathing. Typically, the patient will take deep, rapid breaths, often heaving or sighing. This rapid breathing may appear to be hyperventilation.
- Dry, warm skin. Sometimes the skin may become reddened.
- Rapid, weak pulse.
- In some cases, the eyes will appear sunken.
- Sweet or fruity odor on the patient's breath, which is called acetone breath. Acetone, the same compound found in fingernail polish remover, is a deadly poison in the body.
- Dry mouth.
- Restlessness and/or stupor.
- Unresponsiveness. ■

FIRST➤ Emergency care for hyperglycemia consists of the following:

1. Perform scene size-up, including taking BSI precautions.

2. Have someone activate the EMS system. This patient will have to be transferred to a medical facility.

3. Administer oxygen per local protocols.

4. Keep the patient at rest. If the patient is alert, try to gain additional information through a focused history and physical examination. Ask if the patient is diabetic. Find out if the patient has taken insulin and has eaten recently.

5. If the patient is alert and you are not certain if the problem is too much sugar (hyperglycemia) or too little sugar (hypoglycemia), give the patient sugar, candy, orange juice, or a soft drink (make certain that the substance contains real sugar, not an artificial sweetener). Some jurisdictions may allow First Responders to give oral glucose. Check local protocols and always call for medical direction before assisting a patient with medications (see Appendix 3). ■

NOTE: *Do not give any liquids to patients unless they are fully alert. Even though guidelines still exist in some EMS systems that allow for granulated sugar to be placed under the tongue of a patient who is unresponsive, many systems have withdrawn this as part of the*

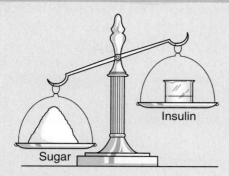

Hyperglycemia

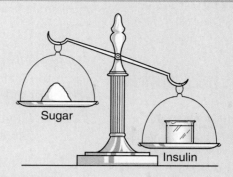

Hypoglycemia

HYPERGLYCEMIA

Causes

- Diabetic's condition has not been diagnosed or treated.
- Diabetic has not taken his insulin.
- Diabetic has overeaten, flooding the body with a sudden excess of carbohydrates.
- Diabetic suffers an infection or other stress that disrupts his glucose/insulin balance.

Signs and Symptoms

- Gradual onset of signs and symptoms over days.
- Patient complains of dry mouth and intense thirst.
- Abdominal pain and vomiting common.
- Gradually increasing restlessness, confusion, followed by stupor.
- Unresponsiveness with these signs:
  —Air hunger, or deep, sighing respirations.
  —Weak, rapid pulse.
  —Dry, red, warm skin.
  —Eyes that appear sunken.
- Breath smells of acetone—sickly sweet, like nail polish remover.

Emergency Care

Immediately transport to a medical facility.

HYPOGLYCEMIA

Causes

- Diabetic has taken too much insulin.
- Diabetic has not eaten enough to provide her normal sugar intake.
- Diabetic has over exercised or overexerted herself, thus reducing her blood glucose level.
- Diabetic has vomited a meal.

Signs and Symptoms

- Rapid onset of signs and symptoms in minutes.
- Dizziness and headache.
- Abnormal, hostile, or aggressive behavior, which may appear to be alcohol intoxication.
- Fainting, convulsions, and occasionally coma.
- Full rapid pulse that may develop into a weak rapid pulse.
- Patient intensely hungry; drooling.
- Skin pale, cold, clammy; profuse perspiration.

Emergency Care

- *Responsive patient with gag reflex:* Administer sugar, granular sugar, honey, hard candy or other candy placed under the tongue, or orange juice.
- *Unresponsive patient:* Avoid giving liquids. Give oral glucose per local protocols and medical direction.
- Place patient in the recovery position.
- Transport to the medical facility.

When faced with a patient who may be suffering from either hyperglycemia or hypoglycemia:

- Determine if the patient is diabetic. Look for a medical identification device or information cards. Interview patient and family members.
- If the patient is a known or suspected diabetic, and hypoglycemia (insulin shock) cannot be ruled out, conclude that it is possible hypoglycemia and administer sugar.

Often a patient suffering from these conditions may appear drunk. Always check for underlying conditions—such as diabetic complications—when caring for someone who appears to be intoxicated.

care for diabetics. There is a fear that some patients will vomit from this procedure and could breathe in (aspirate) their vomitus. If allowed to sprinkle sugar under the tongue of an unresponsive patient, you must sprinkle a few granules at a time from your fingers and constantly monitor the patient to ensure an open airway. ALWAYS follow your local EMS system guidelines.

Hypoglycemia (Low Blood Sugar) The diabetic who has taken too much insulin, has eaten too little sugar, or is overexerted may develop **hypoglycemia**, which usually comes on suddenly.

FIRST Signs and symptoms of hypoglycemia and developing **insulin shock** include:

- Pale, moist skin, often cold and clammy.
- Full and rapid pulse. However, some patients may have a weak pulse that is of normal or slow rate.
- Dizziness. The patient may become disoriented, faint, and go into convulsions or a coma.
- Headache.
- Normal or shallow breathing with no unusual odors.
- Being very hungry.
- Some patients will develop seizures if they do not receive early care.
- Some patients develop stroke-like symptoms, including weakness or numbness.
- As the hypoglycemia becomes more severe, the patient's mental status may become altered with dizziness, confusion expressed through behavior or speech, and repeated short-term loss of awareness. ■

FIRST Emergency care for hypoglycemia and developing insulin shock consists of the following:

1. Perform a scene size-up, including taking BSI precautions.
2. Keep the patient at rest.
3. If the patient is alert, provide sugar in the form of granulated sugar, sugar cubes, candy, orange juice, or soft drink. Make certain that the substance contains sugar and not an artificial sweetener. Do not give liquids or foods to the patient who is not responsive. The patient should be fully alert, with no signs of stupor expressed in his speech.
4. Have someone activate the EMS system. If you are not sure that you are dealing with severe hypoglycemia or insulin shock, if the patient does not respond to sugar, if this is his first case of a diabetic-related emergency, or if he began experiencing seizures or became unresponsive, be sure that dispatch has this information.
5. Care for shock, including oxygen per local protocols. ■

ABDOMINAL PAIN

FIRST The sudden onset of severe abdominal pain is sometimes called an **acute abdomen** or acute abdominal distress. The presence of pain alone is enough to indicate that the patient must be seen as soon as possible by someone with more advanced training. ■

The cause of the pain may be anything from simple indigestion to a very serious medical problem. Your role is to assess the patient and provide the needed

remember

When in doubt about a patient being hyperglycemic or hypoglycemic, follow the "sugar for everyone" rule. (See Scan 9–4.)

care, making certain that the EMS system has been activated. Do not attempt to diagnose the patient's problem. If the pain is severe enough for the patient to seek emergency care, then his problem must be considered serious.

Many medical problems are associated with severe abdominal pain. Some examples include appendicitis, ulcers, inflamed abdominal cavity membranes, aortic aneurysm, pancreatitis, obstruction of the intestine, serious liver disease, gallstones, and kidney stones. Female patients, who do not know they are pregnant, may have severe abdominal pain related to problems with the pregnancy. Detecting the exact nature of the pain is not possible at the First Responder level of care.

Do not assume that pain over the top of a specific organ means that this organ is the location of the patient's problem. Abdominal pain is usually *referred*, or spread out over one or more areas (Figure 9.10).

Signs and Symptoms

FIRST➤ Signs and symptoms associated with acute abdomen may include:

- Abdominal pain.
- Back pain.
- Nausea and vomiting.

remember

The location of abdominal pain may not be the actual site of the patient's problem.

REFERRED AND ACTUAL PAIN AREAS

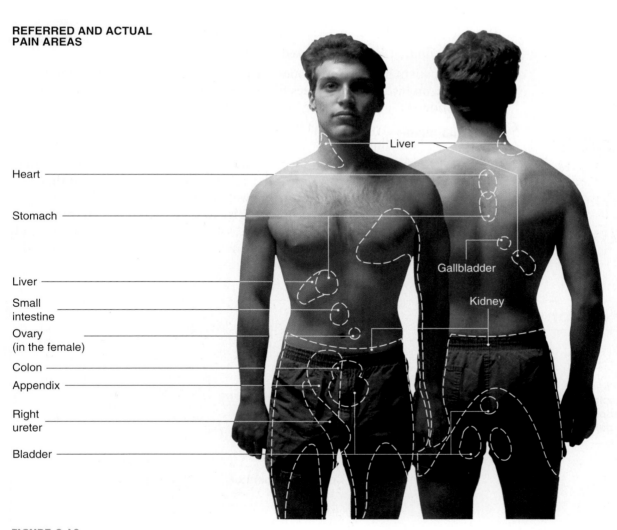

Heart

Stomach

Liver

Small intestine

Ovary (in the female)

Colon

Appendix

Right ureter

Bladder

Liver

Gallbladder

Kidney

FIGURE 9.10
Patterns of abdominal pain.

- Rapid pulse.
- Rapid and shallow breathing.
- Fever.
- Signs of developing shock.
- Guarding the abdomen. That is, the patient may fold his arms across his abdomen and draw up his knees. Usually, the patient tries not to move.
- Bulging (distention) and/or rigid abdominal wall.
- Abdominal tenderness.
- Protrusion, lump, or mass is seen or felt.
- Rectal bleeding; dark, tarry stools or changes in stools; blood in the urine; or nonmenstrual vaginal bleeding. ■

As you gather signs and symptoms, carefully watch the patient. Does he appear ill? Does he continue to guard the abdomen? Is he reluctant to move?

Emergency Care

FIRST➤ Basic care for patients with abdominal complaints requires you to (Figure 9.11):

1. Perform scene size-up, including taking BSI precautions.
2. Maintain an open airway. Stay alert for vomiting.
3. Provide care for shock, including oxygen per local protocols.
4. Make certain that EMS is activated.
5. Keep the patient at rest. Sometimes the patient's pain may be reduced if he is positioned on his back with knees flexed. Do not force the patient to assume this position.
6. Save all vomitus. Avoid contact with the vomitus, discharges, mucous membranes, and body fluids.
7. Reassure the patient and continue to gather information. Ask if the pain came on suddenly, the nature or *quality* of the pain (sharp, dull, stabbing), if there were any fevers or chills, any unusual bowel movements (dark, light, tarry, bloody, loose, or hard), or any problems with urination (inability to urinate, frequent urination, or blood in the urine). Ask the patient when he last ate and what was consumed. Make sure you document his answers. Ask the female patient about her menstrual history. ■

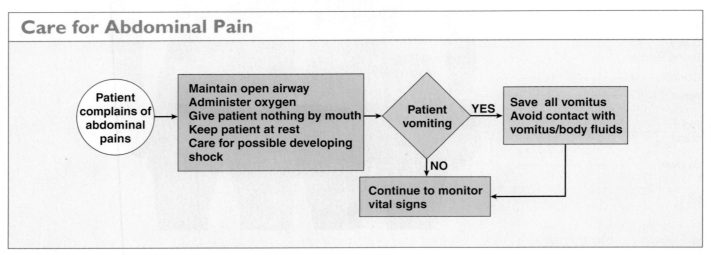

Care for Abdominal Pain

FIGURE 9.11

WARNING: *Do not give the patient anything by mouth. To do so may cause the patient to vomit.*

POISONINGS, BITES, STINGS

Any substance that can be harmful to the body is known as a poison. There are more than one million incidents of poisoning reported annually in the United States. While some cases might be related to murder or suicide attempts, most are accidental and often involve children.

ROUTES OF POISONS

We usually think of a poison as a liquid or solid chemical that has been ingested (swallowed), but there are actually four routes of exposure, or ways that a poison can enter the body. The following is a description of each:

- *Ingestion*—poisons taken into the body by way of the mouth. Ingested poisons can include various household and industrial chemicals, certain foods and improperly prepared foods, plant materials, petroleum products, medications (particularly if taken in improper doses), and poisons made specifically to control rodents, insects, and crop diseases.

- *Inhalation*—poisons taken in by breathing. Inhaled poisons take the form of gases, vapors, and sprays, including carbon monoxide (from car exhaust, kerosene heaters, and wood-burning stoves), ammonia, chlorine, volatile liquid chemicals (including many industrial solvents), and insect sprays.

- *Absorption*—poisons absorbed through the skin and through body tissues. Poisons absorbed through the skin may or may not damage the skin. Many contact poisons will do harsh damage there and then be slowly absorbed into the bloodstream. Some insecticides and agricultural chemicals can be absorbed through the skin. Corrosive chemicals may damage the skin and then be absorbed by the body. Contact with a wide variety of plant materials and certain forms of marine life can cause allergic reactions and/or damage to the skin, with the poison (toxin) being absorbed into tissues under the skin.

- *Injection*—poisons delivered directly into the bloodstream. Insects, spiders, snakes, and certain marine life are able to inject poisons into the body. Injection might be self-induced by way of a hypodermic needle. Unusual industrial accidents producing cuts or puncture wounds also can be a source of poisons being injected into the body.

Table 9-2 lists some of the types of poisons that could require emergency care. This information is provided so that you may learn more about various poisons as part of your continued training. The table is not meant to be memorized as part of your basic course.

POISON CONTROL CENTERS

There are approximately 62 regional poison control centers in the United States, most of which are staffed 24 hours a day. The staff at each center is trained to advise you on what should be done for most cases of poisoning. There are several ways the First Responder can access one of these poison control centers. The first is by calling the local poison control center directly. Your instructor can provide you with the location and phone number of the regional poison control center serving your

TABLE 9-2 COMMON POISONS

POISON	SIGNS AND SYMPTOMS
Acetaminophen (Tylenol, Comtrex, Bancap, Datril, Excedrin P.M.)	Nausea, vomiting, altered mental status (late).
Acids	Burns on or around the lips. Burning in the mouth, throat, and stomach, often followed by heavy vomiting.
Alkalis (ammonia, bleaches, detergents, lye, washing soda, certain fertilizers)	Check mouth to see if the membranes appear white and swollen. There may be a soapy appearance in the mouth. Abdominal pain is usually present. Vomiting may occur, often full of blood and mucus.
Arsenic (most rat poisons and now warfarin)	"Garlic breath," with burning in the mouth, throat, and stomach. Abdominal pain can be severe. Vomiting is common.
Aspirin	Delayed reactions, including ringing in the ears, rapid and deep breathing, dry skin, and restlessness.
Chloroform	Slow, shallow breathing with chloroform odor on breath. Pupils are dilated and fixed.
Corrosive agents (disinfectants, drain cleaners, household acids, iodine, pine oil, turpentine, toilet bowl cleaners, styptic pencil, water softeners, strong acids)	(See Acids.)
Food poisoning	Difficult to detect since signs and symptoms vary greatly. Usually, you will note abdominal pain, nausea and vomiting, gas and bowel sounds, and diarrhea.
Iodine	Upset stomach and vomiting. If a starchy meal has been eaten, the vomitus may appear blue.
Metals (copper, lead, mercury, and zinc)	Metallic taste in mouth, with nausea and abdominal pains. Vomiting may occur. Stools may be bloody and dark.
Petroleum products (some deodorizers, heating fuel, diesel fuels, gasoline, kerosene, lighter fluid, lubricating oil, naphtha, rust remover, transmission fluid)	Cough, altered mental status. Note characteristic odors on patient's breath and clothing or in vomitus.
Phosphorus	Abdominal pain and vomiting
Plants: Contact (poison ivy, poison oak, poison sumac)	Swollen, itchy areas on the skin, with quickly forming blister-like structures
Plants: Ingested (azalea, castor bean, poison, elder, foxglove, lily of the valley, mountain laurel, mushrooms, nightshade, oleander, mistletoe and holly berries, rhododendron, rhubarb leaves, rubber plant, some wild cherries)	Difficult to detect, ranging from nausea to coma. Always question in cases of apparent child poisoning.
Strychnine	Face, jaw, and neck will stiffen. Strong convulsions occur quickly after ingesting.

area. Another way is by contacting the EMS dispatcher who, in most cases, can put the First Responder in direct contact with the local center. Finally, there is a nationwide poison control number, which when called will automatically redirect the caller to the closest or most appropriate poison control center (Figure 9.12).

In some EMS systems, rescuers must receive directions for the care of poisoning patients from a physician. This is not always the case for every poison control

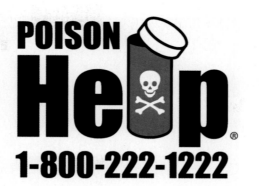

POISON
He**p
1-800-222-1222

FIGURE 9.12
The American Association of Poison Control Center number redirects the caller to the closest or most appropriate poison control center.

center. If directions must come from a physician, the First Responder should phone or radio the emergency department or EMS dispatch. You are to follow the method used by your EMS system. Remember, a nurse or the dispatcher may relay the physician's directions. You may not have a chance to speak directly to a physician.

In your jurisdiction, First Responder care for ingested poisons may include giving the patient syrup of ipecac or activated charcoal. Check local protocols and always call for medical direction before assisting a patient with these medications (see Appendix 3).

To aid the poison control center or medical direction, note and report any containers at the scene of the poisoning. Let them know if the patient has vomited and describe the vomitus (check for pill fragments). When possible, and if it can be done quickly, gather information from the patient or from bystanders before you call the center.

TYPES OF POISONS

Ingested Poisons

In cases of possible ingested poisoning, you must gather information quickly. If at all possible, do so while you are doing the focused history and physical exam. Note any containers that may hold poisonous substances (Figure 9.13). See if there is any vomitus. Check if there are any substances on the patient's clothes or if the patient is wearing clothing that indicates the nature of work (farmer, miner, and so on). Can the scene be associated with certain types of poisonings? Question the patient and any bystanders.

Signs and Symptoms

FIRST➤ The signs and symptoms for ingested poisons can be gathered during the initial and focused assessments. They can include any or all of the following:

- Burns or stains around the patient's mouth.
- Unusual breath odors, body odors, or odors on the patient's clothing or at the scene.
- Abnormal breathing.
- Abnormal pulse rate and character.
- Sweating.
- Dilated or constricted pupils.
- Excessive saliva formation or foaming at the mouth.
- Burning in the mouth or throat, or painful swallowing.
- Abdominal pain.

FIGURE 9.13
Common household poisons.

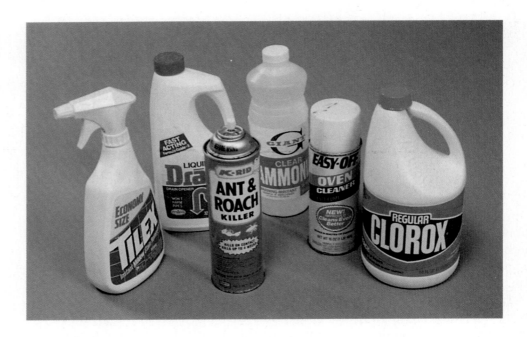

- Upset stomach or nausea, vomiting, diarrhea.
- Convulsions.
- Altered mental status, including unresponsiveness. ■

Emergency Care Contact your local poison control center to obtain advice on appropriate care for specific poisons. But do not provide any care, other than the ABCs to ensure control of life-threatening situations until you have contacted medical direction.

Emergency care directions from a poison control center may consist of diluting the poison in the patient's stomach or using activated charcoal to absorb the poison. Never attempt to dilute the poison or give activated charcoal (see Appendix 3) if the patient is not fully alert. The patient who is not responsive may not have an *intact* gag reflex. Follow your local guidelines and the instructions given by the poison control center.

FIRST> Providing liquids by mouth to ingested poisoning patients may be dangerous for some victims. This is especially true if the patient has been convulsing, or if the source of the poison is a strong acid, alkali, or petroleum product. Included in these groups of substances are oven cleaners, drain cleaners, toilet bowl cleaners, lye, ammonia, bleaches, kerosene, and gasoline. Always check for burns around the patient's mouth and the odor of petroleum products on the patient's breath. Follow the poison control center's instructions. ■

FIRST> For responsive patients, the typical procedures include:

1. Perform scene size-up, including scene safety and BSI.
2. Ensure an open airway and adequate breathing.
3. Call the poison control center or medical direction.
4. You may be directed to dilute the poison by having the patient drink one or two glasses of water or milk, or you may be directed to give syrup of ipecac or activated charcoal. Check local protocols, and always call for medical direction before assisting a patient with medications. The poison control center or medical direction may tell you to have the patient consume the fluids in sips to

warning

Always follow the poison control center's instructions before giving liquids by mouth to ingested poisoning patients.

prevent vomiting. Do not give anything by mouth if the patient is having convulsions or is gagging, unless otherwise directed by a physician or the poison control center.

5. Administer oxygen as per local protocols. Assisted ventilations may be required.

6. If supplies are available and you are directed to do so, give activated charcoal. For an adult, give 25 to 50 grams. For a child, give 12.5 to 25 grams (see Appendix 3).

7. In case of vomiting, position the patient so that no vomitus will be aspirated (inhaled). Put him on one side or in a semi-sitting position with the head turned to the side.

8. Save all vomitus. ■

In cases of ingested poisons, be realistic about the limits of emergency care. Some poisons kill quickly. Some patients can be helped only by very special antidotes, and there are no antidotes at all for some poisons. Understand that you may do your best and the patient may still die from an ingested poison.

In addition to the usual risks, if the patient has ingested a highly concentrated dose of certain poisons, such as arsenic or cyanide, and if deposits remain on the patient's lips, there is a chance the rescuer may be harmed. The current recommendation is to use a pocket face mask with HEPA filter, a bag-valve mask, or your EMS system's approved protective barrier (see Chapter 3) on all poisoning patients who need rescue breathing. Keep in mind that patients receiving a high dose of these poisons may die within minutes.

Inhaled Poisons

Gather information from the patient and bystanders as quickly as possible. Look for indications of inhaled poisons. Possible sources can be automobile exhaust systems, stoves, charcoal grills, industrial solvents, and spray cans.

Signs and Symptoms

FIRST➤ Signs and symptoms of inhaled poisons vary depending on the source of the poison. Shortness of breath and coughing are common indicators. Pulse rate is usually fast or slow. Often, the patient's eyes will appear irritated. ■

Emergency Care

FIRST➤ Emergency care consists of safely removing the patient from the source of the inhaled poison, maintaining an open airway, giving oxygen (see Appendix 2), providing needed life-support measures, contacting the poison control center or medical direction, and making certain that the EMS system has been activated. Remember to gather information from the patient and bystanders (substance inhaled, length of time exposed, early care measures, patient's initial reactions and appearance).

It may be necessary to remove contaminated clothing from the patient. Avoid touching this clothing since it may cause skin burns. Wear latex or vinyl gloves to protect yourself. ■

Fire presents problems other than thermal burns. One such problem is smoke inhalation. The smoke from any fire source contains poisonous substances. Modern building materials and furnishings often contain plastics and other synthetics that release toxic fumes when they burn or are overheated. It is possible for the

warning

Do not attempt to rescue the victim of an inhaled poisoning unless you are absolutely certain that the scene is safe. This is true even when the incident occurs outside or in a well-ventilated area. Unless you are trained to enter such a scene and have the proper equipment, do not try to provide care for a patient in a poisonous atmosphere. Do only what you have been trained to do.

substances found in smoke to burn the skin, irritate the eyes, injure the airway, cause respiratory arrest, and, in some cases, cause cardiac arrest. Do not attempt a rescue unless you have been trained to do so and have all the required personnel and equipment.

As a First Responder, you will probably see irritation to the eyes and injury to the airway associated with smoke. Irritations to the skin and eyes may be cared for by flushing with water. But your first priority will be the patient's airway. In cases of smoke inhalation, you should:

1. Move the patient to a safe, smoke-free area.

2. Perform an initial assessment and supply life-support measures as needed.

3. Provide oxygen if you have been trained and your jurisdiction permits First Responders to do so.

4. If the patient is responsive and without signs of neck or spine injury, place him in a sitting or semi-sitting position. The patient may find it easier to breathe in a different position, so let him assume a position of comfort. Always provide support for the back and be prepared if the patient becomes unresponsive.

Carbon monoxide poisoning is often present at fire scenes. This gas enters the patient's bloodstream, where it is picked up by red blood cells that should be carrying oxygen. The patient's nervous system is affected. He will complain of headache and dizziness. Other signs and symptoms include confusion, seizures, and coma. Other inhaled gases from combustion can cause injuries to the respiratory system.

Proper care requires moving the patient away from the source and the same basic procedures as would be provided for any smoke inhalation or inhaled poison victim. EMT-level care and transport are required in all cases of carbon monoxide poisoning.

Absorbed Poisons

As mentioned earlier in this chapter, absorbed poisons usually irritate or damage the skin or eyes. However, there are cases in which a poison can be absorbed through the skin with little or no damage to the skin. The patient, bystanders, and the scene will help you determine if you are dealing with such rare cases. In First Responder care, most cases of absorbed poisoning will be detected because of skin reactions related to chemicals or plants at the scene.

Signs and Symptoms

FIRST▸ Signs and symptoms of absorbed poisoning include any or all of the following:

- Skin reactions, ranging from mild irritations to severe burns.
- Itching.
- Eye irritation.
- Headache.
- Increased skin temperature.
- Anaphylactic (allergy) shock. ■

Emergency Care

FIRST▸ Emergency care for absorbed poisons includes moving the patient from the source of the poison (when safe to do so) and immediately flooding with water all the areas of the patient's body (including the eyes) that have been exposed to the poison. After flushing with water, remove all contaminated clothing (including shoes and jewelry), and wash the affected areas of the patient's skin with soap and water. If no soap is available, continue to flush the exposed areas of the patient's skin. Be certain to have someone contact the poison control center and activate the EMS system or medical direction.

If the poison is in the form of a powder, you may have to brush it from the patient's clothing, skin, and hair. It is best done with you wearing gloves and eye protection. If available, protect the patient's eyes as well. Take precautions so that the powder is not inhaled by you, the patient, and onlookers. Some inhaled powders can set off asthmatic events or anaphylactic (allergy) shock. More specific directions for chemical burns appear in Chapter 10. ■

Injected Poisons

Insect stings, spider bites, stings from marine life, and snakebites can all be sources of injected poisons. Some of these poisons cause very serious emergencies for all patients. Others are only problems for those patients sensitive to the poison. In all cases of injected poisons, be alert for anaphylactic shock (see page 261).

Poisons can also be injected into the body by a hypodermic needle. Drug overdose and drug contamination can produce serious medical emergencies. This topic will be covered later in this chapter.

Signs and Symptoms

FIRST➤ Gather information from the patient, bystanders, and the scene. Signs and symptoms of injected poisoning may include:

- Noticeable stings or bites to the skin.
- Puncture marks to the skin. Pay careful attention to the fingers and hands, forearms, toes and feet, and lower legs.
- Pain at or around the wound site.
- Itching.
- Weakness, dizziness, or collapse.
- Difficulty breathing and abnormal pulse rate.
- Headache.
- Nausea.
- Anaphylactic (allergy) shock. ■

Emergency Care

FIRST➤ Since a patient may go into anaphylactic (allergy) shock, alert the poison control center and the EMS system or medical direction as soon as possible for all cases of injected poisoning. Emergency care for injected poisons (except snakebite) includes:

1. Perform scene size-up, including taking BSI precautions.
2. Administer oxygen as per local protocols.
3. Scrape away bee and wasp stingers and venom sacs. Do not pull out stingers. Always scrape them from the patient's skin. A plastic credit card works well as a scraper.
4. Place an ice bag or cold pack over the bitten or stung area. ■

NOTE

You are responsible for all clothing, jewelry, documents, and money removed from the patient. Obtain an official receipt for these items when you turn them over to the proper authorities and include it in the patient's medical records. Your instructor will inform you of the forms used in your state.

Some patients sensitive to stings or bites carry medication to help prevent anaphylactic shock. Help all such patients to take their medications (see Appendix 3). (Your First Responder course may include training in how to administer medications by injection when the patient cannot do so. Do only what you have been trained to do.) Remember to look for medical identification devices.

SNAKEBITES

Thousands of people in the United States are bitten by poisonous snakes each year, with fewer than 10 deaths being reported annually. (In the U.S., more people die each year from bee and wasp stings than from snakebites.) Signs and symptoms of poisoning may take several hours to develop. Death from snakebite is usually not a rapidly occurring event unless anaphylactic shock also occurs. Staying calm, as well as keeping the patient calm, is critical. There is time to activate the EMS system and to provide care for the patient.

Consider all snakebites to be from poisonous snakes. The patient or bystanders may indicate that the snake was not poisonous. They could be mistaken. If you see the live snake, do not approach it to determine its species. Only if safe to do so from a distance, note its size and coloration. Unless you are an expert in capturing snakes, do not try to catch the snake. However, if possible, do contact animal control authorities.

Signs and Symptoms

FIRST➤ Signs and symptoms of snakebite may include:

- Noticeable bite to the skin. This may appear as nothing more than a discoloration.
- Pain and swelling in the area of the bite. This may be slow to develop, taking 30 minutes to several hours.
- Rapid pulse and labored breathing.
- Weakness.
- Vision problems.
- Nausea and vomiting. ■

Emergency Care

FIRST➤ Emergency care for snakebite includes:

1. Perform a scene size-up, including taking BSI precautions.
2. Keep the patient calm and lying down.
3. Have someone activate the EMS system.
4. Locate the fang marks and clean this site with soap and water.
5. Remove from the bitten extremity any rings, bracelets, and other constricting items.
6. Keep any bitten extremities immobilized. Try to keep the bitten area at the level of the heart, or when possible, below the level of the heart.
7. Provide care for shock, conserve body heat, and monitor vital signs. ■

If you know that the patient will not reach a medical facility within five hours after having been bitten, or if the signs and symptoms of the patient begin to worsen, apply a constricting band above and below the fang marks (Figure 9.14). Each band should be about 1-1/2 to 2 inches wide, placed about two inches from the wound, or above and below the swelling. (Never place one band on each side of a joint, such as above and below the knee.) The constricting bands should be from a snakebite kit or made of wide, soft rubber. If only one band is available, place it above the wound (between the wound and the heart). If no bands are available, use a handkerchief.

Constricting bands should be placed so that you can slide your finger underneath them. Do not place them so that they cut off arterial flow. Monitor for a distal pulse at the wrist or ankle, depending on the extremity involved.

Many EMS systems recommend constricting bands for all cases of snakebite. Check with your instructor.

Do not place an ice bag or cold pack on the bite unless you are directed to do so by a physician or the poison control center. Do not cut into the bite and/or apply suction unless you are directed to do so by a physician. Never suck the venom from the wound using your mouth.

NOTE

The coral snake has a small mouth. Usually, its bites are limited to the patient's finger or toe. When the bite is known to be from a coral snake, apply one constricting band above the wound site.

ANAPHYLACTIC SHOCK

Anaphylactic (allergy) shock occurs when people come into contact with a substance to which they are allergic. The body considers the substance an invader and reacts to counteract it. This is a life-threatening emergency. There is no way of knowing if patients will stabilize, grow worse slowly or rapidly, or overcome the reaction on their own. Many patients decline rapidly. For some, death is a certain outcome unless special care is provided quickly.

Many different things can cause anaphylactic shock, such as:

anaphylactic (AN-ah-fi-LAK-tik) **shock** a severe allergic reaction in which a person goes into shock. Also called allergy shock.

- Insect bites and stings, including bee stings.

- Foods (nuts, spices, shellfish).

- Inhaled substances, including dust and pollens.

- Chemicals, inhaled or when in contact with the skin.

- Medications, injected or taken by mouth, including penicillin.

Signs and Symptoms

FIRST➤ Signs and symptoms of anaphylactic shock are:

- Skin—burning, itching, or breaking out (such as hives or some type of rash).
- Breathing that is difficult and rapid, with possible chest pains and wheezing.

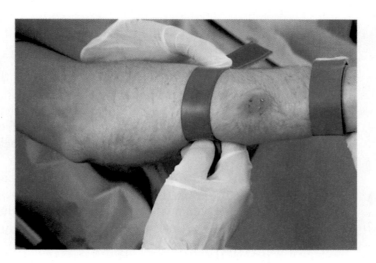

FIGURE 9.14
Constricting bands must not be too tight.

- Pulse that is rapid, very weak, or not detected.
- Lips often turn blue (cyanosis), and the face and tongue may swell.
- Restlessness.
- Changes in mental status, such as fainting or unresponsiveness. ■

REMEMBER: *When you interview patients, ask if they are allergic to anything and if they have been in contact with that substance. Look for a medical identification device, which may indicate that there is an allergy problem. If you are in the patient's residence, look for a "Vial of Life" or similar type sticker on the main entrance, the closest window to the main door, or the refrigerator door. This sticker indicates the presence of patient information and medications in a vial kept in the refrigerator.*

Emergency Care

FIRST▶ To care for patients in anaphylactic shock, follow the same procedures used for shock. (See Chapter 10.) Even though the danger to the patient may be immediate, do not attempt to transport him unless you are allowed to do so. It is usually better to wait for the EMTs to respond. In many cases, EMTs can respond to the scene and administer the medications required to stabilize the patient before transport. Some jurisdictions may allow First Responders to give medications to counteract the effects of allergic reaction or anaphylactic shock. Check local protocols, and always call for medical direction before assisting a patient with medications. ■

Patients in anaphylactic shock need medications as soon as possible. In some states, certain First Responders are allowed to transport anaphylactic shock patients immediately to a hospital. Dispatch in those areas may decide that the EMT response time is too long and recommend that the First Responder provide transport. The First Responder may be allowed to transport anaphylactic shock patients to a medical facility only if they have no injuries. Your instructor can tell you the policy for your own state or certain areas within your state. If you do transport anaphylactic shock patients, be prepared to provide ventilations or CPR.

Some people who are sensitive to bee stings or have other allergy problems carry prescribed medications to take in case of an emergency. These medications, usually epinephrine and/or antihistamines, can be administered by the patient (see Appendix 3). Your jurisdiction may allow First Responders to help the patient take medications. State laws and protocols will govern if you can assist the patient in administering the medication. Your instructor will inform you of local policies for the care of these patients.

HEAT EMERGENCIES

Exposure to hot and humid environments can cause the body to generate too much heat, which can create an abnormally high body temperature known as **hyperthermia**. Such a condition could result from a patient being outside on a hot, humid afternoon for a prolonged period of time, or from exposure to excessive heat while indoors, such as a boiler room. Left unchecked, this condition could lead to death.

The body generates heat by creating energy during digestion and metabolism. Heat is lost through the lungs and skin. The entire process is controlled by a structure in the brain (hypothalamus) that acts as the body's thermostat. It is responsible for regulating all processes to maintain a normal body temperature (98.6°F, or 37°C).

hyperthermia an increase in body core temperature above its normal temperature.

Sweating is one of the body's ways of ridding itself of excess heat. On a really hot day, you can lose up to one liter (about two pints) of sweat per hour. The sweat, in turn, is evaporated from the motion of the wind or gentle breeze. Heat is then lost at the same time. The problem develops on humid days or days without breezes, which inhibit the evaporative process.

Dry heat can often fool individuals, causing them to continue to work in or be exposed to heat far beyond the point that can be accepted by their bodies. For this reason, the problems caused by dry heat exposure are often far worse than those seen in moist heat exposure.

When dealing with problems created by exposure to excessive heat, you must perform patient interviews and assessments (Figure 9.15). A history of blood pressure or heart or lung problems may have quickened the effects of heat exposure. What appears to be a problem related to heat exposure could be a heart attack. Also, remember that certain types of patients are at risk for heat emergencies. Children, the elderly, the chronically ill, and alcoholics are especially susceptible to temperature extremes. Individuals who are taking certain heart or other medications may also be prone to such conditions along with anyone with a pre-existing illness or condition (Scan 9-5).

HEAT EXHAUSTION

The typical heat-emergency patient with moist, pale, normal-to-cool skin is a healthy individual who has been exposed to excessive heat while working or exercising. The circulatory system of the patient begins to fail because of fluid and salt loss. During this process, sometimes known as **heat exhaustion**, the individual perspires heavily, often drinking large quantities of water.

heat exhaustion prolonged exposure to heat, which creates moist, pale skin that may feel normal or cool to the touch.

Signs and Symptoms

FIRST➤ Signs and symptoms of heat exhaustion include:

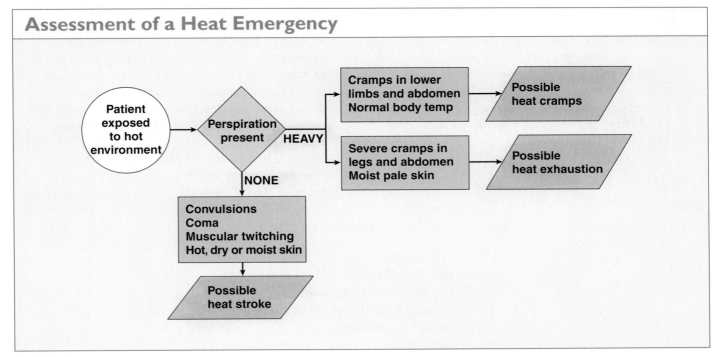

Assessment of a Heat Emergency

FIGURE 9.15

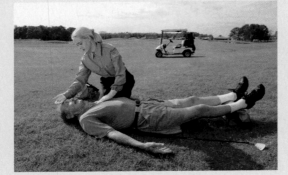

Heat cramps/exhaustion.

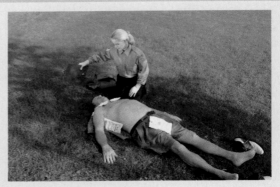

Heat stroke.

HEAT CRAMPS/EXHAUSTION

Heat emergency patient with moist, pale, normal-to-cool skin (heat cramps, heat exhaustion)

Signs and Symptoms

- Severe muscle cramps in legs and abdomen.
- Exhaustion, possible altered mental status (dizziness, faintness, and unresponsiveness).
- Weak pulse and rapid, shallow breathing.
- Heavy perspiration.

Emergency Care

- Move patient to nearby cool place. Loosen or remove clothing. Do not chill. Watch for shivering.
- Provide oxygen at 15 liters per minute by nonrebreather mask if allowed.
- Give water to the responsive patient.
- Position the patient—responsive patient on his back with legs elevated; unresponsive patient on the left side, monitoring airway and breathing.
- Help ease cramps by applying moist towels over cramped muscles or, if the patient has no history of circulatory problems, apply gentle but firm pressure on the cramped muscle.

HEAT STROKE

Heat emergency patient with hot, dry or moist skin (heat stroke).

Signs and Symptoms

- Rapid, shallow breathing.
- Strong and rapid pulse.
- Weakness, unresponsiveness.
- Scant or no perspiration.
- Large (dilated) pupils.
- Seizures or muscular twitching.
- Altered mental status.

Emergency Care

- Rapidly cool the patient in any manner. Move to a cool place. Remove clothing. Keep skin wet by applying wet towels. Fan the patient.
- Wrap cold packs or ice bags, if available, and place them at the neck, armpits, wrists, and groin (latest protocols often request only positions that touch trunk). Fan the patient to increase heat loss.
- If transport is delayed, find tub or container and immerse patient in cool water. Monitor to prevent drowning.
- Continue to monitor the patient's vital signs.
- Provide oxygen at 15 liters per minute via nonrebreather mask if allowed.

- Heavy perspiration.
- Moist, pale skin that may feel normal or cool.
- Weakness, exhaustion, or dizziness.
- Muscle cramps (usually in legs or abdomen).
- Rapid, shallow breathing.
- Rapid, weak pulse.
- Altered mental status. ■

Emergency Care

FIRST➤ Emergency care for heat exhaustion includes (Figure 9.16):

1. Complete a scene size-up, including taking BSI precautions.
2. Make sure the EMS system has been activated.
3. Perform an initial assessment. Provide oxygen as per local protocol.
4. Remove the patient from the hot environment and place him in a cool area.
5. Loosen or remove clothing.
6. Cool the patient by fanning. Be careful not to chill the patient.
7. Place the patient in the recovery position.
8. Provide emotional support and reassure the patient. ■

HEAT CRAMPS

Heat cramps are painful muscle spasms following strenuous activity in a hot environment, usually caused by an electrolyte (such as salt) imbalance. Sometimes, these cramps are accompanied by signs and symptoms of heat exhaustion. In most cases, however, the patient will be mentally alert and sweaty with a normal body temperature. The care for these victims is to simply remove them from heat and replenish fluids by having them drink water. If symptoms persist, activate the EMS system for an EMT or more advanced response.

heat cramps common term for muscle cramps in the lower limbs and abdomen associated with the loss of fluids and salts while active in a hot environment.

HEAT STROKE

Sometimes, the body's temperature-regulating mechanism fails and is unable to rid the body of excess heat. The temperature then rises significantly, causing the patient to become very hot. This condition is known as **heat stroke** and should be considered a life-threatening condition. A patient's body temperature may increase to 105°F or higher and the patient may experience a decreased level of responsiveness. The skin will be hot and dry.

heat stroke prolonged exposure to heat, which creates dry or moist skin that may feel warm or hot to the touch.

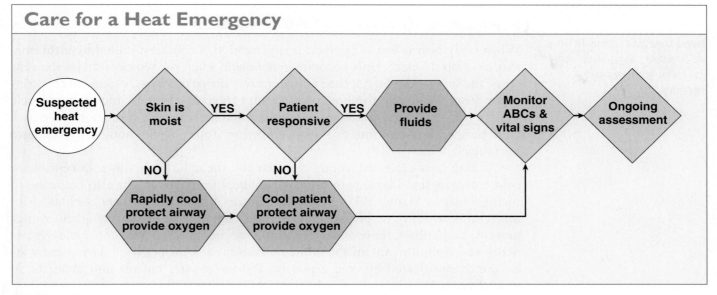

Care for a Heat Emergency

FIGURE 9.16

Signs and Symptoms

FIRST➤ Patients suffering from heat stroke may have the following signs and symptoms:

- Rapid, shallow breathing.
- Full and rapid pulse.
- Generalized weakness.
- Hot, dry skin.
- Altered mental status.
- Little or no perspiration. ■

Emergency Care

FIRST➤ Emergency care for heat stroke (hot, dry skin) includes the following:

1. Complete a scene size-up, including taking BSI precautions.
2. Make sure EMS has been activated.
3. Perform an initial assessment. Provide oxygen as per local protocol.
4. Remove the patient from the hot environment and place him in a cool area.
5. Loosen or remove clothing. Pour cool water over wet wrappings.
6. Cool patient by fanning. Be sure not to chill the patient.
7. Wrap cold packs or ice bags, if available, and place one under each of the patient's armpits, one on each wrist and ankle, one on the groin, and one on each side of the neck. Note that testing indicates that cold packs at wrists and ankles may not be useful. Follow your local protocol.
8. Place patient in the recovery position.
9. Monitor vital signs.
10. Provide emotional support and reassure patient. ■

COLD EMERGENCIES

HYPOTHERMIA (GENERALIZED COLD EMERGENCY)

hypothermia (HI-po-THURM-e-ah) a general cooling of the body. Also called generalized cold emergency.

When body heat is lost faster than it is generated, a condition called **hypothermia** may develop. Hypothermia becomes generalized when the temperature at the center of the body—the body's core temperature—drops too low. To prevent this condition from occurring, the body will attempt to compensate by increasing muscle activity (shivering) to increase metabolism and maintain body heat. But as the core body temperature continues to drop, shivering stops and the body can no longer warm itself.

As with heat exposure, young children and the elderly are more susceptible to cold emergencies. Those with previous medical problems might also be prone to such problems. Many cold exposures are more obvious than others, such as a victim who is working or playing outside in a cold environment during the winter months. Sometimes, however, the exposure can be subtle. For example, elderly patients who do not maintain the home thermostat at a proper level during the winter are often affected by cold exposure. Refrigeration accidents and incidents in mild climates also occur.

The patient experiencing a generalized cold emergency will present with cool or cold abdominal skin temperature. Place the back of your hand against the patient's abdomen to assess the general temperature of the patient. In healthy adults, the abdomen should be warm, dry, and pink.

REMEMBER: *The environmental temperature does not have to be below freezing for hypothermia to occur.*

Signs and Symptoms

FIRST➤ Signs and symptoms of a generalized cold emergency may include the following:

- Cool or cold skin temperature.
- Shivering.
- Decreased mental status.
- Initially rapid, then slow pulse.
- Lack of coordination.
- Stiff or rigid posture.
- Muscle rigidity.
- Impaired judgment.
- Complaints of joint/muscle stiffness. ■

Emergency Care

FIRST➤ Emergency care for generalized cold emergencies includes:

1. Perform a scene size-up, including taking BSI precautions.
2. Make sure that someone activates the EMS system.
3. Perform an initial assessment. Administer oxygen as per local protocols.
4. Remove the patient from the cold environment, but do not allow the patient to walk or exert himself in any way.
5. Protect the patient from further heat loss.
6. Remove any wet clothing and place a blanket over the patient. If there are no indications of possible spinal injuries, place a blanket under the patient using a log roll. Remember to handle the patient gently.
7. Monitor vital signs.
8. Comfort the patient and reassure him. While awaiting additional EMS resources, do not give the patient anything to eat or drink (including hot coffee or tea or alcohol). ■

Some cases of generalized cold emergency are extreme. The patient might be unresponsive and show no vital signs, with skin cold to the touch. You cannot assume that this patient is dead. Assess the pulse for 30–45 seconds. If there is no pulse, begin CPR immediately. Arrange for transportation to an emergency department. The doctors at the hospital will pronounce a patient biologically dead only after they have rewarmed the tissues and there is still no response.

LOCALIZED COLD INJURY

Another environmental emergency that is characterized by the freezing or near freezing of a body part is known as **frostbite**, or a localized cold injury. It is caused by a significant exposure to cold temperature (below 0°F). It mainly occurs in the extremities and in areas of the fingers, toes, ears, face, and nose (Scan 9-6).

frostbite localized cold injury in which the skin is frozen.

Cold-Related Emergencies

CONDITION	SKIN SURFACE	TISSUE UNDER SKIN	SKIN COLOR
Early, Superficial	Soft	Soft	White
Late, Deep	Hard	Initially soft, progressing to hard	White and waxy progressing to blotchy white, then to yellow-gray to blue-gray

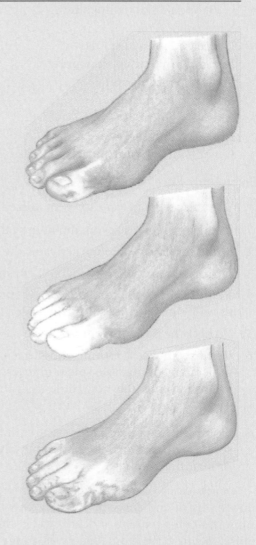

EARLY, SUPERFICIAL

Slow onset with numbing of affected part. Have the patient rewarm the part with his own body heat. Tingling and burning sensations are common during rewarming.

LATE, DEEP

Tissues below the surface initially will have their normal bounce. Protect the entire limb. Handle gently. Keep the patient at rest and provide external warmth to injury site. Untreated, this will progress to where the tissue below the surface will feel hard. Provide the same care you would for early superficial cooling. Immediate EMS transport is recommended.

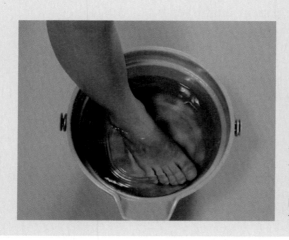

Rewarming: Only if transport is delayed in case of late or deep local cooling and if medical direction allows, rewarm the affected part by immersing it in warm water (100°F to 105°F). Do not allow the body part to touch the container bottom or side. After re-warming, gently dry the part and pad between fingers or toes. Dress the affected area, cover and elevate the limb, and keep the patient warm. **DO NOT REWARM** if there is any chance that the tissue may refreeze, usually due to extended exposure.

A classic example of a victim of a cold emergency is someone who is outdoors during the winter for a prolonged period of time. Perhaps he is unprotected by scarves, gloves, or boots. The core of the body continues to be warmed by metabolism, but the exposed areas are susceptible to the impact of cold and wind. Most patients will describe a localized cold injury as starting with a cold sensation to the extremities that leads to pain, followed by numbness. This is the classic progression of symptoms.

Signs and Symptoms

FIRST➤ Signs and symptoms of a localized cold injury may include the following:

Early

- Blanching of the skin (after palpation of the skin, color does not return).
- Feeling of cold, pain, or loss of feeling and sensation to the injured area.
- Skin remains soft.
- If thawed, tingling sensation is present.

Late

- White, waxy skin.
- Firm to frozen feeling upon palpation.
- Swelling may be present.
- Blisters may be present.
- If thawed, may appear flushed with areas of purple and blanching. ■

Emergency Care

FIRST➤ Emergency care for a localized cold injury is as follows:

1. Perform a scene size-up, including taking BSI precautions.
2. Perform an initial assessment.
3. Make sure that someone activates the EMS system.
4. Remove the patient from the cold environment.
5. Protect the patient from further cold exposure.
6. Remove any wet or constrictive clothing.
7. If it is an early injury,
   —Manually stabilize the extremity.
   —Cover the extremity.
   —Do not rub or massage.
   —Do not re-expose to cold.
8. If it is a late injury
   —Remove jewelry.
   —Cover with dry, sterile dressings.
   —Do not break blisters.
   —Do not rub or massage area.
   —Do not apply heat.
   —Do not rewarm. (Some jurisdictions allow rewarming. Check with medical direction.)
   —Do not allow the patient to walk on the affected extremity.
9. Comfort and reassure the patient. ■

remember
Do not allow the patient to smoke or drink alcohol or caffeine. These substances may affect blood vessels and worsen the patient's condition.

BEHAVIORAL EMERGENCIES

Behavior is the manner in which a person acts or performs. This includes any or all of a person's activities including physical and mental activity. The behavior of most people is considered typical or normal because it is accepted by our families and society. It does not interfere with our daily activities of life. Behavior that is unacceptable or intolerable to others is known as *abnormal (atypical) behavior.* While caring for this type of patient might be challenging, it is crucial that you remain professional and provide appropriate care.

CAUSES

A **behavioral emergency** exists in situations where the patient exhibits abnormal behavior that is unacceptable or intolerable to the patient, family, or community. Such behavior may occur because of extremes of emotion or a psychological or medical condition. Other causes of behavioral change include:

- Situational stress (patient reacting to events at the scene).
- Mind-altering substances.
- Psychiatric problems.
- Psychological crises, including panic or paranoia.

ASSESSMENT

FIRST▶ Remember, when performing an assessment on behavioral emergency patients (Figure 9.17):

FIGURE 9.17
Evaluate the scene and maintain a safe distance as you begin to ask questions and reassure the patient.

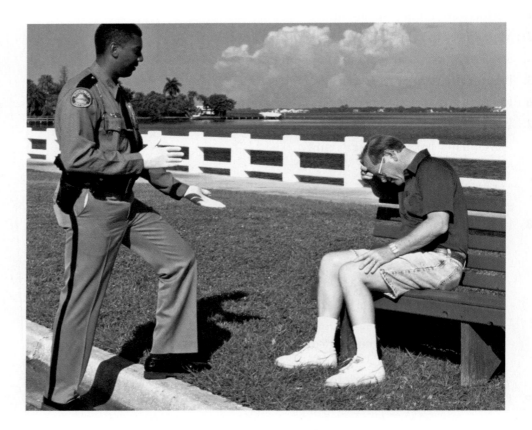

- Identify yourself and let the person know you are there to help.
- Inform the person of what you are doing.
- Ask questions in a calm, reassuring voice.
- Without being judgmental, allow the patient to tell what happened.
- Show you are listening by rephrasing or repeating part of what is said.
- Assess the patient's mental status:
  — Appearance.
  — Activity.
  — Speech.
  — Orientation to person, place, time, and event. ■

EMERGENCY CARE

FIRST➤ Emergency care of a patient with a behavioral emergency includes the following:

- Perform a scene size-up, including taking BSI precautions and considering the need for law enforcement.
- Make sure that someone has activated the EMS system.
- Perform an initial assessment by observing the patient from a safe distance.
- Acknowledge that the patient seems upset and restate that you are there to help.
- Inform the patient of what you are doing.
- Ask questions in a calm, reassuring voice.
- Maintain a comfortable distance.
- Encourage the patient to state what is troubling him or her (Figure 9.18).
- Do not make quick moves.
- Answer questions honestly.
- Do not threaten, challenge, or argue with disturbed patients.
- Do not "play along" with hallucinations or auditory disturbances.
- Involve trusted family members or friends, if appropriate.
- Be prepared for an extended scene time.
- Avoid unnecessary physical contact.

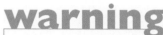

warning

If the patient creates an unsafe scene and you are not a trained law enforcement officer following SOPs, get out and find a safe place until the police arrive.

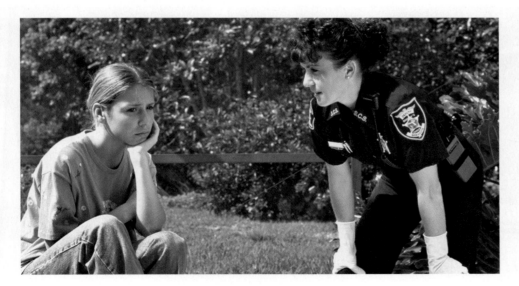

FIGURE 9.18
Encourage the emotionally distraught patient to tell you what is troubling her.

- Maintain eye contact.
- Leave yourself a way out. Never let the potentially violent patient come between you and your exit. ∎

ASSESSING THE POTENTIAL FOR VIOLENCE

Sometimes patients experience conditions that cause them to become violent and uncooperative. As a First Responder, your priority is to prevent the patient from harming himself or others while protecting yourself. Consider contacting law enforcement (Figure 9.19). You should also utilize the following when assessing the potential violence of patients:

- *Scene size-up.* Use caution when approaching a scene. Observe the patient and the surroundings for any indication that he might be a danger to himself or others. Ensure that he has no weapons or anything that may be used as a weapon.

- *History.* Often, patients who have exhibited violent behavior in the past will repeat it again. Take such past history into consideration during your assessment.

- *Posture.* How is the patient standing? Is he in an offensive stance? What does his body language tell you? Are you positioned at a safe distance?

- *Verbal activity.* Often, verbal abuse is a precursor to violence. If a patient continues to use foul language or raise his voice, consider such action as a possible warning sign for violent behavior.

- *Physical activity.* Patients may begin to pace or wave their arms in the air with increased activity. Such movements may escalate into more violent behavior.

RESTRAINING PATIENTS

In some cases, behavioral emergency patients might become violent to the point that it is necessary to physically restrain them. While this task should be avoided, it is often necessary to protect the patient, yourself, and others. In these situations, follow your local guidelines for contacting police and consulting medical direction. Remember that there may be a medical condition causing the emotional disturbance that the patient is not aware of, does not understand, or cannot control. Because of this, emotionally disturbed patients may threaten those who are trying to help and will often resist emergency care.

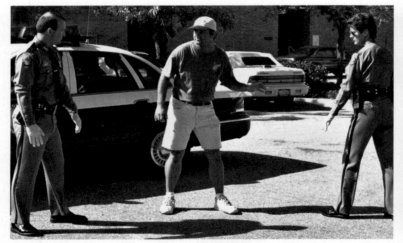 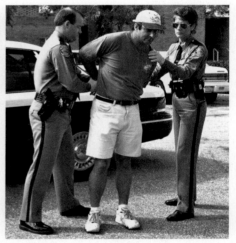

FIGURE 9.19
Law enforcement officers may be needed to approach and control a behavioral patient who may become violent.

You cannot provide emergency care to a patient without proper consent, so you must have a reasonable belief that the patient will harm himself or others and would want help if he were able to understand and consent to it. Contact medical direction for guidance before attempting to provide care for a patient without consent. In these cases, local protocols may direct you to contact law enforcement for assistance.

Do not approach a violent patient alone. While waiting for assistance, try the following:

- Talk and listen to the patient to divert his focus and keep him from harming himself and others.

- Sit or stand passively but remain alert to the patient's actions and responses.

- Avoid any action that may alarm the patient and cause him to react violently.

- Wait for law enforcement assistance to arrive if restraining the patient is necessary and let police officers take the lead in restraining the patient.

- Use reasonable force only to defend yourself against attack.

ALCOHOL AND OTHER DRUGS

For all situations involving patients with alcohol or other drug emergencies, perform your scene size-up. Your safety is especially important. Once you can approach the patient, let him know who you are and what you are going to do before you start the initial assessment and focused history and physical exam. You may have to modify your approach and communication techniques as you try to determine whether the situation also involves a medical or a trauma problem. It may be difficult to perform the detailed physical exam, the ongoing assessment, or any care procedures until you can calm the patient and gain his confidence.

ALCOHOL ABUSE

Alcohol is a drug, socially acceptable in moderation, but still a drug. Abuse of alcohol, as with any other drug, can lead to illness, poisoning of the body, antisocial behavior, and even death. A patient under the influence of alcohol is not funny. He may have a medical problem or an injury requiring your care. The patient may become injured or could hurt others while under the influence of alcohol.

As a First Responder, try to provide care to the patient suffering from alcohol intoxication as you would any other patient. It is often very difficult to determine that the problem has been caused by alcohol and if alcohol abuse is the only problem. Even trained mental-health professionals can miss making a dual diagnosis. Do not depend on the smell of alcohol on the patient's breath or clothing to be a meaningful sign, especially if the source of alcohol is vodka.

If the patient allows you to do so, conduct a patient assessment that includes a thorough history. In some cases, you will have to depend on bystanders for meaningful information. Also, remember that diabetes, epilepsy, head injuries, high fevers, and other medical problems can make a patient appear drunk.

Signs and Symptoms

FIRST➤ The signs of alcohol abuse in an intoxicated patient may include:

- Odor of alcohol on the patient's breath or clothing. This is not enough by itself unless you are sure that this is not "acetone breath," a sign of the diabetic patient.
- Swaying and unsteady, uncoordinated movement.

- Slurred speech and the inability to carry on a conversation. Do not be fooled into thinking that the situation may not be serious because the patient jokes or clowns around.
- Flushed appearance, often with sweating and complaining of being warm.
- Nausea and vomiting or feeling the need to vomit. ■

FIRST➤ A patient suffering from alcohol abuse may be going through withdrawal from having been without alcohol. Delirium tremens (DTs) may result from sudden withdrawal. In such cases, look for:

- High blood pressure, rapid heart rate.
- Confusion and restlessness.
- Atypical behavior, to the point of being "mad" or demonstrating "insane" behavior.
- Some DT patients will hallucinate.
- Gross tremor (obvious shaking) of the hands.
- Convulsions. ■

As you see, some of the signs displayed in alcohol intoxication are similar to those found in some medical emergencies. **Be certain that the only problem is alcohol intoxication.** Remember, persons who abuse alcohol may also be injured or ill. The effects of the alcohol may mask the typical signs and symptoms observed during assessment. Also, be on the alert for other signs, such as depressed vital signs, because of the patient mixing alcohol and drugs. Never ask if the patient has taken any "drugs." The patient may think that you are gathering evidence of a crime. Ask if any "medications" have been taken while drinking. Most patients, however, will not report recreational drugs or even over-the-counter medications.

Emergency Care

FIRST➤ The basic care for the alcohol abuse patient consists of the following:

- Perform scene size-up, and take appropriate BSI precautions.
- Perform a proper history and physical exam to detect any medical emergencies or injuries. Remember, alcohol may mask pain. Look carefully for mechanisms of injury and the signs of illness.
- Monitor vital signs, staying alert for respiratory problems.
- Talk in an effort to keep the patient alert.
- Help the patient when vomiting so the vomitus will not be aspirated (inhaled).
- Protect the patient from further injury without the illegal use of restraint.
- Alert dispatch and let them decide if the police must be alerted or if EMTs are to respond on their own. ■

DRUG ABUSE

uppers stimulants that affect the central nervous system to excite the user.

downers depressants that affect the central nervous system to relax the user.

narcotics a class of drugs for the relief of pain. Illicit use is to provide an intense state of relaxation.

hallucinogens mind-altering drugs that act on the central nervous system to excite the user or to distort perception of surroundings.

volatile chemicals vaporizing chemicals that cause excitement or produce a "high" when they are inhaled by the abuser (huffing).

FIRST➤ Drugs may be classified as uppers, downers, narcotics, hallucinogens (mind-affecting drugs), or volatile chemicals. **Uppers** are stimulants affecting the nervous system to excite the user. **Downers** are depressants meant to affect the central nervous system to relax the user. **Narcotics** affect the nervous system and change many of the normal activities of the body. Often they produce an intense state of relaxation and feelings of well-being. **Hallucinogens**, or mind-altering drugs, act on the nervous system to produce an intense state of excitement or distortion of the user's surroundings. **Volatile chemicals** give an initial rush, but then depress the central nervous system. ■

Some courses that train rescuers, EMTs, and others in the EMS system have spent considerable time in the past teaching specific drug names and reactions. As a First Responder, you will not need such knowledge. For you, it is important to be able to detect possible drug abuse at the overdose level and to relate certain signs to certain types of drugs. Your care for the drug-abuse patient will be basically the same for any drug that may have been used. Your care will not change unless you are ordered to do something by medical direction or a poison control center. Figure 9.20 and Table 9-3 list some of the names of common drugs that are abused, though you do not need to memorize them.

Signs and Symptoms

The signs and symptoms of drug abuse and drug overdose can vary from patient to patient, even for the same drug. The scene, bystanders, and the patient may be your only sources of finding out if you are dealing with drug abuse and the substance involved. When questioning the patient and bystanders, you will get better results if you ask if the patient has been taking any medications, rather than using the word "drugs." If you have any doubts, then ask if the patient has taken drugs or is "using anything." Patients may not give information about their drug use.

FIRST➤ Some significant signs and symptoms related to specific drugs include:

- *Uppers*—excitement, increased pulse and breathing rates, rapid speech, dry mouth, dilated pupils, sweating, and the complaint of having gone without sleep for long periods.
- *Downers*—sluggish, sleepy patient lacking normal coordination of body movements and speaking with slurred speech. Pulse and breathing rates are low, often to the point of a true emergency.
- *Hallucinogens*—fast pulse rate, dilated pupils, and a flushed face. The patient often sees things and hears voices or sounds that do not exist, has little concept of real time, and may not be aware of the true environment. Often, the patient makes no sense when speaking. Many show signs of anxiety and fearfulness. They have been described as *paranoid*. Some patients become very aggressive, while others tend to withdraw.

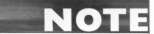

NOTE

Many drug abusers will abuse more than one drug, often mixing several at one time. It may be impossible through simple physical examination to tell what drugs are causing the patient's problem.

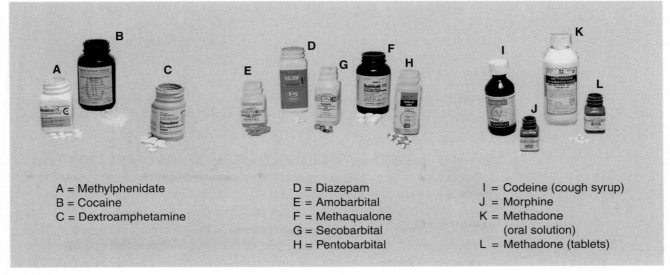

A = Methylphenidate
B = Cocaine
C = Dextroamphetamine

D = Diazepam
E = Amobarbital
F = Methaqualone
G = Secobarbital
H = Pentobarbital

I = Codeine (cough syrup)
J = Morphine
K = Methadone
  (oral solution)
L = Methadone (tablets)

FIGURE 9.20
Commonly abused substances.

TABLE 9-3 COMMONLY ABUSED SUBSTANCES

Uppers

Amphetamine (Benzedrine, bennies, pep pills, ups, uppers, cartwheels)
Biphetamine (bam)
Cocaine (coke, snow, crack)
Desoxyn (black beauties)
Dextroamphetamine (dexies, Dexedrine)
Methamphetamine (speed, meth, crystal, diet pills, Methedrine)
Methylphenidate (Ritalin)
Preludin

Downers

Amobarbital (blue devils, downers, barbs, Amytal)
Barbiturates (downers, dolls, barbs, rainbows)
Chloral hydrate (knockout drops, Noctec)
Ethchlorvynol (Placidyl)
Glutethimide (doriden, goofers)
Methaqualone (Quaalude, ludes, Sopor, sopors)
   Nonbarbiturate sedatives (various tranquilizers and sleeping pills; Valium or Diazepam,
   Miltown, Equanil, meprobamate, Thorazine, Compazine, Librium or chlordiazepoxide,
   reserpine, Tranxene or chlorazepate, and other benzodiazepines)

Narcotics

Codeine (often in cough syrup)	Meperidine
Demerol	Morphine
Dilaudid	Opium (op, poppy)
Heroin (H, horse, junk, smack, stuff)	Paregoric (contains opium)
Methadone (dolly)	Fentanyl
	Oxycodone (perc), OxyContin

Hallucinogens and Mind-Altering Drugs

Hallucinogenic	Psilocybin (magic mushrooms)
DMT	STP (serenity, tranquility, peace)
LSD (acid, sunshine)	*Nonhallucinogenic*
Mescaline (peyote, mesc)	Marijuana (grass, pot, weed, dope)
Morning glory seeds	Hash
PCP (angel dust, hog, peace pills)	THC

Volatile Chemicals

Amyl nitrate (snappers, poppers)	Glue
Butyl nitrate (locker room, rush)	Hair spray
Cleaning fluid (carbon tetrachloride)	Nail polish remover
Furniture polish	Paint thinner
Gasoline	

REMEMBER: *The most commonly abused substance in the United States is alcohol (ethanol). In addition to its direct effects, alcohol is often mixed with other abused substances, worsening effects on the body.*

- *Narcotics*—reduced rate of pulse and breathing, often seen with a lowered skin temperature. The pupils are constricted, muscles are relaxed, and sweating is heavy. The patient is very sleepy and does not wish to do anything. In overdoses, coma is a common event. Respiratory arrest may occur.
- *Volatile chemicals*—dazed or showing temporary loss of contact with reality. The patient may go into a coma. The inside of the nose and mouth may show swollen membranes. The patient may complain of a numbness or tingling inside the head or a headache. The face may be flushed and the pulse rate accelerated. There may be a chemical odor to the patient's breath, skin, or clothing. ■

These signs and symptoms have a lot in common with many medical emergencies. Never assume drug abuse or drug abuse occurring by itself.

FIRST➤ Withdrawal varies from patient to patient and from drug to drug. In most cases of drug withdrawal, you will see shaking, anxiety, nausea, confusion, irritability, sweating, and increased pulse and breathing rates. ∎

Emergency Care

FIRST➤ When providing care for drug-abuse patients, you should:

1. Provide life-support measures if required.
2. Alert dispatch as soon as possible. They should be informed that the problem may be caused by drugs.
3. Administer oxygen as per local protocols.
4. Monitor vital signs and be alert for respiratory arrest.
5. Talk to the patient to gain his confidence and to maintain his level of responsiveness.
6. Protect the patient from further harm.
7. Continue to reassure the patient throughout all phases of care. ∎

Medical direction in your area may require you to induce vomiting if an overdose is suspected within 30 minutes of your arrival at the scene. Your instructor will give you the protocols and exceptions for your area. For all cases of possible drug overdose, it is good practice to contact medical direction and your local poison control center.

CAUTION: *Many drug abusers may appear calm at first and then become violent as time passes. Always be on the alert and be ready to protect yourself. If the patient creates an unsafe scene and you are not a trained law enforcement officer, get out and find a safe place to wait until the police arrive.*

CAUTION: *Always consider PCP users dangerous, even when they appear to be calm. PCP usage leads to aggressive behavior. The drug can build up in the body and cause a violent reaction without warning. If PCP is the cause of the problem, wait for police to arrive, unless the patient is unresponsive or in need of life-support measures.*

remember
For all cases of possible drug overdose, first contact medical direction. Then contact your local poison control center if protocol directs you to do so.

Chapter Review

Various illnesses and conditions can bring about a **medical emergency.** The signs and symptoms gained from patient assessment and history-taking will help you recognize a medical emergency. Abnormal pulse, breathing, skin color, and temperature are some of the important signs in determining a medical emergency. Note lip color, any odors of the breath, abdominal tenderness, nausea, vomiting, bleeding, and altered mental status, which are also important signs. Listen to the patient and bystanders for reports of other symptoms, including pain, fever, nausea, dizziness, shortness of breath, problems with bowel and bladder activities, burning sensations, thirst, hunger, and odd tastes in the mouth. Look for medical identification devices and question the patient. There may be medication that should be taken during medical emergencies.

If the patient appears or says he feels unusual or has unusual vital signs and there is no injury present, conclude that there is a medical emergency. An injury can mask a medical emergency or problem. Always check for medical emergencies.

Consider chest pain in any patient as a possible **heart attack.** Ask if the patient has chest, arm, neck, or jaw pain. Nausea, shortness of breath, sweating, and weakness also may indicate a heart attack. Alert dispatch. Keep the patient at rest and in a position to ease difficult breathing. Loosen restrictive clothing and prevent chill. Monitor vital signs and provide emotional support.

Respiratory difficulties, including those seen in **congestive heart failure,** may produce the same signs and symptoms regardless of the cause of the distress. Check for labored breathing, unusual breath sounds, rate, and quality. Make sure there is no airway obstruction. Skin color change is an important sign in serious cases. Check for altered mental status. Look for swelling at the ankles and engorged neck veins, which may indicate congestive heart failure.

In all cases of respiratory difficulty, have someone call dispatch. Care for all respiratory difficulty cases by maintaining an open airway and making sure the patient is breathing adequately. Place the patient in a sitting position and conserve body heat. Keep the patient at rest and provide emotional support.

Numerous conditions can cause a patient to experience an **altered mental status:** seizures, strokes, diabetic emergencies, poisonings, breathing problems, and cardiac events. Signs and symptoms of an altered mental status include dizziness, impaired speech, hearing loss, confusion, or rapid mood changes. To check patient status, use the AVPU scale to categorize a patient's level of responsiveness.

A **stroke** patient may complain of nothing more than a headache. Consider all headaches to be a serious complaint. In cases of possible stroke, you may notice altered mental status, numbness or paralysis, speech or vision difficulty, confusion, convulsions, breathing difficulty, or unequal pupils. Maintain an open airway, keep the patient at rest, and place in the recovery position. Protect all paralyzed limbs. Provide emotional support and monitor vital signs.

A seizure patient may have a sudden loss of responsiveness and collapse. The body will stiffen and there may be a loss of bowel and bladder control. Convulsions may occur, followed by body limpness. On regaining responsiveness, the patient is usually confused and tired. Protect the patient from physical harm during the seizure and from embarrassment after the seizure. Keep the patient at rest.

Diabetics may have trouble with **hyperglycemia** or **hypoglycemia.** In both cases, the patient may become unresponsive and go into a coma. In severe hyperglycemia, expect to find labored breathing with a fruity or sweet odor on the breath, rapid and weak pulse, and dry and warm skin. In severe hypoglycemia, there is no labored breathing and no fruity odor, but the pulse is strong and rapid, and skin is cold and moist. The only indication of a diabetes-related problem may be an altered mental status. Activate EMS and keep the patient at rest. When in doubt as to whether the condition is hyperglycemia or hypoglycemia, give the patient sugar.

In the case of an **acute abdomen,** keep the patient at rest and as comfortable as possible. Monitor for vomiting, give nothing by mouth, and activate EMS.

Anaphylactic (allergy) shock is a life-threatening emergency. It is brought about when people come into contact with a substance to which they are allergic (bee stings, insect bites, chemicals, foods, dusts, pollens, drugs). Signs may include burning or itching skin, breaking out (hives), rapid and difficult breathing, very weak pulse, swelling of the face and tongue, blue lips, and sudden loss of responsiveness. Care for anaphylactic shock is the same as for other cases of shock. Transport the patient to a hospital as soon as possible and care for the patient according to local protocol. Ask the patient about allergies during the interview. Be certain to look for a medical identification device.

When dealing with a possible poisoning, look for evidence of the nature of the poison. Signs and symptoms associated with **ingested poisons** include burns or stains around the patient's mouth, unusual breathing and pulse rate, and sweating. Abdominal pain, nausea, and vomiting are common. (Save all vomitus.) **Inhaled poisons** can cause shortness of breath or coughing, irritated eyes, rapid or slow pulse rate, and changes in skin color. **Absorbed poisons** can be severe, irritating or damaging to the skin and eyes. **Injected poisons** usually cause pain and swelling at the site, difficulty breathing, and abnormal pulse rate.

In cases of poisoning, contact the poison control center and medical direction. (Follow your EMS guidelines.) Emergency care of ingested poisons may include diluting with water or milk, or using activated charcoal to absorb the poison. Be prepared for vomiting. If an unresponsive patient vomits or convulses, assure an open airway and alert the EMTs.

In cases of inhaled poisons, remove the patient from the source (when safe to do so), provide life-support measures as needed, and remove contaminated clothing. For absorbed poisons, remove the patient from the source, flush with water all areas of the body that came into contact with the poison, and remove contaminated clothing and jewelry. When providing care for injected poisons other than snakebite, care for shock, scrape away stingers and venom sacs, and place an ice bag or cold pack over the area. For snakebite, keep the patient calm and lying down, clean the site, keep bitten extremities immobilized, alert the dispatcher, and provide care for shock.

A hot and humid environment may cause the body to generate too much heat, which can create an abnormally high body temperature, known as **hyperthermia. Heat exhaustion** results from prolonged exposure to heat, which creates moist, pale skin that may feel normal or cool to the touch. Signs and symptoms include excessive sweating, rapid weak pulse, weakness, and possible altered mental status. **Heat stroke** results from prolonged exposure to heat and causes hot, dry or moist skin, altered mental status, and rapid breathing. This is a life-threatening emergency. Emergency care for heat emergencies includes removing patients from the hot environment, cooling them with water, and fanning them. Alert dispatch.

In cold environments, body heat may be lost faster than it can be generated. Rapid heat loss creates a state of low body temperature known as **hypother-mia,** or a **generalized cold emergency.** Patients will have cool skin temperature, shivering, decreased mental status, stiff or rigid posture, and poor judgment. The environmental temperature does not have to be below freezing for hypothermia to occur. Another environmental emergency that is characterized by the freezing or near freezing of a body part is known as a **localized cold injury,** or **frostbite.** Frostbite patients will experience a feeling of cold followed by pain and finally numbness or tingling. Emergency care includes removing the patient from the cold environment, removing any wet clothes, keeping the patient calm and warm, and stabilizing any cold extremity.

First Responders might encounter patients whose behavior is unacceptable or intolerable to others. This is known as **abnormal** (atypical) **behavior.** There are many causes for a patient to act in this manner, such as stress, mind-altering substances, psychiatric problems, psychological crises, and medical causes. When assessing a patient with abnormal behavior, it is important to use methods of keeping the patient calm.

Patients may experience conditions that cause them to become violent and uncooperative. Exercise caution when approaching these patients. Consider any past history of behavioral difficulties or violence. Remember that a patient's posture and verbal activity may be warning signs of potential violent behavior. Notify law enforcement to assist you in dealing with these patients.

In some cases, behavioral emergency patients might become violent to the point that it is necessary to physically restrain them, but the patient must be endangering himself or others in order for First Responders to have the legal right to restrain him.

Patients suffering from **alcohol abuse** should receive the same professional level of care as any other patient. The problem may be because of alcohol or alcohol withdrawal, but there may be a medical problem or injuries. Try to detect the odor of alcohol, slurred speech, swaying, and unsteadiness of movement. Find out if the patient is nauseated. Be alert for vomiting. In cases of alcohol withdrawal, look for tremors that may indicate the DTs. In all cases of alcohol abuse, monitor vital signs and be alert for respiratory arrest.

Drug abuse can show itself in many ways, depending on the drug, the patient, and whether it is withdrawal or overdose. Withdrawal from most drugs will produce shaking, anxiety, nausea, confusion, irritability, sweating, and increased pulse and breathing rates.

In cases of drug overdose or drug withdrawal, provide life support as needed and alert dispatch. Monitor vital signs and talk to the patient. Protect the patient and provide care for shock. Reassure the patient through the entire process.

Medical emergencies are very common. As a First Responder, you will more than likely encounter many patients with medical complaints. In this chapter and in your classes, you will discuss how to assess these patients and manage certain specific conditions. Remember the overview of medical emergencies and how to approach a victim with a generalized medical complaint or a specific illness.

- What will you do for a victim of a seizure in a public place?

- What are the various causes of an altered mental status?
- Are your CPR skills up to date?
- How do you feel about providing care to a patient who is experiencing a behavioral emergency?

You should feel comfortable answering these questions. Review what you have learned in this chapter and in class and try applying it to your life. How will these things be useful to you, your coworkers, family, friends, and others?

Regardless of where you live or what type of job you have, you should be prepared to handle any medical emergency. Remember, by definition, an emergency happens when and where you least expect it. There are several things you may be able to predict and prepare for ahead of time, based on the area in which you live. For example, many areas in the United States are exposed to extreme heat and humidity conditions.

- What are the major types of medical emergencies you might encounter in your area?
- What can you do to prepare for an emergency in your area or organization?

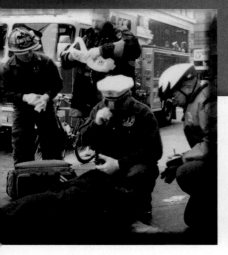
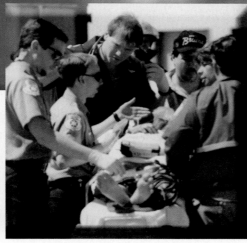
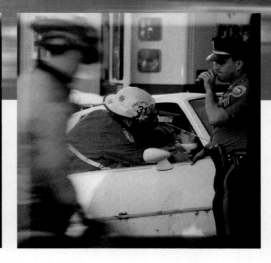

Bleeding, Shock, and Soft-Tissue Injuries

The leading cause of death in the United States for people under forty is trauma. As a First Responder, you will be called upon to provide emergency care to trauma patients with injuries that range from minor to life threatening. Early assessment and intervention is crucial to the proper care of these patients. As a First Responder, you must know how the body responds to bleeding, how to help keep bleeding under control, and how to manage shock.

This chapter covers bleeding, shock, and various soft-tissue injuries and provides descriptions of the skills you will need to care for such emergencies.

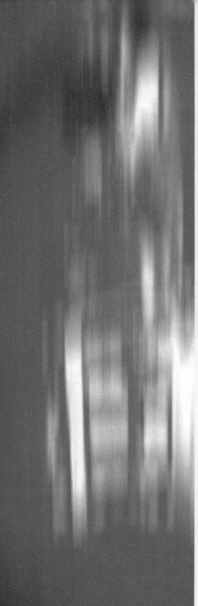

NATIONAL STANDARD OBJECTIVES

This chapter focuses on the objectives of Module 5, Lesson 5-2, of the U.S. DOT's First Responder National Standard Curriculum and serves as an instructional aid to help you meet any specific objectives added to the course by your local EMS system.

By the end of this chapter, you will be able to (from cognitive or knowledge information):

5–2.1 Differentiate between arterial, venous, and capillary bleeding. (pp. 287–288)

5–2.2 State the emergency medical care for external bleeding. (pp. 288–297)

5–2.3 Establish the relationship between body substance isolation (BSI) and bleeding. (p. 287)

5–2.4 List the signs of internal bleeding. (pp. 302–305)

5–2.5 List the steps in the emergency medical care of the patient with signs and symptoms of internal bleeding. (pp. 305–306)

5–2.6 Establish the relationship between body substance isolation (BSI) and soft-tissue injuries. (p. 319)

5–2.7 State the types of open soft-tissue injuries. (pp. 315–317)

5–2.8 Describe the emergency medical care of the patient with a soft-tissue injury. (pp. 318–320)

5–2.9 Discuss the emergency medical care considerations for a patient with a penetrating chest injury. (pp. 335–337)

5–2.10 State the emergency medical care considerations for a patient with an open wound to the abdomen. (pp. 337–338)

5–2.11 Describe the emergency medical care for an impaled object. (p. 337)

5–2.12 State the emergency medical care for an amputation. (pp. 322–323)

5–2.13 Describe the emergency medical care for burns. (pp. 339–347)

5–2.14 List the functions of dressing and bandaging. (pp. 297–301)

Feel comfortable enough to (by changing attitudes, values, and beliefs):

5–2.15 Explain the rationale for body substance isolation when dealing with bleeding and soft-tissue injuries. (p. 287)

LEARNING TASKS

This chapter explains the functions of blood and the blood vessels, and describes the effects bleeding has on the body. You will need to understand the relationship between profuse bleeding and shock. As you work through this chapter, you will also need to know and recognize:

✔ Differences between internal and external bleeding and what actions should be taken for each during the initial assessment.

✔ Methods used to control profuse bleeding versus the methods used to control mild bleeding.

You will learn how to perform the steps of controlling bleeding, including:

✔ How to apply direct pressure.

✔ Use of elevation in controlling external bleeding, including the situations when elevation should *not* be used.

✔ How to apply a pressure dressing.

✔ Use of the two major pressure points.

5–2.16 Attend to the feelings of the patient with a soft-tissue injury or bleeding. (pp. 312, 314–315, 320, 327, 328, 329, 339, 347)

5–2.17 Demonstrate a caring attitude towards patients with a soft-tissue injury or bleeding who request emergency medical services. (pp. 312, 314–315, 320, 327, 328, 329, 339, 347)

5–2.18 Place the interests of the patient with a soft-tissue injury or bleeding as the foremost consideration when making any and all patient-care decisions. (pp. 287, 295, 297, 302, 303, 306–307, 318–319)

5–2.19 Communicate with empathy to patients with a soft-tissue injury or bleeding, as well as with family members and friends of the patient. (pp. 312, 314–315, 320, 327, 328, 329, 339, 347)

Show how to
(through psychomotor skills):

5–2.20 Demonstrate direct pressure as a method of emergency medical care for external bleeding. (p. 289)

5–2.21 Demonstrate the use of diffuse pressure as a method of emergency medical care for external bleeding. (pp. 291–292)

5–2.22 Demonstrate the use of pressure points as a method of emergency medical care for external bleeding. (pp. 293–295)

5–2.23 Demonstrate the care of the patient exhibiting signs and symptoms of internal bleeding. (pp. 305–306)

5–2.24 Demonstrate the steps in the emergency medical care of open soft-tissue injuries. (pp. 318–320)

5–2.25 Demonstrate the steps in the emergency medical care of a patient with an open chest wound. (pp. 335–337)

5–2.26 Demonstrate the steps in the emergency medical care of a patient with open abdominal wounds. (pp. 337–338)

5–2.27 Demonstrate the steps in the emergency medical care of a patient with an impaled object. (p. 337)

5–2.28 Demonstrate the steps in the emergency medical care of a patient with an amputation. (pp. 322–323)

5–2.29 Demonstrate the steps in the emergency medical care of an amputated part. (p. 323)

✔ Why tourniquets are used as a last resort, only after other methods to control bleeding have failed.

✔ Step-by-step procedure for applying a tourniquet, including all precautions relating to the procedure.

✔ Procedures used to care for:
  – Cuts, burns, and foreign objects in the eye.
  – Impaled objects.
  – Injuries to the ear.
  – Nosebleeds and other soft tissue injuries to the face.
  – Injuries to the mouth.
  – Bleeding from the neck.
  – Injuries to the genitalia.

It will be important for you to learn about internal bleeding, what causes it, and how it can affect the body. As you gain knowledge, you will also be able to:

✔ Define shock.
✔ List the signs and symptoms of shock.

☑ Describe the step-by-step procedures used to care for shock.

☑ Describe how to reduce a patient's chances of fainting.

As you work through this chapter, you will learn about the assessment and care of burns and will be able to:

☑ Distinguish among superficial, partial-thickness, and full-thickness burns.

☑ Use the rule of nines.

☑ Demonstrate the appropriate care for burn injuries.

HEART, BLOOD, AND BLOOD VESSELS

THE HEART

The heart is the center of the circulatory system. It pumps blood through the many miles and types of vessels to all the body's tissues, organs, and systems. If the heart stops functioning, as in cardiac arrest, blood does not circulate or carry fuel to the body's parts, and they die.

The heart has four separate chambers (Figure 10.1). The top two are called *atria* (plural), or the right and left *atrium* (singular). The right atrium receives de-oxygenated blood from the body; the left atrium receives oxygenated blood from

FIGURE 10.1
The heart.

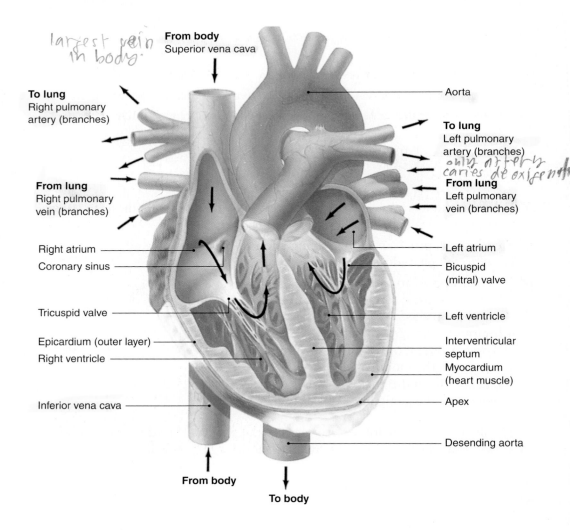

the lungs. The bottom two chambers are called *ventricles* (plural), or the right or left *ventricle* (singular). The right ventricle receives the deoxygenated blood from the right atrium and pumps it to the lungs through the *pulmonary artery* (the only artery that carries deoxygenated blood and is named so because arteries carry blood away from the heart). The left ventricle receives oxygenated blood from the left atrium, which received it from the lungs through the *pulmonary veins* (the only veins that carry oxygenated blood and so named because veins carry blood to the heart).

The ventricles are larger than the atria because they do the more difficult task of pumping blood to the lungs and body. The atria only have to pump blood to the ventricles below them. The left ventricle pumps blood to the body, leaving the heart by way of the *aorta*. The venous system carries blood from the body back to the heart, entering by way of the *superior vena cava* and *inferior vena cava*.

BLOOD

Blood performs many functions necessary to sustain life. Blood carries oxygen to the body's cells and carries away carbon dioxide (Figure 10.2). It transports nutrients to the cells and carries away certain waste products. The blood contains cells that destroy bacteria and cells that produce substances that help resist infection. There are elements in the blood that act with calcium and chemical factors to combine blood cells and form sticky clots around cuts to help control bleeding. Compounds carried in the blood called *hormones*, such as insulin, regulate many body activities. Without blood circulating through your body, you would quickly die.

The functions of blood are to:

- Carry oxygen and carbon dioxide.
- Carry food to the tissues (nutrition).
- Carry wastes from the tissues to the organs of excretion—kidneys, lungs, and liver.
- Carry hormones, water, salts, and other compounds needed to keep the body's functions in balance (body regulation). *Insulin is hormone.*
- Protect against disease-causing organisms (defense).

Blood contains red blood cells, white blood cells, and elements involved in forming blood clots. All of these are carried by a watery, salty fluid called **plasma**. The volume of blood in the typical adult's body is approximately six liters (about 12 pints). When bleeding occurs, the body not only loses blood cells and clotting elements, it also loses plasma and total fluid volume. This loss can be very signifi-

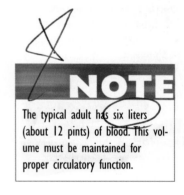

NOTE

The typical adult has six liters (about 12 pints) of blood. This volume must be maintained for proper circulatory function.

plasma (PLAZ-mah) the fluid portion of the blood.

FIGURE 10.2
The blood vessels.

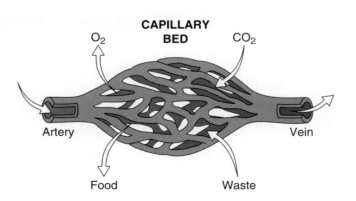

CAPILLARY BED

O₂

CO₂

Artery

Vein

Food

Waste

cant since the volume of blood must be maintained at a certain level in order to have proper heart action, blood flow, and exchange between the blood and the body's cells. The body has more blood than is needed to produce minimum circulation. During bleeding, once this reserve is gone, the patient experiences circulatory system collapse, followed very quickly by death. See Table 10-1 for blood volumes and lethal blood loss volumes for adults, children, and infants.

BLOOD VESSELS

artery any blood vessel that carries blood away from the heart.

Arteries carry blood away from the heart and to the tissues, organs, and systems of the body. The largest artery is the *aorta*. The smallest artery is called an *arteriole*. All other sizes are just referred to as arteries. At certain points on the body, where arteries are close to the skin surface, you can feel the blood pumping through the artery. These points are called *pulse points*, places where you can feel the pumping heart at work and assess pulse rate.

vein any blood vessel that returns blood to the heart.

Veins carry blood from the tissues, organs, and systems of the body back to the heart. The largest veins are the superior and inferior vena cava. The smallest vein is called a *venule*. All other sizes are just referred to as veins. On some parts of the arms (inside the wrist and elbow) and legs (lower leg and ankle), and sometimes the face (temple), you can see the blue of veins showing through skin where they are close to the surface. Veins appear blue because they are carrying deoxygenated blood.

capillary the microscopic blood vessels that connect arteries to veins; where exchange takes place between the bloodstream and the body tissues.

The oxygen and nutrients carried by arteries are passed off to body cells when the blood reaches a small system of vessels called **capillaries**. Capillaries act as an exchange point for nutrients and wastes. Some of our organs act as disposal and maintenance organs, such as the kidneys and liver, but the heart is the organ that works with the lungs to replenish the oxygen. Once the blood has dropped off all its supply of oxygen for the body's cells to use, it travels from the capillary system into the veins and back to the heart, through the lungs to pick up oxygen, and back to the heart again to be pumped through vessels to the body. By the time blood reaches the capillaries, pressure and speed are greatly reduced and the beating action of the heart no longer causes pulsations. Blood moving through the capillaries in a constant flow is called **perfusion**. (A reduction in blood volume can seriously affect perfusion.)

perfusion the constant flow of blood through the capillaries.

FIRST➤ For now, you should know:

- *Arteries*—carry blood away from the heart.
- *Veins*—return blood to the heart.
- *Capillaries*—where oxygen, nutrient, and waste exchange takes place. ■

TABLE 10-1 BLOOD VOLUMES AND SERIOUS BLOOD LOSS

PATIENT	TOTAL BLOOD VOLUME	LETHAL BLOOD LOSS (RAPID)
Adult male (154 pounds)	6.6 liters	2.2 liters
Adolescent (105 pounds)	3.3 liters	1.3 liters
Child (early to late childhood: depends on size)	1.5 to 2.0 liters	0.5 to 0.7 liters
Infant (newborn, normal weight range)	300+ milliliters	30 to 50 milliliters

BLEEDING

Having an idea of how blood and blood vessels work within the body will assist you in assessing patients with bleeding problems. Keep these general considerations in mind while learning how to care for these patients:

- *Body substance isolation (BSI) precautions*—The risk of infectious disease should be kept at the forefront when caring for bleeding patients. BSI precautions must be taken routinely to avoid skin and mucus contact with bodily fluids. Gloves should be worn during every patient encounter. Additional equipment (goggles, gown, mask) should also be used when there is an increased risk of contact with blood or other body fluids (for example, childbirth).

- *Severity of blood loss*—The severity of blood loss should be based on the patient's signs and symptoms and an estimation of blood loss. If signs and symptoms of shock are present, bleeding should be considered serious.

- *Body's normal response to bleeding*—The body's automatic response to bleeding is blood vessel constriction and clotting. In cases of major bleeding, however, clotting might not occur. The factors affecting the body's response will be discussed throughout this chapter.

Uncontrolled bleeding should be taken seriously. If not stopped, it will lead to shock and death.

EXTERNAL BLEEDING

Bleeding can be classified as external or internal. The assessment and care of both kinds of bleeding will be presented in this chapter.

Types of External Bleeding

FIRST▶ External bleeding may be classified as (Figure 10.3):

- *Arterial bleeding*—Blood spurts from an artery, often pulsating as the heart beats. The color of the blood is bright red since it contains oxygen. A great deal of blood can be lost in a short amount of time.
- *Venous bleeding*—Blood flows steadily from a vein. The color of the blood is dark red, often appearing deep maroon (since it contains little oxygen). However, it may look or become a brighter red when exposed to the oxygen in the air. Venous bleeding can also be profuse.

NOTE

Large veins may produce profuse bleeding, but there is no pulsation as is typically seen with arterial bleeding. Rate of flow and pulsation are more significant factors than color in determining if the bleeding is arterial or venous.

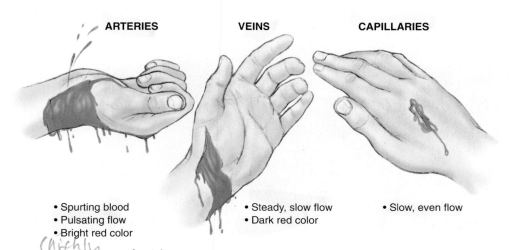

| ARTERIES | VEINS | CAPILLARIES |

- Spurting blood
- Pulsating flow
- Bright red color
  (*highly oxygenated*)

- Steady, slow flow
- Dark red color

- Slow, even flow

FIGURE 10.3
Three types of bleeding.

● *Capillary bleeding*—Blood oozes from a bed of capillaries. The color of the blood is bright red, usually less bright than arterial blood. The flow is slow, as seen in minor scrapes and shallow cuts to the skin. ■

Evaluating External Bleeding

Of the three types of external bleeding, arterial bleeding is usually the most serious. The action of the heart and the pressure in the arteries prevent blood clot formation because of the rapid, pressurized flow. The muscular nature of vessel walls creates problems in stopping the flow of blood. Sometimes the end of a completely severed artery will collapse and seal off the flow. In small arteries, the pulsation of the muscular wall may slow bleeding. In larger arteries, the thickness of the vessel walls prevents this collapse from being complete and the flow remains profuse. Arterial bleeding can take 10 minutes or more to clot. Since arteries are located deep within body structures, capillary and venous bleeding is seen more often than arterial bleeding.

Venous bleeding can range from very minor to very severe, leading to death within minutes. Some veins are located near the body surface. Many of these are large enough to be seen through the skin. Other veins are deep in the body and can be as large as arteries. Bleeding from a deep vein will produce rapid blood loss. Surface bleeding from a vein can be profuse, but blood loss is not as rapid as that seen from arteries and deep veins because of the smaller diameters. Veins have a tendency to collapse as soon as they are cut. This often reduces the severity of venous bleeding.

Most individuals experience little difficulty with capillary bleeding. The blood slowly oozes and clotting is very likely to occur within six to eight minutes. However, the larger the area of the wound, the more likely is the chance of infection. Capillary bleeding requires care to stop blood flow and reduce contamination.

In emergency care, arterial and large vein bleeding are given priority over small vein and capillary bleeding. If bleeding is severe and considered an immediate threat to life, bleeding control has to begin while you are observing for signs of breathing during the initial assessment. Even though it may prove awkward, a First Responder may be faced with the task of stopping severe bleeding while at the same time evaluating airway and pulse.

Determining external blood loss requires some experience (Figure 10.4). It is important in cases where slow bleeding has been occurring for a long time or in cases where both internal and external bleeding are present. To get a good idea of how to estimate blood volume loss, pour a pint of water on the floor next to a fellow student or a manikin. Also, try soaking an article of clothing with a pint of water and then note how much of the article is wet and how wet it feels.

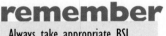

remember

Always take appropriate BSI precautions prior to initiating emergency care for bleeding.

remember

Finding and stopping profuse bleeding is a component of the initial assessment.

FIGURE 10.4
External blood loss of about 1/2 liter (approximately one pint).

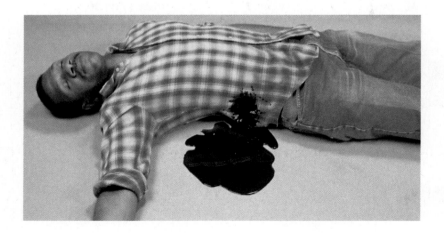

Controlling External Bleeding

FIRST➤ There are four steps to the procedure used by First Responders to control external bleeding (Figure 10.5 and Scan 10-1):

- Direct pressure (including use of pressure dressing).
- Elevation (combined with direct pressure).
- Pressure points (upper arm and groin).
- Tourniquet (used only as a last resort when other bleeding control steps fail. ■

Direct Pressure   Most cases of external bleeding can be controlled by applying **direct pressure** to the site of the wound. Ideally, a sterile **dressing** should be used. However, hunting in your pocket for a sterile dressing, going back to your car, going to a kit found in the next room, or other such activities are a waste of precious time. If profuse bleeding is found during the initial assessment, and you do not have dressings immediately available (Figure 10.6):

1. Place your gloved hand directly over the wound and apply pressure.
2. Keep applying steady, firm pressure.

If dressings are immediately available, then (Figure 10.7):

1. Apply firm pressure using sterile dressings or clean cloth. (You may have to use a clean handkerchief or towel.)
2. Apply pressure until bleeding is controlled. In some cases, this may take 10 minutes, 30 minutes, or longer.
3. Secure the dressing in place with a **bandage** to create a pressure dressing.

Never remove or attempt to replace any dressing once it is applied to the wound. To do so may interrupt clot formation and restart bleeding or cause additional injury to the wound site. If an outer dressing becomes soaked with blood, re-

direct pressure the quickest, most effective way to control most forms of external bleeding. Pressure is applied directly over the wound site.

dressing any material used to cover a wound; helps to control bleeding and reduce contamination.

bandage any material that is used to hold a dressing in place.

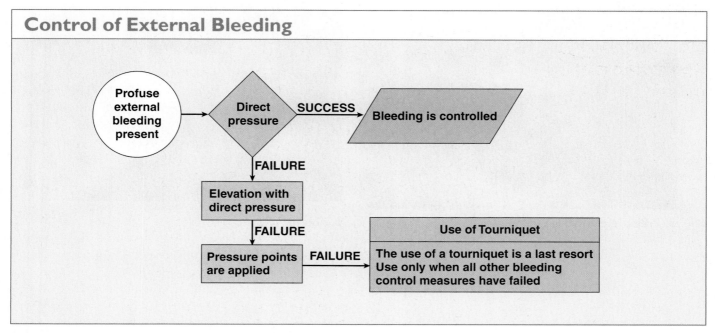

Control of External Bleeding

FIGURE 10.5

Methods of Controlling External Bleeding

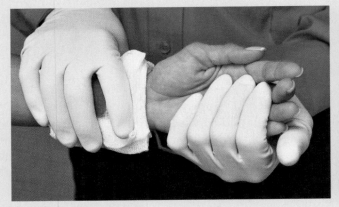

1. Direct pressure.

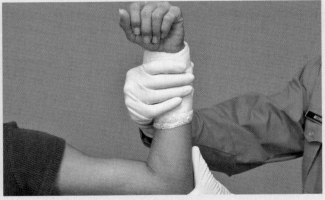

2. Elevation.

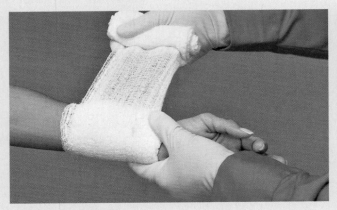

3. Pressure dressing.

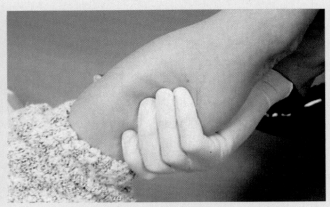

4. Pressure point: arm (brachial artery).

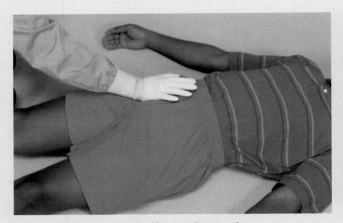

5. Pressure point: thigh (femoral artery).

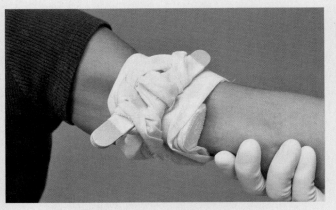

6. Tourniquet.

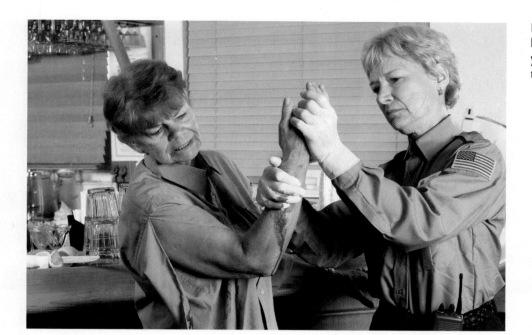

FIGURE 10.6
In cases of profuse bleeding, use your gloved hand. Do not waste time hunting for a dressing.

place it with another dressing. Make sure you do not disturb the dressing that is immediately against the wound.

Most bleeding can be controlled by a *pressure dressing* (Figure 10.8). To apply a pressure dressing:

1. Place several sterile gauze dressings directly on the wound. Maintain pressure with your gloved hand.

2. Place a bulky dressing pad (multi-trauma or universal dressing, sanitary pad, or several handkerchiefs) over the gauze dressing pads. Continue to apply hand pressure.

3. Use a roller bandage or cravat to hold the entire dressing in place. It should be wrapped snugly over the dressing and above and below the wound.

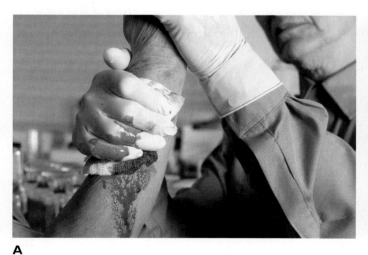

A

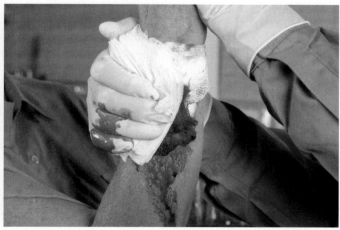

B

FIGURE 10.7

A. To control bleeding, place several (a small stack) of 4 × 4s on the wound and apply direct pressure. **B.** If the wound bleeds through the dressings, apply several more 4 × 4s.

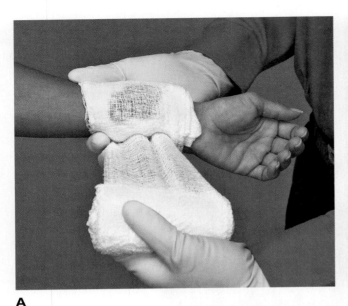
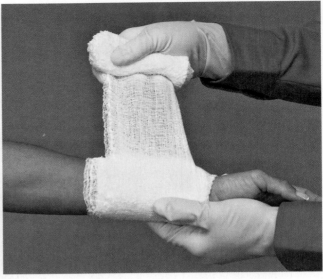

A

B

FIGURE 10.8
A. To use a pressure dressing, maintain direct pressure to the wound site by applying a bulky pad. **B.** Secure the entire pressure dressing in place with a self-adherent roller bandage or cravat.

4. Wrap the bandage to produce enough pressure to control the bleeding.

5. Check for a distal pulse to be certain that the pressure has not restricted blood flow.

A pressure dressing should not be removed once it is in place. If bleeding continues, add more pressure by using the palm of your gloved hand, applying more dressing pads, and continuing the process of bandaging. (Do not remove the bandage to add more pads.) You also may apply more bandages to increase the pressure. In very few cases (amputations and severe tearing injuries), you will have to create more bulk by using additional dressings.

If you use your gloved hand or a dressing to apply direct pressure, you can apply a pressure dressing once the bleeding is controlled. If you are dealing with bleeding from an armpit, the abdominal wall, a large artery, or a deep vein, attempting to apply a pressure dressing may not be of any real use. Your best approach to such situations is to maintain direct pressure on the wound using your gloved hand and a dressing.

Elevation

FIRST➤ Elevation may be used in combination with direct pressure when dealing with bleeding from an arm or leg (Figure 10.9). The effects of gravity will help reduce blood pressure and slow the bleeding. This method should not be used, however, with suspected fractures to the extremities, objects impaled in the extremities, or possible spinal injury.

To use elevation:

1. Lift the injured extremity. When practical, raise it so that the wound is above the level of the heart. If the forearm is bleeding, you do not have to elevate the entire arm. Simply elevate the forearm.

2. Continue to apply direct pressure to the site of bleeding as explained earlier in this chapter. ∎

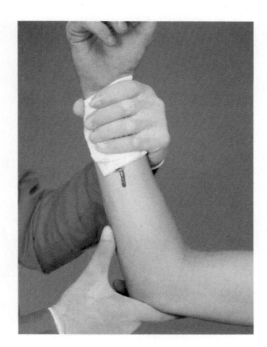

Pressure Points

FIRST➤ Pressure points are sites where an artery that is close to the skin surface lies directly over a bone. The flow of blood through such an artery can be slowed if pressure is applied to the artery. This procedure should be used only after direct pressure or direct pressure with elevation has failed to control the bleeding.

There are 22 pressure point sites that could potentially be used to control bleeding. They occur at 11 sites on each side of the body. Because the combination of direct pressure and elevation is so effective for most areas of the body, only the upper arm and groin pressure points are commonly used to control serious bleeding in the field. These sites are:

● **Brachial artery pressure point** in the upper arm for controlling bleeding from the arm.
● **Femoral artery pressure point** in the thigh for controlling bleeding from the leg. ■

Pressure point techniques are to be used only after direct pressure and elevation have failed to control bleeding.

CAUTION: *Exercise care in the practice of pressure point techniques. A single compression of short duration will not harm a healthy adult. However, repeated practice on someone, applying pressure for more than a few seconds, and too much pressure applied to children all can cause problems. Do not attempt to practice or demonstrate this technique on infants, children, or adults with a history of heart problems, blood clot problems, or inflamed blood vessels.*

FIRST➤ For bleeding from the forearm (Figure 10.10):

1. Make sure someone activates the EMS system.
2. Perform scene size-up.
3. Take appropriate BSI precautions.
4. Perform initial assessment, ensuring the patient's ABCs.

brachial (BRAY-ke-al) **pressure point** a location in the upper arm, where the brachial artery is close to the skin surface and lies over a bone. It can be used to help control serious external bleeding from the upper limb.

femoral (FEM-o-ral) **pressure point** a location at the anterior pelvis in the thigh, which can be used to help control serious external bleeding from the lower limb.

remember
Use pressure point techniques only after direct pressure and elevation have failed.

FIGURE 10.10
Apply pressure to the brachial pressure point to control bleeding from
the forearm.

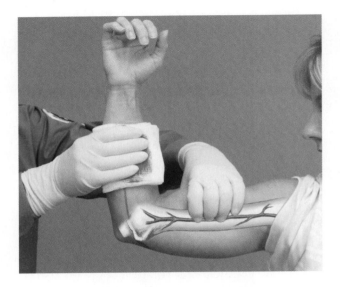

5. Apply direct pressure.

6. Elevate the limb.

7. If necessary, use a pressure point. Extend the patient's arm, placing it at a right angle, lateral to the body. This angle will provide the best results, but may be reduced if a 90-degree extension is not possible. Place the palm of the patient's hand in the anatomical position.

8. Press your fingers in the groove found below the biceps muscle.

9. Apply pressure to the brachial artery by pressing your fingers into this groove. Bleeding should slow and you may no longer be able to feel a radial (wrist) pulse.

10. Provide care for shock. Calm and reassure the patient, maintain normal body temprature, and administer oxygen as soon as possible as per local protocols. ■

FIRST▶ For bleeding from the leg (Figure 10.11):

1. Make sure someone activates the EMS system.

2. Perform scene size-up.

3. Take appropriate BSI precautions.

4. Perform initial assessment, ensuring the patient's ABCs.

5. Apply direct pressure.

6. Elevation the limb.

7. If necessary, use a pressure point. Locate the anterior medial side of the leg where the thigh joins the lower trunk. The femoral artery has a pulse that can be felt at this location.

8. Use the heel of your gloved hand to apply pressure to this site. Keep your arm straight, using your body weight to help apply the pressure. The number of leg muscles, their size, and the fat content of the thigh require that you exert much more pressure than you would use to compress the brachial artery in the arm.

9. Apply the necessary pressure to control bleeding.

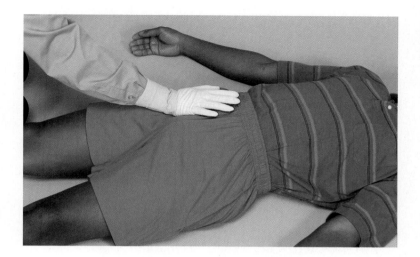

10. Reassure the patient and keep him calm.

11. Provide care for shock. ■

Keep in mind that the brachial (upper arm) and femoral (thigh) pressure points are not to be used if there are possible fractures to the bone under the pressure point site. To do so could produce severe pain and cause serious damage to the bone, soft tissues, nerves, and blood vessels in the area. You could cause more bleeding, rather than reduce the bleeding. If there are no indications of spinal injury or possible fractures of the extremity (remember to consider the mechanism of injury), elevation and pressure point techniques can be combined to control bleeding. Any patient who has suffered moderate to severe blood loss will benefit from receiving oxygen. If you are a First Responder who carries oxygen, administer it as needed. (See Appendix 2.) Follow local protocols.

Tourniquet

FIRST▶ A **tourniquet** is a last resort, used only when the other methods of controlling life-threatening bleeding have failed. In most cases when you think you should use a tourniquet, a pressure dressing would be the better choice. ■

A partial amputation of the arm or leg may leave you with no other choice than to use a tourniquet. However, many total amputations do not have uncontrollable, profuse bleeding since the ends of the blood vessels tend to collapse. In cases in which there is profuse bleeding from an arm or leg wound, a tourniquet should be applied to stop life-threatening bleeding after direct pressure, elevation, and pressure point techniques have failed. If there is no other way to stop bleeding and save the patient's life, then this is an acceptable action.

FIRST▶ If all other methods have failed and you must apply a tourniquet, carefully follow these steps (Figure 10.12):

1. Locate the site for the tourniquet. This should be between the wound and the patient's heart, as close to the wound as possible without being on its edge. The most effective and safest location is about two inches from the wound.

2. Place a tourniquet pad on the site you have selected, over the artery. This pad can be a roll of dressing, a folded handkerchief, or a piece of cloth folded to about the same thickness as a folded handkerchief.

tourniquet a wide, flat band or belt used to constrict blood vessels to help stop the flow of blood.

remember
Use a tourniquet only as a last resort.

warning
Never practice tightening a tourniquet on anyone.

FIGURE 10.12
Application of a tourniquet.

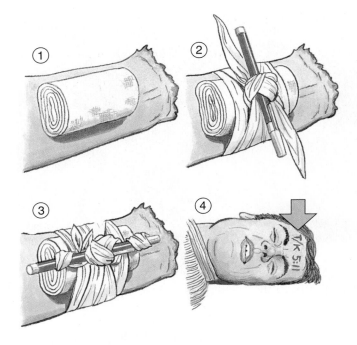

3. If you are using a manufactured tourniquet, carefully place it around the limb just above the wound. Pull the free end of the band through the friction catch or buckle and draw it tightly over the pad. Tighten the tourniquet to the point where bleeding is stopped. Do not tighten it beyond this point.

   If you do not have a commercially manufactured tourniquet or you would have to leave the patient to retrieve one, use a flat belt, necktie, stocking, or long dressing material. Flat materials are best. The band should be at least one inch wide. Do not use any material that could cut into the patient's limb. Carefully slip the tourniquet around the patient's limb and tie a half-knot with the ends of the tourniquet. The knot should be over the pad. A device such as a long stick, wooden dowel, or metal rod should then be placed over the half knot. (Pens and pencils tend to break.) Next, tie a full knot over the stick or rod. Then turn the device until bleeding has been stopped. Do not tighten the tourniquet beyond this point.

4. Once it is in place, *do not loosen the tourniquet.* Tie it or tape it in place.

5. Attach a note to the patient stating that a tourniquet has been applied and the time at which it was applied (for example: T/K—5:11 p.m.). If you do not have a tag, write the information, in ink, on the patient's forehead. If you do not have a pen, write the note in lipstick, crayon, or whatever is available at the scene. This note must be written so that the tourniquet does not go unnoticed and so that the hospital staff will know how long it has been in place.

6. Provide care for shock, but do not cover the tourniquet. This is an additional safeguard to prevent it from being missed by others who provide care for the patient. ■

NOTE

As a First Responder, you have the responsibility to advise the EMTs or other more highly trained personnel about the application of a tourniquet and the time it was applied.

Splinting Splinting is usually not considered a First Responder-level method of controlling bleeding. However, some First Responders are trained to use air-inflatable splints. For long wounds on an arm or leg, the application of an air splint can help to control bleeding. This is actually a form of direct pressure. Using an air splint requires special training in its application and knowledge of its limitations (see Chapter 11). The air splint can be used even when there is no suspected fracture to the bones of the limb.

Combining the use of an air splint and elevation can work well on long, bleeding wounds. The splint also serves to immobilize the limb, helping to reduce the chance of restarting bleeding due to patient movement. Since obtaining and applying air splints consumes time, this procedure is best done in cases of minor bleeding. The skilled rescuer can use air splints to control more serious bleeding if the splint is immediately at hand.

Special Cases of External Bleeding   There are situations in which a deep cut opens a major artery or vein and then the cut partially closes. Such cuts do not always appear to be major, and the bleeding from these cuts is often mild. Be alert for blood flow from wounds to change quickly from mild to profuse. If there is a wound to the arm or leg and you cannot detect a distal pulse, be prepared for profuse bleeding.

In addition, do not let cuts to the chest and abdomen fool you. Some may appear minor, but they could be very deep and have produced internal injuries that are causing a great deal of internal bleeding. When you find an external wound, you must consider the possibility of internal injuries. **Do not open the wound to determine its depth.**

Have someone activate EMS for all patients with external bleeding except for the mildest cases (small areas of capillary bleeding) in which there are no other signs of injury.

NOTE: *Bleeding from the eye, ear, nose, mouth, and around impaled objects requires special consideration. Each area is discussed later in this chapter.*

Dressing and Bandaging

Bandaging is not a difficult skill to learn. In First Responder care, most bandages are simple and easy to apply. If you follow the basic principles of dressing and bandaging wounds, you will provide effective care for the patient.

FIRST➤   To begin, review the following definitions (Figure 10.13):

- *Dressing*—any material (preferably sterile) placed over a wound that will help control bleeding and help prevent additional contamination.
- *Bandage*—any material used to hold a dressing in place. ■

Dressings, whenever possible, should be sterile. This means that they have been processed so that all germs and the spores that can grow into active germs are killed. They are nonfibrous so that material particles do not stick to wounds. Commercially prepared dressings are usually sterile. They come in a variety of sizes, with the most common size being four inches square. They are referred to according to size, such as 2 × 2s, 4 × 4s, 5 × 9s and 10 × 30s.

Throughout this text, you will find reference to **bulky dressings** and multi-trauma dressings. These are thick dressings, often large enough to allow for the complete covering of large wounds. They are used to help control very serious bleeding and to stabilize impaled objects. Sanitary pads can be used in place of these dressings. They are available individually wrapped. While sanitary pads are not sterile, they are very clean. (Avoid applying any adhesive surface directly to the wound.) Bulky dressings can be formed by applying many layers of simple gauze dressings.

Another type of special dressing is the **occlusive dressing**, which is used to create an airtight seal to a wound or body cavity. It is used to close an open wound that penetrates a body cavity. Commercially prepared occlusive dressings are avail-

bulky dressing a thick dressing or a build up of thin dressings used to help control profuse bleeding, stabilize impaled objects, or cover large open wounds.

occlusive dressing a dressing used to create an airtight seal or to close an open wound of a body cavity.

FIGURE 10.13
Dressings cover wounds. Bandages
hold dressings in place.

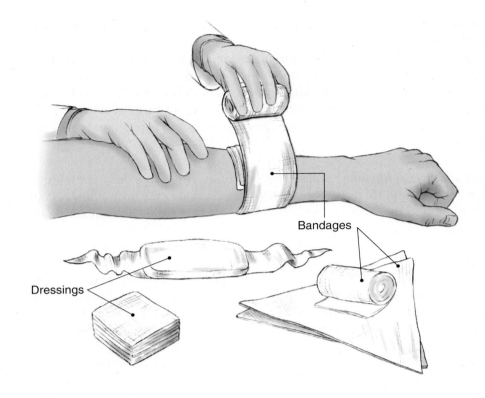

Bandages

Dressings

able. If these are not on hand, you can use folded plastic wrap or a plastic bag to help seal off an open wound to the chest or abdomen.

Often, a First Responder will not have any dressing materials at the scene of an emergency. In such cases, you might have to use clean handkerchiefs, towels, sheets, a piece of clothing, or other similar materials (Figure 10.14). When you improvise a dressing, it will not be sterile, but it can be used to help provide proper care for the patient. Since the patient's wound has already been contaminated, your task is to avoid further contamination by using the cleanest material available. The hospital has special wound-cleansing procedures and antibiotics to care for wound

FIGURE 10.14
Materials used for improvised dressings and bandages.

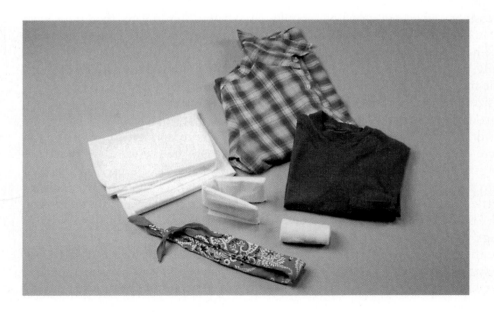

contamination and infection. In the field, you must be concerned with controlling bleeding and minimizing contamination.

Dressings are more effective if they are held in place. The adhesive bandage has a sticky backing that will adhere to the patient's skin. If no such bandaging material is on hand, tie a dressing in place by using a gauze roller bandage, a **cravat**, a handkerchief, strips of cloth, or any other material that will not cut into the patient's skin. *Do not use elastic bandages.* They are often used for injuries to the joints, but they can restrict circulation and apply undesired pressure to injured tissues.

The use of the self-adherent, form-fitting gauze **roller bandage** eliminates the need for highly specialized bandaging techniques (Figure 10.15). It does not have an adhesive backing, yet clings to itself, making the task of wrapping around a dressing easier, quicker, and more efficient.

cravat a piece of cloth that can be used to secure a dressing or splint.

roller bandage a long strip of soft, self-adherent gauze, a few inches wide and some yards long; used to secure dressings in place.

Rules for Dressing and Bandaging

FIRST➤ The following rules apply to dressing wounds:

1. *Control bleeding.* A dressing and bandage are of little value if they do not help to control bleeding. Continue to apply dressing material and pressure as needed to control bleeding.

2. *Use sterile or clean materials.* Avoid touching dressings in the area that will come into contact with the wound.

3. *Cover the entire wound.* A dressing must cover the entire surface of the wound and, if possible, the immediate area surrounding the wound.

4. *Do not remove dressings.* Once a dressing is applied to a wound, it must remain in place. Add new dressings on top of blood-soaked dressings. When a dressing is removed from a wound, bleeding could restart or increase in rate. Removal should be done only in the emergency department. There is an exception to this rule in some EMS systems. (Do only what you have been trained to do.) If a bulky dressing becomes blood-soaked, you may have to remove it so that direct pressure can be re-established or a new bulky pad or dressing can be applied. It is best to apply simple gauze pads to wound sites before applying a bulky dressing. This will allow removal of the bulky dressing if necessary without directly disturbing the wound. ■

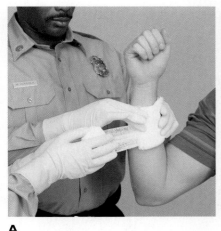 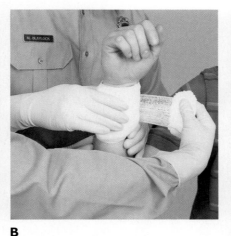 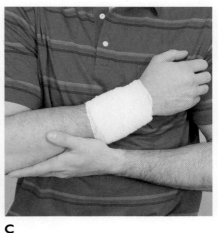

| A | B | C |

FIGURE 10.15

A. While maintaining direct pressure to the wound, hold the end of the roller bandage securely in place. **B.** Then begin to circle the limb, applying the bandage firmly. When complete, the bandage should be snug, but not too tight. **C.** Be sure to secure any loose ends.

FIRST➤ The following rules apply to bandaging (Figure 10.16):

- *Do not bandage too tightly.* Hold the dressing snugly in place, but do not restrict blood supply to the affected area.
- *Do not bandage too loosely.* The dressing must not be allowed to slip from the wound or move while on the wound.
- *Do not leave loose ends.* Loose ends of tape, dressing, or cloth might get caught on objects when the patient is being moved.
- *Do not cover fingers and toes* unless they are injured. These areas must be exposed so that you can watch for color changes that indicate a change in circulation. Blue skin, pale skin, and complaints of numbness, pain, and tingling sensations all indicate that the bandage may be too tight.
- *Bandage from the bottom of a limb to the top* (distal to proximal). The bandage should be wrapped around the limb starting at its far (distal) end and working toward its origin or near (proximal) end. Taking such action will help to reduce the chances of restricting circulation.

Three additional rules for bandaging must be considered when the wound is on a limb:

- Avoid applying the bandage to a narrow area. This can produce enough pressure to restrict circulation. Instead, wrap a large area of the limb, making certain to maintain uniform pressure as you wrap the bandage.
- Do not bend a joint if it is bandaged. Once the bandage is in place, movement of the joint may restrict circulation or cause the bandage and dressing to loosen.
- Always check circulation, sensation, and motor function in the limb receiving care. ■

See Scan 10-2 for examples of general dressing and bandaging techniques.

FIGURE 10.16
The rules of bandaging:
- Do not bandage too tightly or loosely.
- Tuck in loose ends.
- Do not cover fingers and toes.
- Bandage from the bottom to the top of a limb.
- Use sterile or clean materials.
- Cover the entire wound.
- Do not remove dressings.

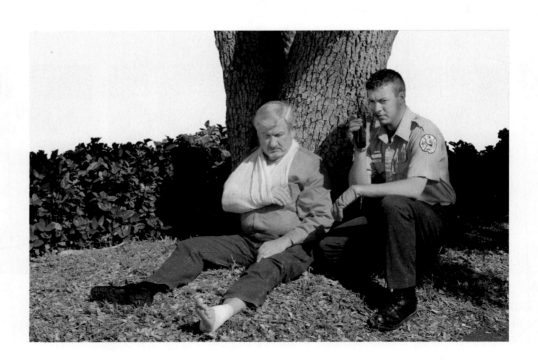

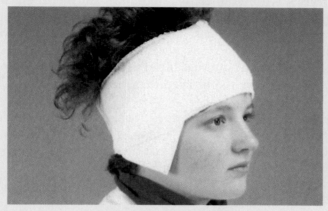

Forehead (no skull injury) or ear. Place dressing and secure with roller bandage.

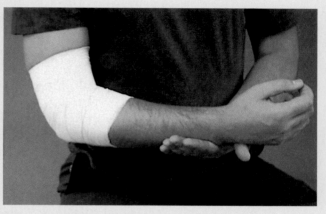

Elbow or knee. Place dressing and secure with cravat or roller bandage. Apply roller bandage in figure-eight pattern.

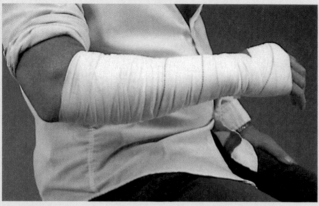

Forearm or leg. Place dressing and secure with roller bandage, distal to proximal. Better protection is provided if palm or sole is wrapped.

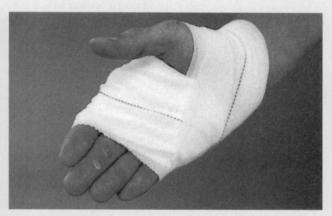

Hand. Place dressing, wrap with cravat, and secure at wrist. Use the same pattern for roller bandage.

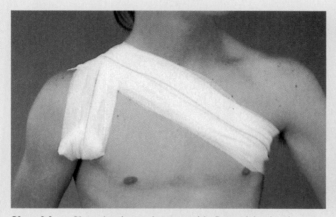

Shoulder. Place dressing and secure with figure-eight dressing made with a cravat or roller bandage. Pad under knot if cravat is used.

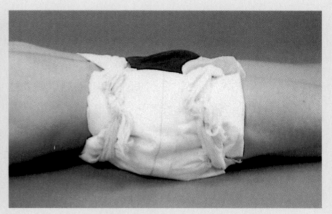

Hip. Place a large dressing to cover hip. Secure with first cravat around waist and second cravat around thigh on injured side.

INTERNAL BLEEDING

Internal bleeding can range from a minor bruise to a major life-threatening problem. Most small, simple bruises are examples of minor internal bleeding. Such minor blood loss is not of great significance. Of primary concern to First Responders is internal bleeding that brings about shock, heart and lung failure, and eventual death. Some cases of internal bleeding are so severe that the patient dies in a matter of seconds. Other severe cases of internal bleeding take minutes to hours before death. First Responder-level care might keep these patients alive until the EMTs arrive.

Even when internal bleeding is not profuse, it does not take very long for serious reactions to occur in the body. The most important, shock, will be covered later in this chapter. The care you provide for internal bleeding and shock, even when the bleeding is not profuse, may save the patient's life.

Detecting Internal Bleeding

Internal bleeding can occur in many ways (Figure 10.17). It can be caused by wounds that are deep enough to sever major blood vessels or the vessels in organs, such as a deep wound to the chest or abdomen. Open wounds that have cut through major vessels to produce profuse internal bleeding may show only minor external bleeding. Many cases of internal bleeding occur even when there are no cuts in the skin. Internal organs and blood vessels may have been ruptured or crushed by a severe blow to the body that did not produce any external wounds. This is an example of **blunt trauma**, an injury caused by an object that was not sharp enough to penetrate the skin. The blunt instrument can be fairly large, such as the steering wheel of an automobile. Even though they do not tend to cause penetrating wounds, blunt instruments can deliver a great deal of force to the body, causing life-threatening internal bleeding.

Pay special attention to bruises on the neck, chest, and abdomen. Severe injury with internal bleeding may show no more than a bruise at first, to be followed by the rapid decline of the patient. Bruise detection can be particularly important in assessing possible internal bleeding when the patient is unresponsive and thus unable to complain of pain that would clearly indicate the problem.

To complicate your assessment of the patient, in some cases a blow to one side of the body can cause internal bleeding on the opposite side of the body cavity. In

blunt trauma an injury caused by an object that was not sharp enough to penetrate the skin.

FIGURE 10.17
Certain types of injuries may indicate serious internal bleeding.

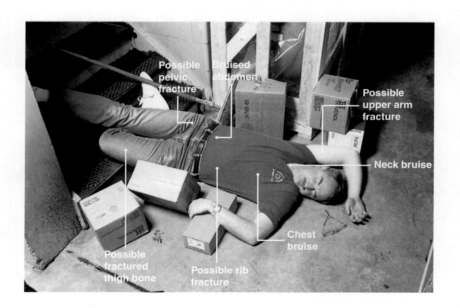

automobile collisions, blunt trauma to the lower right side of the rib cage can cause the spleen, which is on the left side of the body, to rupture and bleed freely, releasing about one liter (two pints) or more of blood.

REMEMBER: *Internal bleeding can be life-threatening. It may be difficult to detect since it can occur in cases where external bleeding is minor, away from the site of noticeable injury, or where there is no obvious external injury. Considering the mechanism of injury (falls, steering wheel injuries, and the like) and conducting a proper patient assessment are of major importance in detecting internal bleeding.*

FIRST ➤ Conclude that there is internal bleeding whenever you detect any of the signs listed below (Figure 10.18). Notice how the signs follow the order of the head-to-toe physical exam:

- Wounds that have penetrated the skull.
- Blood or bloody fluids in the ears and/or nose.
- Patient vomits or coughs up blood (coffee-grounds or frothy red appearance).
- Bruises on the neck.

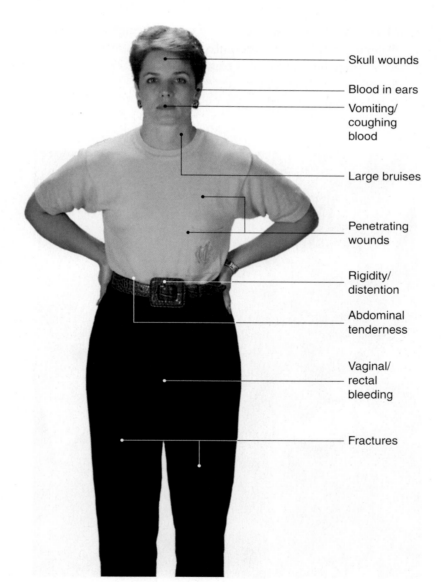

Skull wounds

Blood in ears

Vomiting/ coughing blood

Large bruises

Penetrating wounds

Rigidity/ distention

Abdominal tenderness

Vaginal/ rectal bleeding

Fractures

FIGURE 10.18
Signs and symptoms of possible internal bleeding.

- Bruises on the chest, possible fractured ribs (possible cuts to the lungs and liver), and wounds that have penetrated the chest.
- Bruises or penetrating wounds to the abdomen.
- Rigidity or distention of the abdominal muscles.
- Abdominal tenderness.
- Bleeding from the rectum or vagina.
- Possible fractures (with special emphasis on the pelvis, the long bones of the upper arm and thigh, and the ribs). ■

Always suspect that there is internal bleeding if the patient has been injured and the signs and symptoms of shock are present (Figure 10.19). (More about this later in the chapter.) The symptoms of shock associated with internal bleeding are:

- Weakness or dizziness.

- Thirst.

- Patient may feel cold.

- Anxiety or restlessness.

FIRST➤ The signs of shock associated with internal bleeding include:

- *Mental status*—decreasing level of responsiveness.
- *Behavior*—restlessness or combativeness.
- *Body*—may be shaking and trembling.
- *Breathing*—shallow and rapid.
- *Pulse*—rapid and weak.

FIGURE 10.19
Signs and symptoms of shock associated with internal bleeding.

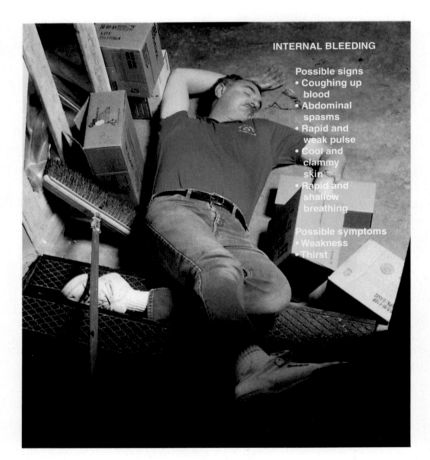

INTERNAL BLEEDING

Possible signs
• **Coughing up blood**
• **Abdominal spasms**
• **Rapid and weak pulse**
• **Cool and clammy skin**
• **Rapid and shallow breathing**

Possible symptoms
• Weakness
• Thirst

- *Skin*—pale, cool, and clammy. (There may be profuse sweating.)
- *Eyes*—sluggish or dilated (enlarged) pupils. ■

Stop now and note how these signs fit into your assessment of the patient during the physical exam. Remember, none of these signs or symptoms may be present in the early stages of internal bleeding. If the mechanism of injury is severe enough to make you think that there may be internal bleeding, assume that there is such bleeding and provide the necessary care.

FIRST➤ You can detect internal bleeding by looking for mechanisms of injury that could cause internal bleeding, wounds, and the signs and symptoms of shock. ■

Medical emergencies that can produce internal bleeding were discussed in Chapter 9.

Evaluating Internal Bleeding

It is very difficult to determine the amount of blood lost in cases of internal bleeding. Special hospital procedures and tests are required. However, estimates can be made. Consider blood loss to be severe if there is penetration of the chest cavity over or immediately above the heart, if the spleen or liver may have been injured, or if you suspect the pelvis is fractured. Estimate blood loss of at least one liter (two pints) if there is a suspected major fracture in the upper arm or thigh bone. Where you find badly bruised skin, assume there is a 10% loss of total blood volume for each bruise the size of the patient's fist (Figure 10.20). For an adult, this is about a one-pint loss. Such estimates will help you evaluate the chance of the patient going into shock, lung or heart failure, or cardiac arrest.

Management of Internal Bleeding

FIRST➤ In general, the steps in the care for patients with suspected internal bleeding include:

1. Make certain that someone activates the EMS system.

2. Take appropriate BSI precautions.

3. Perform a scene size-up.

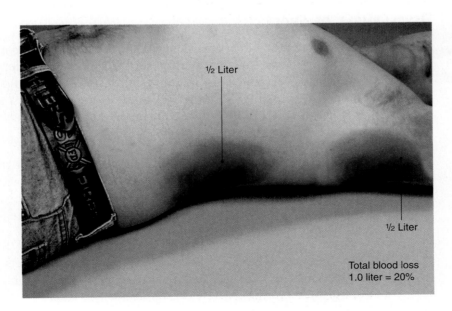

FIGURE 10.20
Estimating internal blood loss.

½ Liter

½ Liter

Total blood loss
1.0 liter = 20%

4. Perform initial assessment. (Maintain the airway and monitor breathing and pulse.)

5. Keep the patient in the proper position and lying still.

6. Loosen restrictive clothing and provide care for shock.

7. Be alert in case the patient starts to vomit.

8. Do not give the patient anything by mouth.

9. Reassure the patient and keep him calm.

10. Report the possibility of internal bleeding as soon as more highly trained EMS personnel arrive at the scene. ■

If you are a First Responder who is allowed to administer oxygen, remember that any patient with possible internal bleeding will benefit from receiving it. Provide oxygen as per local protocols.

Internal bleeding in the abdominal cavity or the chest cavity is a life-threatening situation requiring quick, safe transport to a hospital. Most areas in the country do not consider transport to be a First Responder's duty. Most EMS medical directors believe it is better if First Responders keep patients at the scene. You must recognize that a patient unattended in the back seat of your car could go into cardiac arrest and die while you are trying to rush to the hospital. Improper transport could also aggravate spinal injuries.

Patients with internal bleeding need oxygen as part of their care. By transporting such patients to the hospital without oxygen, you may place them in greater risk than if you waited for EMS personnel to arrive with oxygen and more advanced care.

Internal bleeding is very serious, often leading to death, even in cases in which the bleeding begins once the patient is at the hospital. You may provide excellent First Responder care for a patient with internal bleeding, only to have him die later. To be a good First Responder, accept the fact that there are limits to emergency care at all levels. Some patients will die no matter what you do. The patient has a better chance to survive, however, if you do as you have been trained to do.

SHOCK

DEVELOPMENT OF SHOCK

When providing patients with emergency care, consider the concept of the "golden hour." This is the first hour after serious injury. Providers must make every effort to provide care and assist in delivering seriously injured patients to the hospital as quickly as possible. The first 60 minutes are critical. If shock can be prevented or if its severity can be reduced during this period, the patient's chances for survival are greatly improved.

FIRST➤ Any injury or illness must be considered more severe once the patient enters a state of shock. Keeping patients from going into shock and helping to stabilize patients who are in shock are two of the most important responsibilities of First Responders. If nothing is done for the patient who is in shock, death will almost always result. ■

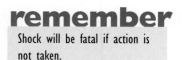

remember

Shock will be fatal if action is not taken.

Whenever the body is hurt, either by injury or illness, it reacts by trying to correct the effects of the damage. If the damage is severe, one consequence is shock, which indicates a problem with the circulatory system. The problem can be related to the:

- *Heart*—The heart should be pumping blood and doing so efficiently. If the heart fails to pump an adequate volume of oxygenated blood, shock will develop.

- *Vessels*—Blood circulates throughout the body through a closed system. If there is any opening in this system, such as a cut or rupture, with enough blood loss, shock will develop. Shock also can develop when blood vessels dilate (enlarge) and there is not enough blood to fill the now larger system.

- *Blood volume*—An adequate amount of blood must be present to fill the vessels. If there is loss of blood volume or if the vessels dilate (enlarge) to a size that no longer allows the system to properly fill, shock will develop.

Basically, **shock** is the failure of the body's circulatory system to provide enough oxygenated blood and nutrients to all vital organs. There must be enough blood being pumped efficiently to allow for a steady flow through the capillaries so that exchange can occur (perfusion). Oxygen and carbon dioxide are exchanged, food and waste are exchanged, and fluid and salt balance must be maintained between the blood and the tissues. When this cannot take place, shock, or hypoperfusion (lack of adequate perfusion), develops.

> **shock** the reaction of the body to the failure of the circulatory system to provide enough blood to the vital organs.

Shock develops, or occurs in a step-by-step progression. The development of shock can be rapid or it can come about slowly. Most new rescuers expect shock to develop rapidly; however, this is not always the case. Some patients can go into shock "a little at a time." Experienced rescuers know that you will often have enough warning to slow down the process. They also know that if you do not continue to monitor patients, you can miss some of the subtle, early signs and symptoms. Shock is a very dynamic process that can be life-threatening.

Care for patients with shock should not be delayed. The problem worsens with time, and early intervention is crucial. Think of shock as a reaction to blood loss. This reaction causes more problems that, in turn, cause more problems. For example, if there is bleeding, the heart rate increases, attempting to circulate blood to all the vital parts of the body. By doing this, more blood is lost. The body's immediate response to this problem is to try to circulate more blood by increasing the heart rate even further. This process will continue until death occurs. This cycle of decline must be stopped (Figure 10.21). The initial problem, such as bleeding, must be corrected, and shock must be managed. First Responder-level care should begin to correct problems and stop the decline.

TYPES OF SHOCK

Shock can be classified into several categories since there is more than one cause of shock. It is not necessary to memorize the following list. It is provided so that you can see the many ways shock develops. A patient in shock may have one or more of the following:

- **Hypovolemic** (HI-po-vo-LE-mic) **shock** is caused by blood loss or by the loss of plasma (a component of blood) as in cases of burns. (The term hypovolemic means low volume.) This term includes all shock caused by fluid loss, such as bleeding, burns, vomiting and diarrhea, and severe dehydration. Shock caused by vomiting and diarrhea is also called **metabolic** (MET-ah-BOL-ic) **shock.**

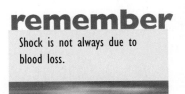

remember

Shock is not always due to blood loss.

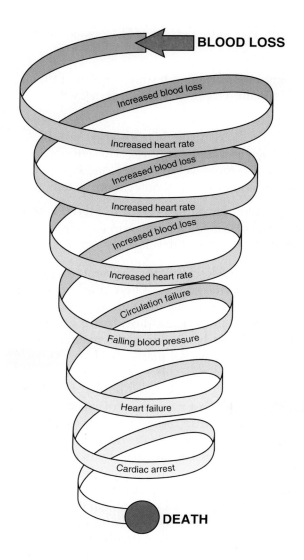

BLOOD LOSS

Increased blood loss

Increased heart rate

Increased blood loss

Increased heart rate

Increased blood loss

Increased heart rate

Circulation failure

Falling blood pressure

Heart failure

Cardiac arrest

DEATH

- **Hemorrhagic shock** is caused when the body loses a significant amount of blood from the circulatory system. It can be caused by either uncontrolled internal or external bleeding.

- **Cardiogenic** (KAR-di-o-JEN-ic) **shock** is heart shock, caused by the heart failing to pump enough blood to all parts of the body. It may be due to the damage of the heart itself as in the case of a heart attack.

- **Neurogenic** (NU-ro-JEN-ic) **shock** is nerve shock, caused when something goes wrong with the nervous system (such as from an injury to the spinal cord) and there is a failure to control the tone of blood vessels. The vessels become dilated. There is not enough blood in the body to fill this increased space, causing inadequate circulation.

- **Anaphylactic** (AN-ah-fi-LAK-tik) **shock** is allergy shock, a life-threatening reaction of the body caused by something to which the patient is extremely allergic. This is such a serious problem that it is covered as a special topic in Chapter 9.

- **Psychogenic** (SI-ko-JEN-ic) **shock** is fainting. It usually occurs when some factor, such as fear, causes the nervous system to react and rapidly dilate the blood vessels. The proper flow of blood to the brain is interrupted. In most cases, fainting is a self-correcting form of shock, with the interruption of

syncope – fainting.

proper blood flow being a temporary condition. Fainting is not the same as neurogenic shock.

- **Septic shock** is caused by infection. Poisons are released that cause the blood vessels to dilate. As in other cases of shock, the blood volume is too low to fill the circulatory system. This type of shock is seldom seen by First Responders.

As a First Responder, you do not have to classify shock, with the exception of anaphylactic, or allergy, shock. For all other cases, report that the patient has the signs and symptoms of shock and any factors you notice usually associated with shock, such as bleeding and loss of body fluids.

SIGNS AND SYMPTOMS OF SHOCK

FIRST➤ The symptoms of shock are (Figure 10.22):

- Weakness.
- Nausea.
- Thirst.
- Dizziness.
- Anxiety, agitation, fear.

The signs of shock are:

- Entire body assessment:
  – Restlessness or combativeness.
  – Profuse external bleeding.
  – Vomiting.
  – Shaking and trembling.
- Altered mental status. The patient may become disoriented, confused, unresponsive (often suddenly), or faint.
- Breathing, shallow and rapid.
- Pulse, rapid and weak.
- Skin, pale, cool, and clammy often with blue color (cyanosis) seen at the lips, tongue, and earlobes (may be profuse sweating).

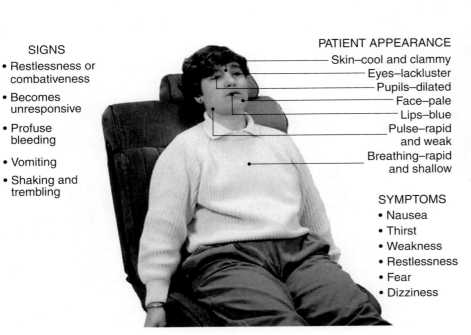

SIGNS
- Restlessness or combativeness
- Becomes unresponsive
- Profuse bleeding
- Vomiting
- Shaking and trembling

PATIENT APPEARANCE
- Skin–cool and clammy
- Eyes–lackluster
- Pupils–dilated
- Face–pale
- Lips–blue
- Pulse–rapid and weak
- Breathing–rapid and shallow

SYMPTOMS
- Nausea
- Thirst
- Weakness
- Restlessness
- Fear
- Dizziness

FIGURE 10.22
Signs and symptoms of shock.

NOTE

Children may compensate for a loss of blood better than adults. This will delay the early indications of developing shock. However, once children and young adults begin to show the first signs of shock, its development may be rapid.

- Eyes, lackluster. Pupils are sluggish and may be dilated. ■

The above lists of signs and symptoms follow the order in which they may be detected during the initial assessment of the patient. However, all the signs and symptoms of shock are not present at once, and they do not necessarily occur in the order listed above. Shock is progressive (becoming worse with time) (Figure 10.23). Look for the following patterns (Scan 10-3):

- *Increased pulse rate*—The body is trying to adjust to the loss of blood and poor perfusion. Unlike the rapid pulse rate associated with the stress of an injury or the fear of needing help during an emergency, this increased rate will not slow down.
- *Increased breathing rate*—When the body is not receiving enough oxygen and the level of carbon dioxide increases, the body tries to compensate by increasing the breathing rate. This increased rate will not slow down as it usually does after experiencing stress.

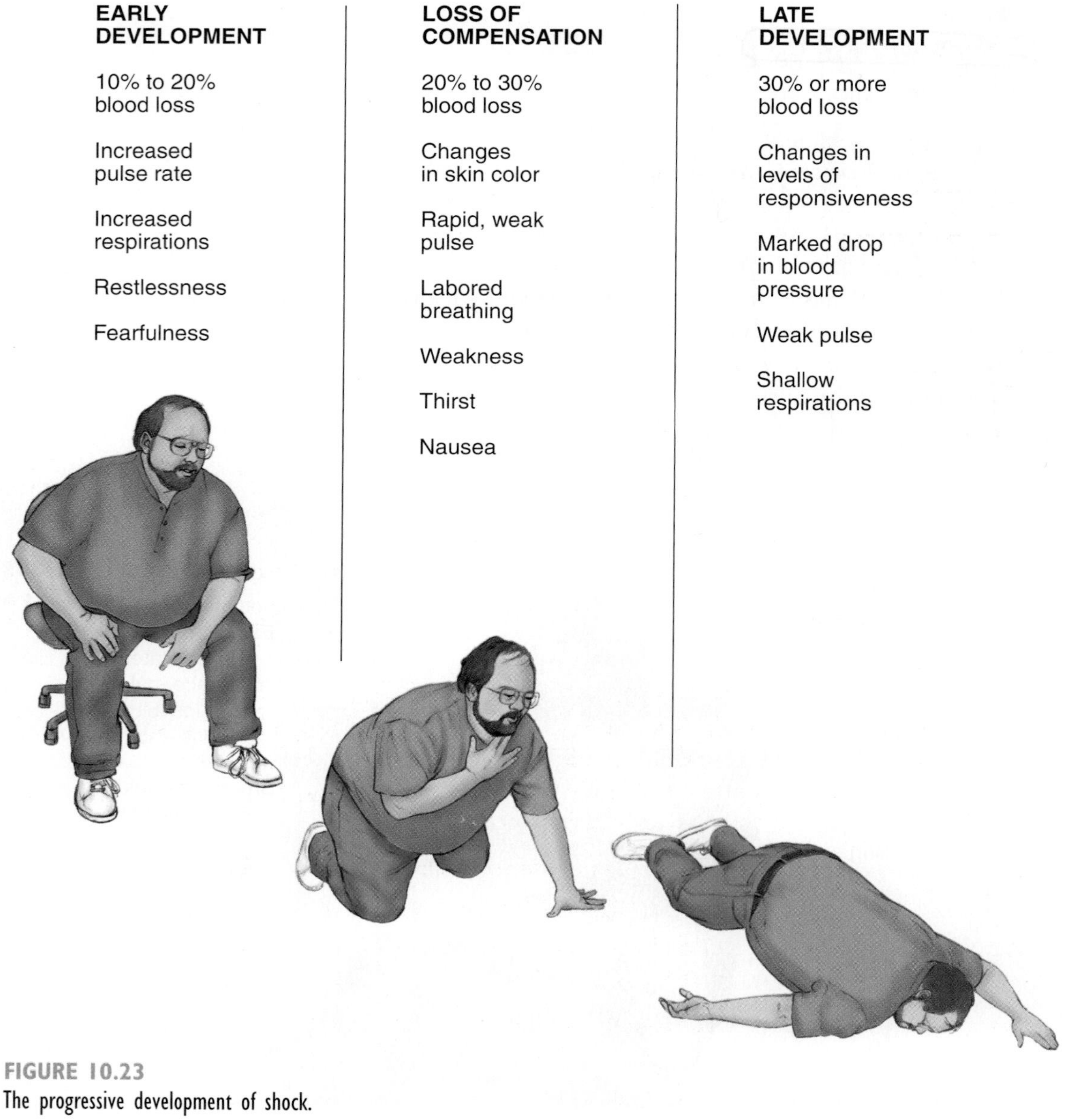

EARLY DEVELOPMENT
10% to 20% blood loss
Increased pulse rate
Increased respirations
Restlessness
Fearfulness
LOSS OF COMPENSATION
20% to 30% blood loss
Changes in skin color
Rapid, weak pulse
Labored breathing
Weakness
Thirst
Nausea
LATE DEVELOPMENT
30% or more blood loss
Changes in levels of responsiveness
Marked drop in blood pressure
Weak pulse
Shallow respirations

FIGURE 10.23
The progressive development of shock.

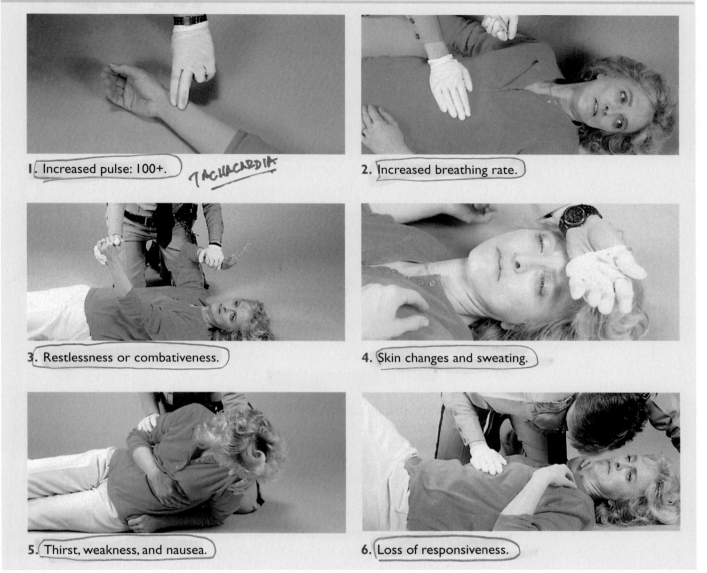

1. Increased pulse: 100+. *TACHACARDIA*

2. Increased breathing rate.

3. Restlessness or combativeness.

4. Skin changes and sweating.

5. Thirst, weakness, and nausea.

6. Loss of responsiveness.

- *Restlessness or combativeness*—The patient is reacting to the body's attempt to adjust to the loss of proper circulatory function. The patient feels that something is wrong and may often look afraid. In some cases, this behavioral change may be the first sign of developing shock.

- *Skin appears pale*—Skin, nail bed, and other color changes occur. The skin feels cool to the touch. Sweating may be profuse.

- *Rapid, weak pulse and labored, shallow respirations*—The body is failing in its attempt to adjust to the circulatory system failure.

- *Changes in mental status*—As adequate circulation to the brain continues to fail, the patient will become confused, disoriented, sleepy, or unresponsive.

- *Respiratory and cardiac arrest* can develop.

FIRST➤ Provide care for all injured patients as if shock will develop. Do the same for all patients with problems involving the heart, breathing, abdominal pain, diabetes, drug abuse, poisoning, and abnormal childbirth. Carefully monitor all patients for the early signs of shock. ■

PREVENTING AND CARING FOR SHOCK

FIRST➤ Help delay the onset of shock by the following (Figure 10.24):

1. Make sure someone activates the EMS system.

2. Perform a scene size-up.

3. Take appropriate BSI precautions.

4. Perform an initial assessment.

5. Control external bleeding. Administer oxygen as per local protocol.

6. Assist the patient in lying down.

7. Provide care for shock. Calm and reassure the patient, and maintain his normal body temperature. Take care not to overheat the patient, because overheating can worsen his condition. Place at least one blanket under and one blanket over the patient, covering all body parts except the head. Do not try to place a blanket under a patient who has possible spinal injuries.

8. Properly position the patient. Regardless of the position used, make certain that the patient has an open airway and be alert for vomiting. If there is no indication of spinal injuries, use one of the following positions (Figure 10.25):

   – *Option 1: Elevate the lower extremities.* This procedure is performed in most cases. Place the patient flat, face up, and elevate the legs 8 to 12 inches. Do not tilt the patient's body. Do not elevate any limbs with possible fractures unless they have been properly splinted. Do not elevate the legs if there are suspected fractures to the pelvis. Remember to consider the mechanism of injury for every patient.

   – *Option 2: Lay the patient flat, face up.* This is the supine position, used for patients with serious injuries to the extremities. If the patient is placed in this position, you must constantly be prepared for vomiting.

   – *Option 3: Slightly raise the head and shoulders.* This position should be used only for responsive patients with no possible neck, spine, chest, or abdominal injuries and only for patients having difficulty breathing, but who have an open

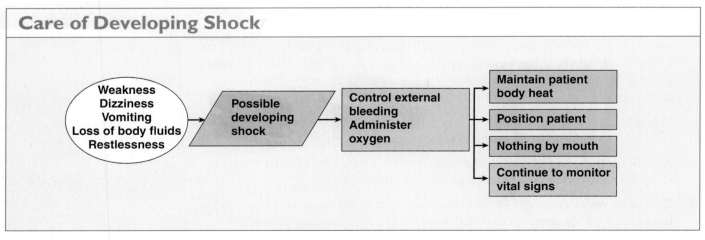

Care of Developing Shock

Weakness
Dizziness
Vomiting
Loss of body fluids
Restlessness → Possible developing shock → Control external bleeding
Administer oxygen →
- Maintain patient body heat
- Position patient
- Nothing by mouth
- Continue to monitor vital signs

FIGURE 10.24

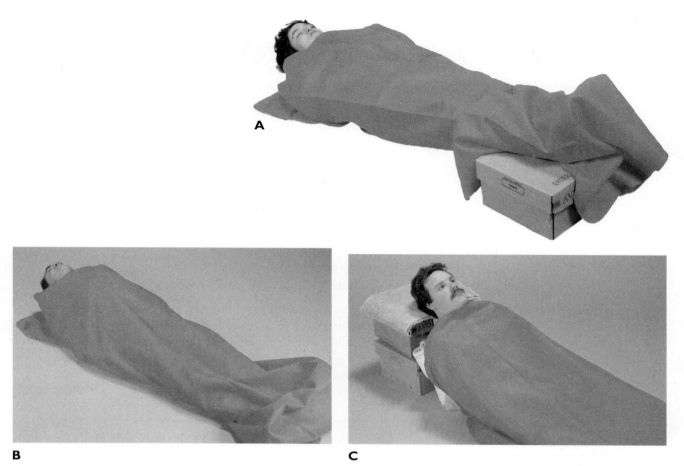

FIGURE 10.25

Properly position the patient in shock. **A.** In most cases, the patient should lie flat with lower extremities elevated 8 to 12 inches. **B.** The patient with serious injuries to the extremities should be in a supine position. **C.** The alert patient who has no possible neck, spine, chest, or abdominal injuries, but has difficulty breathing, may be placed in a semi-sitting position.

airway. A semi-seated position can also be used for patients with a history of heart problems. It is not recommended for moderate to severe cases of shock. Be certain to keep the patient's head from tilting forward.

9. Do not give the patient anything by mouth. Even if the patient expresses serious thirst, do not give any fluids or food.

10. Monitor the patient's vital signs. This must be done at least every five minutes. Stay alert for vomiting, give nothing to the patient by mouth, and provide emotional support to the responsive patient. ■

Restlessness may be a sign of someone going into shock. The patient may want to assume a sitting position even when there are no problems with breathing. A patient has less chance of going into shock if kept lying down and at rest.

You will not be able to reverse shock, but you may be able to delay the onset of shock or keep it from worsening by following the previous procedures. The care you provide may reverse the severity of certain aspects of shock and may help the patient avoid immediate danger.

If you are trained to do so and if your state laws allows, oxygen can be very significant in helping shock patients. Administer oxygen as per local protocols.

remember

Keeping a patient lying down and at rest reduces the risk of developing shock.

FAINTING

Fainting is usually a self-correcting form of mild shock. However, the patient may have been injured in a fall due to fainting. Be certain to examine the patient for injury. Even if no other problems are apparent, keep the patient lying down and at rest for several minutes.

In some cases, fainting is caused by a sudden drop of blood pressure. If you are trained to do so and have the needed equipment, check the patient's blood pressure. Otherwise, have the patient's blood pressure checked by an EMT or a nurse.

Fainting can also be a warning of some serious condition, including brain tumors, heart disease, undetected diabetes, and inner ear problems. Always recommend that the patient see a physician as soon as possible. In a polite but firm manner, tell anyone who has fainted not to drive or operate any machinery until after having been seen by a physician. Make certain that you have witnesses to this warning.

Your patient may have fainted because of fear, stress from problems, bad news, the sight of blood. Be ready to provide emotional support when the patient is alert.

FIRST➤ You can often prevent a person from fainting by lowering the patient's head. Assist the patient to the floor and have him lie down with his feet slightly elevated. This will increase blood flow to the brain and will often prevent fainting (Figure 10.26). ■

SOFT-TISSUE INJURIES

soft tissues the tissues of the body that make up the skin, muscles, nerves, blood vessels, fat, and the cells that line and cover organs and glands.

This section of the chapter describes injuries to the **soft tissues** of the body—skin, muscles, nerves, blood vessels, fatty tissues, and cells (Figure 10.27). Since childhood, we have learned about soft-tissue injuries such as bruises, scratches, and cuts. The idea of amputations and crush injuries are at least known, if not witnessed, before we enter our teens. Our own experiences and those of the people around us lead to our general understanding of injuries.

FIGURE 10.26
For some patients, lying down with feet slightly elevated plus emotional support can prevent fainting.

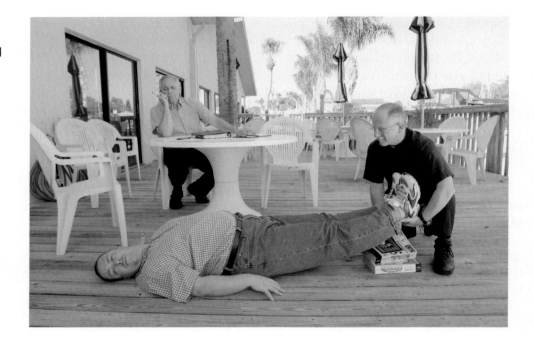

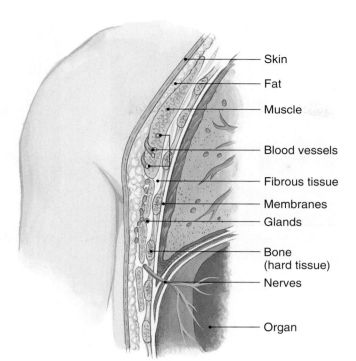

FIGURE 10.27
Soft tissues and associated underlying structures.

Skin
Fat
Muscle
Blood vessels
Fibrous tissue
Membranes
Glands
Bone (hard tissue)
Nerves
Organ

This prior knowledge will be useful to you. To be a First Responder, you will have to refine this knowledge, learning how to recognize and provide care for various injuries. However, you should not forget your basic understanding of injuries. Most of your patients will, at best, have the same level of understanding that you had when you started this course. Remembering this will help you with patient interviews and in providing explanations and reassurance. Also, recalling what you knew about injuries as you went through childhood will help when dealing with children who have suffered injuries.

Except for cases of spinal injury and certain types of internal injury, most adults can look at someone and often tell if there is an injury. Your training will build upon this ability so that you will not miss detectable injuries. This is why there has been so much emphasis on patient assessment. As you progress through this course, you will be trained to determine the extent of an injury and the emergency procedures needed to care for it.

TYPES OF INJURIES

When considering soft-tissue injuries, two general classifications—closed wounds and open wounds—can be used.

Closed Wounds

FIRST▶ A **closed wound** is an injury in which the skin is not broken. Such injuries are usually caused by the impact of a blunt object. Bleeding can range from minor to major, while the extent of injury can range from a simple bruise to the rupturing of internal organs. ■

Most closed wounds detected during First Responder care are **bruises** (contusions) (Figure 10.28). There is always some internal bleeding associated with a bruise. Since the skin is not broken, the blood leaks between tissues, causing discoloration over time ranging from black and blue to a brownish-yellow. Keep in mind that large bruises can mean serious blood loss and that there may be fractures or extensive tissue damage under the site of the bruise.

closed wound an internal soft-tissue injury in which the skin is not broken.

bruise a simple closed wound in which blood leaks between soft tissues, causing a discoloration; a *contusion* (kun-TU-zhun).

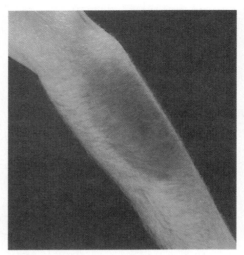

FIGURE 10.28
Bruises are the most common form of closed wounds.

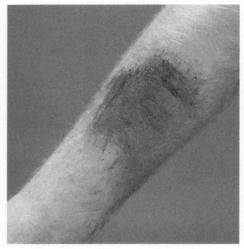

FIGURE 10.29
Abrasions are the least serious form of all open wounds.

Open Wounds

open wound an injury to the body in which the skin or its outer layers are opened.

FIRST➤ In cases of **open wounds**, the skin is opened. The extent of injury can range from a mild scrape (abrasion) to a tearing or cutting open of the skin (laceration). A simple scraping of the skin may produce no bleeding, while more severe open wounds may be associated with minor to life-threatening bleeding. ■

Open wounds may be classified as:

abrasion (ab-RAY-zhun) the simplest form of open wound that damages the skin surface but does not break all the layers of skin; scratches and scrapes.

- **Abrasions.** Wounds such as skinned elbows and knees, "road rash," "rug burns," and thorn scratches are minor open wounds known as abrasions (Figure 10.29). Although such scratches and scrapes may be painful, tissue injury is usually not serious since the skin is not fully penetrated and the force causing the injury does not crush or rupture underlying structures. There may be no detectable bleeding or only minor capillary bleeding. Wound contamination tends to be the most serious problem faced when caring for abrasions to the skin.

laceration a soft-tissue injury in which all the layers of skin are opened and the tissues immediately below the skin are damaged.

incision a laceration with smooth edges, usually caused by very sharp objects such as a razor blade, knife, or broken glass.

- **Lacerations.** In cases of lacerations, the skin is fully penetrated, with injury also occurring to tissues lying under the skin. Lacerations may be classified as:
  - *Smooth cuts*, also called **incisions** (Figure 10.30), are produced by very sharp objects, such as razor blades, knives, and broken glass. The edges of a smooth cut appear straight, with no apparent tears or jagged areas. Deep incisions can cause severe tissue damage and life-threatening bleeding.
  - *Jagged cuts* are torn with rough edges (Figure 10.31). Sometimes jagged cuts can be produced from the impact of a blunt object. Usually, they occur when the skin is cut by an object that does not have a very sharp edge.

puncture an open wound that tears through the skin and damages tissues in a straight line.

- **Punctures.** Objects such as knives, nails, and ice picks can produce puncture wounds. An object puncturing the body will tear through the skin and usually proceed in a straight line, damaging all the tissues in its path. A puncture wound may be a **penetrating wound,** ranging from shallow to deep (Figure 10.32). A penetrating wound may also have both an entrance and an exit

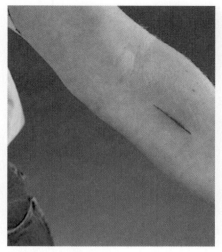

FIGURE 10.30
The edges of a smooth cut (incision) are straight.

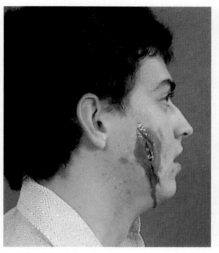

FIGURE 10.31
Tissues along the edges of a jagged cut (laceration) will be torn and rough.

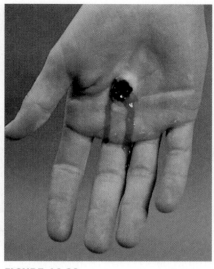

FIGURE 10.32
Puncture wound.

wound, as the object, such as a bullet, passes through the body. Often, the exit wound is the larger and more serious of the two (Figure 10.33).

- **Avulsions.** These wounds most frequently involve the tearing loose or the tearing off of large flaps of skin (Figure 10.34). A torn ear, an eyeball removed from its socket, and the loss of a tooth are also examples of avulsions.

- **Amputations.** These wounds involve the cutting or tearing off of the fingers, toes, hands, feet, arms, or legs (Figure 10.35). Since amputation can be done as a surgical procedure, this injury is often called a traumatic amputation.

- **Crush injuries.** Most of the time, when people see an incident in which a body part has been crushed, their first thoughts are of fractures. Soft tissues and internal organs are also crushed, often rupturing (Figure 10.36). Both external and internal bleeding can be profuse.

avulsion (ah-VUL-shun) a soft-tissue injury in which flaps of skin are torn loose or torn off.

amputation a soft-tissue injury that involves the cutting or tearing off of a limb or one of its parts. Often, hard tissues are also injured.

crush injury a soft-tissue injury produced by crushing forces. Soft tissues and internal organs are crushed, and hard tissues are usually damaged.

FIGURE 10.33
A penetrating wound can have both (A) an entrance wound and (B) an exit wound. Often the exit wound is the more serious of the two.

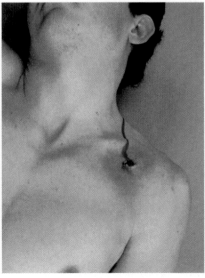

A

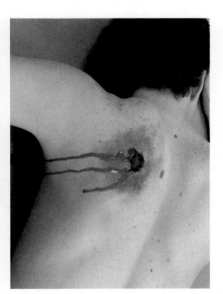

B

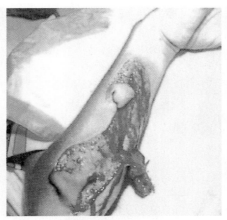

FIGURE 10.34
Avulsions are open wounds.

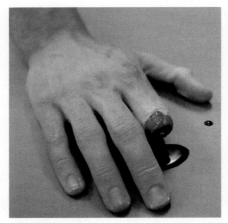

FIGURE 10.35
Amputation.

BASIC EMERGENCY CARE

Bystanders at emergency scenes may begin care before First Responders or other members of the EMS system arrive to provide professional-level assessment and care. Untrained individuals often focus on soft-tissue injuries. Your EMS system may require that you do not attempt to undo what has been done before your arrival until EMTs or other more highly trained personnel arrive. Usually, EMS system protocols state that obviously harmful care must be stopped and corrected. For example, people at the scene may have applied a very tight bandage and stopped circulation in an extremity. In such a situation, you may be required to re-establish distal circulation. Your instructor will alert you to specific protocols for your EMS system.

A special problem associated with soft-tissue injuries and sporting events involves the application of ice or ice and pressure to injury sites before EMS assessment. Even though the RICE method (a memory aid that stands for rest, ice, compression, and elevation) is a time-honored procedure used by many coaches and trainers, it is usually not part of EMS protocols. Improperly done, the RICE method may contaminate wounds, expose the patient to excessive cold, injure tissue, or reduce circulation. The RICE method typically employs elastic bandages to hold a bag of ice to the injury site. Removal of this bandage may cause additional

FIGURE 10.36
Both soft tissues and internal organs are damaged in crush injuries.

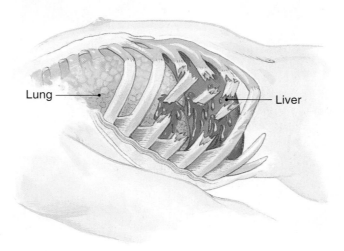

Lung

Liver

problems, especially if the RICE method was used over a fractured bone or dislocated and/or fractured joint.

In situations where care has been rendered by individuals having less training than a First Responder, follow your EMS protocols for assessment and care. If there is any doubt, call or have someone call 9-1-1.

Care During Assessment

A limited amount of care may be initiated during the patient assessment. Immediately care for injuries involving airway, breathing, and circulation (major bleeding and arrest). As a First Responder, you may begin certain types of soft-tissue injury care during assessment (Figure 10.37), but take care to avoid a tunnel-vision approach.

Remember, each patient is different. Follow local protocols and begin care when safe to do so. You should care for any life-threatening injuries as you encounter them, but always remember to continue to monitor the ABCs, as they take precedence. Do not be in such a hurry to start patient care that you miss detecting serious injuries.

Care of Closed Wounds

As mentioned earlier in this chapter, the most frequently seen closed wound is the bruise or contusion. Generally, bruises do not require emergency care in the field. However, bruises can be a warning sign of possible internal injuries and related bleeding. Look for large bruises or large areas of the body covered with bruises. Remember that a deep bruise the size of the patient's fist equals a blood loss of about 10%. Be certain to look for swelling and deformities that may indicate suspected fractures. Note if the patient's abdomen is rigid, if the patient is coughing up blood, or if there is blood in the mouth, nose, or ears.

Care of Open Wounds

FIRST▶ To care for open wounds, you should (Figure 10.38):

1. *Expose the wound.* Clothing over and around an open wound must be cut away. Avoid aggravating the patient's injuries. Do not try to remove clothing by pulling the items over the patient's head or limbs. Simply lift aside or cut the clothing away from the site of injury.

2. *Clear the wound surface.* Remove superficial foreign matter from the surface of the wound with a sterile gauze pad. This method will reduce the chances of contamination from your gloved fingers and will protect your fingertips. Do not try to clean the wound or pick out any particles or debris. If bleeding from the wound is controlled, take care not to restart or increase the flow of blood.

remember
Providing care for soft-tissue injuries may place you in contact with blood and body fluids. Take BSI precautions. Also, remember to wash your hands after each patient contact.

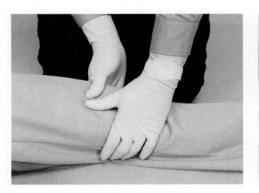
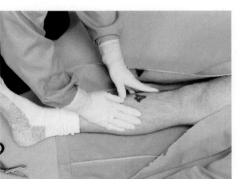

FIGURE 10.37
A limited amount of care for soft-tissue injury may be started during patient assessment.

FIGURE 10.38
Emergency care for open wounds.

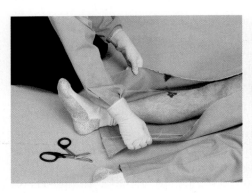

A. Expose the wound.

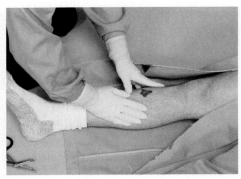

B. Clear the wound surface.

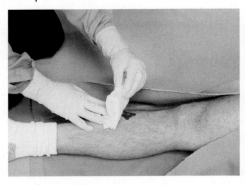

C. Control bleeding with direct pressure or direct pressure and elevation.

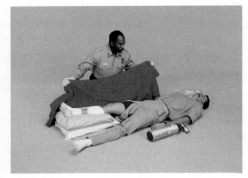

D. Keep the patient lying still, and provide emergency care for shock.

3. *Control bleeding.* Start with direct pressure or direct pressure and elevation. If the bleeding continues, try pressure point control. A tourniquet should be used only as a last resort for life-threatening bleeding from a limb. Administer oxygen as per local protocols.

4. *Prevent further contamination.* Use a sterile dressing, clean cloth, or clean handkerchief to cover the wound. After the bleeding has been controlled, bandage the dressing in place.

5. *Keep the patient lying still.* Any patient activity increases circulation. Keep the patient lying down, using a blanket or other form of covering to provide protection from the elements.

6. *Reassure the patient.* This will reduce patient movement and may help to lower the patient's blood pressure toward a normal level.

7. *Care for shock.* This applies to all but the simplest of wounds. Do not elevate a limb if there is the possibility of a fracture, unless the limb is immobilized. ■

remember

Do not remove a dressing once it is in place.

If you have to control bleeding from an extremity or if the wound on a limb is long, dress the wound and immobilize the limb with a splint (see Chapter 11). If an air splint is part of your First Responder equipment, use it to help control the bleeding.

CARE OF SPECIFIC INJURIES

Care for certain soft-tissue injuries is summarized in Figure 10.39.

Puncture Wounds

FIRST▸ When dealing with any puncture wound, assume that there is extensive internal injury and internal bleeding. Always check for an exit wound,

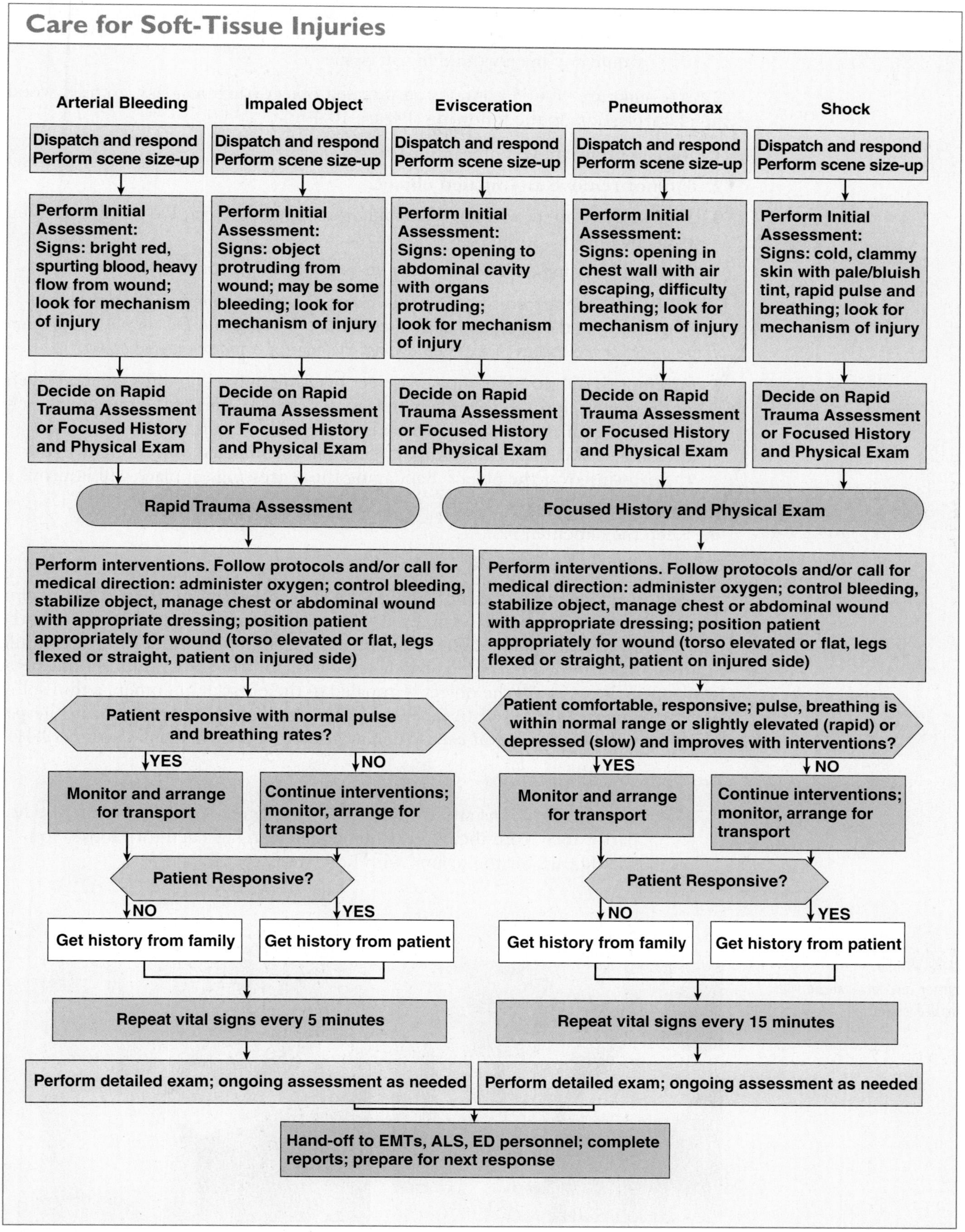

Care for Soft-Tissue Injuries

Arterial Bleeding	Impaled Object	Evisceration	Pneumothorax	Shock
Dispatch and respond Perform scene size-up	Dispatch and respond Perform scene size-up	Dispatch and respond Perform scene size-up	Dispatch and respond Perform scene size-up	Dispatch and respond Perform scene size-up
Perform Initial Assessment: Signs: bright red, spurting blood, heavy flow from wound; look for mechanism of injury	Perform Initial Assessment: Signs: object protruding from wound; may be some bleeding; look for mechanism of injury	Perform Initial Assessment: Signs: opening to abdominal cavity with organs protruding; look for mechanism of injury	Perform Initial Assessment: Signs: opening in chest wall with air escaping, difficulty breathing; look for mechanism of injury	Perform Initial Assessment: Signs: cold, clammy skin with pale/bluish tint, rapid pulse and breathing; look for mechanism of injury
Decide on Rapid Trauma Assessment or Focused History and Physical Exam	Decide on Rapid Trauma Assessment or Focused History and Physical Exam	Decide on Rapid Trauma Assessment or Focused History and Physical Exam	Decide on Rapid Trauma Assessment or Focused History and Physical Exam	Decide on Rapid Trauma Assessment or Focused History and Physical Exam

Rapid Trauma Assessment

Focused History and Physical Exam

Perform interventions. Follow protocols and/or call for medical direction: administer oxygen; control bleeding, stabilize object, manage chest or abdominal wound with appropriate dressing; position patient appropriately for wound (torso elevated or flat, legs flexed or straight, patient on injured side)

Perform interventions. Follow protocols and/or call for medical direction: administer oxygen; control bleeding, stabilize object, manage chest or abdominal wound with appropriate dressing; position patient appropriately for wound (torso elevated or flat, legs flexed or straight, patient on injured side)

Patient responsive with normal pulse and breathing rates?

Patient comfortable, responsive; pulse, breathing is within normal range or slightly elevated (rapid) or depressed (slow) and improves with interventions?

↓YES — Monitor and arrange for transport

↓NO — Continue interventions; monitor, arrange for transport

↓YES — Monitor and arrange for transport

↓NO — Continue interventions; monitor, arrange for transport

Patient Responsive?

↓NO — Get history from family

↓YES — Get history from patient

Patient Responsive?

↓NO — Get history from family

↓YES — Get history from patient

Repeat vital signs every 5 minutes

Repeat vital signs every 15 minutes

Perform detailed exam; ongoing assessment as needed

Perform detailed exam; ongoing assessment as needed

Hand-off to EMTs, ALS, ED personnel; complete reports; prepare for next response

FIGURE 10.39

realizing that exit wounds can be more serious than entrance wounds (in the case of gunshot wounds). Care for entrance and exit wounds as you would any open wound in soft tissue.

If a puncture wound contains an impaled object (such as glass, a knife, wood, metal, or plastic), do the following (Figure 10.40):

1. Take appropriate BSI precautions.

2. **Do not remove an impaled object.**

3. Expose the wound, without disturbing the impaled object. Do not lift clothing over the object.

4. Control bleeding. Administer oxygen as per local protocols.

CAUTION: *Take special care not to cut your gloves or hand on an impaled object. Spread your fingers around the object and apply pressure to the wound site. Do not put any pressure on the object or the tissues that are up against the edge of a sharp impaled object.*

5. Attempt to stabilize the impaled object by using bulky dressings. Several layers of dressings, cloths, or handkerchiefs placed on the sides of the object will help stabilize it. An alternative approach is to cut a hole in the center of a bulky dressing, making the cut slightly larger than the impaled object. Gently pass the dressing over the object. Bandaging these dressings in place will improve stability.

6. Keep the patient at rest.

7. Provide care for shock. ■

Adhesive tape often does not stick to the skin around an impaled object wound site. Blood and sweat on the skin, even when the surface is cleared, may cause the tape to slip. Cravats can be used to tie the dressings in place. These cravats should be made from folded triangular bandages. Once folded, the cravats should be at least two inches wide. If the object is impaled in the chest or abdomen, a thin splint or coat hanger can be used to push the cravats under the natural void in the patient's back so that the cravat can be tied around the patient's trunk (Figure 10.41).

Avulsions and Amputations

FIRST➤ Care for avulsions and amputations is the same. If skin or another body part is torn from the body, or if a flap of skin has been torn loose, you should care for the wound with bulky pressure dressings:

FIGURE 10.40
Emergency care for a wound with an impaled object.

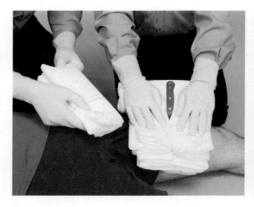

A. Control bleeding.

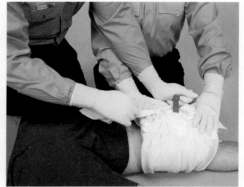

B. Stabilize the object in place.

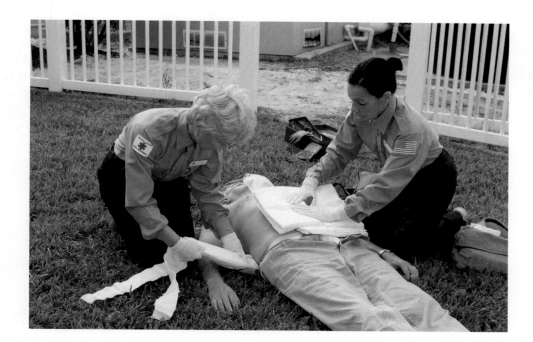

1. Take appropriate BSI precautions.

2. Clear the surface of the wound.

3. If there is an avulsion, gently fold the skin back to its normal position. Follow local protocols for procedures.

4. Control bleeding and care as you would for any open wound, using bulky pressure dressings.

5. Provide care for shock. Administer oxygen as per local protocols. ■

Save and preserve an avulsed or amputated part. This is best done by wrapping the part in a slightly moistened sterile dressing, if available, and placing it into a plastic bag or wrapping it in plastic wrap. If possible, keep the part cool (not cold, avoid freezing). Do not place the avulsed or amputated part in water or in direct contact with ice. Be certain that the bag with the part in it gets transported with the patient. It may be helpful to label the bag with the patient's name.

FIRST> In most cases of avulsion or amputation, bleeding can be controlled by direct pressure, elevation, and a pressure dressing held firmly over the stump or area of avulsion. Use pressure point techniques if the bleeding continues. Should this fail, apply a tourniquet. ■

Protruding Organs

FIRST> A deep open wound to the abdomen may cause organs to protrude through the wound opening. This is known as an *evisceration* (e-VIS-er-a-shun). In such cases:

- Do not try to replace the organ(s).
- Place a plastic covering over the exposed organs. If possible, apply a thick, moist dressing over the top of this covering to help conserve heat.
- Provide care for shock. Do not give the patient anything by mouth. ■

Scalp Injuries

Injuries to the scalp can be difficult to care for because of the numerous blood vessels found there. Many of these vessels are close to the surface of the skin, producing profuse bleeding even from minor wounds. Additional problems arise if the bones of the skull are involved.

Injuries to the scalp (and face) require an extra effort on the part of the First Responder to provide emotional support for patients. These injuries tend to be very painful, produce bleeding that frightens many patients, and are in a body region where people have concern for their appearance. Talk to patients in a calm, professional manner. Always let them know what you are going to do before you do it. Make certain that they know additional help is on the way.

FIRST➤ The procedures for the care of soft-tissue injuries covered earlier in this chapter apply to the care you should provide for injuries to the soft tissues of the scalp. However, there are three exceptions:

- *Exception 1:* Do not attempt to clear the surface of a scalp wound. This will often cause additional bleeding and may cause great harm if there are fractures to the skull.
- *Exception 2:* Do not apply firm pressure to the wound if there is any chance of skull fracture.

Care of scalp wounds includes the following (Figure 10.42):

- Do not clear foreign matter or dirt from the wound. It will cause more bleeding.
- Control bleeding with a dressing held in place with gentle pressure. Avoid exerting excessive pressure if there are signs of a fractured skull or the injury site feels spongy.
- Adhesive bandages will not work well. A roller bandage or gauze can be wrapped around the patient's head to hold dressings in place once bleeding has been controlled. If there is any indication of neck or spine injuries, do not attempt to wrap the patient's head. Do not wrap the bandage around the patient's lower jaw or neck.
- If there are no signs of skull fracture or injuries to the spine, neck, or chest, you may position the patient so that the head and shoulders are elevated. ■

An optional approach to holding a dressing in place over a scalp wound is to use a commercially prepared triangular bandage or one made from gauze or some other cloth. The steps for this procedure are shown in Figure 10.43.

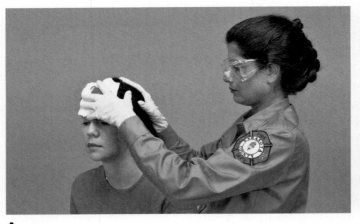
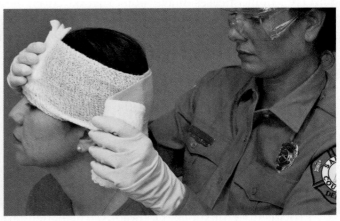

A **B**

FIGURE 10.42
Emergency care for a scalp wound. **A.** Use a dressing to apply controlled pressure. **B.** When bleeding is controlled, wrap a roller bandage around the patient's head to hold dressings in place.

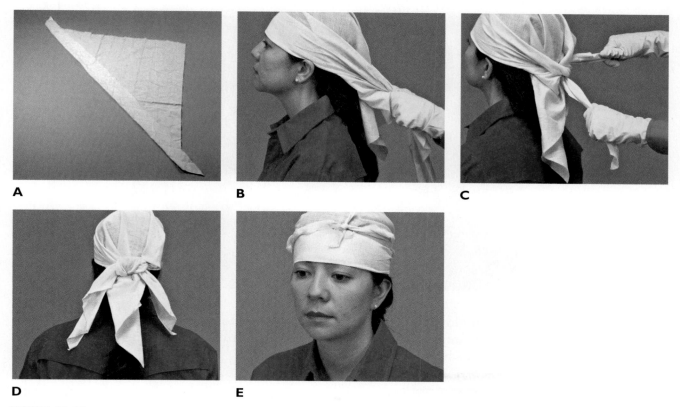

FIGURE 10.43

Using a triangular bandage to hold dressings for a scalp wound in place. **A.** Fold the bandage to make a two-inch hem along its base. **B.** Have the folded edge face out when you position the bandage on the patient's forehead, just above the eyes. Make certain that the point of the bandage hangs down behind the patient's head. **C.** Draw the ends of the bandage behind the patient's head. **D.** Then tie the ends over the point of the bandage. **E.** Pull the ends to the front of the head and tie them together. Finally, bring the point of the bandage down and tuck it into the crossed folds.

Facial Wounds

The first concern when caring for facial injuries is to make certain that the patient's airway is open and breathing is adequate. Even though bleeding may appear to be the only problem, check the airway and establish the presence of a carotid pulse. Continue to watch the patient to be sure that the airway remains open and clear of fluids and obstructions (tongue, teeth, blood clots).

FIRST➤ When caring for patients with facial injuries, you should (Figure 10.44):

1. Correct breathing problems, taking care to note and properly care for neck and spine injuries.

2. Control bleeding by direct pressure, taking care not to press too hard since many facial fractures are not obvious.

3. Apply a dressing and bandage.

If you find the patient has an object that has passed through the cheek wall and is sticking into the mouth, you may have to remove it. This should be done if the object blocks the airway or is loose and may fall into the airway.

To remove an impaled object from the cheek (Figure 10.45):

1. Look into the mouth and probe to see if the object has passed through the cheek wall.

2. If you find penetration, pull or safely and carefully push the object out of the cheek wall, back in the direction from which the object entered. Avoid cutting

FIGURE 10.44
Care of soft-tissue injuries to the face.

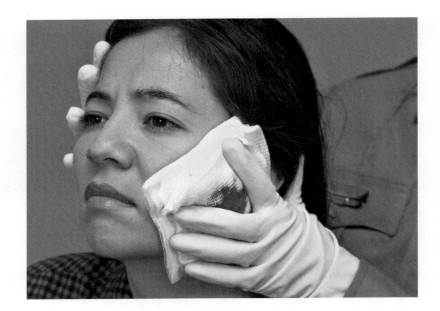

your gloves and yourself. If the object has not penetrated the cheek wall, or if you cannot easily remove the object, stabilize it with dressings applied to the outer surface of the cheek.

3. In all cases, except for neck and spine injuries, turn the patient so that blood will drain from the mouth. If there are neck or spine injuries, do not turn the patient. Use dressing material packed against the inside wound to control the flow of blood.

4. If you remove an impaled object, place the dressing material between the wound and the patient's teeth, leaving some of the dressing outside the mouth so that it can be held to prevent swallowing it. Watch closely to be sure that the dressing does not work its way loose and into the airway. Do not assume that the patient's gag reflex will prevent the dressing from becoming an airway obstruction.

5. Dress and bandage the outside of the wound.

6. Provide care for shock. ■

Eye Injuries

Two rules of soft-tissue injury care apply when caring for an eye injury: do not remove any impaled objects, and do not try to put the eye back into its socket. When

FIGURE 10.45

Removing an impaled object impaled in the cheek. **A.** Look into the mouth and probe to see if the object has passed through the cheek wall. If it has, remove it. **B.** Use dressing material packed against the inside wound to control the flow of blood.

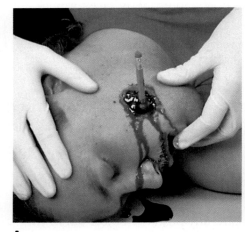

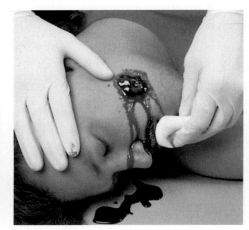

A   B

caring for a cut eyeball, there is one major exception to the procedures listed for soft-tissue injury care.

EXCEPTION: *Do not apply direct pressure to a cut eyeball. There are jelly-like fluids inside the eyeball that cannot be replaced. A loose bulky dressing will help the formation of blood clots to control the bleeding.*

Problems resulting from foreign objects in the eyes are common. These problems can range from minor irritations to permanent injury. If the patient's own tears do not wash away a foreign object, use running water to remove it (Figure 10.46). **Do not apply the wash if there are impaled objects or cuts in the eye.** Apply the flow of water at the corner of the eye socket closest to the patient's nose. You may have to help the patient hold open the eyelids. As you pour the water, direct the patient to look from side to side and up and down. Before completing the wash, have the patient blink several times. When possible, continue the wash for at least 20 minutes or for the time recommended by medical direction.

NOTE

After debris is washed from the eye, the patient must be examined by someone with more advanced training. A physician or qualified eye care specialist should see the patient.

First➤ It is critical that you:

● Do not remove impaled objects (including what may appear to be small pieces of glass impaled in the globe of the eye).
● Do not probe into the eye socket.
● Reduce the patient's eye movements. If there are sharp objects in the patient's eye, do not direct the patient to move the eyes during the wash. After the wash, keep the patient's eyes shut. Cover both eyes, bandaging the materials in place. ■

Whenever you are caring for a patient with eye injuries, you will have to cover both of the patient's eyes. In most cases, only one eye will actually be injured. However, when one eye moves, the other eye will also move (sympathetic movement). If you cover the injured eye and leave the uninjured eye uncovered, the uninjured eye will continue to react to activities and movement. Each time the uninjured eye moves, so will the injured eye. Having both of the patient's eyes covered reduces eye movements.

Having both eyes covered can cause fear and anxiety in the patient. Tell him why you are covering the uninjured eye. Keep close to him or have someone else stay close. Try to maintain contact with him through conversation and touch. If a friend or loved one of the patient also has been injured, reassure the patient that care is being provided for others.

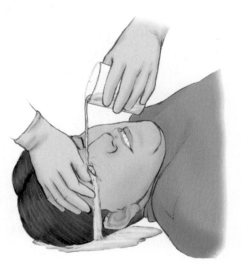

FIGURE 10.46
Foreign objects can be washed from the eye. Flush with water from a medial to lateral direction.

If the patient is unresponsive, it is best to keep someone with him at all times. This person can reassure him if responsiveness returns and can help prevent him from reaching for his covered eyes. Should the unresponsive patient have to be left unattended, you may tie his hands at the waist to prevent grabbing at the eyes should responsiveness be regained. Even though this may produce a fearful moment for the patient, it is better than the additional injury that could take place. Any procedure that requires the tying of a patient's hands must be approved by your EMS system.

FIRST➤ Always remember to close the eyelids of unresponsive patients. Since unresponsive people do not blink, moisture is quickly lost from the eye surface, damaging the eye. If you notice that the patient is wearing contact lenses, be sure to point this out to the EMTs who take over the care of the patient. ■

FIRST➤ Burns to the eye must always be considered serious, requiring special in-hospital care. As a First Responder, you may have to care for burns to the eyes caused by heat, light, or chemicals (Figure 10.47). Your actions can make the difference as to whether or not the patient's sight can be saved.

- *Thermal (heat) burns*—Do not try to inspect the eyes if there are signs of thermal burns to the eyelids. With the patient's eyelids closed, cover the eyes with loose, moist dressings. If you have no means to moisten the dressings, then apply loose, dry dressings. Do not apply any burn ointment to the eyelids.
- *Light burns*—"Snow blindness" and "welder's blindness" are two examples of light burns. Close the patient's eyelids and apply dark patches over both eyes.

FIGURE 10.47
Emergency care for burns to the eye.

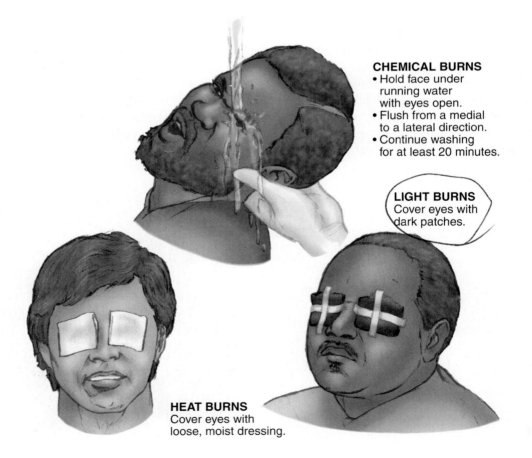

CHEMICAL BURNS
- Hold face under running water with eyes open.
- Flush from a medial to a lateral direction.
- Continue washing for at least 20 minutes.

LIGHT BURNS
Cover eyes with dark patches.

HEAT BURNS
Cover eyes with loose, moist dressing.

If you do not have dark patches, then use thick dressings or dressings followed with a layer of an opaque material such as dark plastic.

- *Chemical burns*—Many chemicals cause rapid, severe damage to the eyes. Flush the eyes with water. Do not delay care by trying to locate sterile water. Use any source of clean drinking water. If possible, continue the washing flow for at least 20 minutes. After washing the patient's eyes, close the eyelids and apply loose, moist dressings.

If you find an object impaled in the globe of a patient's eye, you should (Figure 10.48):

1. Use several layers of dressing or small rolls of gauze to make thick pads. Place them on the sides of the object. If you have only enough material for one thick pad, cut a hole, equal to the size of the eye opening, in the center of this pad. Set the pad over the patient's eye, allowing the impaled object to stick out through the opening cut into the pad.

2. Fit a disposable cardboard drinking cup or paper cone over the impaled object. (Do not use foam cups since they can break and send flakes into the eye.) This will serve as a protective shield. Rest the cup or cone onto the thick dressing pad, but do not allow this protective shield to come into contact with the impaled object.

3. Hold the pad and protective shield in place with a self-adherent roller bandage or with a wrapping of gauze or other cloth material.

4. Use dressing material to cover the uninjured eye, and bandage this dressing in place. This will reduce sympathetic eye movements.

5. Provide care for shock.

6. Provide emotional support to the patient. ■

Wrapping a paper cup or cone with gauze is very tricky and cannot be done easily unless you practice. Ideally, you should wrap around the cup and then continue around the patient's head and wrap around the cup again. This procedure is repeated until the cup is stable. Do not wrap the gauze over the top of the cup. Take great care not to push the cup down onto the impaled object or pull the cup out of place.

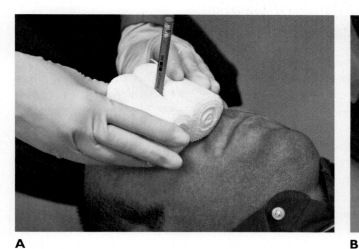
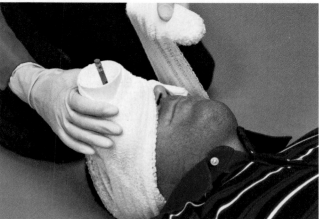

A **B**

FIGURE 10.48
Emergency care for a patient with an object impaled in the globe of the eye includes (A) stabilizing the object and (B) securing it in place.

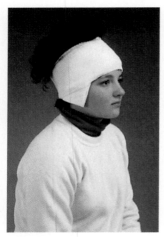

FIGURE 10.49
When caring for injuries to the external ear, apply a dressing and bandage.

remember

Consider any bleeding from the ear as a sign of a possible head injury.

NOTE

Most nosebleeds are minor, requiring very little attention. However, they can be serious. Care for them accordingly.

FIRST➤ If the eye is pulled out of the socket (avulsed eye), the care provided is the same as for an object impaled in the eye. ■

Ear Injuries

External ear injuries include (Figure 10.49):

- *Cuts*—Apply dressings and bandage in place.

- *Tears*—Apply bulky dressings, beginning with several layers behind the torn tissue.

- *Avulsions*—Use slightly moistened bulky dressings, bandaged into place. Save the avulsed part in a plastic bag or plastic wrap. Keep the part dry and cool. If no plastic is available, then wrap in dressing material. Be certain to label the bag, wrap, or dressing with the patient's name.

Internal ear injuries may appear as bleeding from the ears. Any such bleeding must be considered a sign of serious head injury. Bloody or clear fluids draining from the ear may indicate the presence of cerebrospinal fluid (a clear watery fluid that helps to protect the brain and spinal cord). For such cases, assume there is serious injury and provide the necessary care. (More about head injuries in Chapter 11.)

Do not pack the external ear canal. To do so can cause increased internal injury. If there is bleeding or clear fluid leaking from the ears, apply external dressings, sterile if possible, and hold them in place with bandages. Report this bleeding to the EMTs.

Do not attempt to remove foreign objects from inside the ear. Apply external dressings, if necessary, and provide emotional support to the patient.

If the patient tells you he feel his ears are "clogged" or "stopped up," suspect possible damage to the eardrum, fluids in the middle ear, or objects in the ear canal. Do not probe into the ears. Many of these problems will clear up quickly after hospital care. As a First Responder, your main duty in such cases is to prevent the patient from hitting the side of the head in an effort to clear the ears. These blows may cause severe internal ear damage.

Nose Injuries

FIRST➤ When dealing with any nasal injuries—and there are no suspected skull fractures or spine injuries—you will have two duties: maintain an open airway and control bleeding. ■

For a nosebleed in a responsive patient, maintain an open airway. Have the patient assume a seated position, leaning slightly forward. This position will help prevent blood and mucus from obstructing the airway or draining down the throat and into the stomach, which can cause nausea and vomiting. Next, have the patient pinch the nostrils. Bleeding is usually controlled when the nostrils are pinched shut. If the patient cannot pinch them shut, you will have to do so (Figure 10.50). However, if other patients are in need of your help, do not delay their care while you sit pinching someone's nose. Have a bystander put on gloves, pinch the patient's nose, and inform you of any problems as you continue to care for the other patients. Do not pack the patient's nostrils.

For a nosebleed in an unresponsive patient or in a patient injured in such a way that he cannot be placed in a seated position, place him on one side with the head turned to provide drainage from the nose and mouth. Attempt to control bleeding by pinching the nostrils shut. In addition, do not pack the nose. Do not remove ob-

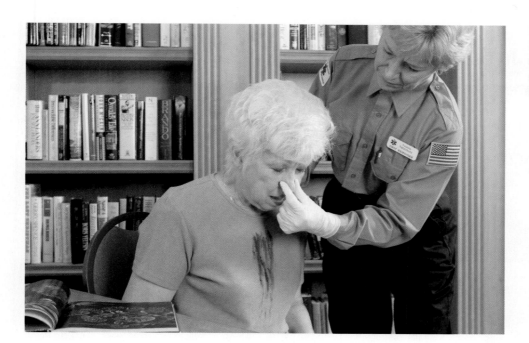

jects or probe into the nose. Do not allow the patient to blow his nose if he is bleeding from the nostrils or has recently controlled a nosebleed.

For an avulsion of the nose, apply a pressure dressing to the site. Save the avulsed part in plastic or a sterile or clean dressing. Keep the part cool.

(See Scan 10-4 for a summary of care for soft-tissue injury to the head.)

Injury to the Mouth

FIRST➤ As with all injuries that occur along the pathway of respiration, your first concern will be to ensure an open airway. If there are no suspected skull, neck, or spine injuries, position the patient in a seated position with the head tilted slightly forward to allow for drainage. If the patient cannot be placed in a seated position, position him on one side with the head turned slightly downward to provide some drainage for blood and other fluids.

For cut lips, use a rolled or folded dressing. Place the dressing between the patient's lip and gum. Take great care that the patient does not swallow this dressing.

For avulsed lips, apply a pressure bandage to the site of injury. Save the avulsed part in plastic or a sterile or clean dressing. Keep the avulsed part cool.

For cuts to the internal cheek, position a dressing between the patient's cheek and gum. (Do not pack the mouth with dressings.) Hold the dressing in place with a gloved hand. Always leave three to four inches of dressing material outside the patient's mouth to allow for quick removal. This is necessary to prevent the patient from swallowing the dressing. If possible, position the patient's head to allow drainage. ■

Neck Wounds

FIRST➤ Blunt and sharp injuries can occur to the neck. As a First Responder, be aware of the following signs that indicate soft-tissue wounds to the neck:

● Difficulty speaking, loss of voice.
● Airway obstruction when the mouth and nose are clear and no object can be dislodged from the airway. This is often due to swollen tissues.

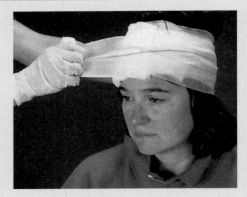

Scalp. Control bleeding, dress, and wrap with roller bandage.

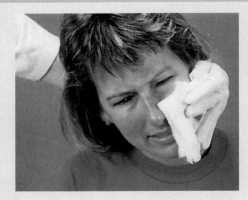

Facial. Ensure airway, control bleeding, dress, and wrap with roller bandage.

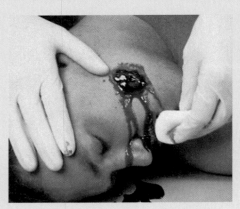

Cheek. Ensure airway, remove impaled object, and control bleeding. Dress and bandage the external wound.

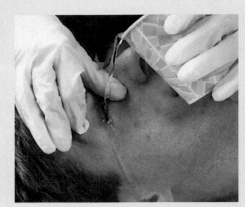

Debris in eye. If eye is not cut, wash objects from surface.

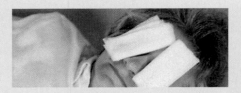

Eye burns. Flush chemical burns (20 minutes). Loosely dress heat burns. Apply dark patches for light burns.

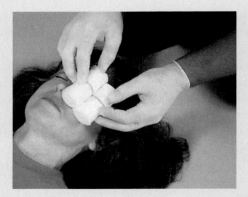

Impaled object in the eye. Stabilize the object and apply rigid protection.

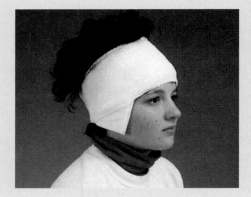

Ear. Do not pack canal. Dress and bandage.

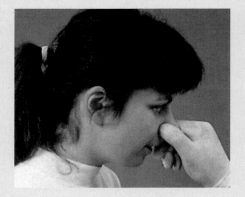

Nosebleed. Pinch nostrils shut.

- Obvious swelling or bruising of the neck.
- Pain upon swallowing or speaking.
- Trachea pushed off to one side (tracheal deviation).
- Depressions in the neck.
- Obvious cuts or puncture wounds.

For all profuse bleeding from the neck, make certain that someone activates EMS and reports the problem and the need for immediate EMS transport.

Cut or severed arteries in the neck require the following procedure:

1. Take appropriate BSI precautions.

2. Immediately apply direct pressure over the wound, using the palm of your gloved hand.

3. Try controlling the bleeding with a pressure dressing, taking care not to close the airway and not to apply pressure to both sides of the neck.

4. Once the bleeding is controlled, place the patient on his left side (Figure 10.51). If possible, lay the patient on a surface that can be slanted (spine board, table, long bench, plywood) so that the entire body can be tilted into a head-down position. The slant should be no more than 15 degrees. This will help trap any air bubbles that may have entered the bloodstream.

5. Provide care for shock. Administer oxygen as per local protocols.

Bleeding from a large cut or severed neck veins usually cannot be controlled by pressure dressings. For such emergencies, you should (Figure 10.52):

1. Immediately apply direct pressure to the wound, using the palm of your gloved hand.

2. Apply an occlusive dressing or some type of plastic over the wound. Use tape to seal this dressing on all sides. When complete, the dressing must be air-tight. If you do not have the materials to make an occlusive dressing, use any sterile or clean dressing material and attempt to control bleeding by direct pressure.

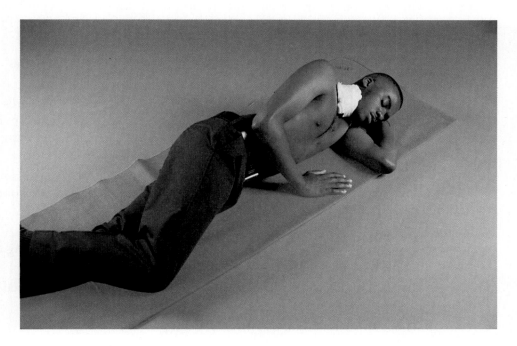

FIGURE 10.51
With open wounds to the neck, place the patient on the left side.

FIGURE 10.52
Use an occlusive dressing to help
control bleeding from the neck.

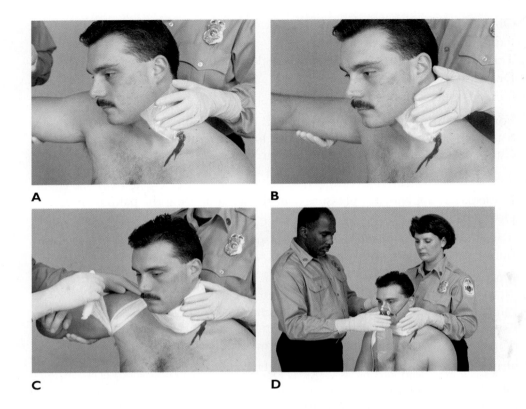

3. To help trap any air bubbles that may have entered the bloodstream, place the patient on the left side for transport, with the body slanted as described above.

WARNING: *Do not attempt to reposition the patient if there are indications of spinal injury, if the bleeding was very difficult to control, or if you have difficulty carrying out the dressing and bandaging procedures.*

4. Care for shock by maintaining body warmth and providing oxygen. ■

An alternative method of securing a dressing to the neck is as follows. Your instructor will tell you if the technique is approved for use in your state. This method uses the same procedure for both arterial and venous bleeding of the neck:

1. Immediately apply direct pressure over the wound, using the palm of your gloved hand.

2. Place a plastic occlusive dressing over the wound and continue to apply pressure, using the palm of your hand. Do not use a single layer of plastic wrap. It is too thin and may be sucked into the wound. Ideally, the occlusive dressing should extend one inch beyond the wound on all sides.

3. Place a roll of gauze dressing or dressing materials over the occlusive dressing and continue to apply pressure. Another roll can be placed between the wound and the trachea to help reduce pressure on the trachea.

4. While maintaining pressure, secure the entire dressing with a figure-eight wrap of self-adherent roller bandage. This eliminates the problem of trying to make adhesive tape stick to a bloody surface.

5. Place the patient on his left side for transport, with the body slightly slanted in a head-down position.

6. Care for shock by maintaining body warmth and providing oxygen.

NOTE: *These methods take a great deal of practice and review if they are to be done correctly in the field.*

Should your attempts to control bleeding from a neck wound fail, a last-resort method would be to place your gloved finger or fingers into the wound and attempt to compress the vessel or pinch shut the ends. This is a last resort to be used only when standard First Responder-level care procedures have failed to control life-threatening profuse bleeding.

Penetrating Chest Wounds

Soft-tissue injuries to the chest receive the same basic type of care as you would give to soft-tissue injuries in other areas of the body. Typically, these injuries are cuts, bruises, and puncture wounds.

Serious soft-tissue injuries to the chest include deep puncture wounds, penetrating wounds, and impaled objects. For puncture and penetrating wounds, apply occlusive dressings; impaled objects must be stabilized. Wounds from punctures and impaled objects may go through the chest. If this occurs, you will have to care for both an entrance wound and an exit wound. Deep punctures to the chest are generally serious because of the vital organs located there. In addition, as explained in Chapter 6, breathing causes pressure in the chest cavity. When the chest wall is punctured, this pressure balance is affected. A lung will collapse because air gets between it and the chest wall causing extra pressure to build up inside the chest cavity and breathing to be ineffective.

You must seal an open wound to the chest to prevent air from entering the chest space and causing lung collapse. The seal will also allow the lungs to re-expand.

In some cases, the lung itself will be penetrated (Figure 10.53). As the patient inhales, air from this lung will leak out and enter the chest cavity. If the wound has been tightly sealed on the outside, pressure may still build from the inside as air continues to enter the cavity from the punctured lung during each breath. Unless this pressure is released, it may interfere with heart and lung actions.

FIRST➤ You will be able to tell if a puncture wound has penetrated the lung by noting:

● Open chest wound in which the chest wall is torn or punctured.

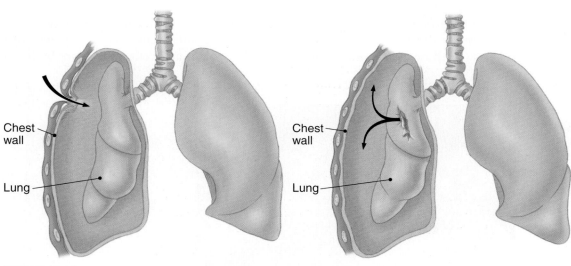

FIGURE 10.53
Penetrating chest wounds.

- Sucking sound each time the patient breathes. This is why this type of wound is sometimes called a **sucking chest wound**. Bubbling may be noted.
- Patient is coughing up bright red, frothy blood. ■

If you find that a penetrating chest wound has both an entrance and an exit wound, assume that at least one lung has been punctured.

FIRST➤ The following method is recommended for open chest wounds free of impaled objects. If there is no puncture to the lung, the method will work. If there is a punctured lung, this method will allow release of air trapped in the chest:

1. Have all dressing materials ready. Take appropriate BSI precautions. Then seal the patient's wound with the palm of your gloved hand as the patient exhales (a forceful exhalation will push trapped air out of the chest cavity). Do not unseal the wound to prepare dressings. Have others at the scene help in preparing the dressings.

2. Place an occlusive dressing under your hand while the patient exhales, and hold it in place.

   – *Taping three sides:* Have someone seal it by placing tape on three sides (Figure 10.54). This will produce a flutter valve effect. That is, when the patient inhales, the free edge will seal against the skin. When the patient exhales, the free edge will break loose from the skin and allow any build up of air in the chest cavity to escape.

   – *Taping four sides:* Some EMS systems prefer that all four sides be taped. The last side is taped as the patient exhales.

   With either taping method, the patient must be monitored. If the patient begins to have trouble breathing again, lift up one side of the plastic and have him forcefully exhale. Then quickly reposition the plastic to reseal.

3. Provide oxygen as soon as possible, and maintain body temperature to prevent shock. ■

A commercial occlusive dressing is the best choice for open chest wounds. Plastic wrap can be used, but it must be folded over several times so that it is thick enough to prevent air from seeping through it and so it will not be sucked into the wound. The occlusive dressing should extend two or more inches beyond the edge of the wound.

If blood or perspiration prevents the tape from sticking to the patient's skin, apply bulky dressings over the occlusive dressing and secure them in place with cravats (cloth ties). You must still monitor the patient and relieve pressure build up

sucking chest wound an open chest wound in which air is sucked through the wound opening and into the chest cavity each time the patient breathes.

remember

Closely monitor the breathing of all patients with open chest wounds.

FIGURE 10.54
Apply an occlusive dressing to an open chest wound. If local protocol allows, tape it only on three sides to allow air to escape.

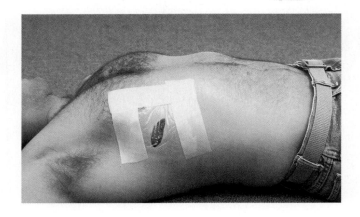

if the patient develops difficulty breathing. In cases when the EMTs will not be delayed in their arrival and tape will not hold the dressing, hold the occlusive dressing in place with the palm of your gloved hand. If the patient's condition declines, periodically release one edge of the seal in order to allow trapped air to escape as described above.

If there is an entrance wound and an exit wound, both wounds will need a dressing. You may have to wait for EMT assistance to roll the patient and apply a dressing to the patient's back.

Penetrating wounds of the chest may also penetrate the heart. When this occurs, there is little that the First Responder can do other than provide care for shock and the open chest wound and provide basic life support as needed.

Impaled Objects

FIRST➤ An impaled object must be left in place. Even though it created the wound, the impaled object is also sealing the wound. If it is removed, the patient may bleed profusely. The object must be stabilized with bulky dressings or pads (Figure 10.55). Begin by placing these materials on opposite sides of the object, along the vertical line (long axis) of the body. Place the next layer perpendicular (opposite direction) to the first. Use tape or cravats to hold all dressings and pads in place. If tape will not hold, carefully apply cravats according to local protocols. ■

Abdominal Injuries

(In Chapter 4, the locations of the various body organs were presented. Before continuing with this section of Chapter 10, study Scan 4-1, page 65, to review the locations of the major hollow and solid organs of the abdomen and pelvis.)

Internal bleeding can be severe when an internal organ ruptures. In addition, hollow organs can rupture and drain their contents into the abdominal and pelvic cavities, producing a very serious and painful reaction. As a First Responder, you should be aware of the following signs, which indicate injury to organs of the abdomen and pelvis:

- Any deep cut or puncture wound to the abdomen, pelvis, or lower back.

- Indications of blunt trauma to the abdomen or pelvis.

- Pain or cramps in the abdominal or pelvic region.

- Patient is protecting the abdomen (guarding).

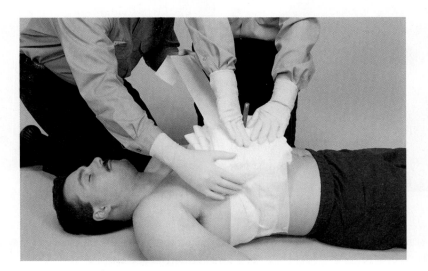

FIGURE 10.55
Never remove an object impaled in the chest. Stabilize it in place.

- Patient is trying to lie still with legs drawn up.
- Rapid, shallow breathing and a rapid pulse.
- Rigid and/or tender abdomen.

FIRST➤ To care for all possible abdominal and pelvic injuries:

1. Take appropriate BSI precautions.

2. Dress all open wounds.

3. Have the patient lie on his back. For open wounds or eviscerations, flex the patient's legs and support them with pillows or a rolled blanket. Do not flex the legs if there are signs of injury to the pelvic bones, lower limbs, or back. For impaled objects, leave the legs in the position found.

4. Care for shock, administer oxygen as per local protocols, and constantly monitoring vital signs.

5. Be alert for vomiting.

6. Do not touch exposed internal organs. Cover them with an occlusive dressing. Maintain warmth to the organ by placing dressings or a towel over the occlusive dressing (Figure 10.56). (Some EMS systems provide sterile materials to allow the First Responder to apply a moist, sterile dressing in place of the occlusive dressing. Follow local protocols.)

7. Do not remove an impaled object. Stabilize it with bulky dressings. ■

Many patients with abdominal pain find some relief by hugging a bulky, soft object such as a pillow against the abdomen.

Injury to the Genitalia

FIRST➤ Because of the location, external reproductive organs are not a common site of injury. The pelvis and the thighs usually prevent injury to these organs, which are known as the external **genitalia**. When injury does occur, two types of soft-tissue injury are commonly seen:

genitalia (jen-i-TA-le-ah) the external reproductive organs.

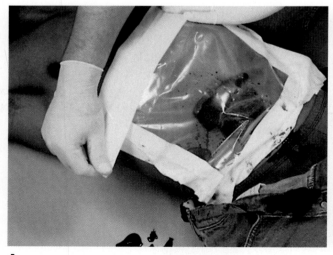
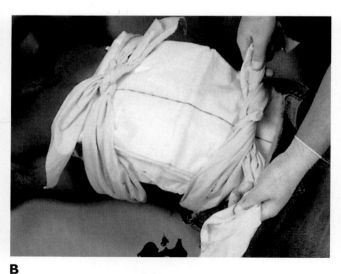

A   **B**

FIGURE 10.56

Emergency care of an open wound to the abdomen. **A.** Cover the wound with an occlusive dressing. **B.** Help maintain body heat by placing dressings or a towel over the occlusive dressing.

- *Blunt trauma*—Such an injury is very painful, but little can be done by the First Responder. An ice pack, if available, will help reduce the pain.
- *Cuts*—Bleeding should be controlled by direct pressure. A sterile dressing or a sanitary pad should be used. If either of these is not available, then use any clean, bulky dressing. Once bleeding is controlled, the dressing can be held in place with a large triangular bandage, applied in the same manner as a diaper (Figure 10.57).

Other soft-tissue injury care procedures also apply when caring for injuries to the genitalia:

- Do not remove impaled objects.
- Save avulsed parts, wrapping them in plastic, sterile dressings, or any clean dressing. ■

First Responders are a part of the professional health-care team. As such, you must carry out your role in a manner that will reduce embarrassment for the patient. Tell the patient what you are going to do. Tell him why you must examine and care for the genitalia. Protect him from the sight of onlookers by having them leave the scene. If this is not possible, have them turn their backs to the patient. Then, provide care without any hesitation. Conduct all procedures in the same manner as you would care for an injury to any other part of the body. This is essential if you are to provide proper total patient care.

Genital injury may be the result of rape. Maintain the patient's privacy and remain professional in your conversation and care. Inform the patient not to wash, urinate, or change clothing. The patient should be transported by EMS to the emergency department.

Many genital injuries are self-inflicted or are the result of abuse. They may also be caused by an attempt to abort an unborn fetus by the mother or some other unlicensed person. Whatever the cause, the patient will need emotional support and understanding.

BURNS

First Responders should consider burns to be very complex soft-tissue injuries that can range from a simple one to the skin's surface (epidermis) to a very serious deep injury that involves nerves, blood vessels, muscles, and bones. Careful patient as-

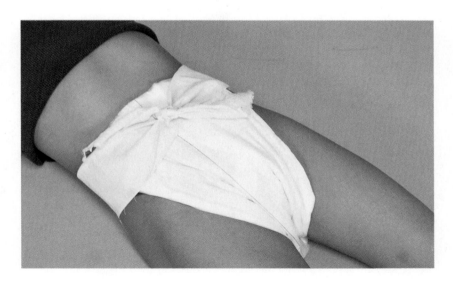

FIGURE 10.57
Dressings applied to the genitalia can be secured with a triangular bandage.

sessment is necessary to avoid missing injuries or medical problems that may be far more serious than obvious burns.

Classifications of burns

FIRST➤ Burns are classified in a number of ways. One way is to categorize burns based on the agent that caused the injury (source of the burn). This information should be gathered and forwarded to more highly trained personnel during transfer of care. Categories of burns based on source include:

- Heat (thermal) burns—may be caused by fire, steam, or hot objects.
- Chemical burns—may be caused by caustics, such as acids and alkalis.
- Electrical burns—originate from outlets, frayed wires, and faulty circuits.
- Lightning burns—occur during electrical storms.
- Light burns—occur with intense light. Light from the arc welder will damage unprotected eyes. Also, ultraviolet light (including sunlight) can burn the eyes and skin.
- Radiation burns—usually result from nuclear sources. ■

Always investigate the source of a burn carefully. Never assume a source. The environment where the patient was burned may be hazardous and may contain hazardous materials. Talk with bystanders and the patient in addition to performing a patient assessment. This information will assist in finding out exactly what happened to cause the injury.

FIRST➤ Most often burns are categorized according to the depth of the burn (Figure 10.58):

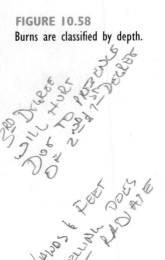
150°# For 1 Second
Enough For 3rd Degree
Burns
120° For 3 Minutes
212° Boiling Point

FIGURE 10.58
Burns are classified by depth.

3rd Degree
Will Hurt Due To Previous
2nd 1st Degree

Hands & Feet
Swelling Does
Not Radiate

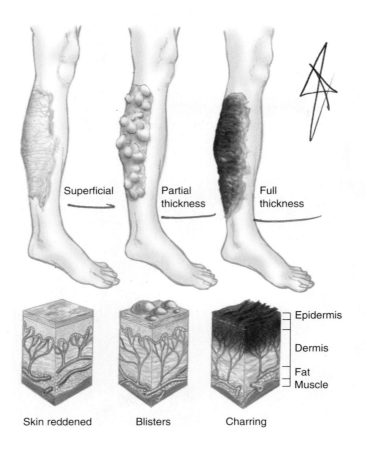

Superficial   Partial thickness   Full thickness

Epidermis
Dermis
Fat
Muscle

Skin reddened   Blisters   Charring

- **Superficial burns** involve the top layer of skin known as the epidermis. Once known as first-degree burns, they involve reddening of the skin and pain at the site. A common example is a sunburn. *← BLISTER*
- **Partial-thickness burns** involve both the epidermis and the dermis (the top two layers of skin). Once known as second-degree burns, they generally involve intense pain, white to red skin that is moist and mottled, and blisters. A classic example is a steam burn.
- **Full-thickness burns** extend through all dermal layers and may involve subcutaneous layers, muscle, bone, or organs. Once known as third-degree burns, they can be dry and leathery and may appear white, dark brown, or charred. Since there is often nerve damage present, there may be no sensation of pain present. ∎

Severity

FIRST➤ An important aspect of care is being able to assess the severity of a burn, or extent of the damage. A superficial or partial-thickness burn that involves less than 9% of the patient's total body surface area is considered a **minor burn**. The exceptions are if the burn involves the respiratory system, face, hands, feet, groin, buttocks, or major joint.

Any burn to the face (other than simple sunburn) is an example of a **major burn**. Other major burns include any superficial burns covering a large area of the body or burns involving the feet, hands, groin, buttocks, or major joint. ∎

One system used for determining the amount of skin surface burned is called the **rule of nines** (Figure 10.59). A quick reference for learning the rule of nines is to keep in mind that a patient's palm is about 1% of his or her body surface area. For example, the front of one leg equals 9% of approximately the same area that nine of the patient's palms would cover. You may also use your own palm to help you make a quick estimate.

For adults, the head and neck, chest, abdomen, each arm, the front of each leg, the back of each leg, the upper back, and the lower back and buttocks are each

superficial burn a burn involving only the outer layer of skin (epidermis). Also called *first-degree burn.*

partial-thickness burn a burn in which the outer layer of skin is burned through and the second layer (dermis) is damaged. Also called *second-degree burn.*

full-thickness burn a burn involving all the layers of skin. Muscle layers below the skin and bones may also be damaged. Also called *third-degree burn.*

minor burn a superficial or partial-thickness burn involving a small portion of the body with no damage to the respiratory system, face, hands, feet, groin, medial thigh, buttocks, or major joints. It does not encircle or cover an entire body part.

major burn any full-thickness burn, or a partial-thickness burn involving an entire body area or crucial area, or a superficial burn that covers a large area, or any burn to the face, hands, feet, neck, or genitals, or any burn that involves the respiratory system.

rule of nines a system used for estimating the amount of skin surface that is burned. The body is divided into 12 regions. For adults, each of 11 regions equals 9% of the body surface and the genital section is classified as 1%.

*rule of palms:
palm = 1% of
body area.*

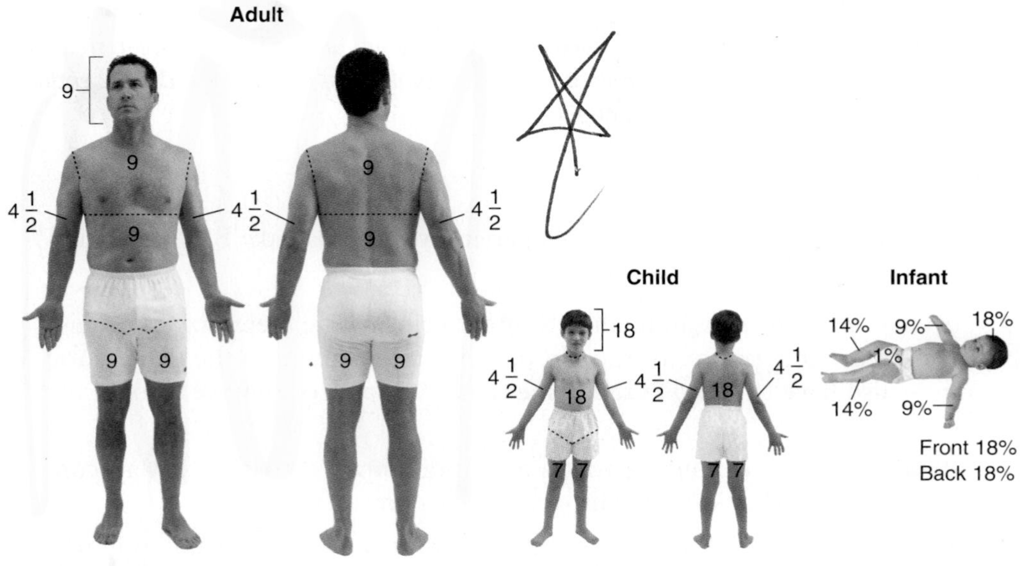

FIGURE 10.59
Rule of nines.

considered equal to 9% of the total body surface area. This gives a total of 99%. The remaining 1% is assigned to the genital area.

For infants and children, a simple approach assigns 18% to the head and neck, 9% to each upper limb, 18% to the chest and abdomen, 18% to the entire back, 14% for each lower limb, and 1% to the genital area. This method adds up to a total of 101% but provides an easy way to make approximate determinations.

By using the rule of nines, you can add up the areas affected by burns to determine how much of the patient's body has been injured. For example, if an adult patient has full-thickness thermal burns to the chest and front of one leg, this 9% + 9% means that 18% of the total body surface area has been burned. Note that burns often overlap different body regions. So when in doubt, always estimate to the higher percentage.

As a First Responder, you may not be required to learn the rule of nines. In most situations, knowing this information will not be necessary to carry out your duties. However, the rule of nines may be useful when communicating patient information to more highly trained EMS personnel.

Rules for First Responders

FIRST➤ Regardless of the system used to evaluate burns, follow these rules:

- Always perform a scene size-up, initial assessment, and provide basic life support as needed.
- Provide care for all burns, even the most minor or superficial ones.
- Any of the following burns should be considered critical and should be evaluated by someone in the EMS system above the level of First Responder:
  – Burns to the hands, feet, face, groin, buttocks, thighs, major joints.
  – Any burn that encircles a body part.
  – Burns estimated at greater than 15% or more of the patient's body.
  – Burns that include respiratory involvement.
- When in doubt, over classify. For example, consider a serious superficial burn to be partial-thickness burn.
- Always consider the effects of a burn to be more serious if the patient is a child, elderly, the victim of other injuries, or someone with a medical condition (for example, respiratory disease). ■

WARNING: *Do not attempt to rescue people trapped by fire unless you have been trained to do so. The simple act of opening a door or window could cost you your life. Do not endanger yourself and risk creating more patients.*

Care of Burns

FIRST➤ For First Responder care of a patient with burns, take BSI precautions. Then follow these steps:

1. *Stop the burning process* immediately after performing a scene size-up. This may require the patient to stop, drop, and roll to extinguish the flames. You might also have to smother the flames and wet down or remove smoldering clothing.

2. *Activate EMS* and, if a burn involves the mouth, nose, throat, or airway, consider it critical. Request assistance as per local protocol.

3. *Flush minor burns* with cool or running water (or saline) for several minutes. **For major burns,** do not flush burns with cool water unless they involve an

area of less than 9% of the total body surface area. Flushing large burn areas may chill the patient and increase the risk of developing shock and infection.

4. *Remove smoldering clothing and jewelry.*

5. *Continually monitor the airway.* Any burns to the face or exposure to smoke may cause airway problems. Administer oxygen as per local protocols.

6. *Prevent further contamination.* Keep the burned area clean by covering it with a dressing. Infection is common with burns.

7. *Cover the burn area* with dry, sterile dressing (Figure 10.60). In some EMS systems, you may be instructed to moisten dressings before placing them on the patient. Otherwise, place dry, sterile dressings onto the burned area. Follow local protocols.

NOTE: *Do not use ointment, lotion, or antiseptic. These items serve to insulate the burn, which may result in more damage. Also, do not break blisters. Breaking blisters will increase the risk of infection.*

8. *Give special care to the eyes.* If the eyes or eyelids have been burned, place sterile dressings or pads over them. Moisten these pads with sterile water if possible.

9. *Give special care to the fingers and toes.* If a serious burn involves the hands or feet, always place a sterile or clean pad between toes or fingers before completing the dressing.

10. *Care for shock.* ■

Special Considerations
Thermal Burns   See Scan 10-5 for a summary of caring for thermal burns.

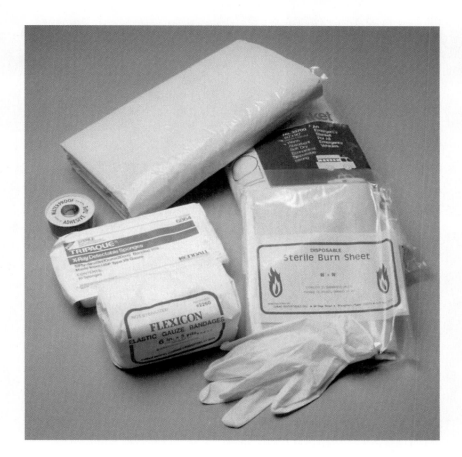

FIGURE 10.60
First Responder supplies for emergency care of burns.

Assessment and Care of Thermal Burns

TYPE OF BURN	TISSUE BURNED			COLOR CHANGES	PAIN	BLISTERS
	Outer Layer of Skin	Second Layer of Skin	Tissues Below Skin			
Superficial	Yes	No	No	Red	Yes	No
Partial-thickness	Yes	Yes	No	Deep red	Yes	Yes
Full-thickness	Yes	Yes	Yes	Charred black or white	Yes	Yes

MINOR: SUPERFICIAL AND PARTIAL-THICKNESS

- Have someone alert dispatch.
- Cool the burn if possible.
- Cover entire burn with dry, sterile dressing.
- Moisten dressing only if burn is less than 9% of skin surface.

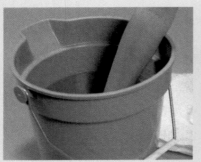
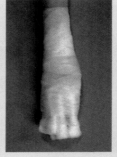

MAJOR BURNS: EXTENSIVE SUPERFICIAL, PARTIAL-THICKNESS, AND ANY FULL-THICKNESS BURNS

- Stop burning process.
- Have someone alert dispatch.
- Maintain open airway.
- Wrap area with dry, clean dressing.*
- Provide care for shock.
- Moisten dressing only if burn is less than 9% of skin surface.

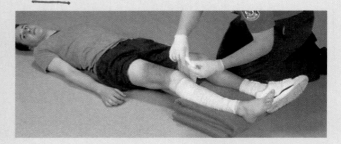

IF HANDS OR TOES ARE BURNED:

- Separate digits with sterile gauze pads.
- When appropriate, elevate the extremity.

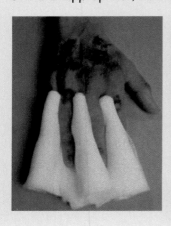
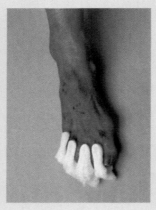

BURNS TO THE EYES:

- Do not open eyelids if burned.
- Be certain burn is thermal, not chemical.
- Apply moist, sterile gauze pads to both eyes.

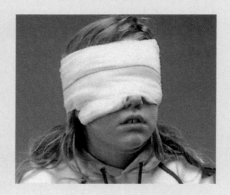

Chemical Burns   Many chemicals are harmless if they are used properly or remain contained. However, if those chemicals come in contact with the human body, they can cause harm. Some irritate the skin and create burns very quickly. Others create a slow, painful burning process. In either case, it is crucial to stop the burning process and remove the irritant.

Scenes involving patients with chemical burns can be very dangerous. Completing a scene size-up and ensuring scene safety is very important. There may be a pool of dangerous chemicals near the patient. Acids may be spurting from containers. Toxic fumes may be in the air. If you believe there are hazards at the scene that will place you in danger, do not attempt a rescue unless you have been trained to do so and have the necessary equipment.

Remember that taking BSI precautions is required for every patient contact. Wear latex or vinyl gloves and additional equipment if required by local protocol.

The primary method of caring for chemical burns is to wash away the chemical with water. A simple wetting of the burned area is not enough. Flush the area of the patient's body that has been exposed. Continue to **flush the area for at least 20 minutes.** Be sure to remove all contaminated clothing, shoes, socks, and jewelry from the patient during the wash.

Once you have flushed the area for at least 20 minutes, apply a dry, sterile dressing, care for shock, and make sure EMS has been notified. If the patient begins to complain of increased burning or irritation once a dressing is in place, remove the dressing and flush the burned area with water for several minutes more. Then, apply a new dry dressing.

Activate EMS for all cases of chemical burns.

FIRST➤   Remember, when providing care for chemical burns:

1. Flush the burned area for at least 20 minutes. If possible and if it can be done quickly, try to identify any chemical powders before applying water. Water could cause a reaction that will produce heat and increase burning of the skin.

2. Apply a dry, sterile dressing.

3. If burning continues, remove dressing and flush again. ■

If dry lime is the agent causing the burn, DO NOT begin by flushing with water. Instead, use a DRY dressing to BRUSH the substance off the patient's skin, hair, and clothing. Also have the patient remove any contaminated clothing or jewelry. Once this is done, you may flush the area with water (Figure 10.61).

Chemical burns to the eyes require immediate attention. Assume that both eyes are involved. When caring for chemical burns to the eyes, you should:

1. Perform a scene size-up, including taking appropriate BSI precautions.

2. Perform initial assessment, ensuring the patient's ABCs.

3. Immediately flood the eyes with water (Figure 10.62).

4. Keep the water flowing from a faucet, bucket, or other source into the eye. You may have to hold the eyelid open to ensure a complete washing.

5. Continue flushing for at least 20 minutes.

6. After flushing the eyes, cover both of them with moistened pads.

7. Remove the pads and flush again if the patient begins to complain about increased burning sensations or irritation.

warning

Scenes involving chemical burns may be hazardous to emergency personnel.

remember

Brush dry lime from the patient's skin before applying water.

Chemical burn—
flood area with
water.

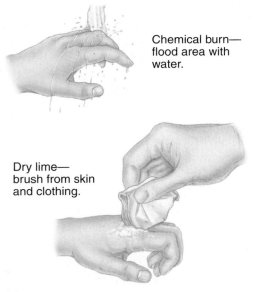

Dry lime—
brush from skin
and clothing.

FIGURE 10.61
Emergency care of chemical burns.

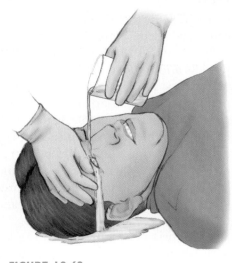

FIGURE 10.62
When caring for a patient with chemical burns to
the eyes, flush the eyes with water, pouring from a
medial to lateral direction.

FIGURE 10.63
Injuries due to electrical incidents.

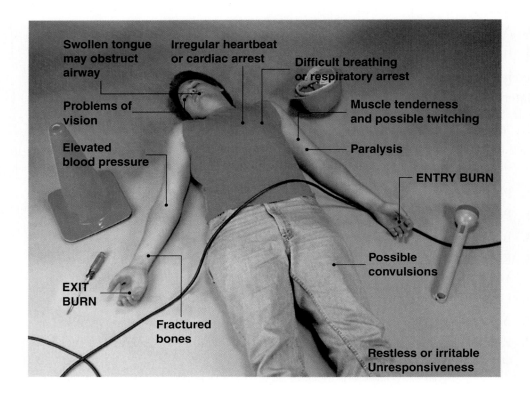

Swollen tongue
may obstruct
airway

Irregular heartbeat
or cardiac arrest

Difficult breathing
or respiratory arrest

Problems of
vision

Muscle tenderness
and possible twitching

Elevated
blood pressure

Paralysis

ENTRY BURN

EXIT
BURN

Possible
convulsions

Fractured
bones

Restless or irritable
Unresponsiveness

Electrical Burns On the scene of an electrical injury, burns are not usually the most serious problem a patient sustains. Cardiac arrest, nervous system damage, and injury to internal organs may occur with these incidents (Figure 10.63). Activate EMS for all cases involving electrical burns.

The scene of an electrical injury is often very hazardous. Make sure that the source of electricity has been turned off before caring for the victim. If the electricity is still active, do not try to attempt a rescue unless you have been trained to do so and have the necessary equipment.

To provide care for a patient with an electrical burn, you should:

1. Perform scene size-up, including taking appropriate BSI precautions.

2. Perform an initial assessment. Electricity passing through a patient's body will cause cardiac arrest. Even if the patient appears stable, be prepared for complications involving the airway and heart. Administer oxygen as per local protocols.

3. Evaluate the burn. Look for two burn sites: an entrance and an exit wounds. The entrance wound (often the hand) is where the electricity entered the body. The exit wound is where the electricity came into contact with a ground (often a foot).

4. Apply dry, sterile dressings to the burn sites. You may apply moistened dressings if transport is delayed, the burn involves less than 9% of the body, and the patient will not be in a cold environment.

5. Provide care for shock.

6. Make certain EMS has been notified. NOTE that external burns do not reflect the true nature of an electrical injury. All such injuries require medical attention.

Infants and Children The extent of burns to infants and young children can be very difficult to assess, because the patient may not understand why he hurts or he may feel the pain is a punishment for something he did wrong. The pediatric patient may be unable to explain how much or exactly where the pain is.

Also, remember that children have a greater skin surface area in relation to total body size. In other words, more areas can be burned. The greater the surface area is, the greater the fluid and heat loss will be. So keep the environment warm whenever possible.

Consider the possibility of child abuse. If the burns are suspicious, do not confront the parents. Report your suspicion to local authorities.

warning

Always make certain the electricity is off before entering the scene of an electrical injury.

Chapter Review

Bleeding can be classified as external or internal. Both types of bleeding can range from minor to life-threatening. The risk of infectious disease must be considered when caring for bleeding patients. Use the appropriate BSI precautions—including gloves, goggles, gowns, and masks—to protect yourself from infectious bodily fluids.

Bleeding may be classified as **arterial, venous,** or **capillary bleeding.** The four major techniques for controlling external bleeding are **direct pressure, elevation, pressure points,** and a **tourniquet.**

Dressings cover wounds. To control bleeding, use sterile or clean materials and cover the entire wound. Do not remove any dressing once it is in place. Occlusive dressings are used when an airtight seal is required.

Bandages hold dressings in place. Secure a bandage so that it is not too loose or too tight. It should have no loose ends. Do not cover the patient's fingertips or toes.

Internal bleeding can be very serious. Look for mechanisms of injury that can cause internal bleeding. Look for wounds associated with internal bleeding, and examine the patient for signs and symptoms of shock. Care for internal bleeding is the same as you would for shock.

Shock (hypoperfusion) is the lack of perfusion to all vital organs. Unless the process is stopped, the patient will die. The symptoms of shock may include weakness, nausea, thirst, dizziness, and fear. The signs of shock may include restlessness, combativeness, profuse external bleeding, vomiting or loss of body fluids, shaking and trembling (rare), altered mental status, shallow and rapid breathing, rapid and weak pulse, pale skin (with the face often turning blue), cool and clammy skin, and lackluster eyes with dilated pupils.

To care for shock, administer oxygen as per local protocols, calm and reassure the patient, keep the patient at rest, maintain an adequate airway, and maintain normal body temperature. Be sure to control external bleeding and splint injuries you suspect are major fractures. For most cases of shock, elevate the lower extremities.

Closed wounds and **open wounds** are soft-tissue injuries. Internal body organs may also be involved. **Bruises** (contusions) are the most common form of closed wound, while **scratches** and **scrapes** (abrasions) and **cuts** (lacerations and incisions) are the most common forms of open wounds. **Puncture wounds** are open wounds. If it is a penetrating puncture wound, it may have both an entrance and an exit wound. **Avulsions** occur when skin or a body part (tip of the nose, fingertip, external ear, tooth, lip) is torn loose or off the body. The cutting or tearing off of fingers, toes, hands, feet, arms, or legs is called an **amputation. Crush injuries** can have open or closed wounds with severe soft-tissue damage. Internal and external bleeding is seen with these injuries.

When caring for closed wounds, assume there is internal bleeding. When providing care for open wounds, ensure personal safety, then expose the wound. Control bleeding by dressing the wound. Care for shock (hypoperfusion). Remember to provide emotional support by reassuring the patient.

For puncture wounds, assume that there are internal injuries and bleeding. Remember to look for exit wounds.

Do not remove **impaled objects.** Control bleeding and stabilize the object. If the object is in the cheek wall, has passed though into the mouth, and causes an airway obstruction, remove the object.

Partially avulsed skin can be placed back in its normal position. If skin is torn loose, preserve the part. Do not try to replace an avulsed eye. Do not try to replace protruding organs. In cases of avulsion, control bleeding and be prepared to care for shock.

Attempt to control bleeding from **amputations** with direct pressure applied to a dressing held firmly over the stump. Elevate and apply pressure point techniques if needed. Your last resort is a tourniquet.

Specific care procedures require you to remember certain rules and exceptions. For example:

- *Scalp wounds*—Do not try to clean the wound. Do not apply finger pressure if there is any chance of a skull fracture.
- *Facial wounds*—Maintain an open airway, control bleeding, dress and bandage the wounds. If there are no skull, neck, or spine injuries, position the patient for drainage.
- *Eye wounds:*
  – Do not apply direct pressure to a cut eyeball.

- Do not remove objects impaled in the eye. Cover with dressing pads and a rigid shield (for example, a paper cup).
- Do not replace an eyeball pulled from its socket.
- Do not open the eyes of a patient with burns to the eyelids.
- Flush foreign objects from the eye.
- Care for chemical burns by flushing the eyes for at least 20 minutes.
- Keep the patient's eyelids closed.
- Always cover both of the patient's eyes.
- *Ear wounds*—Do not probe into the ear. Do not pack the ear canal. For cuts and bleeding from the ear, apply a dressing and bandage. Wrap avulsed parts in plastic.
- *Nose injuries*—Maintain an open airway. Do not pack the nostrils. Control bleeding by pinching nostrils shut. Wrap avulsed parts in plastic.
- *Mouth injuries*—Maintain an open airway and position for drainage. Do not pack the mouth. Use dressings and direct pressure to control bleeding and hold the dressings in place.
- *Neck wounds*—Look for signs of neck wounds. Care for arterial bleeding with pressure dressings and venous bleeding with an occlusive dressing.
- *Open chest wounds*—Place occlusive dressings on open chest wounds. Apply and seal the dressing as per local protocol and monitor the patient for signs of pressure building up in the chest. If you see signs of pressure build up, release the seal and reseal it after the patient has exhaled.
- *Abdominal injuries*—Look for signs of abdominal injury, care for shock, and be alert for vomiting. If there are no injuries to the pelvic bones or lower limbs, flex the patient's legs to reduce pain.
- *Genitalia injuries*—Conduct an examination and provide care in a professional manner. Control bleeding by direct pressure and a pressure dressing. Save avulsed parts.

Burns can be caused by heat, chemicals, electricity, light, or radiation. They may be classified as:

- *Superficial* (first-degree)—involve the top layer of skin known as the epidermis.
- *Partial-thickness* (second-degree)—involve both the epidermis and the dermis (the top two layers of skin).
- *Full-thickness* (third-degree)—extend through all dermal layers and may involve subcutaneous layers, muscle, bone, or organs.

For **minor burns,** flush the burned area with water (or saline) for several minutes. Do not flush **major burns** with water unless they involve less than 9% of the total body area. Cover with dry, sterile dressings.

REMEMBER AND CONSIDER

Bleeding is a common occurence. All of us at some point in our lives have suffered a scraped knee, paper cut, or perhaps a laceration to the palm from a broken glass while washing dishes. The good news is that most wounds are relatively minor and bleeding can be controlled easily. Approximately 95% of the time, direct pressure and elevation can effectively control bleeding. The bad news is that even minor bleeding can, in some cases, become serious. Never assume that a condition is minor simply based on the absence of major bleeding.

In your First Responder classes, you will practice bandaging wounds, controlling bleeding, and caring for patients in shock. Bandages do not have to be neat. They simply have to be functional. Think about the types of wounds you may encounter and how you will care for them.

✔ Do you have personal protective equipment readily available for use?

✔ What will you use to control bleeding?

✔ What equipment will you need to care for bleeding/shock victims?

Remember, the purpose of the initial assessment is to detect and control life-threatening problems. Go back to Chapter 7 and review the steps involved in performing an initial assessment. Relate the detection of developing shock to all stages of the patient assessment.

✔ What might you find during the initial assessment?

✔ What might you see that would indicate shock when you observe the entire patient?

- What will you find when taking vital signs (breathing, pulse, and skin color, temperature, and condition)?
- What should you notice about a patient's eyes if he is going into shock?
- What information related to shock is gained when you examine the head and face of a patient?
- What might have caused this patient to develop shock?

INVESTIGATE...

- Do public places keep emergency care supplies handy for public use?
- Does your employer have a first-aid kit stocked and ready to use?
- How do the contents of the kits relate to the emergency care of problems found during the initial assessment?

First-aid kits vary greatly in contents. Search for kits that contain gloves, pocket face masks, barrier shields, gauze pads, roller bandages.

- Did you find any supplies that you would recommend against and why?

Mishaps and injuries can happen anywhere. They often occur when you least expect them.

- What would you do if you encountered someone who is bleeding or in shock in a public place or at work?
- Are bandages or dressings available that you could use?
- What would you do without supplies? What plan could you have in mind in case you run into such a problem?

You might choose to carry a personal first-aid kit in your car. This would allow you access to first-aid supplies and BSI equipment at any time. While some malls and shopping centers are beginning to have equipment available at a centralized location, many do not. Know where the equipment is or how to gain access to it. Be prepared to render aid at any time and any place.

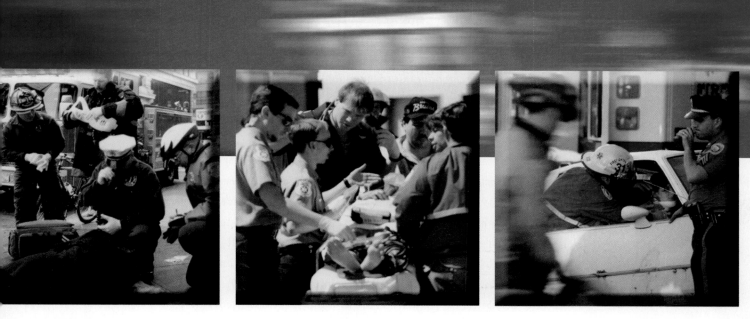

Muscle and Bone Injuries

Bones are the foundation of our body. Like the steel girders that make the foundation of buildings and give the strength to their structure, bones provide the tough, internal structure and support for the demanding activities we put our bodies through daily. But unlike steel girders, bones are made of living tissue. Bones are able to move and bend by the actions of muscles and other tissues and by the messages received from a system of nerves controlled by the brain.

In your career as a First Responder, you will manage many patients with muscle and bone injuries. Such injuries are fairly common. To help you learn to evaluate and care for them, this chapter covers the general causes, types, and signs and symptoms of muscle and bone injuries, as well as First Responder care.

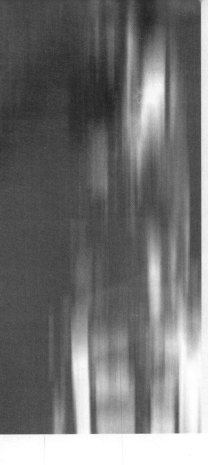

NATIONAL STANDARD OBJECTIVES

This chapter focuses on the objectives of Module 5, Lesson 5-3, of the U.S. DOT's First Responder National Standard Curriculum and serves as an instructional aid to help you meet any specific objectives added to the course by your local EMS system.

By the end of this chapter, you will be able to (from cognitive or knowledge information):

5–3.1 Describe the function of the musculoskeletal system. (pp. 354–356)

5–3.2 Differentiate between an open and a closed painful, swollen, deformed extremity. (pp. 359–360)

5–3.3 List the emergency medical care for a patient with a painful, swollen, deformed extremity. (pp. 364–365)

5–3.4 Relate mechanism of injury to potential injuries of the head and spine. (p. 395)

5–3.5 State the signs and symptoms of a potential spine injury. (pp. 401–403)

5–3.6 Describe the method of determining if a responsive patient may have a spine injury. (pp. 401–405)

5–3.7 List the signs and symptoms of injury to the head. (pp. 397–399)

5–3.8 Describe the emergency medical care for injuries to the head. (pp. 399–401)

Feel comfortable enough to (by changing attitudes, values, and beliefs):

5–3.9 Explain the rationale for the feelings of patients who have need for immobilization of a painful, swollen, deformed extremity. (pp. 365, 367)

LEARNING TASKS

This chapter explains the functions of the muscles and bones and how they are controlled by the nervous system. You will need to understand the relationship between the system of muscles and bones (musculoskeletal system) and the nervous system and apply the knowledge you gain to the assessment and care steps that you will provide to injured patients. As you work through this chapter and meet the objectives, you will also need to keep the following information in mind and be able to perform the skills listed.

You will learn the parts of the skeleton through the pictures in this chapter and from your instructor. As you practice your assessment skills, you must be able to:

✔ Locate and name the major bones of the skeletal system.

While performing a patient assessment, you will look and feel for signs and symptoms of injured extremities. You must be able to:

✔ Describe a painful, swollen, deformed extremity.
✔ Demonstrate how to identify injuries to extremities based on signs and symptoms.

You will also practice stabilizing and immobilizing injured extremities using a variety of splinting techniques. You must be able to:

✔ List five complications related to extremity injuries.
✔ Define immobilization and state its primary purpose.
✔ Define splinting and state its purpose.

You must handle extremity injuries carefully. There are several steps to follow when you splint these injuries. You must be able to:

5–3.10 Demonstrate a caring attitude toward patients with a musculoskeletal injury who request emergency medical services. (pp. 365, 367, 370, 375, 399, 406)

5–3.11 Place the interests of the patient with a musculoskeletal injury as the foremost consideration when making any and all patient-care decisions. (pp. 364, 366, 367, 374, 376, 381, 384, 395, 397, 405)

5–3.12 Communicate with empathy to patients with a musculoskeletal injury, as well as with family members and friends of the patient. (pp. 365, 367, 370, 375, 399, 406)

Show how to
(through psychomotor skills):

5–3.13 Demonstrate the emergency medical care of a patient with a painful, swollen, deformed extremity. (pp. 364–365)

5–3.14 Demonstrate opening the airway in a patient with suspected spinal cord injury. (pp. 401, 403)

5–3.15 Demonstrate evaluating a responsive patient with a suspected spinal cord injury. (pp. 402–403, 404–405)

5–3.16 Demonstrate stabilizing of the cervical spine. (pp. 403, 406)

✔ State the rules for immobilization and the general steps to follow in all cases requiring splinting.

✔ Describe the splinting procedures for injuries to the extremities.

✔ Define manual stabilization and describe how it is applied to an extremity prior to splinting.

Sometimes the mechanism of injury is so severe that its force causes the extremity to become deformed or bent out of its normal position. You must be able to:

✔ Describe a deformed injury and the procedures for straightening a closed deformed injury.

First Responders may not carry much in the way of commercial splints. Painful, swollen, or deformed extremities can be immobilized with a variety of rigid, semi-rigid, and soft items that will support and stabilize the limb. You must be able to:

✔ List objects that can be used as splints when commercial splints are not available.

✔ Perform splinting procedures on "patients" with simulated painful, swollen, or deformed extremity injuries, using improvised or commercial splints.

Depending on the mechanism of injury, bones other than the extremities can also be injured. Many vital organs are protected by bones such as the skull, spine, and rib cage. This central part of the skeleton is referred to as the axial skeleton. You must be able to:

✔ List the parts of the axial skeleton and describe their functions.

Enclosed in the skull and spinal column are the brain and spinal cord, which together form the major portion of the central nervous system. You must be able to assess and recognize injury to the central nervous system by:

✔ Identifying the parts of the central nervous system and describing their functions.
✔ Describing common mechanisms of injury that can affect the function of the axial skeleton and the central nervous system.
✔ Listing the signs and symptoms of head, spine, and chest injuries.

Injuries can sometimes be distracting to the rescuer. Do not let the site of them distract you from your priorities. Remember patient assessment steps and their proper order. You must be able to:

✔ Describe the challenges of airway management for patients with head, spine, and chest injuries.
✔ Describe and demonstrate airway management techniques for head and spine injuries.

Trauma patients with head injuries may be responsive or unresponsive and, depending on the mechanism of injury, may have multiple injuries. In any case, airway management and the assessment steps must be performed carefully. You must be able to:

✔ Describe and demonstrate the steps for assessing responsive and unresponsive patients for head and spine injuries.
✔ Demonstrate the emergency care procedures for a patient with open and closed head injuries.
✔ Describe and demonstrate how to stabilize and care for injuries to the head and spine.
✔ Describe and demonstrate how to stabilize and care for injuries to the chest.
✔ Describe the problems that may result from improper care to head, spine, and chest injuries.

NOTE: *First Responders often focus on the initial assessment and the care needed for life-threatening injuries, so there may not be time to begin immobilizing less critical injuries before more advanced care providers arrive on scene. Usually, EMTs will splint extremities when they arrive, but may need First Responders to assist them. However, First Responders who learn how to assess and recognize extremity injuries, and who can quickly and carefully splint them after stabilizing life-threatening problems, will be able to make the patient more comfortable sooner. Your ability to use scene time wisely to assess and manage trauma patients while waiting for EMTs will also help shorten the time patients must spend on the scene.*

MUSCULOSKELETAL SYSTEM

musculoskeletal system
all the muscles, bones, joints, and related structures such as tendons and ligaments that enable the body and its parts to move and function.

The **musculoskeletal system** is made up of many muscles, bones, joints, connective tissues, blood vessels, and nerves. Trauma, whether minor or major, can cause a variety of injuries to the muscles, bones, and other tissues that make up the musculoskeletal system. When assessing those injuries, First Responders are not expected to determine whether an injury is a fractured bone, a dislocated joint, a ligament sprain, or a muscle strain. The First Responder's job is to carefully assess the patient, looking for signs and symptoms of injury such as pain, swelling, deformity, and discoloration. Sometimes injuries can be easily identified as fractures, dislocations, or both, simply due to the amount of deformity. However, most musculoskeletal injuries are not that obvious and may present with little swelling or deformity.

The extremities include the many bones and joints of the arms and legs. Surrounding the bones and joints are muscles and other soft tissues such as ligaments, tendons, blood vessels, and nerves. These tissues work with the skeletal structures to nourish, support, and move those structures. Figure 11.1 shows the major blood vessels and a few of the major nerves found in the arms and legs. You do not need to remember every vessel and nerve, but you must remember that a large network of vessels and nerves are woven throughout the body. Injuries to these blood vessels and nerves can cause excessive swelling and loss of movement or function. Careful assessment and management is important for minimizing pain, blood loss, and nerve damage. Your actions can promote healing and help restore the function of the musculoskeletal system.

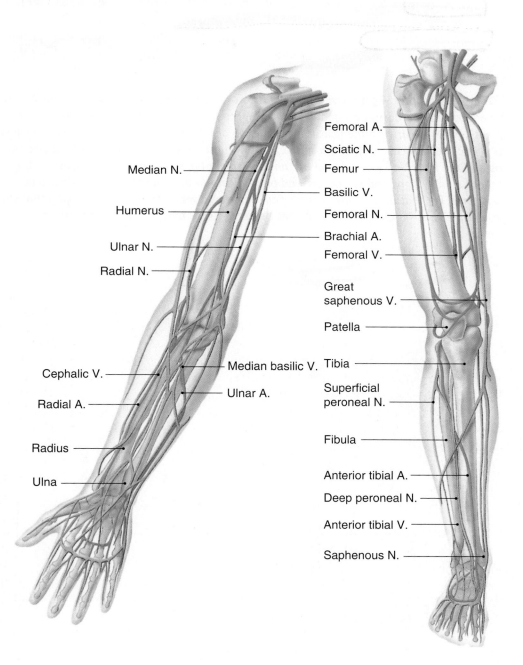

FIGURE 11.1
Anatomy of the extremities.
(A = artery, N = nerve, V = vein)

FIRST➤ The musculoskeletal system has four major functions:

- *Support*—Bones support the soft tissues of the body, acting as a framework to give the body form and to provide a rigid structure for the attachment of muscles and other body parts.
- *Movement*—Muscles, bones, and joints act together to allow for movement.
- *Protection*—Many of the bones in the body provide protection for vital organs: the skull protects the brain; the spine protects the spinal cord; the ribs protect the heart, lungs, liver, stomach, and spleen; the pelvis protects the urinary bladder and internal reproductive organs.
- *Cell production*—Some bones have the special function of producing blood cells.

The bones and joints of the musculoskeletal system are what make up the **skeletal system**. Its two major divisions are the (Figure 11.2):

- *Axial skeleton*—all the bones that form the upright axis of the body, including the skull, spinal column, sternum (breastbone), and ribs.
- *Appendicular skeleton*—all the bones that form the upper and lower extremities including the collarbones, shoulder blades, arms, wrists, hands, hips, legs, ankles, and feet. ■

NOTE: *This chapter will use terms such as fracture, dislocation, strain, and sprain. This is for educational purposes only and in no way suggests that as First Responders you will be diagnosing these injuries in the field. It is not the job of a First Responder to diagnose an injury as a fracture, dislocation, sprain, or strain. Most of these injuries will appear to be the same. Instead, the First Responder should use an assessment-based approach. That is, assess the patient, identify signs and symptoms, and provide care to the patient for those signs and symptoms. For that reason, anyone with pain associated with a mechanism of injury that suggests a possible musculoskeletal injury will be cared for as though they have a fracture until proven otherwise.*

skeletal system all the bones and joints of the body. The skeletal system provides body support and organ protection, enables movement, and produces blood cells.

axial (AK-si-al) **skeleton** bones and joints that form the center or upright axis of the body. It includes the skull, spine, breastbone, and ribs.

appendicular (ap-en-DIK-u-ler) **skeleton** bones and joints that form the upper and lower extremities.

FIGURE 11.2
Two major divisions of the skeletal system are the axial skeleton and the appendicular skeleton.

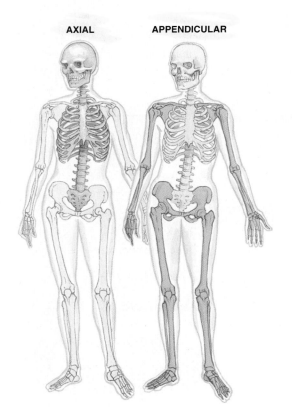

AXIAL   APPENDICULAR

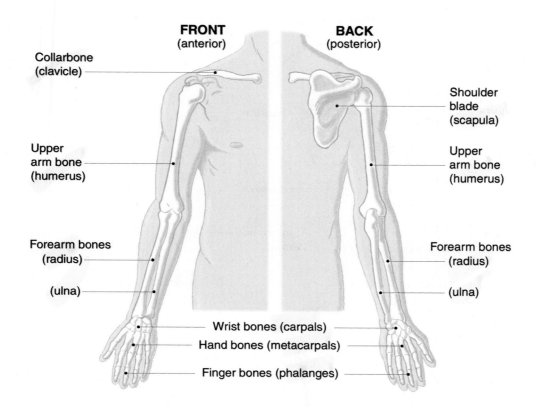

FIGURE 11.3
Bones of the upper extremities.

FRONT
(anterior)

BACK
(posterior)

Collarbone
(clavicle)

Shoulder
blade
(scapula)

Upper
arm bone
(humerus)

Upper
arm bone
(humerus)

Forearm bones
(radius)

Forearm bones
(radius)

(ulna)

(ulna)

Wrist bones (carpals)

Hand bones (metacarpals)

Finger bones (phalanges)

APPENDICULAR SKELETON

As stated above, the appendicular skeleton is made up of the bones that form the upper and lower extremities. The upper extremities are made up of the shoulder girdle and both arms, down to and including the fingers (Figure 11.3). Table 11-1 lists the bones of the upper extremities and the number of bones that form each structure.

The lower extremities are made up of the pelvis and both legs, down to and including the toes (Figure 11.4). Table 11-2 lists the bones of the lower extremities and the number of bones that form each structure.

TABLE 11-1 BONES OF THE UPPER EXTREMITIES

COMMON NAMES	MEDICAL NAMES
Shoulder girdle collarbone (1/side) shoulder blade (1/side)	Pectoral (PEK-tor-al) clavicle (KLAV-i-kul) scapula (SKAP-u-lah)
Upper arm bone (1/arm, from shoulder to elbow)	Humerus (HU-mer-us)
Forearm bones (2/arm, from elbow to wrist: 1 medial and 1 lateral)	Ulna (UL-nah)—medial Radius (RAY-de-us)—lateral
Wrist bones (8/wrist)	Carpals (KAR-palz)
Hand bones (5/palm)	Metacarpals (meta-KAR-palz)
Finger bones (14/hand)	Phalanges (fah-LAN-gez)

FIGURE 11.4
Bones of the lower extremities.

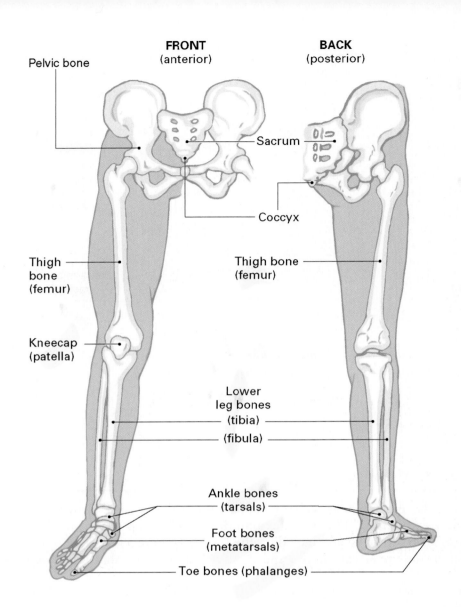

FRONT (anterior)

BACK (posterior)

Pelvic bone

Sacrum

Coccyx

Thigh bone (femur)

Thigh bone (femur)

Kneecap (patella)

Lower leg bones (tibia) (fibula)

Ankle bones (tarsals)

Foot bones (metatarsals)

Toe bones (phalanges)

TABLE 11-2 BONES OF THE LOWER EXTREMITIES

COMMON NAMES	MEDICAL NAMES
Pelvic girdle (pelvis and hips)	Innominate (eh-NOM-eh-nat) or os coxae (os-KOK-se)
Thigh bone (1/leg)	Femur (FE-mer)
Kneecap (1/leg)	Patella (pah-TEL-ah)
Lower leg bones (2/leg: 1 medial and 1 lateral)	Tibia (TIB-e-ah)—medial Fibula (FIB-yo-lah)—lateral
Ankle bones (7/foot)	Tarsals (TAR-salz)
Foot bones (5/foot)	Metatarsals (meta-TAR-salz)
Toe bones (14–15/foot)	Phalanges (fah-LAN-jez)

CAUSES OF EXTREMITY INJURIES

There are three primary forces that cause musculoskeletal injuries. They are *direct force*, *indirect force*, and *twisting force* (Figure 11.5). Extremities are often injured because of the direct force applied to a bone when a person falls and strikes an object (the edge of a step or curb) or when a person is struck by an object (the bumper of a car). Sometimes the energy of a force may be transferred up or down the extremity, which can result in an injury farther along the extremity. Such indirect-force injuries can occur when one puts out the hand to break a fall and dislocates the shoulder instead of breaking the wrist.

An example of an injury caused by a twisting force is when someone gets a hand or foot caught in a wheel or gear. The body remains stationary while the hand or foot turns in the wheel. Twisting injuries can also be caused when the body keeps moving forward while the hand or foot remains trapped.

Aging and disease are also leading contributors to skeletal injuries. As we age, our bones can become weak and brittle, and break more easily. People with certain medical conditions such as bone cancer, kidney disease, or osteoporosis have very fragile bones and the slightest force can result in a fracture.

TYPES OF INJURIES

Skeletal injuries can be categorized into one of two basic types: **closed injuries** or **open injuries** (Figure 11.6). An injury is considered closed when there is no break in the skin. In some cases, the bones and surrounding soft tissue can be damaged extensively even though the skin is unbroken.

NOTE: *There is an exception to the term closed injury when referring to injuries to the head. A closed head injury may indeed have an open wound to the scalp but because the cranium remains intact, it is referred to as a closed injury.*

An injury is considered open when the soft tissues adjacent to an injury are damaged and open. The mechanism of injury causes the bone ends or pieces of bone to tear through the skin from inside out or, in some cases, something enters and opens the skin from the outside and also breaks the bone underneath (for example, a gunshot wound).

closed injury an injury with no associated opening of the skin.

open injury an injury with an associated opening of the skin. The cause of the opening may be from bone ends or fragments tearing out through the skin, a penetrating injury that has damaged a bone and surrounding soft tissue, or a shearing force that results in the tearing off of skin.

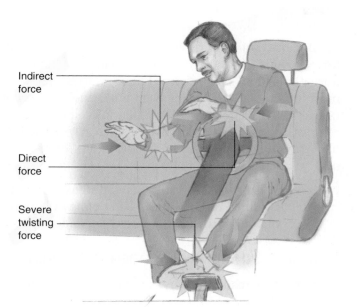

Indirect force

Direct force

Severe twisting force

FIGURE 11.5
There are three basic types of mechanisms of injury to the musculoskeletal system.

FIGURE 11.6
Closed and open injuries.

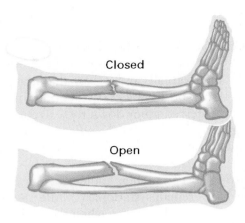

Closed

Open

Any strong force to the extremities can cause damage to bones and surrounding tissues (Scan 11-1). Most such injuries will present with pain, swelling, discoloration, and deformity. Do not try to diagnose the injury as a fracture, dislocation, sprain, or strain. In most cases, the true extent of the injury cannot be determined until X rays are taken and examined by a physician. Instead, you should assess the mechanism of injury and provide care for the worst-case scenario.

Though you will not diagnose specific types of musculoskeletal injury, you probably should know something about each:

- **Fracture**—Any time a bone is broken, chipped, cracked, or splintered, it results in what is commonly referred to as a fracture.

- **Dislocation**—This occurs when one end of a bone that is part of a joint is pulled or pushed out of place. Dislocations often result in serious damage to tendons, ligaments, nerves, and blood vessels because of the way they hold a joint together or weave in and around a joint. Sometimes the force that caused a dislocation of a bone will also cause it or an adjoining bone to fracture resulting in what is referred to as a fracture/dislocation.

- **Sprain**—The tough fibrous tissues called *ligaments* hold together the bones that make up a joint. *Tendons* attach muscle to bones. Excessive twisting forces can cause ligaments and tendons to stretch or tear resulting in a sprain injury.

- **Strain**—A strain is caused by overexerting, overworking, overstretching, or tearing of a muscle.

A more serious type of bone injury is the angulated or **deformed injury**. Deformed injuries occur when an extremity is bulging, bent, or angulated where it normally should be straight. These injuries may be slight, which means you will most likely be able to feel a distal pulse and the patient will have sensation (be able to feel your touch) and motor function (will be able to move the limb). If deformed injuries are extreme or angulated, you may *not* feel a distal pulse and the patient may experience a change in sensation and/or motor function. Deformed injuries may be open or closed (Figure 11.7).

FIRST➤ With all of these injuries, the signs and symptoms are the same: pain, swelling, discoloration, and deformity. In most cases, the emergency care that you provide as a First Responder will also be the same. ■

SIGNS AND SYMPTOMS OF EXTREMITY INJURIES

FIRST➤ The main signs and symptoms to look for in an extremity injury include (Figure 11.8):

fracture any break, crack, chip, split, or splintering of a bone.

dislocation the pulling or pushing of a bone end partially or completely free of a joint.

sprain a partial or complete tearing of a ligament.

strain the overstretching or tearing of a muscle.

deformed injury an injury that causes a bone or joint to take on an unnatural shape or bend. Also called *angulated injury*.

remember

Carefully assess and care for all painful extremities as suspected fractures. Be sure to assess circulation, sensation, and motor function before and after splinting.

mechanism of injury The force or forces that may have caused the patient's injury.

direct force Energy is transmitted directly to an extremity, causing an injury at the site of impact.

indirect force Energy of a direct force blow is transferred along the arm or leg and causes an injury farther along the extremity.

twisting force The energy transmitted to an extremity that is caught in a twisting or circular mechanism, while the rest of the extremity or the body is stationary or moving in another direction.

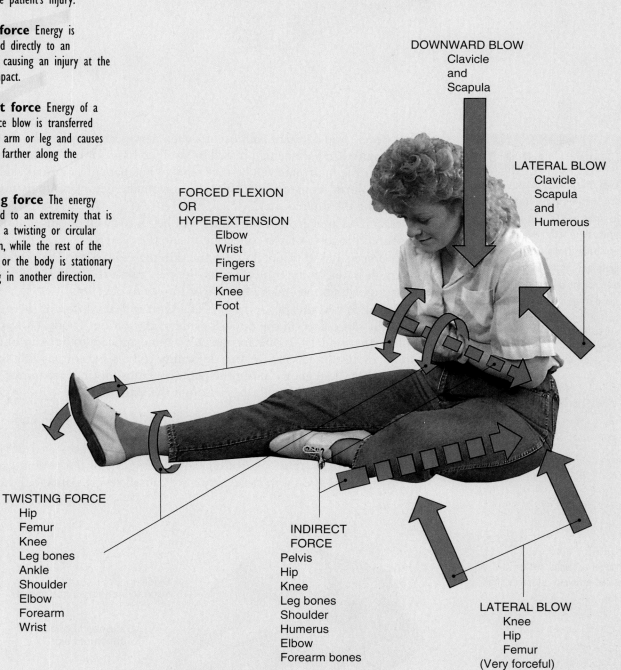

DOWNWARD BLOW
Clavicle
and
Scapula

LATERAL BLOW
Clavicle
Scapula
and
Humerous

FORCED FLEXION
OR
HYPEREXTENSION
Elbow
Wrist
Fingers
Femur
Knee
Foot

TWISTING FORCE
Hip
Femur
Knee
Leg bones
Ankle
Shoulder
Elbow
Forearm
Wrist

INDIRECT
FORCE
Pelvis
Hip
Knee
Leg bones
Shoulder
Humerus
Elbow
Forearm bones

LATERAL BLOW
Knee
Hip
Femur
(Very forceful)

FIGURE 11.7
Deformed injuries may be closed or
open.

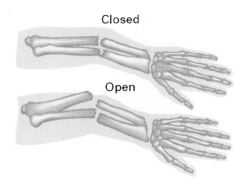

Closed

Open

NOTE

Even though most patients can tell you "where it hurts," some diabetics, spine and/or head injury patients, those with nerve damage, and patients who may be taking prescribed (or illegal) pain killers may not be able to locate or respond to pain at a suspected fracture or dislocation site.

- *Pain.* Severe and constant pain occurs when nerves surrounding the injury have been injured and are being pressed by swelling tissue or broken bone ends. Tissues near the injury site will be very tender. The patient can usually tell you where it hurts. As part of your focused assessment, gently examine (touch) the area along the injured site.
- *Swelling.* The area around the injury will begin to swell because blood from ruptured blood vessels is collecting inside the tissues.
- *Discoloration.* Blood trapped under the skin may cause it to look reddish or discolored. Later, as these blood cells die, they cause the typical black-and-blue bruising, which may take 24 hours or longer to develop.
- *Deformity.* When this occurs, a part of a limb appears different in size or shape than the same part on the opposite side of the patient's body. (Always compare both arms and legs to one another.) If a bone appears to have an unusual angle, bulge, or swelling, consider this deformity to be a sign of possible fracture or dislocation. Feel gently along the patient's limbs, noting any lumps, swelling, discoloration, or ends of bones through the skin. ■

Other common signs and symptoms of an extremity injury include:

- *Inability to move a joint or limb.* Sometimes movement is possible but very painful. If the patient can move an arm but not the fingers, or if a patient can move a leg but not the toes, a fracture may have caused severe damage to nerves and

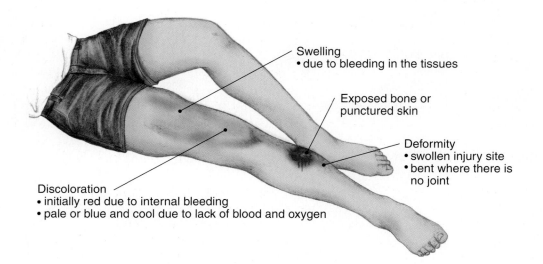

Swelling
• due to bleeding in the tissues

Exposed bone or
punctured skin

Deformity
• swollen injury site
• bent where there is
  no joint

Discoloration
• initially red due to internal bleeding
• pale or blue and cool due to lack of blood and oxygen

blood vessels. The patient will often cradle, or guard, an injured arm, or hold it close to the body to stabilize it in a comfortable position. An injured person will often ask you not to touch or move the injured extremity.

- *Numbness or tingling sensation.* This can be from pressure on nerves or blood vessels caused by swelling or broken bones.

- *Loss of distal pulse.* Bone ends or bone fragments may be pressing against or cutting through an artery. Swelling from internal bleeding may be pressing against an artery. The extremity may be pale and cold because of restricted blood flow, and then turn bluish (cyanotic) because of lack of oxygen.

- *Slow capillary refill,* taking longer than two seconds.

- *Grating.* When the patient moves, the ends of fractured bones rub together, making a grating sound referred to as *crepitus* (KREP-i-tus). Do not ask a patient to move in order to confirm or reproduce this sound.

- *Sound of breaking at the time of injury.* If the patient or bystanders tell you this, suspect a fracture has occurred.

- *Exposed bone.* In cases of open fractures, the fragments or ends of broken bones may be visible where they break through the skin.

All injured extremities should be assessed for adequate circulation, sensation, and motor function.

NOTE: *Circulation, sensation, and motor function must be evaluated on all extremity injuries. Check circulation by assessing distal pulses and capillary refill. In the absence of a pulse, good color can be interpreted as good circulation. If necessary, compare the injured side to the uninjured side. Sensation is assessed by feeling the fingers or toes and asking if they feel tingly or numb. Determine if the patient can tell which digit you are touching without looking. Motor function can be assessed simply by the patient's ability to move the extremity. Strength testing is another way to assess motor function but may be affected by pain.*

Several important signs will tell you the state of circulation to the extremity. They are:

- If the injury site is swollen and discolored, there is bleeding in the tissues.

- If there is no distal pulse and the extremity is pale and cool, there is lack of blood flow.

- If the extremity is blue, there is lack of oxygen in the limb.

To check circulation in pediatric patients, check capillary refill. To do this, press the nail bed or tip of the finger or toe on the injured extremity between your finger and thumb. When you press, the finger or toe turns white, or blanches, because you have pressed the blood out of it. When you release pressure, the blood should flow back into the area in less than two seconds. If it takes more than two seconds, then you must suspect that there is pressure on or damage to a blood vessel and that circulation is restricted in the extremity or that there is significant blood loss in the circulatory system. This procedure is more reliable in children than it is in adults. Blood-flow return time is also affected by cold temperature.

While you are checking distal pulses, you can also check sensation (feeling) and motor function (ability to move). Ask the patient to tell you if he can feel your touch and where you are touching. You can also ask the patient to try to move the fingers or grasp your hand. For the foot, ask the patient to wiggle toes or press a foot against your hand. When assessing motor function of the extremity by having the patient grasp or push against your hands, be sure to assess both extremities simultaneously. This will allow for a more accurate assessment of strength between the injured and uninjured side.

Checking for sensation and motor function gives you information about the nervous system. A lack of feeling or the inability to move may indicate that there is pressure on or damage to a nerve. This nerve damage may be the result of injury to the spinal cord and not just an injury to the extremity. (More later about the signs and symptoms of spinal injury and the precautions to take when managing a spine-injured patient.)

TOTAL PATIENT CARE

In the scene size-up, quickly determine scene safety, take BSI precautions, and don all personal protective equipment. Note the mechanism of injury and the total number of patients. Then determine what additional assistance you may need. If the mechanism of injury suggests a possible spinal injury and the scene is safe to enter, immediately stabilize your patient's head and neck.

During your initial assessment, get an impression of the environment and the patient and determine how quickly the patient needs to be moved and transported. Do not focus on obvious injuries. Instead, assess mental status, then airway, breathing, and circulation. Look for and control all major bleeding. Detect and correct life-threatening problems as quickly as possible.

There is a certain order to caring for injuries. After correcting and stabilizing life-threatening injuries to airway, breathing, and circulation, after you have checked for and stabilized neck and spine injuries, and after you have provided care for shock that develops from major bleeding or serious burns, then you can focus on extremity injuries. Always be sure to note the mechanism of injury as this will give you an idea of the possible extent, type, and location of the injury site.

In the order of care for skeletal injuries, first priority is given to possible injury to the spine. Next is care for possible injuries to the following:

- *Skull*—because it protects the brain and contains a portion of the airway.

- *Rib cage*—because it protects the heart and lungs and broken sections may damage the function of these organs as well as prevent adequate breathing.

- *Pelvis*—because it protects reproductive and urinary organs and major nerves and blood vessels.

- *Thigh*—because it takes major trauma to injure the largest, sturdiest bone (femur) in the body, which is surrounded by major nerves and blood vessels. Blood loss can be life-threatening.

- *Any extremity injury*—where no distal pulse is detected during the initial assessment.

- *Injuries to the arm, lower leg, and individual ribs*—are considered and managed last.

Note the mechanism of injury and be concerned with major bleeding and possible shock whenever there are injuries to the chest, pelvis, and thigh. A great amount of blood can be lost internally in these areas. Watch the patient's signs and symptoms carefully. A slow pulse, pale or blue skin color, slow or no response or confusion, and cold extremities are signs and symptoms that should alert you to manage and transport this patient as soon as possible.

Remember the following emergency care steps when caring for a patient with musculoskeletal injuries (Figure 11.9):

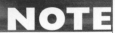

NOTE

Medical direction may allow you to reposition an extremity if there is no distal pulse. Follow local protocol.

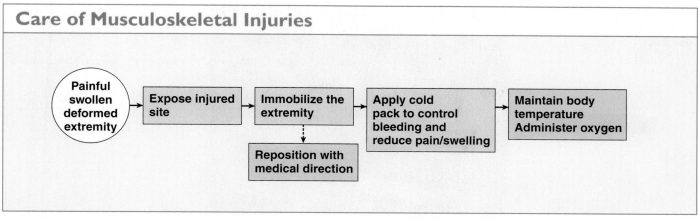

Care of Musculoskeletal Injuries

Painful swollen deformed extremity → Expose injured site → Immobilize the extremity → Apply cold pack to control bleeding and reduce pain/swelling → Maintain body temperature Administer oxygen

Reposition with medical direction

FIGURE 11.9

1. Always perform an initial assessment before focusing on a particular injury.
   – Manage life-threatening problems first.
   – Prioritize and manage other injuries second.

2. Carefully cut away clothing to expose the injury site. Control bleeding if there is an open wound. Check for distal circulation, sensation, and motor function.

3. Immobilize the extremity using manual stabilization or splints if available.
   – Splint the suspected fracture site.
   – Immobilize the joints above and below the suspected fracture site. Use a sling and swathe for an arm to keep it elevated across the chest. Splinted, immobilized legs may be propped up on a folded blanket or pillow if there is no indication of spinal injury.
   – Recheck distal circulation, sensation, and motor function often.

4. Apply a cold pack to the injury site to help reduce the pain and swelling. Never put a cold pack directly on the skin. Wrap it in gauze or a towel first. Then place it gently over the injury site. If the patient experiences pain from this extra pressure on the injury, place the cold pack just above the site.

5. Administer oxygen as soon as possible as per local protocol.

6. Assess the patient's skin color, temperature, and condition. Maintain a comfortable body temperature to help minimize the effects of developing shock.

Emotional support is important when caring for a patient with injuries. Tell the patient what you suspect may be wrong, how you will manage it, and what will be done by other emergency care providers on scene and at the hospital. You may need to remind the patient that fractures can be set at the hospital and bones will heal. Talking with the patient helps to give the patient confidence and relieve anxiety. It may also help lower blood pressure, pulse rate, and breathing rate.

SPLINTING

FIRST► **Splinting** is the process of immobilizing an injury using a device such as a piece of wood, cardboard, or folded blanket (Figure 11.10). Any object that can be used to restrict the movement of an injury is called a splint.
Manual stabilization is the process of restricting the movement of an injured person or body part. You can manually stabilize an injury simply by holding the part still with your hands. ■

splinting applying a device that will immobilize an injured extremity.

NOTE

You cannot learn splinting without proper instruction and supervised practice. You must be trained by a qualified instructor, and you must practice splinting procedures under the guidance of that instructor.

manual stabilization restricting the movement of an injured person or body part with your hands.

FIGURE 11.10
Splinting immobilizes injured
extremities.

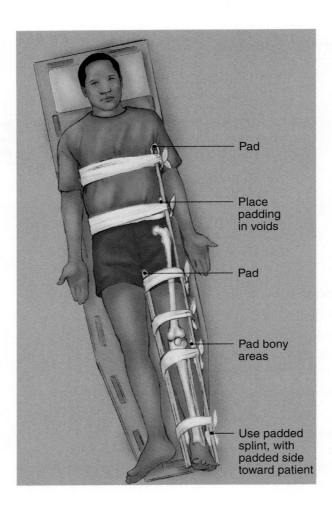

Pad

Place
padding
in voids

Pad

Pad bony
areas

Use padded
splint, with
padded side
toward patient

WHY SPLINT?

FIRST➤ The application of splints allows emergency care providers to reposition
and transfer the patient while minimizing movement of the injury.
Damage to soft tissues can cause complications and prolong recovery
(Figure 11.11). Complications include:

- *Pain*—A splint can reduce much of the patient's pain because it secures the broken
or dislocated bones in place and prevents them from compressing or damaging
surrounding nerves and tissues.
- *Damage to soft tissues*—The movement of an injured extremity may cause blood
vessels, nerves, and muscles to be crushed, ruptured, pinched, or compressed.
Splinting reduces movement of the injured part, the possibility of further damage to soft tissues, and the accompanying pain, internal bleeding, and swelling.
- *Bleeding*—Dislocated bones, ends of fractured bones, and moving bone fragments can damage blood vessels and cause internal and external bleeding.
Splinting immobilizes the bone ends and reduces the possibility of their damaging blood vessels and causing bleeding. (The initial force of injury may have
caused bone ends to damage soft tissues and blood vessels. Splinting will stabilize the injury and apply a steady pressure that can reduce and control bleeding.)
- *Restricted blood flow*—Dislocated joints and fractured bones and fragments also
can press against blood vessels and shut off blood flow. Splinting can help relieve the pressure against blood vessels.

remember

Never delay the transport of a
patient with life-threatening injuries in order to splint an injured extremity.

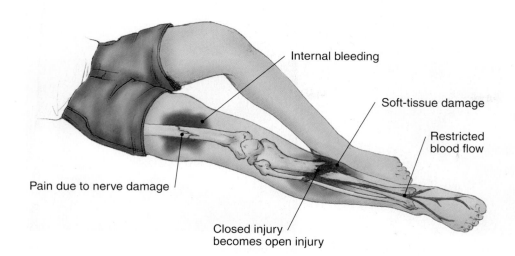

Internal bleeding

Soft-tissue damage

Restricted blood flow

Pain due to nerve damage

Closed injury becomes open injury

- *Closed injuries become open injuries*—The sharp edge of a broken bone can rip through skin to produce an open wound. Immobilizing the injured extremity by splinting it will minimize movement of the broken part and help prevent a closed wound from becoming an open wound. ■

FIRST RESPONDER RESPONSIBILITIES

The primary duties of a First Responder are to detect and control life-threatening problems first. Then, during patient assessment, attempt to find all injuries and care for the worst ones first. Suspected fractures are cared for after neck and spine injuries, which you must stabilize. Open head, chest, and abdominal wounds must be dressed. Shock is managed by administering oxygen and maintaining body temperature. Serious burns are dressed. In the case of major trauma, EMTs will likely arrive before you have an opportunity to apply splints.

Some patients may have indications of neck or spine injuries, and you will not be able to splint extremities until you have additional help and equipment from more advanced care providers. In the meantime, this patient must not be moved but should be kept still while you stabilize his head and neck with your hands (explained later in this chapter). The process of splinting may cause you to move the patient or the injured limb, but even slight movements, without appropriate help to stabilize the body and coordinate the move, could worsen a spinal injury.

FIRST> For all cases involving injured extremities, alert dispatch so you may receive appropriate assistance from EMTs. ■

RULES FOR SPLINTING

For all cases of splinting, you will (Scan 11-2):

- Assess and reassure the patient and explain what you plan to do.
- Splint injuries before moving the patient. Move the patient before splinting only if another injury or the environment is life-threatening.
- Expose the injury site. Cut away clothing if it cannot be easily removed or folded back. Remove jewelry from the injured limb if it can be done without using force, causing pain, or repositioning the patient or the limb.

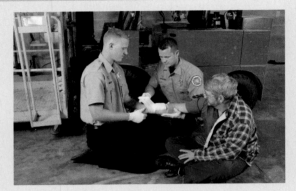

1. After controlling bleeding, dress and bandage open wounds to the injured extremity.

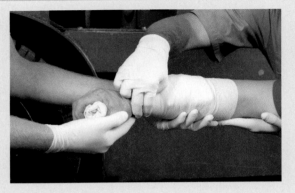

2. Check distal circulation, sensation, and motor function before splinting.

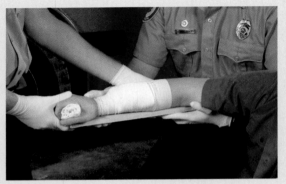

3. Apply a padded splint for comfort and improved contact between limb and splint. If you must use an unpadded splint, wrap it in dressings before application.

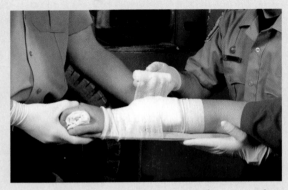

4. Firmly secure the splint, leaving fingertips (or toes) exposed so you can monitor circulation.

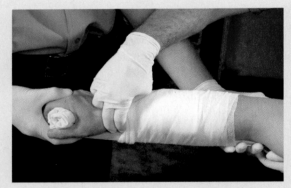

5. After immobilization, reassess distal circulation, sensation, and motor function.

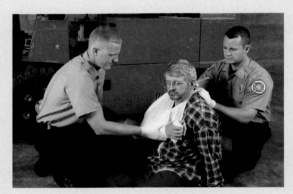

6. Elevate the extremity. For an arm, use the sling to immobilize it against the chest. For a leg, prop it on a pillow or rolled blanket (if there is not indication of spinal injury).

- Control all major bleeding. If necessary, use finger-tip pressure to control bleeding. Avoid applying pressure directly over exposed bone ends. To control major bleeding, use bulky dressings secured snugly with a bandage.

- Dress open wounds. Do not push bone ends back into the wound. Do not try to pick bone fragments from the wound. If the bone ends withdraw into the wound as you care for it, report this to personnel who take over patient care so they can take steps to prevent infection in the patient.

- Check distal circulation, sensation, and motor function before and after splinting.

- Have all materials ready and at hand before splinting. Use padded splints for patient comfort and improved contact between limb and splint. Wrap unpadded splints in dressings before applying them.

- If local protocols allow, gently attempt to realign an angulated limb in the anatomical position before splinting. Attempt to reposition the limb to regain a pulse if the limb is cold and blue and has no pulse.

- Apply gentle manual traction (see next section), and secure the splint firmly but do not restrict circulation. Do not intentionally allow a protruding bone to re-enter the skin.

- Immobilize the suspected fracture site and the joints above and below the injury site. (Secure upper extremities to the torso with a sling and swathe. Secure lower extremities to each other and assist the EMTs in transferring the patient to a spine board or similar device.)

- Secure splints with cravats or roller gauze, starting at the distal end of the extremity. Leave fingertips and toes exposed so you can monitor circulation, sensation, and motor function.

- Elevate the extremity. For an arm, use a sling and swathe. For a leg, prop it on a pillow or rolled blanket if there is no indication of spinal injury. (Otherwise, leave the patient lying flat.)

- Minimize the effects of developing shock by providing oxygen as soon as possible and maintaining body temperature.

APPLYING MANUAL TRACTION

FIRST➤ The effects of splinting may be improved if you apply gentle tension to the injured extremity during the splinting process. In First Responder care, this tension is applied by pulling gently on the injured limb. This is called **manual traction**, which helps to stabilize the injury. ■

manual traction process of drawing or pulling; a stabilizing procedure that precedes the application of a splint.

Most EMS systems do not allow First Responders to straighten deformed injuries. Do only what you have been trained to do and what is allowed in your EMS system. Check your local protocols to find out what you are allowed to do if there is angulation or no distal circulation. If you find no distal pulse, and the skin in the distal extremity is pale or blue and cold, you need to take action immediately. Notify dispatch, the responding EMTs, or the hospital and let them know the patient's status. You may be directed to gently align the limb in an attempt to restore distal pulse. Do not force the limb if you meet resistance or if the patient complains of too much pain. Apply a soft splint and elevate the limb by propping it on a blanket roll or pillow. Provide oxygen and other appropriate emergency care interventions until the EMTs arrive.

NOTE

Not all EMS systems allow First Responders to apply manual traction. You may only be allowed to gently reposition a limb to allow for the application of a splint. Your instructor will inform you of local guidelines.

When you start to apply manual traction, it may cause a temporary increase in pain for the patient. Explain this to him, but also explain that the pain caused by the injury will probably lessen once the traction and the splint are applied.

Do not release manual traction to apply a splint. Traction is of little use if it is not maintained. So, it usually takes two people to properly apply a splint: one to hold and maintain manual traction, while the other applies the splint. If you are the only trained EMS provider on scene, you may be able to direct a bystander to secure a splint while you maintain traction. (Follow local protocol.) If you are working alone, do not try to apply traction unless distal circulation is absent. Once you apply manual traction, you must maintain it until the extremity is secured to a splint.

To apply manual traction, you must (Figure 11.12):

1. Grasp the patient's limb by placing one hand above the injury site and the other hand below the injury site. Position your hands so that the splint can be applied without having to release manual traction.

2. Gently apply steady tension by pulling with your lower hand. The direction of pull should be along the long axis of the limb. If you feel resistance, stop the procedure.

3. Maintain manual traction throughout the splinting process. A rigid splint will maintain traction after it is secured to the patient.

WARNING: *Do not apply manual traction if the injury is to the joints of the shoulder, elbow, wrist, hand, pelvis, hip, knee, ankle, or foot. All extremity injuries that may be dislocations must be splinted in the position in which they are found. Remember, moving dislocated bones may cause further damage to surrounding tissues.*

STRAIGHTENING DEFORMED INJURIES

The main reason for straightening closed deformed injuries is to improve circulation. Straight limbs also make it easier for you to apply a rigid splint. If the limb cannot be straightened or if you are not allowed to straighten it, immobilize the

FIGURE 11.12
Manual traction.

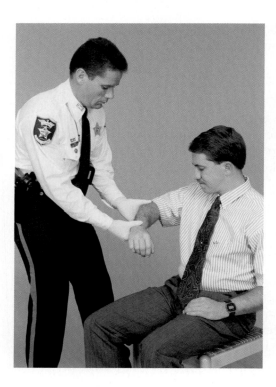

limb in the position found. The procedure for straightening closed deformed injuries is the same as for applying manual traction:

- Straighten closed deformed injuries of the elbow, knee, and ankle if there is no distal circulation. In these cases, do not apply manual traction to the limb. Simply align for splinting.

- Make only one attempt to straighten the angulation.

- Stop if you meet resistance or if the patient complains of severe pain.

Some jurisdictions do not allow for straightening angulated injuries under certain conditions or for certain extremities. Always follow your local protocols.

TYPES OF SPLINTS

Soft Splints

There are two main types of splints: soft and rigid. When properly applied, **soft splints** such as pillows, blankets, towels, cravats, and dressings, may be used to stabilize injuries. Soft splints can provide support to an injury and help decrease pain and swelling. A commonly used soft splint is the **triangular bandage**. It can be folded to any width to fit any part of the body, to secure arms to the torso and legs to each other, or to secure extremities to rigid splints. A triangular bandage is frequently used for a sling and swathe.

A **sling** is a triangular bandage used to stabilize the shoulder and arm. A properly placed sling will adequately immobilize an injured elbow as well as provide support to the lower arm. Once the arm is placed in a sling, a swathe is used to hold the arm against the side of the chest and restrict movement of the shoulder. A **swathe** is made from a triangular bandage, which is folded to about a two-inch by four-inch width so it fits the area of the arm between the shoulder and elbow. (A triangular bandage folded to a width of three or four inches and used to tie soft or rigid splints in place is called a **cravat**.) Together, the sling and swathe work well to immobilize both the elbow and shoulder joints, which is necessary when caring for suspected fractures of the arm.

The sling and swathe are effective for injuries to the following:

- Shoulder girdle.
- Upper arm.
- Elbow.
- Lower arm.
- Wrist, hand, and fingers.
- Ribs.

Roller bandages and wide Velcro fasteners can be used to form a sling and swathe. Any material may be used, as long as it will not cut into the patient's skin and cause further damage. To make and apply a sling and swathe, you should (Scan 11-3):

1. Use a commercial sling, or make one from a piece of cloth or sheet. Fold or cut this material so that it is in the shape of a triangle. The ideal sling should be about 50 to 60 inches long at its base and 36 to 40 inches long on each of its sides.

2. Position the triangular material over the patient's chest. The peak of the triangle should point toward the patient's injured arm and extend beyond the

soft splint a device, such as a sling and swathe or a pillow secured with cravats, which can be applied to immobilize a painful extremity.

triangular bandage a piece of triangular cloth material about 50 to 60 inches long at its base and 36 to 40 inches long on each side. It can be folded and used as a sling, a swathe, or a cravat.

sling a large triangular bandage or other cloth device that is applied as a soft splint to immobilize possible injuries to the shoulder girdle and upper extremity.

swathe a large cravat, usually made of cloth, used to secure a sling or rigid splint and sling to the body.

cravat a triangular bandage that is folded to a width of three or four inches and used to tie soft or rigid splints in place.

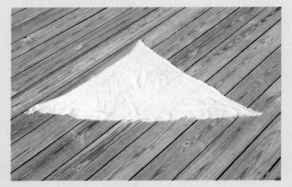

1. A sling and swathe starts with a triangular bandage 50 inches at its base and about 36 inches on each side. Fold it to any width.

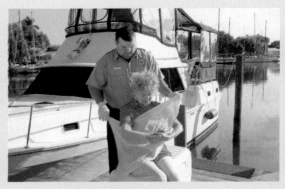

2. After assessing circulation, sensation, and motor function, position the longest side of the bandage over the chest while holding on to the point and one corner.

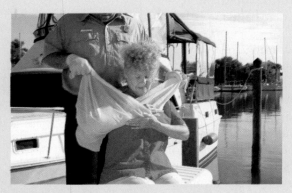

3. Bring the bottom end up and over the patient's injured arm. Keep the hand elevated above the elbow.

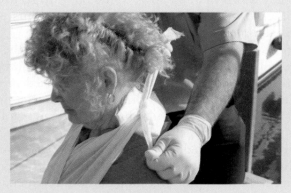

4. Tie the two ends together. Pad the knot and make sure it does not rest on the patient's neck. Reassess circulation, sensation, and motor function.

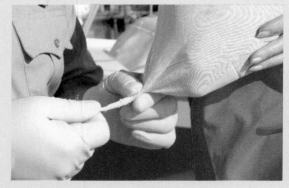

5. Secure the point of the sling to form a pocket for the elbow.

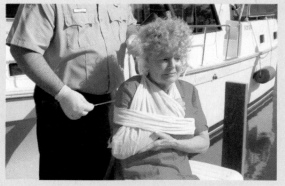

6. Fold another triangular piece of material to form a swathe. Tie it around the patient to support the arm and to maintain elevation.

elbow. The long end should be draped over the opposite shoulder. Have the patient position his arm so the hand is above the elbow. If he cannot hold his arm, have your partner or a bystander support the arm while you prepare and secure the sling.

3. Take the bottom end of the triangle and bring it up and over the patient's arm and shoulder on the injured side.

4. Draw up on the ends of the sling so that the patient's hand on the injured side is about four inches above the elbow. Tie the two ends together and be sure to position the knot so it does not rest on the back of the patient's neck. Place a flat layer of cloth (gauze pads or handkerchief) under the knot for comfort. Leave the patient's fingertips exposed so you can check for circulation, sensation, and motor function. If circulation is absent following immobilization, support the arm while the sling is removed and gently reposition it until you can feel the pulse. (Follow local protocols.) Replace the sling.

5. Take the point of the sling at the patient's elbow and fold it forward. Then tuck it in or pin it in place, or twist and tie the point. (It may be easier to tie the knot before the sling is placed on the patient.) This will form a pocket for the patient's elbow.

6. Take a second piece of triangular cloth and fold it to a two- or four-inch width. Center the widest part on the patient's injured arm. Take one end across the patient's back and one end across the chest and tie on the opposite side under the other arm. Be sure that the swathe is placed as low over the injured arm as possible. This will insure that it stays close to the body and minimize movement of the shoulder.

Rigid Splints

Rigid splints can be made of plastic, metal, wood, or compressed cardboard and have very little give or flexibility. They are applied along an injured extremity to immobilize the entire limb and the joints directly above and below the injury site.

Commercial Splints   A wide variety of commercial splints are available for emergency care. These splints are made of wood, aluminum, cardboard, foam, wire, or plastic. Some come with their own washable pads. Others require padding to be applied before being secured. Most splints are either solid rigid pieces or air-inflatable plastic splints. Figure 11.13 shows some of the commercially available splints you might use in First Responder care. These include air splints, vacuum splints, board-and-wire ladder splints, heavy duty cardboard splints, and flexible aluminum splints. All EMTs and many First Responders carry traction splints for splinting and stabilizing injuries to the femur.

Local protocols may provide guidelines for using a pneumatic anti-shock garment (PASG), a special device for suspected pelvic and femur fractures. You must receive training and use the PASG only as allowed by local protocols.

Inflatable Splints   Inflatable splints, or air splints, are not carried by all First Responder units. If you carry them and your jurisdiction allows you to use them, your instructor will teach you their application. Typically, air splints are used for patients with injuries to the arm or lower leg bones. When using an air splint, slip it uninflated over your forearm. Then grasp the patient's hand or foot and pull gentle traction while you slip the air splint onto the patient's limb. Smooth out the splint and inflate it. The splint is fully inflated and effective when you can make a slight surface indentation with your fingertip (Scan 11-4).

rigid splint a stiff device made of a material with very little flexibility (such as metal, plastic, or wood) that is long enough to immobilize an extremity and the joints above and below the injury site.

FIGURE 11.13
There are many types and sizes of commercial rigid splints.

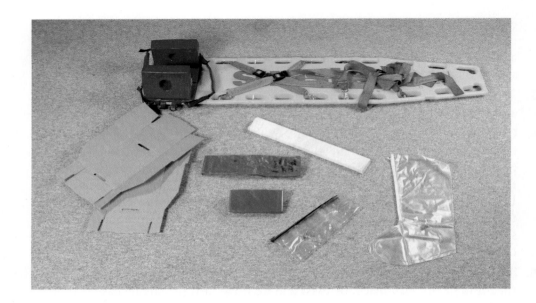

After inflating the splint, you must monitor the limb for changes in circulation, sensation, and motor function. Monitor the splint for changes in pressure. If the patient is moved to a warmer or colder location, the air in the splint will expand or contract with the temperature change. You will have to recheck the pressure in the splint. You may have to remove increased pressure by deflating the splint slightly. The pressure in the splint also will change if the patient is moved to a different altitude. Always monitor the pressure in the splint. Periodically, check the condition of all air splints as old ones may develop leaks.

Once an air splint is applied, you may not be able to assess the distal pulse. Instead, evaluate capillary refill (more reliable in pediatric patients), skin color, sensation, and motor function. The problems with air splints—the inability to check distal pulse and the potential pressure changes—have led some EMS systems to drop them from their approved equipment lists.

Improvising Splints

First Responders may arrive at the scene of an emergency without any splints, or they may use their supply of splints on one patient and have none for another patient. It is helpful to know how to make splints from materials found at the scene. Such an improvised splint may be soft or rigid and may be made from a variety of materials.

First➤ Rigid splints can be made from pieces of lumber, plywood, compressed-wood products, cardboard, rolled newspapers or magazines, umbrellas, canes, broom or shovel handles, sporting equipment (shin guards are an example), and tongue depressors for fingers (Figure 11.14). Soft splints can be made from towels, blankets, pillows, and bulky clothing like sweaters and sweat suits. Most of these items can be found at the scene of a typical incident. Many people carry some of these items in their cars. Ask people at the scene to help you find these items. Give them suggestions and ask if they have any ideas. ■

MANAGEMENT OF SPECIFIC EXTREMITY INJURIES

First➤ In general, when the mechanism of injury and the patient's signs and symptoms indicate possible injuries that require splints:

WARNING: Air splints may leak. When applied in cold weather, an air splint will expand when the patient is moved to a warmer place. Pressure also will change at different altitudes. Monitor the pressure in the splint by pressing with your fingertip. These splints may stick to the patient's skin in hot weather.

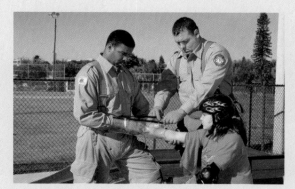

1. Check distal circulation, sensation, and motor function before splinting. Slide the un-inflated splint onto your forearm. Then grasp the patient's hand and pull manual traction.

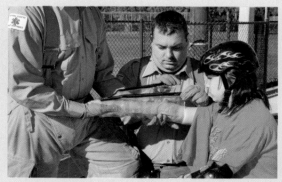

2. Slide the splint from your arm and onto the patient's arm. When applied properly, the lower edge of the air splint should be just above the second joint of the patient's fingers.

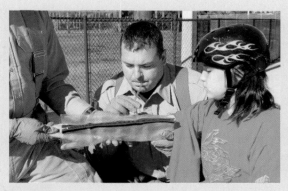

3. Maintain traction and support the arm while your partner inflates the splint to a point where you can make a slight dent when you press your thumb against its surface.

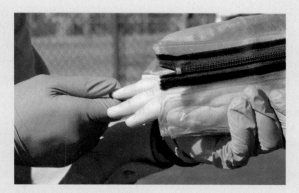

4. Monitor the splint pressure and the patient's distal circulation, sensation, and motor function.

- Apply rigid splints for injuries to the forearm and the lower leg. Rigid splints may be used for injuries to the thigh, but traction splints are more effective. Follow local protocol.
- Use soft splints (blanket, towel, pillow, sling and swathe) if rigid splints are not available (Figure 11.15). Provide further rigid support by securing upper extremities to the torso with a swathe and lower extremities to each other with cravats.
- Use soft or rigid splints for injuries to the arm, elbow, wrist, or hand.
- Use soft splints for injuries to the ankle or foot. ■

remember

As in all emergency care, providing emotional support to the patient is a significant part of total patient care.

FIGURE 11.14
Improvised splints may be made
from a variety of materials.

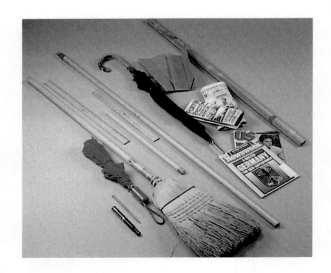

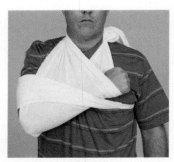

FIGURE 11.15
Sling and swathe.

position of function the
natural position of the body part,
specifically the hand or foot. In the
case of the hand, the natural
position is slightly flexed. In the
case of the foot, the natural
position is slightly extended.

warning

Always wear protective gloves
when providing care for extremity injuries. Face and eye shields
may be necessary if injuries are
spurting blood.

warning

Do not try to realign or reposition angulations or dislocations
of the shoulder. Movement in
this area may cause damage to
nearby blood vessels and nerves.

For an algorithm of assessment and care of patients with specific extremity injuries, see Figure 11.16.

UPPER EXTREMITY INJURIES

Methods for splinting each type of upper extremity injury are summarized in Scan
11-5. For injuries to the upper extremities, be sure to place the hand in a **position
of function**, in which the fingers are slightly flexed and the wrist is cocked slightly
upward, or dorsally. The position of function is a normal and comfortable position
for the patient, especially if the extremity from forearm to hand is secured against a
rigid splint. You may easily secure the hand in its position of function by placing a
roll of gauze in the patient's hand before immobilizing or simply by allowing the
fingers of the hand to extend over the end of the splint. (For upper extremity care,
see Figure 11.17.)

Injuries to the Shoulder Girdle

A common sign of shoulder girdle injury is a condition known as *knocked-down
shoulder* or *dropped shoulder* (Figure 11.18). The patient's injured shoulder will appear to droop. The patient usually holds the arm up against the side of the chest.

Injuries to the shoulder joint often produce what is known as an anterior (to
the front) dislocation. The end of the upper arm bone that forms the shoulder
joint can be felt, or even seen, bulging or protruding under the skin at the front of
the shoulder.

It is not practical to use a rigid splint for injuries to the collarbone, shoulder
blade, or shoulder joint. Place padding between any space between the patient's injured arm and chest, use a cravat to secure the padding in place, and use a sling and
swathe to secure the arm to the chest. Remember to check for distal circulation,
sensation, and motor function before and after splinting. If there is no pulse, attempt to reposition to regain a pulse but do not force the arm.

FIRST➤ When you provide care for patients with shoulder injuries, you will:

1. Take appropriate BSI precautions.

2. Care for life-threatening problems and other injuries that have priority over
   musculoskeletal injuries.

3. Check for a radial pulse (distal pulse at the wrist) and signs of restricted circulation on the injured arm. If there is no pulse, notify the responding EMTs or

Musculoskeletal Injuries to the Extremities

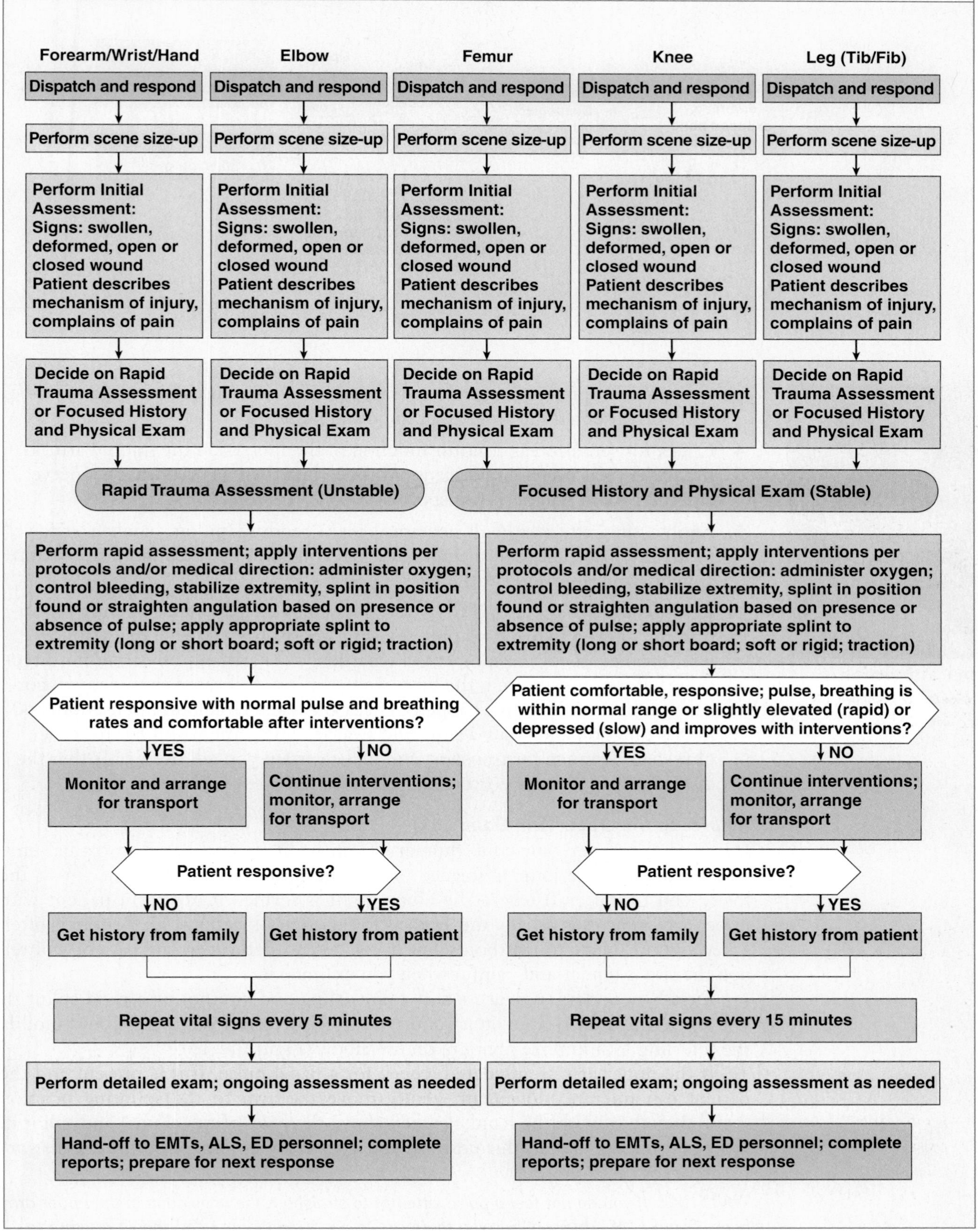

Forearm/Wrist/Hand	Elbow	Femur	Knee	Leg (Tib/Fib)
Dispatch and respond	Dispatch and respond	Dispatch and respond	Dispatch and respond	Dispatch and respond

Perform scene size-up	Perform scene size-up	Perform scene size-up	Perform scene size-up	Perform scene size-up

Perform Initial Assessment:
Signs: swollen, deformed, open or closed wound
Patient describes mechanism of injury, complains of pain
(repeated in all five columns)

Decide on Rapid Trauma Assessment or Focused History and Physical Exam
(repeated in all five columns)

Rapid Trauma Assessment (Unstable)

Focused History and Physical Exam (Stable)

Perform rapid assessment; apply interventions per protocols and/or medical direction: administer oxygen; control bleeding, stabilize extremity, splint in position found or straighten angulation based on presence or absence of pulse; apply appropriate splint to extremity (long or short board; soft or rigid; traction)

Perform rapid assessment; apply interventions per protocols and/or medical direction: administer oxygen; control bleeding, stabilize extremity, splint in position found or straighten angulation based on presence or absence of pulse; apply appropriate splint to extremity (long or short board; soft or rigid; traction)

Patient responsive with normal pulse and breathing rates and comfortable after interventions?

- YES → Monitor and arrange for transport
- NO → Continue interventions; monitor, arrange for transport

Patient comfortable, responsive; pulse, breathing is within normal range or slightly elevated (rapid) or depressed (slow) and improves with interventions?

- YES → Monitor and arrange for transport
- NO → Continue interventions; monitor, arrange for transport

Patient responsive?

- NO → Get history from family
- YES → Get history from patient

Patient responsive?

- NO → Get history from family
- YES → Get history from patient

Repeat vital signs every 5 minutes

Repeat vital signs every 15 minutes

Perform detailed exam; ongoing assessment as needed

Perform detailed exam; ongoing assessment as needed

Hand-off to EMTs, ALS, ED personnel; complete reports; prepare for next response

Hand-off to EMTs, ALS, ED personnel; complete reports; prepare for next response

FIGURE 11.16

Care of Upper Extremity Injuries

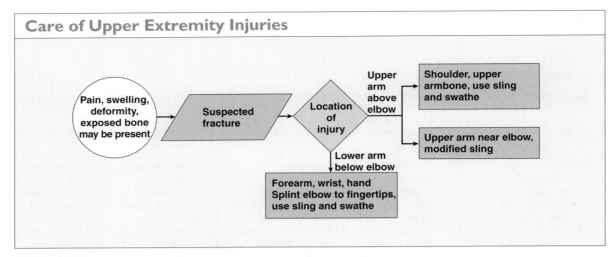

FIGURE 11.17

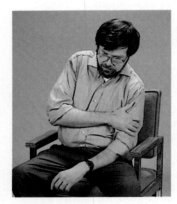

FIGURE 11.18
"Knocked down" or "dropped" shoulder.

notify the hospital and arrange to transport as soon as possible. Note the time that you observed the absence of the distal pulse.

4. Check for sensation and motor function of the fingers on the injured arm. If the patient has no feeling or cannot move, then there is pressure on a nerve and the patient will need transport as soon as possible.

5. Apply a sling and swathe. If necessary, place padding (pillow, blanket, or towel) to fill any space between the patient's arm and chest on the injured side before applying the sling and swathe.

6. Reassess the distal pulse. If the pulse is absent, you may have to gently reposition the injured arm and reapply the sling and swathe. In such cases, follow your local protocols or contact the emergency department physician for directions before repositioning the limb. Sometimes a dislocated shoulder will correct (reduce) itself. If this happens, check the distal circulation, sensation, and motor function and apply a sling and swathe. This patient still has to see a physician. Arrange for transport and make certain you tell the EMTs that the dislocation apparently corrected itself and the time it took place. ■

Injuries to the Upper Arm Bone

Injury to the upper arm bone (humerus) can be at its upper end (proximal end) where the shoulder joint is formed, along the mid-shaft of the bone, or at the lower end (distal end) where the elbow joint is formed. Care for a patient with upper arm injuries is usually the same as for all injury locations. Deformity is often a key sign of injury to this bone, but if you see no deformity, the patient will tell you the site is tender and painful when you examine it.

First Responders may use a soft splint (sling and swathe) or a rigid splint. If you use a sling and swathe on an injury that seems very close to the elbow, modify the full sling to minimize pressure on the elbow (Figure 11.19).

If the upper arm is angulated, check for a distal pulse. If it is present and the patient can tolerate movement, gently move the arm to the splinting position (bend the elbow with the hand elevated above the level of the elbow) and splint it. Do not force the arm to this position and do not try to straighten the angulation. Recheck for distal pulse.

WARNING: *If you do not feel a pulse, attempt to straighten the angulation in the upper arm bone, if your EMS system allows you to do so. Do not force the arm. You should attempt to straighten the angulation only once and stop if there is resistance or severe pain. If straight-*

Splinting an Upper Extremity

NOTE: Place a roll of dressing in the hand to maintain position of function.

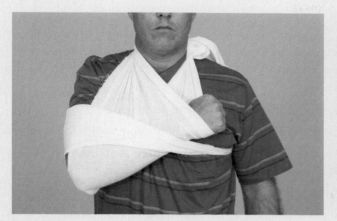

Shoulder —Apply a sling and swathe. Elevate the wrist above the elbow and support it with the swathe.

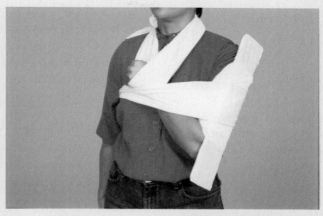

Arm —Immobilize with a rigid splint from the shoulder to below the elbow. Apply a sling and swathe that will elevate and support the limb.

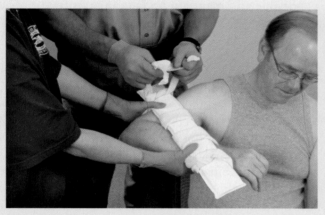

Elbow (bent) —Place the splint from shoulder to wrist. Secure the wrist first. Apply a sling and swathe to elevate and support the limb.

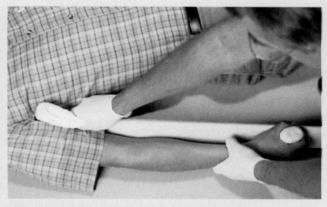

Elbow (straight) —Pad the armpit. Splint should extend from the armpit beyond the fingertips. Use roller bandages to secure the splint to the arm starting at the distal end. Secure the arm to the body with cravats.

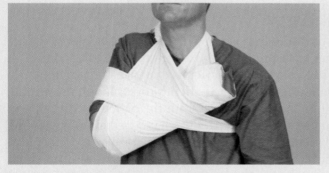

Forearm, wrist, hand —The splint should extend from the elbow to beyond the fingertips. Use a sling and swathe for elevation and support.

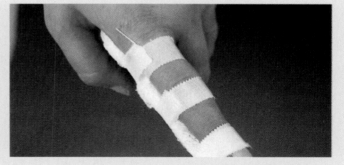

Finger —Use a tongue depressor as a splint or tape the finger to an uninjured finger.

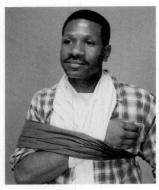

FIGURE 11.19
For an upper arm injury near the elbow joint, gently apply a modified sling so it supports only the wrist.

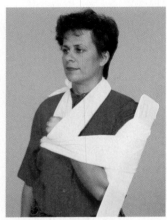

FIGURE 11.20
Wrist sling and swathe.

ening the limb fails to restore a distal pulse, arrange to transport the patient as soon as possible. If the pulse is restored, splint the arm and recheck distal pulse again.

If you use a rigid splint, secure it to the lateral (outside) part of the arm with roller gauze or cravats. Then apply a wrist sling and wide swathe. The swathe will secure the injured arm to the body and immobilize the joints above and below the injury site (Figure 11.20).

FIRST➤ When you apply a splint to an upper arm injury, work with a partner. One of you will maintain manual traction, while the other applies the splint and the sling and swathe. To apply a splint for injuries to the upper arm bone:

1. Check for distal circulation, sensation, and motor function.
2. Select a padded splint long enough for the area between shoulder and elbow.
3. Apply manual traction to the injured extremity. If there is angulation or no distal pulse, gently realign and recheck for pulse.
4. Place the splint against the injured extremity.
5. Secure the splint to the patient with a roller bandage, handkerchiefs, cravats, or cloth strips. Begin securing at the distal end of the splint.
6. Maintain the hand in the position of function and apply a sling and swathe. Recheck distal circulation, sensation, and motor function.
7. Provide oxygen as soon as possible and maintain body temperature to prevent the effects of developing shock. ■

Injuries to the Elbow

The elbow is a joint (not a bone) formed by the lower, or distal, end of the upper arm bone and the upper, or proximal, end of the forearm bones. You can determine if the injury is to the elbow area by placing your hand over the back of the elbow. The elbow includes all the structures that can be covered by the palm of your hand (Figure 11.21). If the injury is above this area, the injury is to the upper arm bone. If the injury is below this area, the injury is to one of the forearm bones.

When caring for elbow injuries, immobilize the elbow in the position in which it is found. Have your partner stabilize the arm while you apply and secure the splint. Check circulation, sensation, and motor function before and after splinting.

FIRST➤ The following methods can be used in caring for a patient with an elbow injury:

- If the elbow is found in a flexed (bent) position natural for the joint, rigid splinting is preferred. However, a wrist sling and a swathe may be effective. Apply a splint as shown in Figure 11.22.
- If the elbow is found in the straight position, and it cannot be placed in the natural flexed or splinting position, immobilize it in the straight position. Rigid splinting is preferred, but body splinting is effective. This is done by tying the injured arm along the side of the patient's torso. If you use a rigid splint, select a padded splint that will extend from the patient's armpit past the fingertips. Place a roll of dressing in the patient's hand to maintain it in the position of function and secure the splint with roller gauze or folded cravats starting at the distal end of the arm (fingertips) (Figure 11.23).
- If the elbow appears to be dislocated and it is in an unnatural or awkward position and cannot be repositioned, place padding around the arm and between the arm and chest if necessary. Secure the arm to the body with a sling and swathe. ■

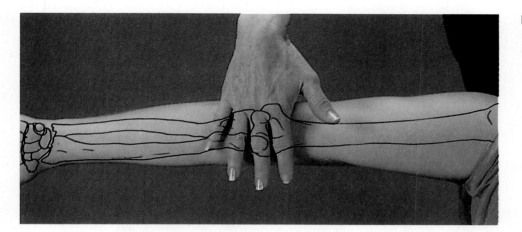

FIGURE 11.21
Consider this area to be the site of elbow injuries.

Injuries to the Forearm, Wrist, and Hand

FIRST▶ The most effective splint for an injured forearm, wrist, or hand is a rigid one. However, the patient can be made comfortable with a pillow splint (Figure 11.24) and a sling and swathe. A sling and swathe used alone is also effective for a forearm. Be sure to check distal circulation, sensation, and motor function before and after splinting.

To use a rigid splint for any injury to the forearm, wrist, or hand, select a padded rigid splint that extends from beyond the elbow to past the fingertips. Place a roll of dressing in the patient's hand to maintain the hand in the position of function. The steps for splinting the forearm, wrist, and hand are the same as steps 3 through 7 listed above for the upper arm. Do not apply manual traction to wrist or hand injuries.

NOTE: *Some jurisdictions permit an alternative method for maintaining the position of function in the hand. They allow the fingers to curve over the end of the rigid splint (Figure 11.25).*

Rolled newspapers, magazines, and creased cardboard make effective rigid splints for injuries to the forearm or wrist (Figure 11.26), but they still should be padded. Apply a sling after splinting to keep the forearm elevated. Add a swathe to

NOTE

Some EMS systems allow First Responders to make one gentle attempt to reposition a limb when there is no distal pulse. Perform this move only if you are allowed to do so. Check with your instructor. Do not try to force the arm, and stop if the limb offers resistance or if the patient complains of increased pain.

warning

Do not attempt to straighten a wrist injury. Keep the wrist in the position in which it is found. Place padding in any space between the wrist and the splint. Your jurisdiction may allow you to try to gently reposition the wrist if there is no distal pulse and the hand is cold and blue.

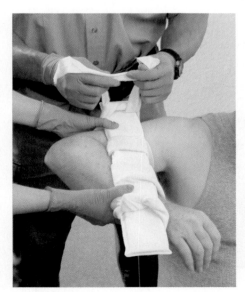

FIGURE 11.22
Splinting an injured elbow in a flexed position.

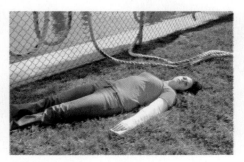

FIGURE 11.23
Splinting an injured elbow in a straight position.

FIGURE 11.24
Soft splinting for wrist and hand injuries.

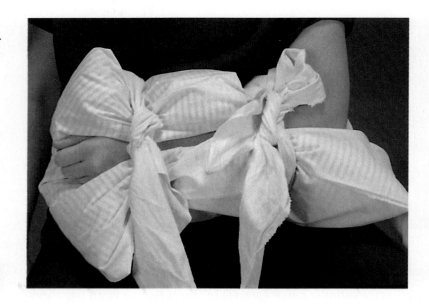

secure the forearm to the chest and immobilize the joint above and below the injury site. ■

Injuries to the Fingers

Not all injuries to the fingers require rigid splinting. You can immobilize a injured finger by taping the finger to an adjacent, uninjured finger (Figure 11.27). You can tape the finger to a tongue depressor, an aluminum splint, or a pen or pencil. You can also make a soft splint by placing a roll of gauze in the patient's hand and wrapping more gauze around the hand and dressing. This soft-splint method immobilizes the hand and fingers and keeps them in the position of function. Some emergency department physicians prefer this type of soft bandage. Check to see if this may be part of your EMS system's protocols.

Apply a sling to keep the forearm elevated. Apply a swathe to immobilize the joints above the injury site and to improve circulation and patient comfort.

Do not attempt to "pop" dislocated fingers back into their sockets. Immobilize dislocated fingers as you would an injured hand.

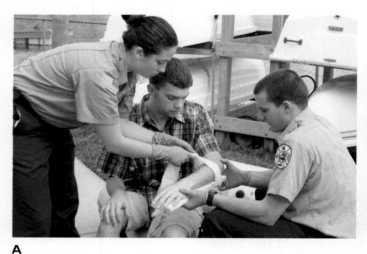

A

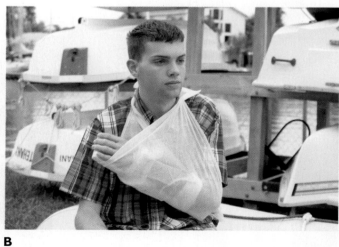

B

FIGURE 11.25
Rigid splinting of an injured forearm, wrist, or hand. **A.** Secure a rigid splint to the limb. **B.** Place the arm in a sling.

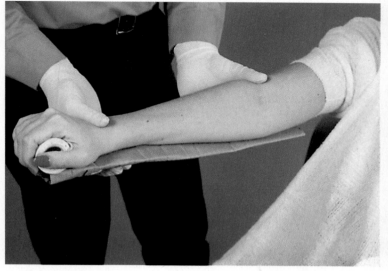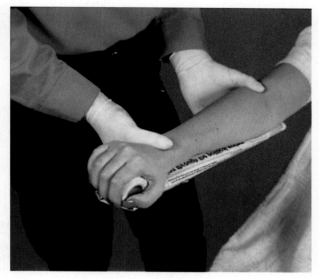

FIGURE 11.26
Rigid splints can be made from cardboard, rolled newspapers, or rolled magazines.

LOWER EXTREMITY INJURIES

NOTE: *When the patient has multiple injuries, it may be best to totally immobilize the patient on a long spine board or a scoop (orthopedic) stretcher rather than to try to immobilize each individual injury. However, do not attempt to use these immobilization devices unless you are trained to correctly move the patient onto them and to properly strap the patient to them.*

Before moving or rolling a patient with suspected spinal injury or with lower extremity injuries, be sure you have the proper equipment ready and a sufficient number of rescue personnel on hand to assist.

For lower extremity care, see Figure 11.28.

Injuries to the Pelvic Girdle

FIRST➤ The patient may have injuries to the pelvic girdle (pelvis and hip joints) if:

- Patient complains of pain in the pelvis, hips, or groin.
- Patient complains of pain when gentle pressure is applied to the sides of the hips or to the hip bones.

remember

Always assess distal circulation, sensation, and motor function before and after splinting. If there is no pulse, and your jurisdiction allows, gently realign an angulation or reposition the leg to regain a pulse.

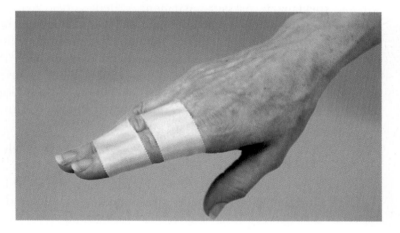

FIGURE 11.27
One way to immobilize an injured finger is to tape it to an adjacent, uninjured finger.

Care of Lower Extremity Injuries

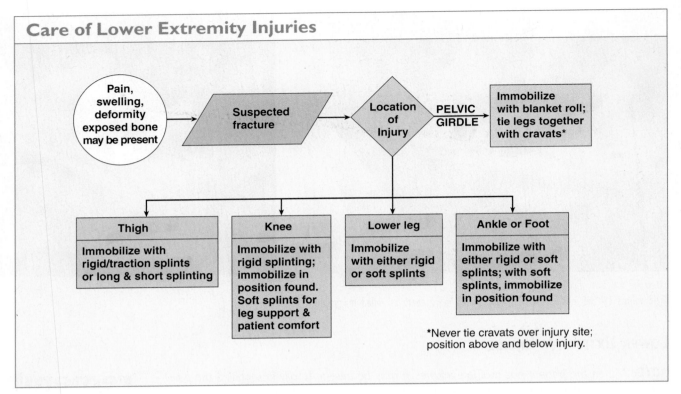

FIGURE 11.28

- Patient cannot lift the legs while lying face up. The patient will usually tell you that "it hurts" or "I can't move my legs." Do not insist.
- Foot on the injured side turns outward more than the uninjured side.
- Injured extremity appears shorter than the uninjured side.
- Pelvis or the hip joint has noticeable deformity. ■

Pelvic injuries are serious because they can damage major blood vessels and internal organs. Injuries to these soft tissues can cause profuse internal bleeding, sterility, and infection. The force that caused the pelvic injury may also have caused spinal injuries. Because of all these critical factors, it may be best to wait for more advanced care to arrive before attempting to immobilize a patient with a pelvic injury. In the meantime, provide oxygen as soon as possible and maintain body temperature to delay the onset of shock. Note the mechanism of injury so you can report it to the responding EMTs.

With certain symptoms, pelvic girdle injuries may be managed at the scene with a specialized pressure garment called a pneumatic anti-shock garment (PASG). Your instructor will know if First Responders are trained and allowed to use or assist more advanced providers with PASGs in your area. Follow your local protocols or medical direction when considering the use of a PASG. Other devices and materials that are effective for immobilizing injuries to the pelvic girdle include: long spine boards, scoop (orthopedic) stretchers, long board splints, and blankets. If you do not carry this equipment, you may continue patient assessment while you are waiting for more advanced care to arrive.

FIRST▸ As a First Responder, you can care for patients with suspected fractures to the pelvic girdle by using a soft splint. Place a blanket roll between the patient's legs and tie them together with cravats. This simple and quick immobilization method will stabilize the injury and provide patient comfort before more advanced care arrives. ■

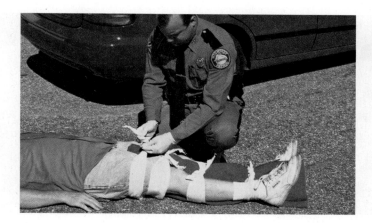

To immobilize a pelvic injury with a blanket roll, do the following (Figure 11.29):

1. Complete a thorough assessment of the injury site.

2. Assess circulation, sensation, and motor function in both distal extremities.

3. Provide oxygen to the patient as soon as possible.

4. Place a folded blanket, large towel, or other thick padding material between the patient's legs from groin to feet.

5. Prepare four cravats (folded triangular bandages) or other strips of material.

6. Use a short splint or coat hanger and drape the ends of all four cravats over the splint or hanger. Slide them under the space behind the knees.

7. Gently slide two cravats above the knees and two below the knees.

8. Starting at the feet (distal end), tie one cravat at the ankles, one just below the knees, one just above the knees, and one just below the hips. Do not tie a cravat over or too near the injury site.

When the EMTs arrive, you can help them place the stabilized patient on a scoop (orthopedic) stretcher or spine board. Remember to provide oxygen to the patient as soon as possible and cover the patient to maintain body temperature and to help reduce the chance of developing shock. If you suspect spinal injury, do not attempt to move the patient until the EMTs arrive with additional help. In the meantime, stabilize the patient's head and neck and continue to talk with and reassure him.

Because the signs and symptoms of musculoskeletal injuries are similar, you will not be trying to determine which type of injury the patient has. Even so, there are certain signs that indicate a possible hip dislocation, and you should look for them because you do not want to attempt to move an injured leg if there is a possible hip dislocation. If you suspect a hip dislocation, there may also be injury to the thigh bone (femur). Do not try to straighten an angulated femur if the hip appears to be dislocated.

FIRST▶ The following points describe two types of hip dislocation. Suspect the patient has a dislocated hip if you find (Figure 11.30):

- *Anterior hip dislocation*—The leg from hip to foot is rotated outward further than the uninjured side. Leg rotation also may be an indication of hip fracture. With hip fracture, the injured leg may appear to be shorter than the other leg. You will probably see or feel the bony end of the femur under the skin at the front or side of the leg where it joins the torso.

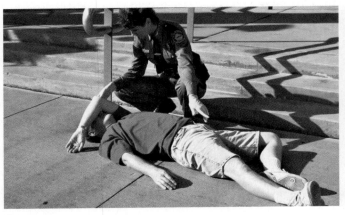
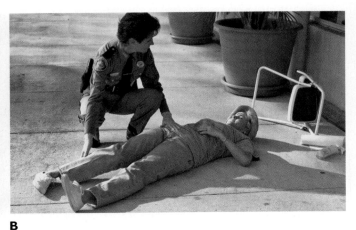

A   **B**

FIGURE 11.30
Classic signs of (A) an anterior hip dislocation and (B) a posterior hip dislocation.

- *Posterior hip dislocation (most common)*—The leg is rotated inward and the knee is usually bent. You may see or feel the bony end of the femur under the skin at the back of the leg where it joins the buttocks.

If the hip is dislocated, wait for more advanced care to arrive. While waiting, provide oxygen as soon as possible and cover the patient to maintain body temperature and help prevent shock. You can immobilize the injured leg by placing and securing pillows or folded blankets or towels around the injured leg, which will support the leg and provide comfort to the patient. Do not reposition or move the patient's leg when you place or secure pillows or blankets. ■

Injuries to the Upper Leg or Thigh

Injuries to the upper leg or thigh bone (femur) are often open. Even when the injury is closed, bleeding inside the tissues can be heavy and life-threatening. There may be a severe and obvious deformity with upper leg fractures. The leg below the injury site may be bent where there is no joint, or it will appear twisted.

To immobilize thigh injuries, use rigid splints or a special device called a traction splint. First Responder units may carry traction splints, and you may be trained and allowed to use them. (Your instructor will advise you if tractions splints are part of your local protocols.) Soft splints are not as effective as rigid or traction splinting, but they will stabilize the injury and provide some pain relief.

While waiting for the EMTs to arrive, provide the patient some relief from pain by securing a blanket roll between the legs in the same way you would for injuries to the pelvic girdle. This is effective once the patient is secured to a spine board or scoop (orthopedic) stretcher, a form of rigid splinting. Provide oxygen as soon as possible and cover the patient to maintain body warmth to help prevent shock.

An alternative approach is to immobilize the leg using a long rigid splint that extends from the patient's buttocks to past the foot. Use cravats to secure the splint. Use a splint or coat hanger to push the cravats under the patient's trunk and legs at the natural voids (lower back and knees) (Figure 11.31). Do not place a tie over the injury site but place one tie above and one tie below the injury.

Injuries to the Knee

FIRST▶ In most cases, you will not be able to tell if the knee is fractured, dislocated, or both. Sometimes a dislocated kneecap (patella) will sponta-

remember

Injuries to the thigh can bleed profusely. Provide oxygen as soon as possible and maintain body temperature to reduce the effects of shock. Monitor the patient's vital signs and comfort level.

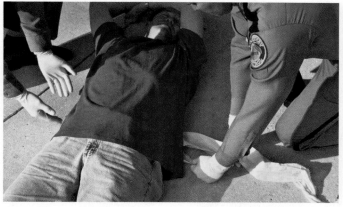
A

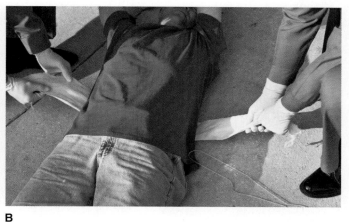
B

FIGURE 11.31

Safely inserting cravats under a patient. **A.** Use a coat hanger or flat splint to push the cravat under the void. **B.** Then reposition the cravat to the proper side.

neously reposition itself. The patient will probably be able to tell you if this has happened. Because of the many nerves and blood vessels and the possibility that soft tissues were damaged, immobilize an injured knee in the position in which it is found (Figure 11.32). Do not attempt to reposition or straighten the injured knee. Some EMS systems allow First Responders to make one attempt at straightening the limb if there is no distal pulse. Your instructor will let you know the requirements of your local protocols. ■

Rigid splinting is the most effective method to use when immobilizing an injured knee, but you can provide support to the leg and comfort to the patient with soft splints. Place and secure pillows or folded blankets around the knee, especially if it is found in the bent position. Do not reposition or move the patient's legs in order to place or secure pillows or blankets. If the injured knee is found in the straight position, you can effectively immobilize it with a blanket placed between both legs and secured with cravats, just as you would for a femur injuries.

For rigid splinting of an injured knee found in the straight position (or straightened because there was no distal pulse), secure a long splint from the patient's buttocks to beyond the foot. You may also use the method described below for splinting the lower leg. In cases where the patient's leg will remain flexed at the knee, you can secure one or two shorter splints at an angle across the thigh and lower leg (A-frame) with cravats (Scan 11-6).

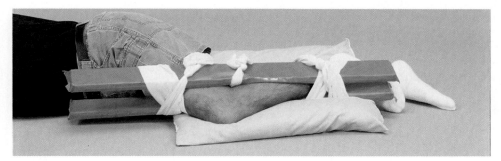

FIGURE 11.32

Splint an injured knee in the position in which it is found.

NOTE: Pillows and blankets can be used to splint injured ankles and feet.

REMEMBER: Check for distal circulation, sensation, and motor function before and after splinting.

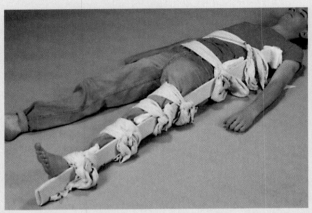

Hip —Tie the legs with a blanket roll or apply a long rigid splint:

- Use a splint from armpit to past the foot.
- Pad the splint and add extra padding at the armpit.
- Use two cravats to secure splint to trunk and four to secure the splint to the leg (two above knee and two below).

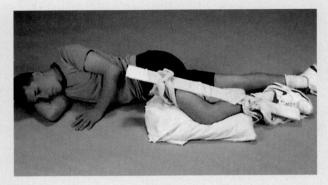

Knee

- If distal pulse present, then splint in position found.
- If no distal pulse, attempt to gently realign or reposition to regain pulse (if your EMS system allows).
- For a bent knee, secure splints behind knee, at the thigh, and at the lower leg.
- For a straight knee, splint using same steps as "Hip" or "Thigh" above, or "Single-splint Method for Lower Leg."

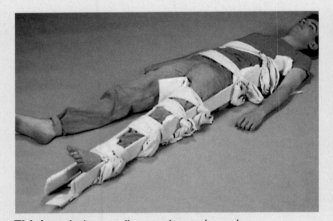

Thigh —Apply two splints, one long and one short:

- Long, from armpit to past foot.
- Short, from groin to past foot.
- Pad armpit, groin, voids between patient and splint, and bony areas.
- Secure the splint to trunk and limb with cravats.

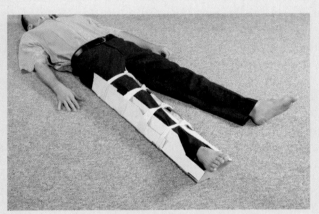

Thigh —Apply a three-sided rigid cardboard splint.

continued

Splinting a Lower Extremity

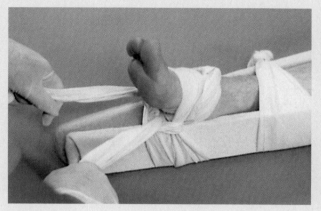

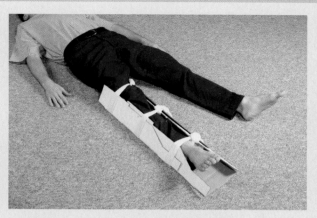

Lower Leg

- Apply two rigid splints, one lateral and one medial.
- Apply a single splint to the back of the leg and secure it with cravats.
- Apply a three-sided cardboard splint and secure it with cravats.

Lower Leg —Apply a three-sided rigid cardboard splint.

Injuries to the Lower Leg

You can provide care for injuries to the lower leg with either rigid or soft splints. A blanket roll between the legs is an effective soft splint. Secure it as you did for pelvic, thigh, and knee injuries described previously. Once you assist the EMTs in placing the patient on the spine board or scoop (orthopedic) stretcher, a form of rigid splinting, you have completed immobilizing all joints above and below the injury site.

If you use a rigid splint, you will need assistance. One person must maintain manual traction while you apply the splint. A single-splint method also can be used to immobilize lower leg injuries. The procedure is shown in Scan 11-7.

Before and after splinting, check for distal circulation, sensation, and motor function. If there is no pulse, remove the splint, realign or reposition the limb, and re-splint.

If you live in an area where skiing is a popular sport, you may have to care for a certain kind of injury, the boot-top injury (Figure 11.33). This is an injury to the tibia and/or fibula (usually both) that typically occurs when a skier falls forward of the ski tips. The leg bends hard over the top of the ski boot, causing a transverse fracture (a break in the bone that is at a right angle to the long part of the bone) of one or both bones. The leg below the fracture is often angulated or rotated, and the fracture is quite painful. Dr. Warren Bowman, author of *Outdoor Emergency Care* and the Medical Director for the National Ski Patrol recommends the following:

- Notify the ski patrol immediately. (Send another skier to an emergency phone or lift shack.)

- Keep the patient warm with others' coats, and place something between the skier and the snow.

- Leave the leg alone or in the position found until the ski patrol arrives; or . . .

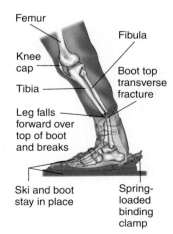

FIGURE 11.33
Boot-top injury.

Single-Splint Method for Lower Leg

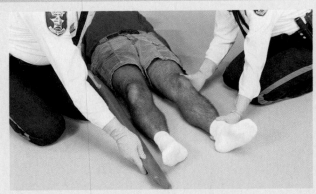

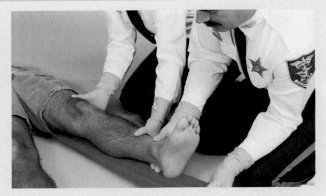

1. Measure the splint. It should extend from mid-thigh to about four inches below the ankle.

2. One rescuer applies and maintains manual traction. The other kneels at the patient's ankle and grips it while sliding the splint under the leg.

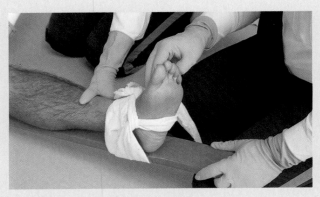

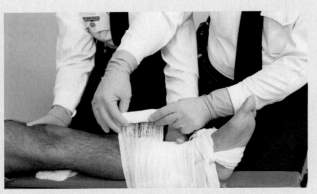

3. The rescuer holding traction grips the splint to the leg and elevates it about 10 inches. Another rescuer applies an ankle hitch.

4. Secure the splint to the leg with a roller bandage starting at the distal end of the extremity.

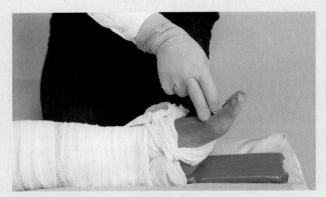

5. After the splint is secured from foot to thigh, check for distal circulation, sensation, and motor function.

- Gently align the injury to see if that will reduce the patient's pain.

- Manually stabilize or splint the injury. (A ski or ski pole will work, or use splints.) Secure with scarves, handkerchiefs, or cravats.

- Do not apply snow to the injury site to prevent swelling. (Swelling is due to bleeding from the damaged soft tissues, and applying cold will not help but will hasten the development or frostbite and/or hypothermia.)

Injuries to the Ankle or Foot

FIRST▶ Rigid splints may be used for injuries to the ankle or foot, but the soft splint is probably the most comfortable for the patient and the quickest for the First Responder to apply. If you apply a rigid splint, use one that extends from above the patient's knee to beyond the foot as described for the single-splint method for the lower leg. ■

When soft splinting an injury to the foot or ankle, immobilize it in the position found with a pillow or folded blanket. Secure the soft splint around the foot and ankle with several cravats or with roller gauze (Figure 11.34), then elevate it by propping it on a blanket roll or pillow.

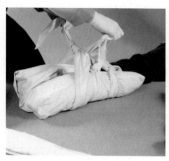

FIGURE 11.34
Emergency care for an injured ankle or foot.

RE-SPLINTING

After splinting, you must always recheck distal circulation, sensation, and motor function. If absent, your protocols may direct you to remove the splint, realign the extremity until distal pulse returns, then re-splint. If you are allowed to realign an extremity, do not force the limb and stop immediately if the movement causes severe pain. Re-splint once the distal pulse returns. One reason for an absent pulse after splinting is because the gauze or cravats may have been applied too tightly. If there is still no distal pulse after removing the splint or realigning the limb, it may be that swelling and pressure have restricted circulation. Arrange for transport immediately if distal pulse does not return.

AXIAL SKELETON

STRUCTURES OF THE AXIAL SKELETON

Remember that the axial skeleton consists of the head (skull), spinal column, and chest (sternum and ribs) (Figure 11.35). It makes up the long axis of the body. Injuries to the axial skeleton can be very serious because trauma can also injure the structures protected by the bones of the axial skeleton. Your concern is not just with the bones, but also with the brain, spinal cord, airway, lungs, and heart—all vital organs protected by the axial skeleton. When the head, spine, or chest is injured, you must also assess the patient for the signs and symptoms that indicate injuries to the underlying vital organs protected by these structures.

Head

The head, or skull, is divided into two major structures: the **cranium** and the face (Figure 11.36). Flat, irregularly shaped bones make up the floor, back, top, and sides of the skull and the forehead. The bones are fused together into immovable joints, which form a rigid, protective case for the brain.

In infants, fusion of the skull bones is not complete. Places called *soft spots* (fontanelles) can be felt at the top, sides, and back of the baby's skull. The smaller soft spots at the sides and back close in the first few months, but the largest soft

cranium (KRAY-ne-um) the bones that form the forehead and the floor, back, top, and upper sides of the skull.

FIGURE 11.35
Axial skeleton.

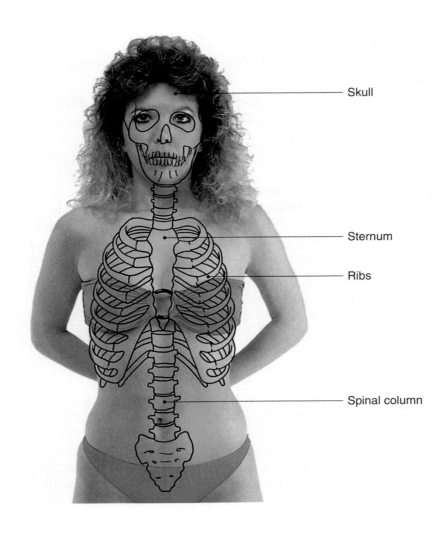

—— Skull

—— Sternum

—— Ribs

—— Spinal column

FIGURE 11.36
The head (skull) consists of the cranium and the face.

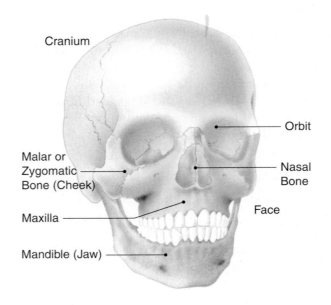

Cranium

Orbit

Malar or Zygomatic Bone (Cheek)

Nasal Bone

Maxilla

Face

Mandible (Jaw)

spot at the top of the skull does not close completely until about 18 to 24 months. When caring for an infant with possible head injuries, avoid applying point pressure to the skull with your fingertips. Instead spread your fingers and hold or stabilize the head with your entire hand.

The face is made up of strong, irregularly shaped bones. The face bones include part of the eye sockets, the cheeks, the upper part of the nose, the upper jaw, and the lower jaw. These bones also are fused into immovable joints except for the lower jaw bone, or **mandible**, which is the only movable joint in the head.

Spinal Column

The spinal column includes the neck bones and the back bones (Figure 11.37). The neck is made up of seven bones called the **cervical spine**. The rest of the spine is commonly known as the backbone. The spine protects the spinal cord as it runs from the brain down through the back. Many of the body's major nerves run into and out of the spinal cord and connect most areas of the body to the brain. In addition, the spine supports the entire body. The skull, shoulder bones, ribs, and pelvic bones connect to the spine.

mandible (MAN-di-bl) the lower jaw bone.

cervical (SER-vi-kal) **spine** the neck bones.

FIGURE 11.37
The spinal column.

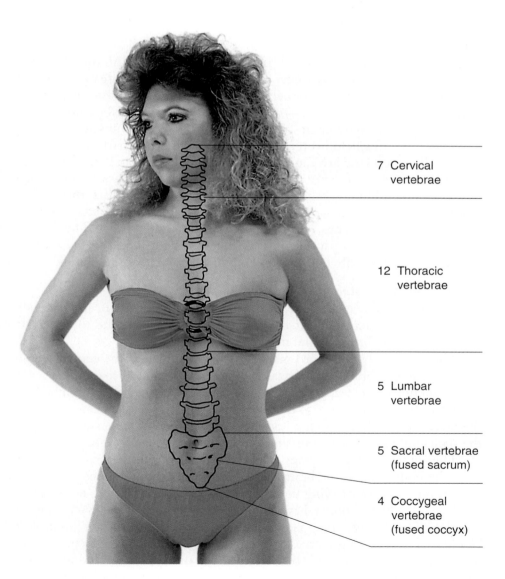

7 Cervical vertebrae

12 Thoracic vertebrae

5 Lumbar vertebrae

5 Sacral vertebrae (fused sacrum)

4 Coccygeal vertebrae (fused coccyx)

FIGURE 11.38
The chest.

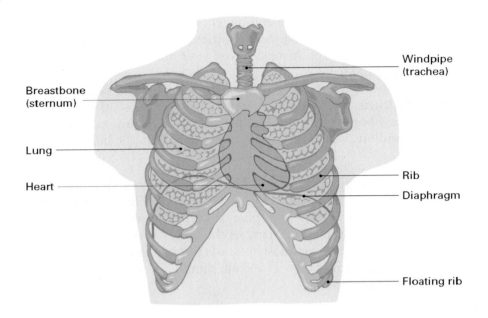

Chest

There are 12 ribs on each side of the chest (Figure 11.38). All the ribs connect with the spine. Most of the ribs attach directly to the sternum (breastbone) by pieces of cartilage. Some of the ribs connect to other ribs by a common cartilage strip. The bottom two ribs on each side—sometimes called floating ribs—do not connect to the breastbone or to other ribs. They are held in place by muscles.

The lower ribs help protect the organs in the upper part of the abdomen: the liver, gallbladder, stomach, and spleen. The upper ribs and sternum help protect the organs in the center or middle part of the chest. These organs include the heart and major blood vessels leading into and out of the heart, the trachea (windpipe) leading to the lungs, and the esophagus leading to the stomach. The upper ribs also protect the lungs, which lie on each side of the heart. The muscles of the back and chest, along with the muscles found between the ribs, give added strength to the spine and the ribs and further help protect the heart and lungs.

Central Nervous System

Injuries to the head and spine can involve much more than just the bones that make up these structures. Soft-tissue injuries to outer skin and to underlying muscles, organs, blood vessels, and nerves can occur as well.

central nervous system (CNS) the brain and spinal cord.

The brain and spinal cord make up what is known as the **central nervous system (CNS)**. The brain not only takes care of thinking, it also controls many of our basic functions, including heart activity and breathing. The brain tells muscles when to contract and relax so that we can move. It receives messages from all over the body and decides how the body will respond to these messages. Any injury to the skull could injure the brain and cause vital body functions to fail.

The spinal cord carries messages along nerves from the brain to the body and from the body back to the brain. Injury to the spine could damage the spinal cord and prevent it from carrying messages to or from a part of the body. That part of the body would no longer have contact with the brain and would be unable to function. The damage could be temporary, caused by pressure or swelling that may be corrected with proper care, or the damage could be permanent so that part of the body would never again be able to move or function. In addition, the spinal cord is the site of many reflexes, which allow us to react quickly to such things as

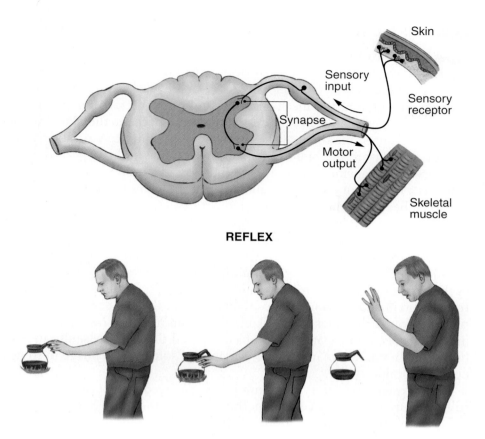

FIGURE 11.39
Reflexes allow for swift reactions to stimuli.

Skin

Sensory input

Sensory receptor

Synapse

Motor output

Skeletal muscle

REFLEX

pain and heat (Figure 11.39). Damage to the spinal cord can take away these reflex abilities.

MECHANISMS OF INJURY

You will not always be able to find and determine all patient injuries. Most of the time, you will conclude that the patient is injured based on the mechanism of injury (MOI). Be highly suspicious of injury if the patient has been involved in or reports the following situations:

- Falls, diving, and motor-vehicle collisions that result in swelling or pressure on a body part.

- Direct or indirect forces that caused excessive flexion (bending) or extension (stretching) of a body part.

- Twisting forces that caused rotation or excessive twisting of a body part.

- Pulling or hanging forces that caused spinal stretching.

- Compression of the spinal column.

- Blunt trauma such as that caused by blows, a car striking a pedestrian, or a driver striking a steering wheel or windshield.

- Penetrating trauma such as that caused by gunshots or stabbings.

- Blows in assault and battery or abuse incidents and the rapid forceful shaking of infants and children.

- Any trauma situation where the patient is unresponsive.

INJURY TO THE HEAD

Types of Injuries

Injuries to the head can be caused by a variety of mechanisms that result in pain, swelling, discoloration, and deformity similar to what was described for extremity injuries. In addition, the mechanism of injury may be forceful enough to cause a patient to experience a loss of responsiveness. Because the skull surrounds the brain on all sides, the force of the mechanism of injury can also be transmitted to the brain. Injury to the brain can affect the patient's ability to breathe. Because of this, airway management is always the first consideration in the care of any patient who has a head injury. Keep the airway open. In addition to skull and brain injury, there can be cuts to the scalp and other soft tissues.

There are certain signs and symptoms that will help you determine if a head injury is an open or a closed one. In an open head injury, you may be able to see or feel that the skull is cracked (fractured) or depressed (deformed), that there is blood and clear or yellow watery fluid leaking from the ears or nose, and that the eyelids are swollen shut and beginning to discolor or bruise. The fluids that protect the brain and are normally contained within the skull are leaking out into the tissues through the crack in the skull. The brain may also be injured in open head injuries. Broken bones or foreign objects forced through the skull can cut, tear, or bruise the brain. There may be no evidence of soft-tissue damage in some cases of open head injury.

In a closed head injury, the skull is not damaged or cracked, but the brain can still be injured by the force of something striking the skull. Such a force can cause the brain to bounce off the inside of the skull. The resulting injuries to the brain include (Figure 11.40):

- **Concussion**—when a blow to the head does not cause an open head injury but does cause damage to the brain. The injury may be so minor it does not cause a loss of responsiveness; or it may be mild, causing a headache after a brief loss of responsiveness; or it may be severe, causing lengthy unresponsiveness and abnormal vital signs. Sometimes short-term memory is lost. Any signs and symptoms of concussion are an indication of brain injury.

- **Contusion** (bruising)—when the force of a blow is great enough to rupture blood vessels on the surface or deep within the brain. In a closed head injury,

concussion (kon-KUSH-un) injury to the brain that results from a blow or impact from an object but does not cause permanent neurological damage.

contusion (kon-TU-zhun) bruising; in the case of the brain, bruising caused by a force of a blow great enough to rupture blood vessels on the surface or deep within the brain.

FIGURE 11.40
Closed head injuries.

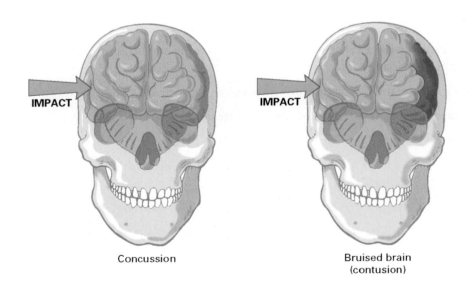

Concussion

Bruised brain (contusion)

the blood has no opening from which to drain. The blood builds up inside the skull, presses on the brain, and affects or impairs its function or ability to send messages to the body.

Signs and Symptoms of Head Injury

FIRST➤ Many injuries to the skull are obvious. Also consider the possibility of head injury when the mechanism of injury suggests it and when you find the following in your assessment (Figure 11.41):

- Unresponsiveness or a decreased mental status.
- Deep cuts or tears to the scalp.
- Exposed brain tissue.
- Penetrating injuries such as gunshot wounds and impaled objects.
- Swelling ("goose eggs") and discoloration of the skin of the scalp.
- Edges or fragments of bones seen or felt through the skin of the scalp.
- Deformity of the skull, such as depressed or sunken-in areas.
- Swelling and discoloration behind the ears—Battle's sign (late sign).
- Swelling or discoloration of the eyelids or the tissues under the eyes (Raccoon's eyes).
- Unequal or unresponsive pupils or both pupils are dilated; one or both eyes appear sunken.
- Bleeding from the ears and/or the nose.
- Clear or bloody fluid flowing from the ears and/or nose. This fluid—called cerebrospinal (ser-e-bro-SPI-nal) fluid (CSF)—surrounds the brain and spinal cord and cannot flow from the ears or nose unless the skull has been fractured.
- Weakness or numbness on one side of the body.
- Deterioration of vital signs. Each time you assess the patient's pulse and respirations, the results are progressively worse. ■

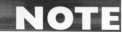

NOTE

Since many of the signs of head and brain injury can be produced by drug or alcohol abuse, take great care in assessing the patient. Never assume alcohol or drug abuse, and always assess and care for possible injuries.

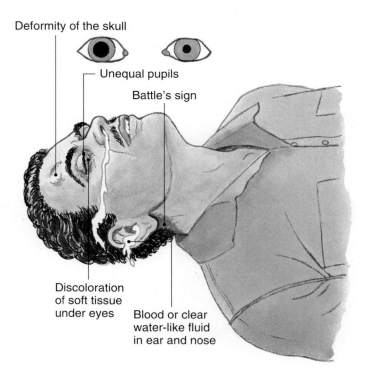

Deformity of the skull

Unequal pupils

Battle's sign

Discoloration of soft tissue under eyes

Blood or clear water-like fluid in ear and nose

FIGURE 11.41
Signs of head injury.

Signs and Symptoms of Brain Injury

FIRST➤ In cases of head injury, consider the possibility of a brain injury if you find the following in your focused assessment:

- Headache (mild to severe) following the incident.
- Any sign of head trauma.
- Unresponsiveness, or altered mental status.
- Confusion or personality changes.
- Unequal, unresponsive, or dilated pupils.
- Paralysis or loss of function, usually to one side of the body and opposite the side of head injury (also an indication of spinal-cord injury).
- Loss of sensation, which may be to one side of the body (also an indication of spinal-cord injury).
- Bilateral weakness or numbness (an indication of spinal-cord injury).
- Paralysis of facial muscles, which may interfere with airway and speech.
- Disturbed or impaired vision, hearing, and/or sense of balance.
- Nausea and/or vomiting.
- Any changing patterns in respiration that include cycles of rapid, slow, shallow, and stopped breathing, and efforts to breathe with the diaphragm but no other chest movement.
- Seizures. ■

Signs and Symptoms of Facial Injury

Facial injuries can be very serious because of the potential for airway obstruction and associated head injury. Blood and other fluids, blood clots, bone, and teeth may cause partial or complete airway obstruction. The force that caused injury to the face can also be transferred to the base, or floor, of the skull and cause an open head injury. If this has happened, you will see cerebrospinal fluid (CSF) leaking from the ears and nose.

Consider the possibility of facial injuries when you find the following in your focused assessment (Figure 11.42):

- Blood in the airway (nose or mouth).

- Facial deformities.

- Swelling and discoloration of the eyelids or discoloration of the tissues below the eyes.

FIGURE 11.42
Signs of facial injury.

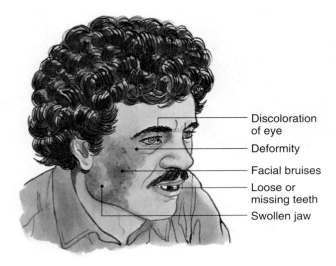

Discoloration of eye

Deformity

Facial bruises

Loose or missing teeth

Swollen jaw

- Swelling or discoloration of any part of the face.

- Swollen lower jaw, poor function of or inability to close jaw.

- Deformity or depression of any part of the face.

- Teeth that are loose or have been knocked out, broken dentures.

- Any mechanism of injury that indicates a blow to the face.

Care for Head Injuries
Injuries to the Cranium

FIRST➤ When caring for patients with injuries to the cranium, always conclude that neck and spine injuries also exist. Always don personal protective equipment, then take the following steps:

1. Maintain an open airway. Use the jaw-thrust maneuver and stabilize the head.

2. Provide resuscitative measures as needed.

3. Keep the patient still. This can be a critical factor. Do not let the patient move or change position.

4. Control bleeding. Do not apply direct pressure over the injury site, because you may cause further damage to the brain or soft tissues. Use a bulky dressing. Do not attempt to stop the flow of blood or cerebrospinal fluid (CSF) from the ears or nose—it needs to flow out, so as to not build up pressure inside the skull. Secure a loose dressing to absorb flow and prevent this now contaminated fluid from flowing back into the brain.

5. Talk to the responsive patient. Try to keep him calm.

6. Dress and bandage open wounds and stabilize penetrating objects. Do not remove any objects or bone fragments.

7. Provide care for shock. Maintain body warmth but avoid overheating. Provide 100% oxygen and give nothing to eat or drink.

8. Monitor and record vital signs. Watch for and record changes.

9. Monitor the level of responsiveness.

10. Provide emotional support.

11. Be prepared for vomiting, and have suction ready.

12. Arrange to transport as soon as possible. ■

Do not reposition any patient with an open head wound or any other possible serious injury to the cranium unless you must do so to provide CPR or assist ventilations. If the mechanism of injury and the patient's mental status indicate the possibility of spinal injury, do not reposition the patient. Suspect that any patient who is unresponsive and has trauma above the collarbones has a spinal injury. Stabilize the head and open the airway using the jaw-thrust maneuver.

For responsive patients with apparently minor closed injuries to the cranium and no sign of spinal injury, you have two choices for positioning the patient. Both methods are also suitable for patients with facial injuries. The methods are:

- Option 1: Elevate head and shoulders (Figure 11.43). Place the patient's upper body at a 45-degree angle, using several pillows or a blanket roll as needed.

- Option 2: Place the patient in the recovery position (on the side) as shown in Figure 11.44. Position the lower shoulder behind the patient and the hand of

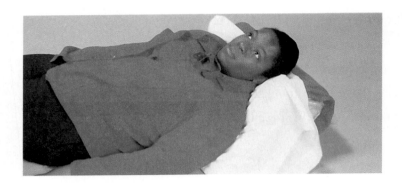

the upper shoulder under and supporting the cheek. Tilt the head slightly back and the face downward to allow for drainage of fluids.

Injuries to the Face

FIRST > As in all cases of facial injury, make certain that the patient has an open airway. If you must assist ventilations, use the jaw-thrust maneuver and stabilize the head in case there is injury to the spine. Apply only gentle pressure to bleeding wounds. Use a bulky dressing to care for soft-tissue injuries. ■

The lower jaw can be dislocated or fractured. Because it is a joint, dislocations can occur where the lower jaw attaches to the skull just in front of the ears. Look for the mechanism of injury—a force that could have struck the jaw from the front or side. The signs and symptoms to look for include:

- Pain and tenderness.
- Swelling and discoloration.
- Deformity, or facial distortion or disfigurement.
- Loss of use or inability to control jaw movement or to open or close mouth.
- Difficulty in speaking.

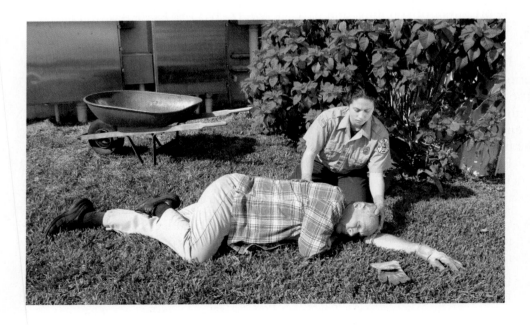

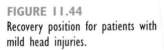
FIGURE 11.44
Recovery position for patients with mild head injuries.

- Bleeding from the nose, mouth, or around the teeth.
- Missing or broken teeth or broken dentures.

To care for possible fracture or dislocation of the lower jaw:

1. Maintain an open airway. Be prepared to suction blood, secretions, and vomitus.
2. Control bleeding and dress any open wounds. Do not tie the patient's mouth shut since there may be vomiting.
3. Keep the patient at rest and provide care for shock.
4. Closely monitor the patient and stay alert for vomiting.
5. Monitor and record vital signs.

Injuries to the face can damage teeth, crowns (caps), bridges, and dentures. Always look for and remove avulsed (dislodged) teeth and parts of broken dental appliances. Be careful not to push these down the patient's airway. When a tooth is avulsed, there is bleeding from the socket. Have the responsive patient bite down on a pad of gauze placed over the socket, but leave several inches of gauze outside the mouth for quick removal. For the unresponsive patient, hold the gauze over the socket. This will control the bleeding and prevent the airway from becoming obstructed with blood.

Wrap the avulsed tooth in a dressing. If you have a source of clean water, keep the dressing moist. (Milk can also be used.) Do not attempt to clean the tooth. Your efforts could damage microscopic structures needed to replant the tooth.

INJURY TO THE SPINE

Types of Spinal Injuries

Soft tissues of the neck can be injured by a number of mechanisms. The forces that cause soft-tissue injury can also injure underlying bones of the spinal column in the vertebrae of the neck (cervical spine). Injuries to and improper care of cervical-spine injuries can impair breathing and lead to paralysis or death. Injuries along the rest of the spinal column also can cause paralysis and reduce normal body movement and function.

Spinal injuries are caused by forces to the head, neck, back, chest, pelvis, or legs. Often, you will find patients with head injuries who also have cervical-spine injuries. Injuries to the upper leg bones or to the pelvic bones may also cause spinal injury through indirect force. Motor-vehicle crashes (including those causing whiplash), falls, diving, and skiing mishaps are common causes of spinal injuries.

If a patient has numbness, loss of feeling, or paralysis in the legs with no problems in the arms, the injury to the spine is probably below the neck. If numbness, loss of feeling, or paralysis involves the arms and the legs, the injury is probably in the neck. Numbness, loss of feeling, and paralysis may be limited to only one side of the body, but usually both sides are involved.

Injuries to the spine can include fractured or displaced spinal bones (vertebrae) or swelling that presses on nerves. These injuries can produce the same signs and symptoms. In some cases, the loss of function associated with spinal injuries may be temporary if the loss is caused by pressure or swelling that may eventually go away. But if the spinal cord was cut, even the best surgery and care cannot restore function.

Signs and Symptoms of Spinal Injury

FIRST➤ The most common signs and symptoms of spinal injury include:

- Weakness, numbness, or tingling sensations, or loss of feeling in the arms or legs.

remember

Consider every unresponsive injured patient to have spinal injuries. Stabilize the patient's head and open the airway with the jaw-thrust maneuver.

- Paralysis to arms and/or legs.
- Painful movement of arms and/or legs (or no pain or sensation).
- Pain and/or tenderness along the back of the neck or the backbone.
- Burning sensations along the spine or in an extremity.
- Deformity of the spine (the angle of the patient's head and neck may appear odd to you). You also may feel pieces of bone that have broken off the spine, though such findings are rare.
- Loss of bladder and bowel control.
- Difficult or labored breathing with little or no movement of the chest and slight movement of the abdomen.
- Positioning of the arms. You may find the patient lying face up with arms stretched out above the head or with arms and hands curled to the chest (Figure 11.45).
- Persistent erection of the penis called priapism (PRY-ah-pism), which indicates spinal injury affecting nerves to the external genitalia. ■

Focused Assessment

FIRST➤ As you read in Chapter 7, you should conduct a thorough SAMPLE history during your focused assessment of a responsive patient (Figure 11.46 and Scan 11-8). You may learn things about the emergency that will help determine the mechanism of injury:

- Question the patient. Do his arms or legs feel numb? Can the patient feel you touch his hands and feet? Can he squeeze your hand or push your hand with his foot? Do not ask the patient to repeat any movement that causes pain.
- Look and feel gently for injuries and deformities.
- See if the patient can move his arms and legs. Do not do this if you have noted any mechanism of injury or other signs that indicate possible injury to the spine.

For the unresponsive patient, remember to:

- Ask bystanders for information on the emergency and what they saw happen to the patient. This may help you to determine the mechanism of injury.

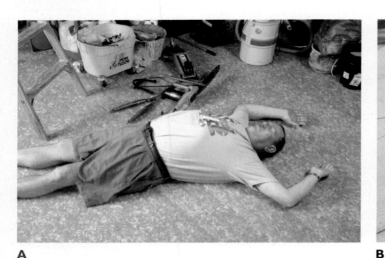 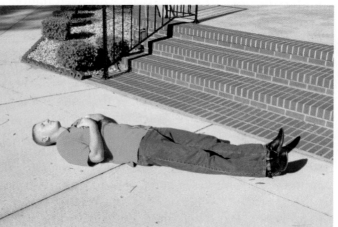

A **B**

FIGURE 11.45
Suspect spine injury if you find the patient **A.** face up with arms stretched above the head or **B.** with arms and hands curled onto the chest (toward the midline).

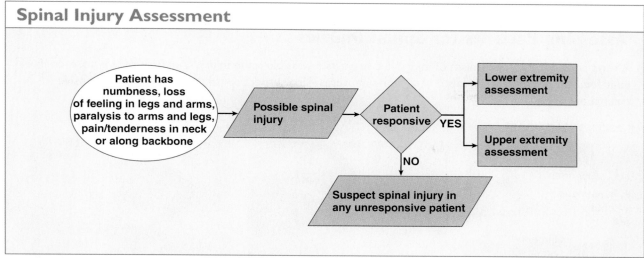

FIGURE 11.46

- Look and feel for injuries and deformities.
- See if the patient responds to pressure on or pinching of the feet and hands. Never probe palms and soles with sharp objects. ■

Rules for Spinal-Injury Care

FIRST➤ Always follow these rules for First Responder care of patients with possible spinal injuries:

- Make certain the airway is open. Assist ventilations or perform CPR as needed, even though the patient may have spinal injuries. Use the jaw-thrust maneuver when ventilating the patient.
- Attempt to control serious bleeding. Avoid moving the injured part of the patient and any of the limbs when applying dressings.
- Always conclude that an unresponsive trauma patient has spinal injuries.
- Do not attempt to splint long-bone injuries if there are indications of spinal injuries until you have appropriate help.
- Never move a patient with suspected spinal injuries unless you must do so to provide CPR or assist ventilations, need to reach and control life-threatening bleeding, or must protect yourself and the patient from immediate danger at the scene.
- Keep the patient still. Tell him not to move. Position yourself to stabilize the patient's head, neck, and as much of the body as possible.
- Continuously monitor patients with possible spinal injury. These patients will often go into shock. Sometimes, their chest muscles will be paralyzed and they will go into respiratory arrest. ■

Stabilizing the Patient's Head and Neck

Suspect that any patient with head injury also has a spinal injury. Suspect that a patient with chest trauma has injuries to the neck. Work carefully and gently as you immobilize the patient. Do not apply traction to the patient's head and neck. Just grip the head with your hands as you would to perform the jaw-thrust maneuver. Do not try to place an extrication collar on the patient or position the patient on a spine board unless you have had training in these procedures and there is enough help to move the patient properly.

A patient with spinal injuries may be able to move the head, neck, arms, trunk, or legs but movement can cause more injury. For this reason, keep the patient

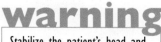

warning

Stabilize the patient's head and neck and wait for more advanced care to arrive before attempting to immobilize further.

Assessing Patients for Spinal Injuries

NOTE: Always consider the mechanism of injury. If it suggests a possible spine injury, then assume it is so, even if your focused assessment reveals no signs or symptoms. Also suspect spinal injury in any unresponsive trauma patient.

SIGNS AND SYMPTOMS

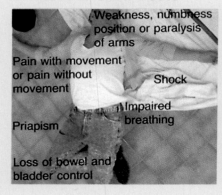

Weakness, numbness position or paralysis of arms

Pain with movement or pain without movement

Shock

Impaired breathing

Priapism

Loss of bowel and bladder control

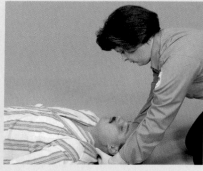

Cervical point tenderness and deformity.

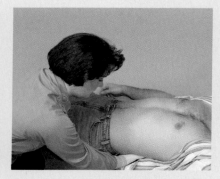

Spinal column tenderness and deformity.

RESPONSIVE: LOWER EXTREMITIES ASSESSMENT

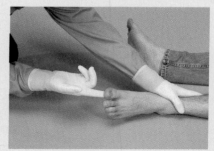

Touch toe.

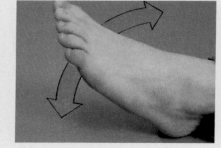

Foot movement.

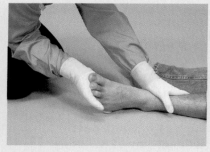

Foot push.

RESULTS: If the patient can perform these tasks, there is little chance of injury to the spinal cord. However, this test does not rule out all injuries, including spinal fractures. If the patient can perform only to a limited degree and with pain, there may be pressure somewhere on the spinal cord. When a patient is not able to perform any of the tests, suspect that there is spinal injury.

RESPONSIVE: UPPER EXTREMITIES ASSESSMENT

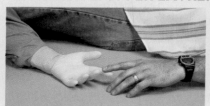

Touch finger.

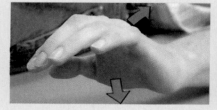

Hand movement.

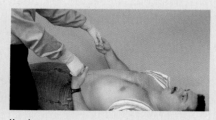

Hand squeeze.

RESULTS: If the patient can perform these tests, there is little chance of damage in the cervical area, but you cannot rule out all injuries. Limited performance and pain: pressure on spinal cord in cervical area. Failure to perform any: suspect severe spinal-cord injury in neck.

continued . . .

Assessing Patients for Spinal Injuries

UNRESPONSIVE PATIENTS

Test the responses to painful stimuli by pinching the back of the hand, the ankle, or the top of the foot or by squeezing a toe. Removing shoes may aggravate injuries.

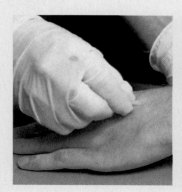

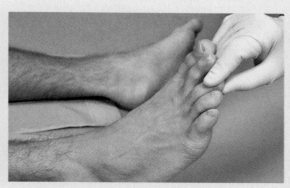

REMEMBER: It is difficult to accurately assess an unresponsive patient. If the mechanism of injury indicates possible spinal damage, or if the patient is unresponsive, care for spinal injury.

RESULTS: Slight pulling back of foot: spinal cord usually intact. No foot reaction: possible damage anywhere along the spinal cord. Hand or finger reaction: usually no damage to spinal cord. No hand or finger reaction: possible damage to the spinal cord. Suspect damage to the spinal cord if you find no reactions, failure to perform any test, limited performance, or performance with pain.

SUMMARY OF OBSERVATIONS AND CONCLUSIONS

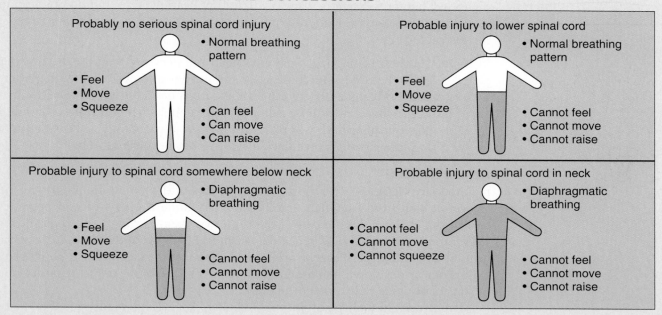

Probably no serious spinal cord injury
- Feel
- Move
- Squeeze
- Normal breathing pattern
- Can feel
- Can move
- Can raise

Probable injury to lower spinal cord
- Feel
- Move
- Squeeze
- Normal breathing pattern
- Cannot feel
- Cannot move
- Cannot raise

Probable injury to spinal cord somewhere below neck
- Feel
- Move
- Squeeze
- Diaphragmatic breathing
- Cannot feel
- Cannot move
- Cannot raise

Probable injury to spinal cord in neck
- Cannot feel
- Cannot move
- Cannot squeeze
- Diaphragmatic breathing
- Cannot feel
- Cannot move
- Cannot raise

WARNING: If the patient is unresponsive or the mechanism of injury indicates spinal injury, provide care for spinal injury.

FIGURE 11.47
Manual in-line stabilization of the patient's head and neck.

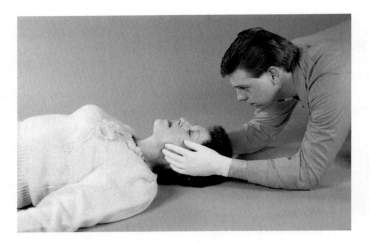

from moving by verbally reassuring him and by physically stabilizing the head and neck.

Follow these guidelines when you manually stabilize a patient's head and neck, (Figure 11.47):

1. Kneel at the top of the patient's head.

2. Place your hands on each side of the head and position your fingers under the lower jaw.

3. Keep the patient's head and neck steady (stable) in this position. Do not allow the patient to move his head and neck. Explain your actions to the patient and offer reassurance while you are keeping his head stable. Do not apply traction or turn or lift the patient's head.

4. Maintain your position until a rigid cervical or extrication collar is applied. (See Chapter 5, Scans 5-9 and 5-10, for application steps, but do not attempt to apply a collar to a patient until you have received proper training from your instructor.)

FIRST➤ It is best to stabilize a patient's head and neck and wait for the EMTs to arrive before trying to proceed any further in immobilizing the patient. Immobilizing a patient on a backboard is not a required First Responder skill. However, your jurisdiction may require that you learn this skill. If so, your instructor will teach you the proper techniques. Do not attempt to place a patient on a backboard without proper training. ■

Helmet Removal

Helmets are designed to absorb energy forces and prevent injury to the head. However, well-fitting helmets—even the most modern ones—cannot prevent the brain from striking the interior of the skull in extreme or high-speed crash forces. When the brain rapidly and repeatedly strikes the inside of the skull, brain tissue is bruised and blood vessels tear and bleed. The patient can suffer a concussion, a contusion, or develop a hematoma (blood clot) in the brain tissue or under one of the layers of tissue that protect the brain.

The American College of Sports Medicine (ACSM) has made recommendations for managing sports injuries, particularly injuries incurred in football. For injured or unresponsive athletes, the college advises against removing the helmet. For an unresponsive athlete (or any injured patient wearing a helmet), suspect a spinal injury, properly immobilize the spine, and initiate safe transport to the hospital. When it is necessary to assess the patient's face to manage the airway, to assist breathing, or to provide CPR, the ACSM advises removing only the face guard of the football helmet. Removing the face guard gives emergency care providers access to the face and airway and allows them to assess vital signs, provide care for face injuries, or begin resuscitation. The ACSM emphasizes that the helmet should be removed only if the rescuers are unable to gain access to the airway by any other means.

For football players who are wearing shoulder pads, the helmet left in place keeps the cervical spine in a midline position. Removing the helmet but keeping the shoulder pads in place causes the head to hyperextend or fall back in an overextended position, which pulls the spinal column out of alignment. Helmets do not prevent neck injuries. The majority of sports-related neck injuries are caused by flexing of the neck either too far forward (hyperflexion) or too far backward (hyperextension) or by a sudden compressing force to the top of the head, which compacts the spinal column.

There are many types of helmets (Scan 11-9). They are made in half-size, three-quarter size, and full-size. Full-size helmets cover the mouth and sometimes part of the nose and usually have a face shield. Bicycle helmets are usually half-size and open in the front and have no face shield or face guard. Football helmets are full-size and have face guards. Motorcycle helmets are available in all three sizes, with the full-size helmets having a clear face shield or visor that moves up and down and is easy to remove. Motorcyclists who wear the half-size or three-fourths size helmets will usually wear glasses or goggles to protect their eyes. If the helmet has a face guard or face shield, remove it to gain access to the patient's airway. If any patient who is not breathing is wearing a helmet with a face guard or face shield that cannot be removed, remove the helmet to gain access to the airway. If a helmet is removed, it must be done cautiously and by two people.

Before removing a helmet, perform the following steps:

1. Remove the face piece or face shield while your partner stabilizes the head. Do not cut the chin strap. Remove glasses or goggles.

2. Check to see if the patient is breathing by placing your ear and/or hand in front of the nose and mouth. Even with full-size, snugly fitting helmets, there is room to slip your hand under the protective face portion to check breathing.

3. If the patient is breathing, check the helmet for fit. A First Responder can stabilize the head by grasping the patient's lower jaw under the helmet while a partner gently pulls on the helmet.

   An alternative method is to have a partner stabilize the head by placing her hands on either side of the helmet while you slide both hands under the helmet on either side of the jaw to check the helmet for fit and snugness. A well-fitting helmet can stay in place as long as the patient is breathing.

4. Determine if you can gain access to the patient's airway without removing the helmet if airway care and breathing assistance are necessary.

5. If you cannot gain access to the airway and you must clear the airway or assist the patient with breathing, remove the helmet. If the patient is wearing shoulder pads, leave them in place. While your partner is maintaining the head in line with the body, place a similar amount of padding under the patient's head to help your partner keep the patient's head in line with the body while you perform airway, ventilation, or resuscitation measures.

Check local protocols for helmet removal procedures. Work with local coaches to learn and practice them. Check with helmet vendors to become familiar with the types of helmets and their fit. Note that the half-size and three-quarter-size

SCAN 11-9 Types of Helmets

To be effective, all helmets must fit the wearer properly, be worn correctly, and meet helmet criteria based on testing by the Snell Memorial Foundation, the only helmet-testing lab accredited to ISO 25 in the United States by the American Association for Laboratory Accreditation. Snell also tests helmets for removability. Emergency care providers must be able to quickly remove headgear from injured patients in order to check for vital signs and to perform emergency procedures.

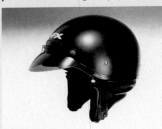

Half-size motorcycle helmet Provides head protection from impact but may not provide face and eye protection, even with a face shield. Easier to remove than a full helmet. (AFX North America, Inc).

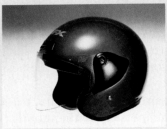

Three-quarter-size motorcycle helmet Provides head protection from impact and may provide face and eye protection. Somewhat easier to remove than the full-size helmet. (AFX North America, Inc.)

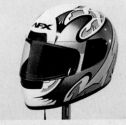

Full-size motorcycle helmet In addition to head-impact protection, provides a measure of facial protection with a face shield. Properly fitting helmets have room beneath the chin bar for a hand to slide under and check for airway and breathing. (AFX North America, Inc.)

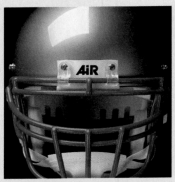

Football helmet Provides a measure of facial protection with a face shield in place as well as head-impact protection. (Schutt Sports)

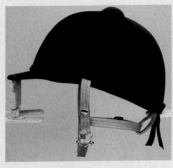

Horseback riding helmet Provides head protection from impact but may not provide face and eye protection. (International Riding Helmets)

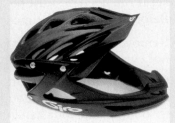

Mountain bike helmet Provides head protection and, with a chin bar, some face protection. (Giro Sport Design)

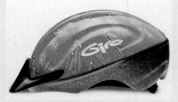

Youth's bicycle helmet Provides head protection if it fits properly and is worn correctly. (Giro Sport Design)

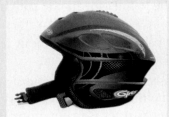

Snowboarding helmet Provides head protection and, with a chin bar, some face protection. (Giro Sport Design)

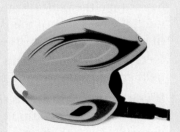

Downhill skiing helmet Provides head protection and, with a chin bar, some face protection. (Giro Sport Design)

helmets give easy access to airway and breathing, but if they are left in place, you may have to place extra padding behind the patient's shoulders.

Remember: provide care to any unresponsive patient as if there is a spinal injury. When you find any helmeted patient face down or on one side, log roll him on to his back (supine). Your instructor will show you how to log roll a patient if First Responders are allowed to do this in your jurisdiction.

Leave the helmet in place if you find or suspect the following:

- Helmet fits well, and the patient's head does not move (or moves very little) inside of it. A well-fitting helmet keeps the head from moving and should be left on if there are no airway or breathing problems and the helmet does not interfere with assessment and management of the airway and breathing.

- Patient is breathing adequately and has no airway problems (fluids, obstructions).

- Patient can be placed in a neutral, in-line position for immobilization on a spine board.

- Helmet does not interfere with your ability to reassess and maintain the patient's airway or assist breathing.

- Patient is wearing shoulder pads. If the helmet is removed, place a similar amount of padding under the head, or remove the shoulder pads also. Removing the shoulder pads may cause further harm to the patient.

Remove the helmet if you find the following:

- Helmet interferes with your ability to assess or manage the patient's airway and breathing.

- Helmet does not fit snugly, and the patient's head moves inside the helmet.

- Helmet interferes with placing the patient on a spine board in a neutral, in-line position. When the helmet rests on the spine board, its size may force the patient's head forward (hyperflexion) and close the airway. Padding can be placed under the patient's shoulders to prevent hyperflexion and maintain an in-line position.

- Patient is in cardiac or respiratory arrest. Quickly remove the helmet while a partner stabilizes the head. Proceed with CPR steps, using the jaw-thrust maneuver.

If you must remove the helmet, consult with medical direction and remove it according to local protocol. The steps listed below provide general directions for removal of full-size helmets (Scans 11-10 and 11-11). Your instructor will demonstrate them. Practice with all three sizes of helmets.

1. Rescuer #1 will kneel at the head of the patient and stabilize the patient's head by placing his hands on each side of the helmet with fingers on the patient's jaw to prevent movement.

2. Rescuer #2 will kneel on one side of the patient at the patient's shoulders, unfasten the chin strap, remove the face guard or face shield (if not yet done), and remove the patient's glasses or goggles if present.

3. Rescuer #2 will place one hand on the mandible at the angle of the jaw and the other hand behind the neck at the base of the skull and stabilize the head while rescuer #1 removes the helmet.

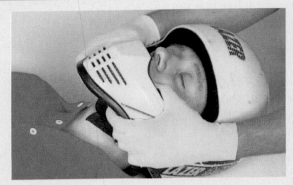

1. Rescuer #1: kneel at the head of the patient. Stabilize the patient's head.

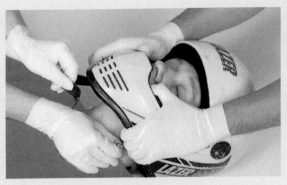

2. Rescuer #2: kneel at the side of the patient's shoulders. Unfasten the chin strap. Remove the face guard, face shield, goggles, or glasses if present.

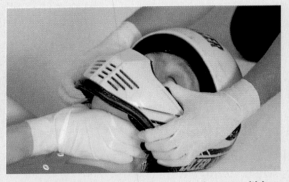

3. Rescuer #2: place one hand on the mandible at the angle of the jaw and the other hand behind the neck at the base of the skull to stabilize the patient's head.

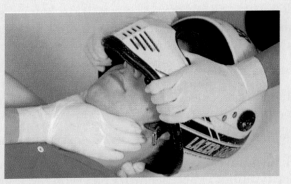

4. Rescuer #1: pull sides of helmet apart and carefully slip helmet halfway off.

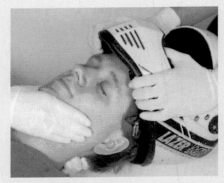

5. Rescuer #2: maintain position of hand stabilizing the jaw. Reposition at the back of the neck slightly higher on the back of the head to maintain in-line stabilization.

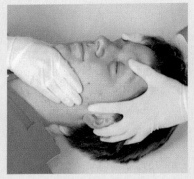

6. Rescuer #1: finish removing the helmet and then place hands on either side of the patient's head to take over in-line stabilization.

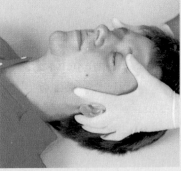

7. Rescuer #2: check and clear airway, provide ventilations, and apply a collar.

Helmet Removal—Alternative Method

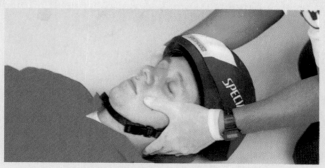

1. Apply steady stabilization to the neck in neutral position.

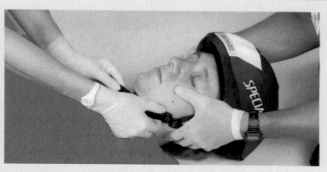

2. Remove the chin strap.

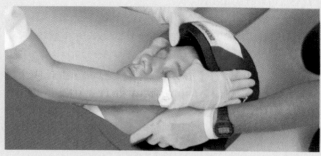

3. Remove helmet by pulling the sides apart (laterally).

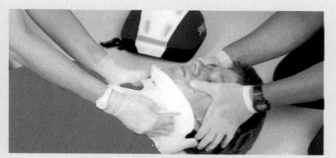

4. Apply a suitable cervical-spine immobilization collar and secure the patient to a long board.

4. Rescuer #1 will pull sides of the helmet apart and slowly and carefully slip the helmet halfway off the patient's head until rescuer #2 can reposition the hand behind the head and neck.

5. Rescuer #2 will maintain the hand position that is stabilizing the jaw. Reposition the hand at the back of the neck a little higher on the back of the head to maintain stabilization of the head and its in-line position of the body, particularly if the patient is wearing shoulder pads.

6. Rescuer #1 will finish removing the helmet, place padding under the patient's head if needed (the patient is wearing shoulder pads), and then place his hands on either side of the patient's head to take over in-line stabilization.

7. Rescuer #2 will check and clear the airway, provide ventilations with supplemental oxygen, and apply a collar.

Remember, you do not have to remove a helmet from a patient if the patient has an airway and is breathing, if the helmet is snug, and if the patient can be secured to a spine board with the helmet on and the head in a neutral, in-line position with the spine.

INJURIES TO THE CHEST

Chest injuries can damage the lungs, heart, major vessels, and upper abdominal organs protected by the ribs. Ribs can be fractured or crushed or the sternum may become fractured or completely separated from the ribs. Broken and crushed ribs and sternum can cause punctures and tears to organs and vessels underneath. The force of the trauma may also directly or indirectly damage the section of the spine where the ribs are attached. Because of these problems, it is important to stabilize the head and neck of a chest trauma patient. Wounds to the chest need immediate attention and care.

Rib Injuries

FIRST➤ Signs and symptoms of suspected fractured ribs include (Figure 11.48):

- Pain and tenderness at the site of the injury.
- Deformity at the site of the injury, which may be slight swelling or obvious rib displacement.
- Increased pain at the site upon moving or breathing.
- Shallow breathing, sometimes with the patient reporting a crackling sensation at or near the site of injury.
- Characteristic stance. Often, the patient will lean toward the side of the injury, with a hand or forearm pressed over the injury.
- Guarding the injury site. Often the patient will hold his hand across the injured side to help support and stabilize the injury. This is called self-splinting. ■

If it appears that no underlying organs have been damaged, you do not need to take any immediate action other than keeping the patient at rest in a comfortable position. But if there are signs that the lungs have been damaged by the fractured rib (for example, frothy blood in the mouth) or several ribs are apparently fractured, you must provide additional care for the patient.

FIRST➤ The care for injured ribs requires you to wear personal protective, equipment and:

1. Ensure an open airway. Suction or clear the mouth if necessary. Keep the patient at rest and monitor breathing.

2. Provide oxygen as soon as possible as per local protocols. Maintain body temperature to help minimize the possibility of shock.

FIGURE 11.48
Possible fractured ribs. **A.** Characteristic stance. **B.** Other signs and symptoms.

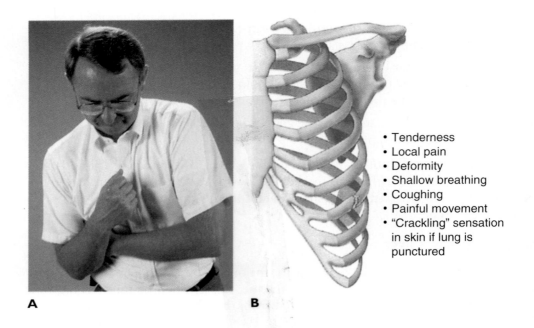

- Tenderness
- Local pain
- Deformity
- Shallow breathing
- Coughing
- Painful movement
- "Crackling" sensation in skin if lung is punctured

A　　　　　　　　**B**

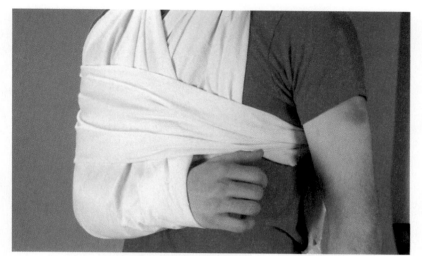

3. Place the forearm of the injured side in a sling so that it rests across the patient's chest. Apply a swathe to provide additional support (Figure 11.49).

4. Initiate transport to the hospital to be examined by more highly trained personnel. ■

Flail Chest

When three or more consecutive ribs on the same side of the chest are fractured in two or more places, it creates a section of chest that moves in the opposite direction of the rest of the chest wall during breathing. The same type of chest wall movement is seen when the breastbone is broken away from the ribs. This type of injury is referred to as a **flail chest** (Figure 11.50). First Responders see flail chests most often at motor-vehicle collisions, where the patient, who is not wearing a seat belt, is thrown against the steering wheel during sudden deceleration (sudden stop).

FIRST➤ The signs and symptoms of flail chest include (Figure 11.51):

● Same signs and symptoms as fractured ribs.

flail chest the condition that results when there are two or more ribs fractured in two or more places, or the breastbone separates from the chest and produces a loose segment of the chest wall. This segment will move in the opposite direction of the chest during breathing.

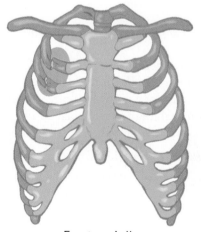

Fractured ribs

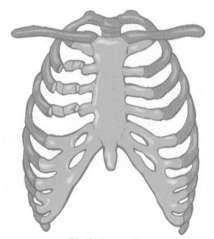

Flail chest ribs

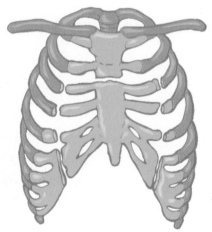

Flail chest sternum

FIGURE 11.50
Rib fractures and flail chest.

FIGURE 11.51
Signs and symptoms of flail chest.

MECHANISMS OF INJURY

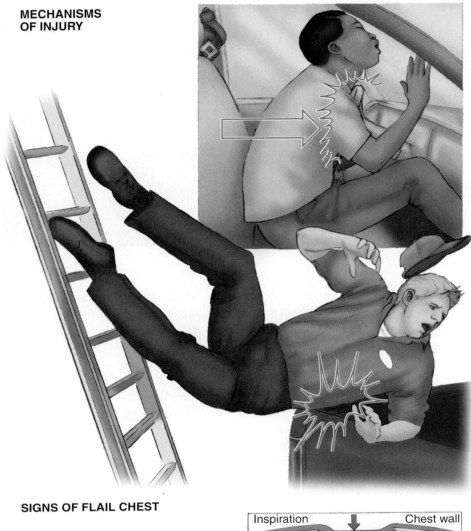

SIGNS OF FLAIL CHEST

- Pain
- Shallow breathing
- Deformity
- Painful movement

- Tenderness
- Crackling sensation
- Irregular chest movement

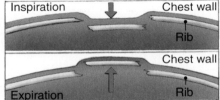

- Section of the chest wall that moves in the opposite direction of the rest of the chest when the patient is breathing. This motion may be slight and can be seen as you watch the patient inhale (the chest expands), when the flail section will slightly depress or sink inward. As the patient exhales (chest relaxes), the flail section will slightly push out from the rest of the chest wall.

To care for a flail chest and stabilize the loose segment: (Figure 11.52):

1. Locate the flail section by gently feeling the injury site. In the majority of cases, the injury will be at the side of the chest.

2. Apply a bulky pad of dressings, several inches thick, over the site or use a small pillow that is soft and lightweight.

3. Use large strips of tape to hold the pad in place. Do not tape entirely around the chest; it would restrict breathing efforts. If you do not have tape:

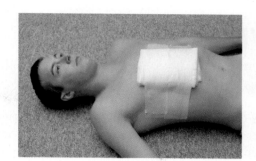

FIGURE 11.52
Emergency care of a patient with flail chest.

- Position the patient on the injured side. Body weight against the surface will help splint the injury. (Do not do this if spinal injuries are suspected.) Or . . .
- Hold the pad in place by hand. When doing so, position your body so that you will not have to shift your weight and move the pad.

4. Provide 100% oxygen via nonrebreather mask as soon as possible and maintain body temperature to minimize the effects of shock.

5. Monitor vital signs and assure adequate breathing and look for signs of heart and lung injury. ■

When the ribs and breastbone are injured, so can the lungs and the heart be injured. Always look for frothy blood in the patient's mouth and signs of difficult or labored breathing, which indicate injury to the lungs. In cases of flail chest, make certain to examine the patient for the following (Figure 11.53):

- Distended (bulging) neck veins.

- Blue coloration of the head, neck, and shoulders.

- Bulging, bloodshot eyes.

- Blue coloration and swelling of the lips and tongue.

- Obvious chest deformity.

These signs indicate that the heart has been injured and that blood has been forced back out of its right side and up through the major veins that lead to the heart from the neck. These patients need oxygen as soon as possible and must be transported immediately.

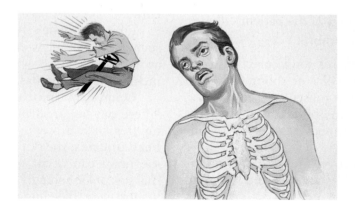

FIGURE 11.53
In cases of flail chest, examine the patient for:
- Distended neck veins.
- Blue coloration of the head, neck, and shoulders.
- Bulging, bloodshot eyes.
- Blue coloration and swelling of the lips and tongue.
- Obvious chest deformity.

Chapter Review

When caring for patients with suspected musculoskeletal injuries, remember that scene safety, mechanism of injury, and patient environment are important factors to consider before patient care may begin. Assess and care for all life-threatening problems first. Before focusing on extremity injuries, provide care for injuries to the head and spine, open injuries to the chest and abdomen, and all serious burns. Provide oxygen, and maintain body temperature to help prevent shock.

The **musculoskeletal system** provides body support and movement, protects organs, and produces blood cells. **Soft tissues** such as muscles, nerves, and blood vessels are damaged when bones are injured. Manage them as part of total patient care.

An **open injury** occurs when a bone tears through the skin or the mechanism of injury causes a puncture to the outer skin and damages the bone inside. If the bones do not tear through the patient's skin, the injury is called a **closed injury.** Apply sterile dressings to all open injuries. A bone that is broken and bends at a place other than a joint is called a **deformed or angulated injury.**

Typical signs and symptoms for musculoskeletal injuries include pain, swelling, discoloration, and deformity. Other signs and symptoms include loss of use, tenderness, guarding, loss of distal pulse, slow capillary refill (in pediatric patients), numbness, tingling, grating, the sound of breaking bone, and exposed bone.

Some special signs to look for with injured extremities include:

- Guarding of the injured extremity.
- Bulging where there is a joint or where the extremity joins the torso.
- Pelvic pain on compression of the patient's hips.
- Leg rotating outward or inward.

Emergency care procedures for injured extremities include applying a rigid or soft splint. When in doubt about the extent of a musculoskeletal injury, splint. All splinting must immobilize the injured extremity and the joints directly above and below the injury site.

Soft splinting can effectively immobilize an injured extremity without rigid splints. Use a sling and swathe for:

- Injuries to the collarbone or shoulder blade.
- Dislocation of the shoulder. Add padding in the space between arm and chest and the sling and swathe.
- Injuries to the upper arm bone and forearm. Modify the full sling to a wrist sling if the injury is in the elbow area. Add a swathe.
- Injuries to the elbow. Use a wrist sling and a swathe.
- Injuries to the wrist, hand, or fingers. NOTE: Always place the hand in the position of function.

Use padding such as folded blankets or towels for injuries to the pelvis or hip, thigh, knee, or leg. Secure the blanket or towels with four cravats, two above and two below the knees. Then, with EMT assistance, place the patient on a spine board or scoop (orthopedic) stretcher.

Use a pillow for injuries to the ankle or foot. Secure the pillow with cravats and elevate.

Applying a splint can prevent or reduce complications, such as pain, soft-tissue damage, bleeding, restricted blood flow, and can prevent closed injuries from becoming open injuries.

To apply a splint, first cut away or remove clothing from the injury site. Control bleeding and dress open wounds. Check for distal circulation, sensation, and motor function before and after splinting. If there is no distal pulse, realign deformed (angulated) injuries or reposition extremities until pulse is regained, if allowed to do so by your EMS system.

Pad all rigid splints before they are secured to the patient. **Manual traction** is applied by pulling gently on an injured limb along its long axis. If manual traction is applied, maintain it until the rigid splint is secured.

First Responders may use noncommercial splints, such as lumber, plywood, rolled newspapers and magazines, compressed wood products, sporting equipment, canes, umbrellas, cardboard, and tool handles.

Open head injuries involve fractures of the skull. There can be direct injury to the brain in open head injuries such as cuts, tears, and bruising. In **closed head injuries,** the skull is not damaged but injuries to the brain can occur and include concussions (brain shaking or bouncing), contusions (brain bruises), and hemorrhage (bleeding inside skull).

Head injuries may be obvious, or they may be difficult to detect. Always look for wounds to the head, deformity of the skull, bruises behind the ear, black eyes, sunken eyes, unequal pupils, and blood or clear fluids flowing from the ears and/or nose. Brain injury can occur with head injuries. Look for signs of possible skull fracture, loss of awareness, confusion, unequal or unresponsive pupils, and paralysis.

When caring for a patient with injuries to the head, maintain an open airway using the jaw-thrust maneuver and manually stabilize the head. Assist ventilations or provide CPR if needed. Keep the head-injury patient at rest and talk to him. Control bleeding but avoid pressure over the site of the injury. Do not remove impaled objects, bone fragments, or other objects from head wounds.

Facial injuries often cause airway obstruction. Maintain an open airway with the jaw-thrust maneuver. The mechanism of injury that causes facial injuries can also cause spinal injury. Be sure to stabilize the head when managing the airway.

Spinal injuries can be very serious and can result in permanent paralysis or disability. Keep the patient from moving. Suspect that all unresponsive trauma patients have spinal injuries. If the mechanism of injury indicates possible spinal injuries, proceed as if the injuries are present.

The focused assessment is very important in determining if the patient has spinal injuries. Always look for weakness, numbness, loss of feeling, pain, or paralysis to the limbs of a patient. Remember to press or pinch the feet and hands of the unresponsive patient and look for reactions.

Follow certain rules when caring for a patient who may have spinal injuries. Even though a patient has spinal injuries, provide ventilations or CPR, if needed, and control bleeding. Do not attempt to splint suspected fractures without help. Never move a patient with spinal injuries without help unless absolutely necessary. Stabilize the patient's head and neck and as much of the body as possible. Continuously monitor the patient.

Injuries to the chest can include soft-tissue injuries, crushing injuries, and penetrating injuries that can cause fractured ribs, flail chest, spinal injuries, lung injuries, and heart injuries. Pain at the site may indicate rib fractures; apply a sling and swathe, placing the forearm of the injured side across the chest. Opposite motion in the ribs or breastbone may indicate **flail chest;** apply a thick pad over the site and tape it in place.

REMEMBER AND CONSIDER

When you are at the scene of any injury, listen to what other care providers are saying and how they care for the emotions of their patients. When people are injured, they are concerned with the pain and how soon you can relieve it. Children want to stop hurting and want you to make the pain go away.

✔ Think about what you will tell your injured patients as you provide care for their injuries.

Sometimes when you have to move a patient during the assessment or while you dress a wound or splint an extremity, the movement will cause additional pain. You must let your patients know what you are doing and why, if it will hurt and for how long, and what the result will be when you are finished.

✔ Keep in mind that most patients will cooperate with your care if they know what to expect. You must respect their concerns, answer their questions, and provide them with as much information about their injury as possible.

If you have not had a chance to look through your First Responder vehicle and see what equipment and supplies are carried, take some time to do so. Ask another department member to work with you to show you where splinting items are kept, or to suggest to you what items can be used as improvised splints.

☑ What materials for securing splints are carried on the unit?

☑ Are the splinting materials in places where they are easily reached, or will you have to take a few minutes to access them?

Practice using items in your unit for splinting. Work with other department members or with friends.

☑ As you hold traction, can you direct your friends to properly apply a commercial or an improvised splint?

☑ As you work with more experienced department members, can you follow their directions to hold traction or to splint while they hold traction?

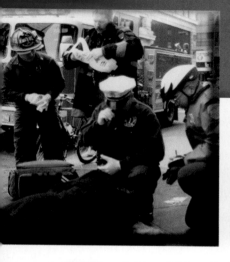
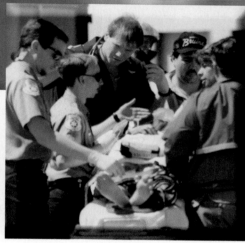
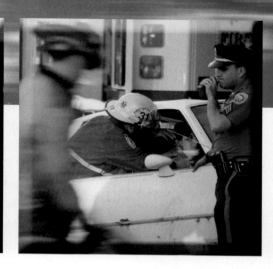

Childbirth

CHAPTER
12

Most expectant mothers know they need to care for themselves and for their unborn infants during pregnancy. Usually, expectant mothers are under the care of a physician, so they do not often have to call for emergency services to assist with the delivery of their babies. Sometimes, though, physiological or environmental situations cause birth to occur unexpectedly or with complications and before the mother can get to the hospital. In addition, trauma to the mother also affects the fetus; therefore, providing care for the mother also helps the infant.

When the unexpected happens, the First Responder must recognize signs and symptoms and know what to do. This chapter will introduce you to the terms, events, stages, and complications of pregnancy and childbirth, the steps for delivery, and how to care for the mother and fetus during and after delivery.

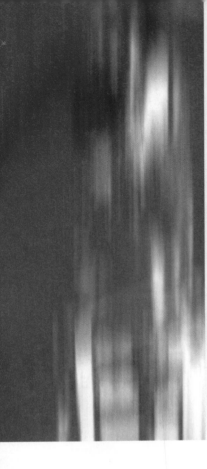

NATIONAL STANDARD OBJECTIVES

This chapter focuses on the objectives of Module 6, Lesson 6-1, of the U.S. DOT's First Responder National Standard Curriculum and serves as an instructional aid to help you meet any specific objectives added to the course by your local EMS system.

By the end of this chapter, you will be able to (from cognitive or knowledge information):

6–1.1 Identify the following structures: birth canal, placenta, umbilical cord, and amniotic sac. (p. 423)

6–1.2 Define the following terms: crowning, bloody show, labor, and abortion. (pp. 423, 442)

6–1.3 State indications of an imminent delivery. (pp. 426–427)

6–1.4 State the steps in the predelivery preparation of the mother. (pp. 425–428)

6–1.5 Establish the relationship between body substance isolation and childbirth. (pp. 425, 428)

6–1.6 State the steps to assist in the delivery. (pp. 428–432)

6–1.7 Describe care of the baby as the head appears. (pp. 428, 431)

6–1.8 Discuss the steps in delivery of the afterbirth. (pp. 432, 439)

6–1.9 List the steps in the emergency medical care of the mother post-delivery. (pp. 439–440)

6–1.10 Discuss the steps in caring for a newborn. (pp. 432–438)

LEARNING TASKS

Emergency care providers assist with the delivery of thousands of babies each year in the United States. You must be able to remember the steps involved in childbirth and be able to assist in delivery. The mother will go through several stages of labor, which may happen very quickly. You must recognize these stages and, if needed in the meantime, prepare the mother for delivery. You must be able to:

✔ List and describe the three stages of labor.
✔ List and explain the use of the materials needed for preparation and delivery.

The mother is not the only patient. If the baby arrives before the mother can get to the hospital, you must also know what to do for the newborn. Be able to:

✔ Describe assessment steps for an infant and how to determine the need for resuscitation.

Sometimes the mother will go through a prolonged birth process, which is not only distressing to the mother, but also stressful for the baby. You must be able to:

✔ Recognize meconium staining in the birth fluids, understand its seriousness, and know what to do for the baby.
✔ Discuss the significance of a stressful birth in which meconium is present.

In an emergency involving a pregnant woman, you will care for most medical and trauma situations as you would for any other patient, but you must be aware of special problems that some expectant mothers may have. Be able to:

✔ List basic care procedures for predelivery emergencies including seizures, vaginal bleeding, and trauma.

Feel comfortable enough to
(by changing attitudes, values, and beliefs):

6–1.11 Explain the rationale for attending to the feelings of a patient in need of emergency medical care during childbirth. (pp. 422, 440)

6–1.12 Demonstrate a caring attitude toward patients during childbirth who request emergency medical services. (pp. 426, 428, 439–440, 442, 446)

6–1.13 Place the interests of the patient during childbirth as the foremost consideration when making any and all patient care decisions. (pp. 426, 427)

6–1.14 Communicate with empathy to patients during childbirth, as well as with family members and friends of the patient. (pp. 426, 428, 440, 442, 446)

Show how to
(through psychomotor skills):

6–1.15 Demonstrate the steps to assist in the normal cephalic delivery. (pp. 428–432)

6–1.16 Demonstrate necessary care procedures of the fetus as the head appears. (pp. 428, 431)

6–1.17 Attend to the steps in the delivery of the afterbirth. (pp. 432, 439)

6–1.18 Demonstrate the post-delivery care of the mother. (pp. 439–440)

6–1.19 Demonstrate the care of the newborn. (pp. 432–438)

Most mothers will progress through the birth process without any problems. Others will have medical or physical problems that will cause an unusual or complicated birth. Be able to:

✔ Describe common delivery complications including prolapsed cord, breech birth, limb presentation, premature births, miscarriages, and stillbirths and state the care for each.

Even more unusual than delivering an infant in the field is delivering two. Once you have delivered one baby, you need to recognize the signs of another delivery, which are slightly different. Be able to:

✔ Describe First Responder steps for delivery in multiple-birth situations.

Trauma is critical for anyone, especially for an expectant mother. Pregnancy conditions may mask signs and symptoms of shock. Not only is the mother an injured patient, but so too is the fetus. In the event of a trauma or any type of assault, be able to:

✔ Describe the care for shock and explain reasons for starting early care.
✔ Describe special care considerations for patients who have been victims of trauma or sexual assault.

As you practice skills with classmates, frequently review and practice the steps for neonatal resuscitation. You must practice these skills frequently so that you can perform them automatically and effortlessly when needed. Be able to:

✔ Demonstrate resuscitation steps for an infant with an inadequate respiratory and/or heart rate.

UNDERSTANDING CHILDBIRTH

You may have noticed that this chapter is called "Childbirth" and not "Emergency Childbirth." As a culture, we have arrived at the point where any birth away from a hospital delivery room is considered an emergency, which is just not true. In many parts of the world, babies are born away from medical facilities. Birth is a natural process. The anatomy of the human female, the unborn child, and the structures formed during pregnancy enable the birth process to occur with few problems. Assistance from the medical community reduces the chances of problems for the mother and the child, but in most deliveries, high-tech medical skills and equipment are not needed.

FIRST➤ Mothers do all the work of delivering their babies. First Responders assist. Your role, then, will be one of helping the mother as she delivers her child. ■

The presence of a First Responder at the scene of a birth that takes place away from a medical facility can be the key factor in a baby's survival if something should go wrong. The mother may need the skills of a First Responder during the birth process to ensure safe delivery if there are complications. The care provided after delivery is just as important. The first hour of life after birth can be a difficult time for some babies and mothers. Your assistance can make a difference.

ANATOMY OF PREGNANCY

A baby is called a **fetus** as it develops and grows inside of its mother. The average period of development for the fetus is from 36 to 40 weeks, or from 9 to 10 months. This development period is divided into three-month segments called *trimesters*. The fetus develops inside a muscular organ called the *womb*, or **uterus** (Figure 12.1). The mother and the developing fetus are normally physiologically ready to deliver sometime after 37 weeks of pregnancy. Then labor will begin.

fetus (FE-tus) the developing unborn baby. The fertilized egg is an embryo until the eighth week after fertilization, when it becomes a fetus.

uterus (U-ter-us) the womb. The muscular structure in which the fetus develops.

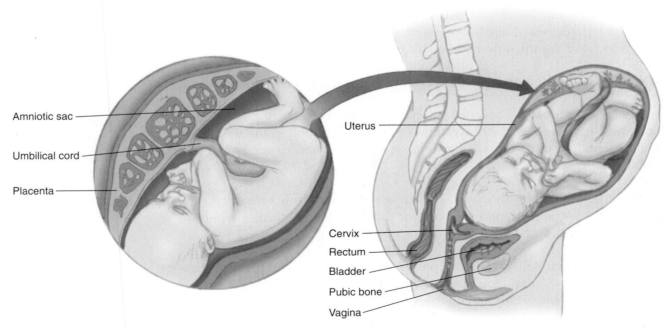

Amniotic sac

Umbilical cord

Placenta

Uterus

Cervix

Rectum

Bladder

Pubic bone

Vagina

FIGURE 12.1
Structures of pregnancy.

During labor, the muscles of the uterus contract and push the baby down through the neck of the uterus, which is called the **cervix**. As the cervix expands to allow the head of the fetus through, the mother may notice a slight staining of blood or blood-tinged mucus. This is called "bloody show" and is normal. The fetus passes through the cervix and enters the *birth canal*, or **vagina**, through which it moves to the outside world to be born. During your assessment of the mother, you must examine her for **crowning**. Crowning is the showing of the baby's presenting part, normally the head. However, any part of the baby may present first, including the buttocks or feet. Once the baby passes into the birth canal, more of the head (or other presenting part) will show, or appear to grow larger, with each contraction. This means that birth is *imminent* (about to occur).

The fetus grows inside a special sac, the **amniotic sac**, which is filled with fluid (amniotic fluid) that surrounds and protects the baby. Although the sac may have ruptured earlier, it usually breaks during labor, and the fluid, or *water*, flows out of the vagina. This is called the *rupture of membranes* and is an important milestone of active labor. When you are assessing the mother, you will ask her if her "water has broken." She will know and be able to tell you if it has or not. Sometimes the sac will break very early in the labor process. Sometimes it will break much later. The fluids help lubricate the birth canal for the passage of the baby.

During pregnancy, a special organ called the **placenta** develops in the womb. Oxygen and nourishment from the mother's blood pass through the placenta and enter fetal circulation through the **umbilical cord**. Fetal wastes pass back through the umbilical cord and the placenta to the mother's circulation to be eliminated.

STAGES OF LABOR

Usually, the process of labor lasts about 16 hours for the first-time mother. In some cases, labor may take longer, or it may take a much shorter time. The time will vary with each mother. You may also expect that, typically, the labor process will be shorter with each successive birth. There are three stages of labor:

- *First stage*—begins with contractions and ends when the cervix is fully dilated so the baby can enter the birth canal.

- *Second stage*—begins when the baby enters the birth canal and ends when he is born.

- *Third stage*—begins when the baby is born and ends when the **afterbirth** (placenta, umbilical cord, tissues from the amniotic sac, and some tissues from the lining of the uterus) is delivered.

It is normal to have vaginal discharges throughout labor. During the first stage of labor, the first type of discharge to appear should be a watery, bloody mucus. Later, the discharge will appear as a watery, bloody fluid. This is normal and not the same as bleeding. If there is bleeding from the vagina prior to delivery rather than the normal bloody fluids, then something is wrong. This could be a serious problem and requires assistance from a higher level of EMS provider and transport as soon as possible.

Contractions of the uterus cause labor pains, and they occur in cycles of contraction and relaxation. At first, contractions are far apart. As the fetus is pushed into the birth canal, and the time of birth gets closer, the time between contractions becomes shorter. The first contractions are about 30 minutes apart and become closer and closer until they are 3 minutes apart or less. Pain during labor is normal and usually starts as an ache in the lower back. Then, as labor progresses, the pain is felt in the lower abdomen. As the muscles of the uterus contract, the

cervix (SUR-viks) the neck of the uterus; the lower portion of the uterus, where it enters the vagina.

vagina (vah-JI-nah) the birth canal.

crowning the bulging-out of the vagina caused by exposure of the baby's head or other presenting part during contractions.

amniotic (am-ne-OT-ik) **sac** the fluid-filled sac that surrounds the developing embryo and fetus.

placenta (plah-SEN-tah) an organ of pregnancy that is composed of maternal and fetal tissues. Exchange between the circulatory systems of the mother and fetus can take place without the mixing of their blood. It makes up most of the afterbirth that delivers after the baby's birth.

umbilical (um-BIL-i-kal) **cord** the structure that connects the fetus to the placenta. It contains fetal blood vessels.

afterbirth the tissues that deliver after the birth of the baby; consists of placenta, umbilical cord, tissues from the amniotic sac, and some tissues from the lining of the uterus.

pain begins. When the muscles relax, the pain is usually relieved. During the relaxation time, the mother rests. Labor pains will normally come at regular intervals and last for about 30 seconds to one minute. It is not unusual for these pains to start, stop for a period of time, and then start again.

First Responders can time labor pains for two characteristics (Figure 12.2):

contraction time the period of time that a contraction of the womb lasts during labor. It is measured from the start of the uterus contracting until it relaxes.

interval time the period of time from the start of one contraction until the beginning of the next.

- **Contraction time**—how long it takes from the time the uterus begins to contract until it relaxes.

- **Interval time**—the time from the start of one contraction to the beginning of the next contraction. As labor progresses, the interval time will decrease.

Sometimes the mother will experience light, painless, irregular contractions throughout her pregnancy, which may increase gradually in intensity and frequency during the third trimester. About four weeks prior to delivery, as the uterus begins to change its size and shape, some women begin to experience these types of contractions and have the sensation that labor has begun. This is known as *false labor,* also referred to as *Braxton Hicks contractions.* False labor pains are not as regular and rhythmic as true labor contractions.

It may be difficult for you and the mother to distinguish false labor pains from true labor. Even when you are certain that the patient is having false labor, it is still recommended that you arrange for EMTs to transport the patient. Any pregnant woman who is having contractions should be evaluated by her obstetrician.

Remember that your primary role is to help the mother deliver the baby if birth is imminent. You will need to make sure that you have the necessary supplies and materials to do this.

SUPPLIES AND MATERIALS

The items you will need for preparing the mother for delivery and initial care are provided in a commercial obstetric (OB) kit (Figure 12.3). If your response unit does not carry a commercial OB kit, assemble and store the required items in a special kit and keep it on your unit. Some of these items are available at the patient's home, but during the emergency is not the time to find supplies. The items that you will need include the following:

FIGURE 12.2
Determining contraction and interval times.

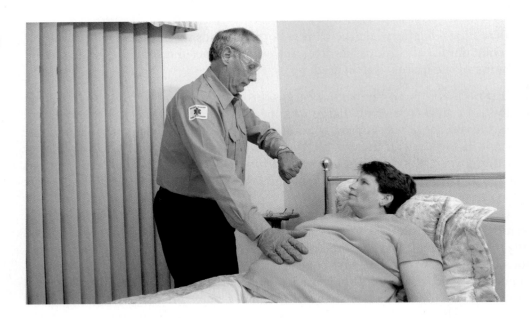

- Personal protective equipment for BSI precautions such as protective gloves. (Caution: the mother may be allergic to latex.) Face masks, eye shields, and gowns are also included.
- Towels, sheets, and blankets for draping the mother, for placing under her, and for drying and wrapping the baby.
- Gauze pads for wiping mucus from the baby's mouth and nose.
- Rubber bulb syringe for suctioning the baby's mouth and nose.
- Clamps and ties for use on the umbilical cord before cutting.
- Sterile scissors or a single-edged razor for cutting the cord.
- Sanitary pads or bulky dressings for vaginal bleeding.
- Basin and plastic bags for collecting and transporting the afterbirth.
- Red, plastic biohazard bags for storing and disposing soiled linens and dressings.

Your initial and focused assessments will help you to determine if the mother is ready to deliver. If birth appears likely before EMTs can transport her to the hospital, place supplies so they are within your reach during the delivery process, don your personal protective equipment, and prepare the mother for delivery.

DELIVERY

PREPARING FOR DELIVERY

Due to the nature of childbirth, it is important for you to wear appropriate face and eye protection, in addition to protective gloves, to minimize exposure to the mother's body fluids during delivery. Then, after taking BSI precautions, introduce yourself to the mother and let her know that you are a trained First Responder. Make sure that EMS (9-1-1) has been activated. Let the mother know that you have called for additional assistance and that you will stay with her to help if she starts to deliver the baby. Provide emotional support throughout the entire process of birth. Talk with the mother to help her remain calm and, if needed, remind her that birth is a natural process.

If the expectant mother complains that she feels as if she needs to go to the bathroom, tell her that this is normal and that it is caused by pressure on her bladder and intestine. Encourage her to remain lying down. Explain that her body is reacting normally to all the changes taking place. It is important that you keep her calm and begin assessing her status as soon as possible. Place layers of newspaper covered with layers of linens under her. If she does have a bowel movement or urinates, tell her that this is normal. Remove soiled linens and replace them with fresh ones.

Fear of delivering away from a hospital can lead some people to try to delay birth. The mother, family, or onlookers may suggest the mother hold her knees together, which you should not allow. It will not slow delivery, but it may complicate the birth or harm the fetus. Have unneeded family members find supplies if you are at the home. Have unneeded onlookers form a privacy shield with blankets, coats, or their bodies if you are in a public place. Your task is to reassure the mother, begin your assessment, and provide care.

FIRST➤ Begin to evaluate the mother by asking for the following information (Figure 12.4):

- Her name, age, and expected due date.
- If she has been seeing a doctor during her pregnancy. If so, ask for the contact phone number.
- If this is her first pregnancy. The typical first delivery lasts about 16 hours. Labor time is usually shorter for subsequent babies.
- If she has any known complications, particularly a multiple birth.
- If she has discharged any watery or bloody mucus.
- How long she has been having labor pains.
- If her water has broken, when, and what color (clear, which is normal, or cloudy or green, which indicates a stressed fetus and requires immediate transport).

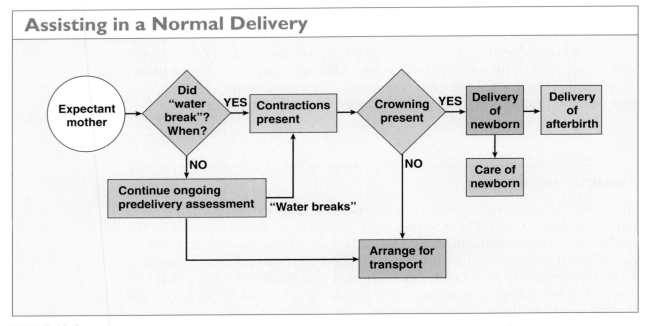

Assisting in a Normal Delivery

FIGURE 12.4

- If she feels strain in her pelvis or lower abdomen, if she feels as if she needs to move her bowels, and if she can feel the baby beginning to move into her vaginal opening.
- If she has any significant medical information such as a history of seizures, diabetes, or vaginal bleeding during the pregnancy. ■

If the mother says she feels the baby trying to be born or that she has the urge to bear down, birth will probably occur before the EMTs arrive. If the mother is having contractions about two minutes apart, birth is near. Should she also be straining, crying out, and complaining about having to go to the bathroom, prepare to deliver very shortly. Even a first-time mother will have some understanding of what is going on. When she says she feels the baby coming, believe her.

Find out if she has taken a childbirth preparation class or natural childbirth classes. In these classes, the expectant mother works with someone she chooses to be her coach. Use her coach if this person is present or tell her that you will work with her to help her follow the procedures she learned in her class with her coach or partner. Though you must follow standard EMS system practices for assisting with the delivery and for providing care afterwards, you or her coach can help the mother with breathing and timing contractions as she was taught in her classes. In addition, you or her coach can also offer the encouragement and support she will need throughout labor. You or her coach can make suggestions on how she can breathe and when to push or relax. Following are a few simple coaching steps.

- As each contraction begins, have the mother take a deep breath and encourage her to gently bear down, or push. She can push with several breaths during each contraction.
- The mother should rest until the next contraction.
- As the baby's head emerges, ask the mother to stop pushing and to start panting so that the baby's head can slide slowly out of the birth canal.

FIRST➤ After evaluating and examining the mother and finding that birth may occur shortly, immediately prepare her for delivery. You will:

1. Take BSI precautions. Put on your personal protective equipment (gloves, mask with eye shield, gown), if you have not already done so.
2. Control the scene so that the mother will have privacy. Ask unneeded bystanders to leave. If you are in a public place, ask some bystanders to turn their backs and help shield the mother. If she appears to be in early labor and this is her first child, her labor pains typically will have long contraction and interval times. You may have to move her a short distance to a more private place.
3. Position the mother on her back with her knees bent, feet flat, and legs spread wide apart. If this position causes her to feel dizzy and faint, it is because the weight of the baby is pressing on the inferior vena cava, the vessel that returns blood from the lower part of the body to the heart, and restricting blood flow back to the heart. If the mother feels dizzy and faint, position her slightly on her left side with one knee bent and foot flat, the other leg extended, and her legs spread wide apart. Place pillows or blankets under her right side to support in the raised position during birth.
4. Feel the abdomen for contractions when the patient says she is having labor pains. Explain what you are going to do and place the palm of your hand on her abdomen above the navel. It is not necessary to remove any of the patient's clothing to feel for contractions. If the mother says that she can feel the baby coming, skip this step. Do not delay other procedures to wait for a contraction. Feel for and time several contractions to help determine if birth is near.

As birth nears, the interval time will decrease and you will feel the uterus and the abdomen become more rigid.

5. Prepare the mother for examination. Tell her that you need to see if her baby has entered the birth canal. Help her remove clothing or underclothing that obstructs your exam of her vaginal opening. Use clean sheets, towels, or table-cloths to cover the mother. If you have an obstetrical pack (OB kit), use the materials provided. Make sure you have enough light to see what you are doing. It may be necessary to supply portable lighting or to move lamps in the home to enable you to evaluate the mother and to deliver the baby.

6. Check for crowning. See if any part of the baby is visible at the vaginal opening. In a normal cephalic (head-first) birth, you will see the top of the baby's head. As you learned earlier, this is called *crowning*, though any part of the baby may present first. The area of the head (or other presenting part) that you see on your first inspection may be less than the size of the dollar coin. If more of the baby's head (or presenting part) becomes visible with each contraction, birth is occurring. The mother is now in the second stage of labor because the baby is in the birth canal. Determine that the birth is in progress. Do not try to transport the mother yourself or in your first response unit. Wait for EMT or ALS personnel to respond.

    The mother, father, or anyone assisting may be embarrassed when you check for crowning. You can minimize this embarrassment by maintaining your professional manner and by explaining what you are going to do and why before you begin. Your professional appearance and approach will generate confidence and trust.

7. Do not attempt any type of internal or vaginal exam. Touch the vaginal area only as necessary during the delivery process. ■

REMEMBER: *During the entire process of assessment and delivery, it is essential for you to take BSI precautions, including gloves, mask with eye shield, and gown. This will help protect you and both mother and baby from potential infection.*

NORMAL DELIVERY

During the delivery, talk to the mother. Ask her to relax between contractions. If her water breaks, remind her that this is normal. Consider the delivery to be normal if the baby's head appears first.

FIRST➤ Perform the following steps when assisting the mother in a normal delivery (Figure 12.5 and Scan 12-1):

1. Wash your hands with soap and water, or use a commercial hand wash. Don personal protective equipment (gloves, mask with eye shield, gown), if you have not already done so.

2. Drape the mother and place her on top of layers of newspapers and clean sheets or towels (Figure 12.6). Place a folded blanket, towels, or sheets under her buttocks to lift her pelvis about two inches. You may place a pillow under her head and shoulders for comfort.

3. Place someone near the mother's head or use the mother's coach to reassure and offer her encouragement and to turn her head in case she vomits. If no one is on hand to help, talk with the patient during the delivery process and be alert for vomiting.

4. Place one hand below the baby's head as it delivers. Spread your fingers evenly around the head to support it but avoid pressing the soft areas at the top, back, and sides of the baby's skull. Apply a slight pressure on the baby's head as it

remember

Showing a professional de-meanor and giving explanations of the care you are going to provide will help to minimize the patient's embarrassment.

Childbirth

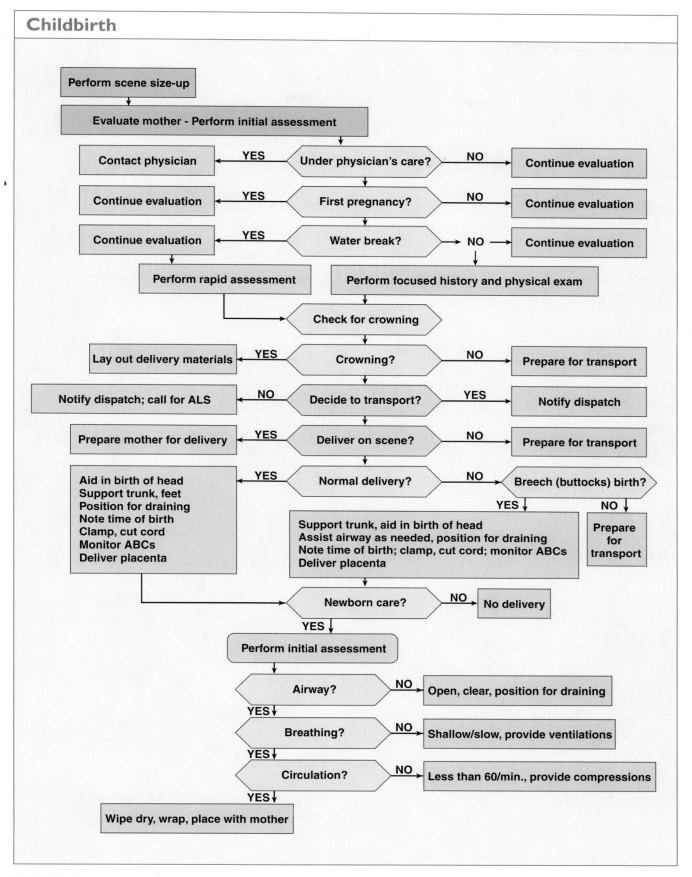

FIGURE 12.5

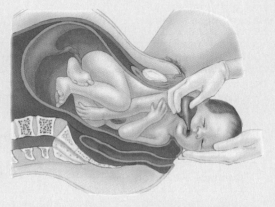

1. Support the head.

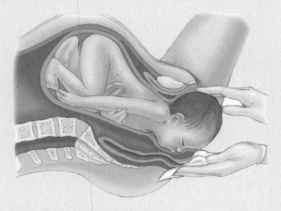

2. Suction the mouth and nose and check for the position of the cord.

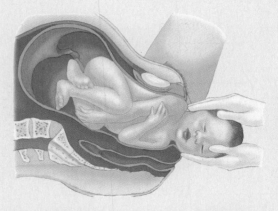

3. Assist in the birth of the head and shoulders.

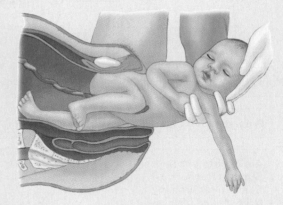

4. Support the head and trunk.

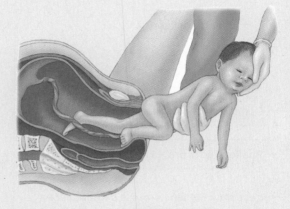

5. Support the head, trunk, and legs.

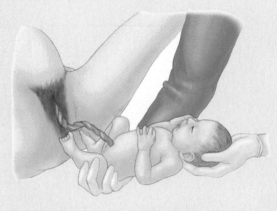

6. Keep the infant level with the vagina until the umbilical cord stops pulsating.

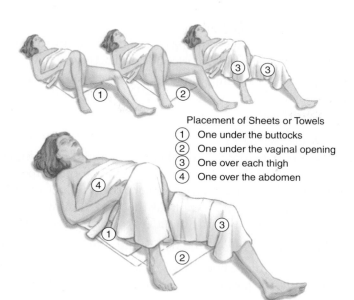

FIGURE 12.6
Preparing the mother for delivery.

Placement of Sheets or Towels
1. One under the buttocks
2. One under the vaginal opening
3. One over each thigh
4. One over the abdomen

emerges to control the delivery speed. Sometimes the head "explodes" from the birth canal quickly, which can badly tear the skin at the vaginal opening. (Some stretching and tearing is normal.) Use your other hand to help cradle the baby's head. **Do not pull on the baby.**

As the baby's head emerges, you may notice that it has caused the skin area between the vaginal and rectal openings (called the *perineum*, per-i-NE-um) to tear. This is normal and will be treated at the hospital. After the delivery, place a sanitary pad at the vaginal opening, which will also help control bleeding from torn tissues. Replace sanitary pads as needed.

5. If the amniotic sac has not yet ruptured, use a cord clamp or your gloved fingers to tear the membrane and pull it away from the baby's mouth and nose. An unbroken sac will prevent the baby from breathing.

6. If the umbilical cord is wrapped around the baby's neck, place your finger under the cord and gently pull it over the baby's head.

   You will have some time before the shoulders emerge. If it is possible for you to do so, clear the airway of fluids by suctioning the baby's mouth first, and then the nose (see step 8). It is especially important that you suction the airway if meconium staining (green or brownish-yellow discoloration) was present in the amniotic fluid.

7. Most babies are born face down as the head emerges, and then they rotate to the right or left. The upper shoulder (usually with some delay) delivers next, followed quickly by the lower shoulder. Continue to support the baby throughout the entire birth process. Gently guide the baby's head downward, which will assist the mother in delivering the baby's upper shoulder. Scan 12-1 illustrates hand placement during delivery.

8. Once the baby's feet deliver (the end of the second stage of labor), lay the baby on his side with his head slightly lower than his body. This position will enable blood, other fluids, and mucus to drain from the mouth and nose. Wipe the baby's mouth and nose with gauze pads. If you have not yet cleared the airway, suction the mouth first, then the nose.

   Standard procedures call for clearing the baby's airway once the head delivers, but First Responders may not carry the rubber bulb syringe (unless it is in an OB kit) for this procedure. Even if you have one, do not try to stop the birth process or release your support of the baby to clear the airway. Since you will

NOTE
Tearing of the perineum is normal.

remember
Maintain support of the baby throughout the birth process.

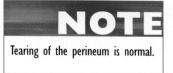

not be delivering babies every day, it is normal to find you lack the confidence to try to assist with the birth and clear the airway at the same time. Most babies can wait the few more seconds of delivery to have their airways cleared.

9. Note the exact time of birth. In many systems, the normal procedure is to notify dispatch or medical direction, where birth time is recorded manually or electronically.

10. Keep the baby at the level of the vagina until the cord is cut.

11. Clamp or tie the umbilical cord. It should be clamped or tied first at about 10 inches from the baby's belly and again about three inches closer to the baby. (More about this later.) Then cut the cord between the ties. If you do *not* have sterile equipment, do not cut the cord. Simply clamp it. (Some jurisdictions may not allow First Responders to cut the cord. Follow local protocol.)

12. Monitor and record the baby's and mother's vital signs (ABCs).

13. Watch for more contractions, which signal the delivery of the placenta. The placenta is a part of the afterbirth, and it is important to save it for examination. If any part of it remains attached inside the uterus, it can cause bleeding and an infection. Wrap it and other birth tissues in a towel, place them in a plastic bag, and give it to EMT or ALS personnel to transport to the hospital.

14. Place a sanitary pad over the mother's vaginal opening. Lower her legs, and place them together. Label the bag with the mother's name. ■

CAUTION: *Babies in the process of being born are slippery. Make certain you have a good but gentle grip and provide proper support throughout the delivery process. Some deliveries are explosive. Do not squeeze or counter-push the baby too much. Remember, you can use one hand to place slight pressure on the baby's head to help prevent an explosive delivery.*

CARING FOR THE BABY

FIRST➤ As you assist the mother with the delivery of her baby (Figure 12.7):

1. Clear the baby's airway. Position the baby on his side with head slightly lower than his body to allow for drainage. Keep the baby's body at the level of the vagina until the cord is clamped. Use a sterile gauze pad or a clean handkerchief to clear mucus and blood from around the baby's nose and mouth (Figure 12.8). Use a rubber bulb syringe, if one is available, to clear the airway. The correct steps for using the bulb syringe are as follows:
   — Squeeze the bulb first.
   — Insert the tip about one inch into the baby's mouth.
   — Gently release the pressure to allow the syringe to take up fluids from inside the baby's mouth (Figure 12.9).
   — Remove the tip of the filled syringe from the baby's mouth and squeeze out any fluids onto a towel or gauze pad.
   — Repeat this process two or three times for the mouth and for each nostril.
   Throughout the rest of your care steps, be sure that the baby's nose is clear. Babies are nose breathers. Plugged nostrils may prevent adequate breathing.

2. Make certain that the baby is breathing. Usually the baby will be breathing on his own by the time you clear the airway, which will take about 30 seconds.
   If the baby is not breathing, then you must encourage him to do so. Begin by vigorously but gently rubbing the baby's back. If this fails to stimulate

Assessment of the Newborn

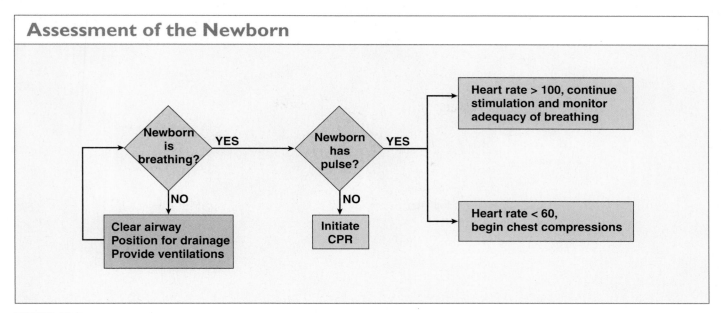

FIGURE 12.7

breathing, snap one of your index fingers against the soles of the baby's feet (Figure 12.10). (Care for the nonbreathing newborn is covered later in this chapter.)

3. Once you are sure the baby is breathing, perform a quick assessment. Note skin color (blue, pale), any deformities, the strength of his cry (loud or weak) and whether he moves on his own or just lies still. After a few minutes, note if there are any changes in these conditions. It is important to give this information to the transport personnel for relay to the hospital physician, who will base the baby's subsequent exam on the original assessment.

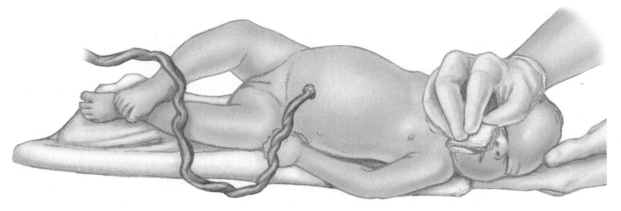

FIGURE 12.8
Use a sterile pad or clean handkerchief to wipe blood and mucus from around the baby's mouth and nose.

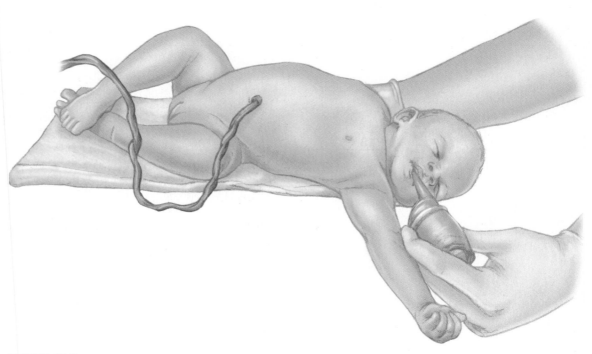

FIGURE 12.9
If you have an OB kit, use the rubber bulb syringe to clear the baby's airway.

4. Clamp or tie off the cord, if protocols allow. (Details are provided later in this chapter.)

5. Keep the baby warm. Dry the baby and discard the wet material in a biohazard bag. Wrap the baby in a clean, dry towel, sheet, or baby blanket and place him on the mother's abdomen (Figure 12.11). Keep the baby's head covered to help reduce heat loss.

   The mother may wish to nurse the baby. You may suggest and encourage the mother to do so because it helps contract the uterus and control bleeding.

6. If tape is available, write the mother's last name and the delivery time on a long piece of it. Place a slightly shorter piece of tape on the back of the first one so the adhesive does not come in contact with the baby's skin. Leave an end exposed to tape to itself in a loop. Place it loosely around the baby's wrist. ■

Caring for the Nonbreathing Newborn

In step #2 above, you helped the baby to breathe. If you are unsuccessful, provide two gentle but adequate breaths using a mouth-to-mask or bag-valve-mask technique (Figure 12.12). Then assess breathing and heartbeat. Remember to check the heartbeat of a newborn by listening at the chest with your ear or a stethoscope or by feeling for a pulse by lightly grasping the base of the umbilical cord. Do *not* use a bag-valve mask or airway adjuncts designed for older children or adults to resuscitate a newborn. Do not use any device unless you have been trained and your jurisdiction allows First Responders to use it. Be careful not to hyperextend the head and neck of the baby, which would close off the airway.

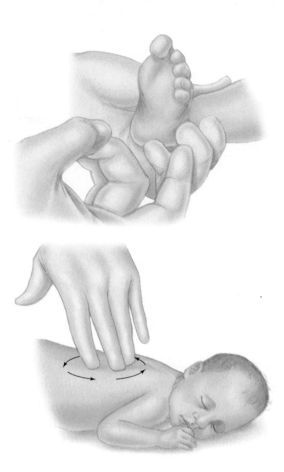

Provide ventilations if breaths are:

- Shallow.

- Slow.

- Absent.

Ventilate at 40 to 60 breaths per minute (about a breath every second) with 100% oxygen. Watch for the chest to rise, which is the best indication of adequate ventilation. Reassess breathing after 30 seconds of assisted ventilations. The next step depends on the heart rate:

- If the heart rate is 100 beats per minute or greater and the infant is breathing adequately, stop ventilations but continue to provide gentle stimulation (rub

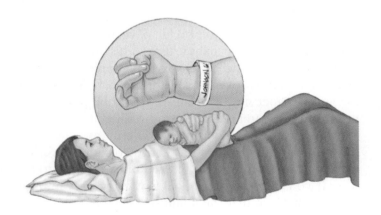

FIGURE 12.11
Wrap the infant and place him on the mother's abdomen. Use tape to make an ID bracelet for the infant. Write the mother's last name and time of delivery on it.

FIGURE 12.12
Resuscitate the newly born baby
with bag-valve-mask resuscitator
that is an appropriate size.

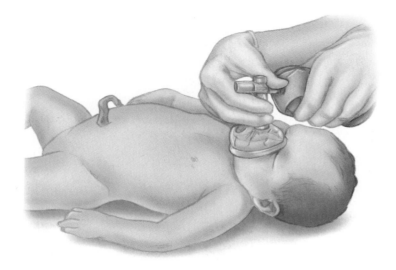

the back) to help maintain and improve the baby's breathing. Continue to provide oxygen.

- If the baby's heart rate is below 100 beats per minute and respirations are inadequate, continue to assist ventilations with a bag-valve-mask.

- If the heart rate is less than 60 beats per minute, continue to assist ventilations and begin chest compressions. Remember, perform infant CPR with either your fingertips or your thumbs with your hands encircling the chest, not the heels of your hands.

If there is a pulse but you:

See this:	**Then do this:**
Breathing rate is inadequate . . .	Ventilate at 40 to 60 breaths per minute for 30 seconds and reassess breathing.
Heart rate is at least 100 beats per minute and spontaneous breathing is present . . .	Stop ventilations but continue to gently stimulate the baby by rubbing the skin.
Heart rate is less than 60 beats per minute . . .	Continue to assist ventilations. Start chest compressions.

Continue resuscitation until the baby has spontaneous heart and lung actions or when a higher level of EMS provider relieves you. Alert dispatch to the baby's status. Dispatch will contact and send appropriate assistance. Your instructor will advise you if protocols allow you to provide oxygen to the baby.

If you are allowed to provide oxygen to the baby, do *not* blow a stream of oxygen directly into the baby's face. This may cause him to react by holding his breath. In addition, the rich oxygen supply can cause medical problems. Instead, direct a stream of oxygen toward the baby's face, either through a face mask or through a paper cup with an oxygen tube placed through the bottom. Hold the mask or cup several inches from the baby's face (Figure 12.13).

Research has found that withholding oxygen may be more damaging than delivering too much. Follow local protocols for delivering oxygen, but *never* withhold oxygen from a sick baby or one who is struggling to breathe in the prehospital setting. If your response unit does not carry oxygen, notify EMT or ALS personnel through dispatch that the infant will need it.

remember

Always provide oxygen to a baby who is sick or struggling to breathe.

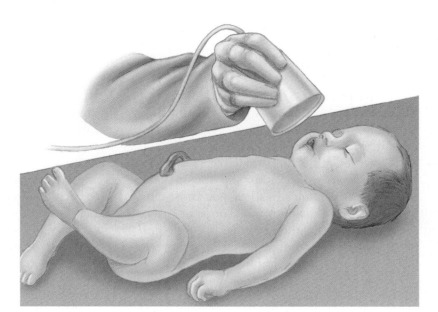

The above few steps of ventilation and chest compression will usually revive the baby, but it is still important to have him and the mother transported as quickly as possible to the hospital.

Most first response units are not designed for transport. Protocols in some states do not allow First Responders to transport. Check your protocols about transporting childbirth patients.

The primary role of the First Responder during such an emergency is to provide basic life support until EMT or ALS units arrive. If you are asked to assist during transport and the afterbirth has not delivered yet, carefully move mother and baby as a unit. Keep the mother on her back and the baby between her legs. If you are resuscitating the baby, coordinate your moves so you do not have to stop resuscitation while moving them. Continue to monitor the baby's breathing and pulse during transport and continue resuscitation as needed. Do not stop resuscitation to tie and cut the umbilical cord; someone else can do this. If you have cut the cord, monitor both ends for bleeding.

If you are assisting EMTs during transport, keep in mind that the mother may still be in labor if she has not delivered the afterbirth. She still carries the placenta, which has the other end of the umbilical cord attached to it. Move the mother carefully. If you have not tied and cut the cord, both mother and baby are still connected as a unit, and they have to be moved with great care to avoid tearing the afterbirth from the uterine wall.

Umbilical Cord

Your instructor will tell you if local protocol allows First Responders to clamp and cut the umbilical cord. If you are allowed to do so, remember that the baby can get an infection through the cord, so cut it only if you have sterile conditions. If you must cut the cord, you will need a sterile pair of scissors, a single-edged razor blade, or a sharp-edged knife. If you do not have sterile items from an OB kit, gather them from the home and soak them in isopropyl alcohol for 20 minutes or sterilize them in boiling water. There will be plenty of time to sterilize these items while you are delivering the baby. Do not touch the cutting edges or lay them on unsterile surfaces after they have been sterilized.

Cutting the umbilical cord is a usually a low priority and First Responders may provide other care until EMT or ALS personnel arrive. In most cases, if dispatch has alerted EMT or ALS personnel, they should arrive before the cord needs to be clamped or tied.

Usually, it is not necessary to tie and cut the cord until the afterbirth is delivered and the cord is empty of blood and stops pulsating. If you see or feel the cord pulsating, it is still delivering oxygen to the baby from the mother. The baby will benefit from this oxygen.

However, if during the delivery, you see that the umbilical cord is around the baby's neck, you must either slip one or two fingers under the cord and try to slip it back over the infant's head or you must cut it. If the cord cannot be slipped over the head, then quickly place clamps or ties on it and cut it. If this is not done, and the infant delivers, the cord may strangle him.

If you are allowed, take the following steps in a normal delivery when the cord has stopped pulsating (Figure 12.14):

1. Use sterile clamps or umbilical tape found in the OB kit. If you do not have a kit, then use clean shoelaces. Never use wire or string because it is too narrow and will slice the cord rather than clamp it. Tie the umbilical tape or shoelace in a square knot.

2. Apply one tie or clamp to the cord about 10 inches from the baby's belly.

3. Place a second tie or clamp about three inches closer to the baby.

4. Cut between the two ties or clamps. Never untie or unclamp a cord once it is cut. Examine the cut ends of the cord. After trapped blood drains, bleeding should stop if the clamps or ties are secure. If bleeding continues, apply another tie or clamp as close to the original as possible.

If the afterbirth delivers while you are still providing care to the baby and you are *not* allowed to cut the cord, then place the afterbirth at the same level as the baby, or slightly higher. The placenta is still the baby's blood source, and blood can continue to flow to him if the placenta is positioned as described. If the placenta is placed lower than the baby, blood can also flow away from him back into the placenta.

If the afterbirth delivers and you *are* allowed to clamp and cut the cord, do so. Advise dispatch and medical direction of the baby's delivery status.

FIGURE 12.14
Cutting the umbilical cord.

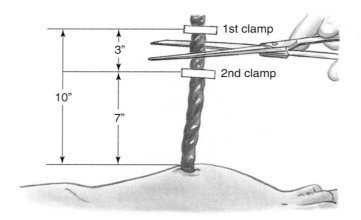

CARING FOR THE MOTHER

Care for the mother includes helping her deliver the afterbirth (the placenta and other birth tissues), controlling vaginal bleeding, making her as comfortable as possible, and providing reassurance.

Delivering the Afterbirth

The delivery of the afterbirth is the third stage of labor. It delivers anywhere from a few minutes to 20 minutes or longer after the baby is born. Some women wish to get up or assume a seated position after they deliver their babies. You may have to remind them that they will have to remain at rest until they deliver the afterbirth. Make the mother as comfortable as possible and wait for the delivery. You will both know it will be soon when she begins to have more contractions. These contractions will be milder with little discomfort.

FIRST➤ Save the placenta, all attached membranes, and all soiled sheets and towels. A physician must examine these items to ensure the entire organ and its membranes were expelled from the uterus. Try to position a basin or container at the vaginal opening so the afterbirth will deliver into it (Figure 12.15). Once you collect it, place the container in a biohazard bag. If no container is available, allow the afterbirth to deliver directly into a biohazard bag and place the bag into another biohazard bag. Always label the bag with the mother's name. ■

Controlling Vaginal Bleeding After Delivery

Bleeding from the uterus is normal after the mother has delivered the afterbirth. Blood is discharged through the vagina, is seldom a problem, and is usually easy to care for.

FIRST➤ Perform the following steps to care for vaginal bleeding after delivery:

1. Place a sanitary pad or clean towel over the vaginal opening. Do not place anything in the vagina.

2. Have the mother lower her legs and keep them together. (She does not have to squeeze them.) Elevate her legs.

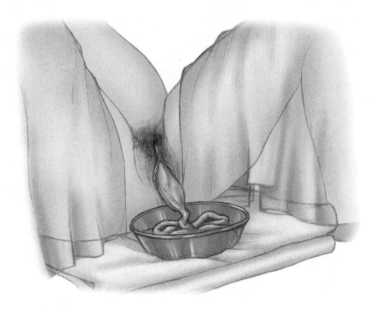

FIGURE 12.15
Collect the afterbirth and have it transported with the mother and infant. A physician must examine the placenta.

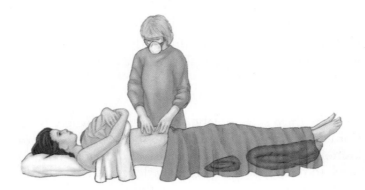

3. Feel the mother's abdomen until you find a grapefruit-size object. This is the uterus. Gently, but firmly massage from the pubis bone at the front of the pelvis upward only and toward the naval (Figure 12.16).

4. If bleeding continues, provide oxygen and maintain normal body temperature to reduce the effects of shock. Arrange transport as soon as possible and continue to massage the uterus. If the mother wishes to nurse, allow her to do so. Nursing stimulates contraction of the uterus and helps control bleeding. ■

Providing Comfort to the Mother

Talk with the mother throughout the entire birth process, explaining what you are doing and what is happening. She will especially want to know about the baby. Once you have completed your duties with the afterbirth, replace any soiled towels or sheets with clean, dry ones. If possible, wipe and dry the mother's face and hands. Make sure that both she and the baby remain warm and comfortable.

COMPLICATIONS AND EMERGENCIES

Some of the common complications and emergencies of childbirth include bleeding and other predelivery emergencies, miscarriages, prolonged labor, abnormal deliveries, premature deliveries, multiple births, and stillbirths. Keep in mind that most births are normal. Those births that produce complications often do not present with immediate problems at the scene. First Responders can often care for some of the difficulties that arise with unusual deliveries. However, some severe complications must be handled by ALS personnel and require immediate transport to a medical facility.

The risk of complications before, during, and after delivery increases when the patient has one or more of the following factors:

- Age under 18 or over age 35.

- First pregnancy or more than five pregnancies.

- Swollen face, feet, or abdomen from water retention.

- High or low blood pressure.

- Diabetes.

- Illicit drug use during pregnancy.

- History of seizures.

- Predelivery bleeding.

- Infections.

- Alcohol dependency.
- Injuries from trauma.
- Premature rupture of membranes (water broke more than a few hours before delivery).
- Using medications such as lithium carbonate, magnesium, or reserpine.

You will find out this information while taking the patient's history during the focused history and physical exam. As you assess the patient, ask her the questions necessary to see if she is in a high-risk group.

FIRST➤ Some pregnant patients develop medical problems long before they are ready to deliver. Some patients will require care for these problems before they show any outward signs of pregnancy. You may improperly assess the patient if you do not know she is pregnant. Be certain to ask the patient if she is pregnant when the patient tells you, or you notice, any of the following:

- Any new medical complaint in women of childbearing age.
- Unusual vaginal bleeding or missed menstrual period(s).
- Swelling of the face, hands, and feet.
- Headache, visual problems, apprehension, and shakiness along with upper abdominal pain.
- Nausea, vomiting, or severe abdominal pain that had a sudden onset.

Other pregnancy-related medical emergencies may present as:

- Chest pain.
- Difficulty breathing.
- Seizure. ■

Infections of the reproductive organs, especially infection by sexually transmitted diseases (STDs), may be transmitted to the baby and to you during birth. Remember to take BSI precautions and wear all personal protective equipment, which will protect you as well as the mother and the infant. Report to the hospital any information you receive from the mother about a history of infection.

PREDELIVERY EMERGENCIES

Prebirth Bleeding

FIRST➤ When a pregnant woman has vaginal bleeding early in pregnancy, it may be that she is having a miscarriage. Light, irregular discharges of blood, called *spotting*, are normal in early pregnancy but may concern the patient. If bleeding occurs late in pregnancy or while the patient is in labor, the problem may be with the placenta. Regardless of the cause of bleeding or stage of pregnancy, you will:

1. Make certain that dispatch has been advised of the situation and that additional resources are on the way.
2. Take BSI precautions and don all personal protective equipment, if you have not already done so.
3. Place the patient on her left side, but do not hold her legs together (Figure 12.17).
4. Provide care for shock, monitor the patient's airway, and administer oxygen as per local protocol.

remember

Protect yourself and the baby from STDs during childbirth by using personal protective equipment.

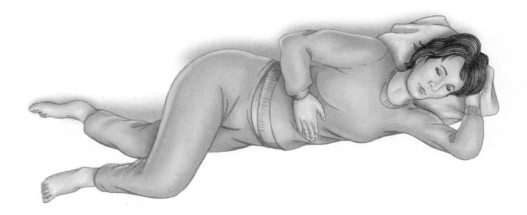

FIGURE 12.17
Position the patient to control excessive prebirth bleeding.

5. Place a sanitary pad or bulky dressings over the vaginal opening.

6. Replace pads or dressings as they become soaked. Do not place anything in the vagina.

7. Save all blood-soaked pads and dressings and any tissues that the mother passes. Place them in a biohazard bag for transport to the hospital and examination by a physician.

8. Monitor and reassure the patient while you wait for EMT or ALS personnel. ■

Miscarriage and Abortion

If the fetus delivers before it can survive on its own (before the twenty-eighth week), it is considered a **miscarriage**. The correct term for a miscarriage is a *spontaneous abortion*. However, since the word **abortion** has other meanings in our society, never use the word with a woman who is having a miscarriage or premature signs of labor.

miscarriage the natural loss of the embryo or fetus before the twenty-eighth week of pregnancy. Also called a *spontaneous abortion*.

abortion a spontaneous miscarriage or induced loss of the embryo or fetus.

FIRST➤ Miscarriage and abortion patients typically have abdominal cramps and pains. Vaginal bleeding is to be expected and can be mild to severe. In many cases, there will be vaginal discharges of bloody mucus and tissue particles.

When caring for a woman having a suspected miscarriage or following an abortion, first get a general impression of the environment and the patient, perform your initial assessment, then focus on the physical exam and patient history. Take the following steps to care for the patient:

1. Place the patient on her side, provide care for shock, and administer oxygen as per local protocols.

2. Take an initial set of vital signs and repeat them every few minutes.

3. Place a sanitary pad or bulky dressing over the vaginal opening. Do not place anything into the vagina.

4. Save all blood-soaked pads and any tissues that are passed. Place them in a biohazard bag.

5. Provide emotional support.

6. Arrange for EMT or ALS personnel to transport immediately. ■

Regardless of the cause of the emergency, the patient will need emotional support. Provide professional care, show concern, and reassure the patient.

ABNORMAL DELIVERY

See Figure 12.18 for the steps to take in the assessment of a mother in labor with signs of a complication of childbirth.

Meconium Staining

A stressful or difficult delivery affects both the mother and the baby. When the baby is stressed during delivery, he may defecate (empty the bowel). The fecal material is called *meconium*. When this material mixes with amniotic fluid, the normally clear fluid is stained green or brownish-yellow and is called **meconium staining**. If the baby inhales this fluid on his first attempt to breathe, he will develop aspiration pneumonia, a lung infection caused by aspirating (breathing in) the meconium.

Sometimes the amniotic sac will rupture many hours before delivery. You will have to rely on information from the mother to determine if the fluids were clear or stained. Ask the mother if she noticed the color of the fluid when her water broke. If you witness the rupture, look for meconium staining. Be prepared to wipe the baby's mouth and nose and to suction.

BREECH BIRTH

In a **breech birth**, the buttocks or both feet (not just one) present and deliver first. Even in this position, the baby can be born without complications. As the buttocks and trunk deliver together, place one hand and forearm under the baby for support. Be sure to also support the head as it delivers. A breech birth can be a complication if the baby's head will not deliver.

FIRST➤ In a breech birth, when the baby's head does not deliver within **three minutes** after the buttocks and trunk, you must immediately notify dis-

meconium staining amniotic fluid that has a green or brownish-yellow color from fetal fecal contamination, which occurs when the fetus is stressed.

remember

In your focused history and physical exam, ask about and look for meconium staining after the amniotic sac has ruptured.

breech birth a birth in which the buttocks or both feet deliver first.

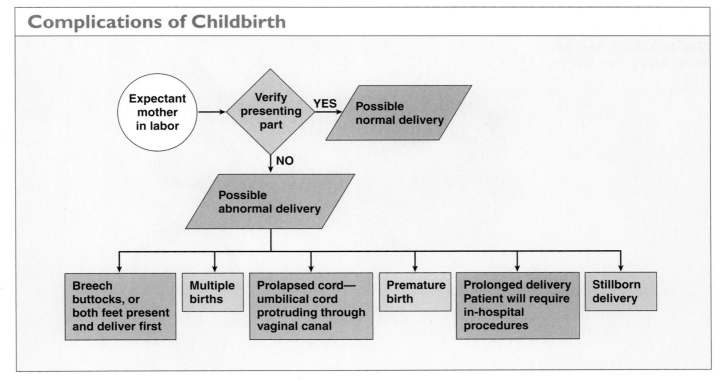

Complications of Childbirth

FIGURE 12.18

patch to alert responding EMT or ALS personnel. They must transport the mother and infant as soon as possible. While waiting for them to arrive, do the following:

1. Place the mother on a high concentration of oxygen.

2. Create an airway for the baby because the umbilical cord will be compressed between the infant and vaginal wall, shutting off blood flow. Tell the mother what you must do and why. Insert your gloved hand into the vagina, with your palm toward the baby's face. Form a "V" by placing one finger on each side of the baby's nose (Figure 12.19). Push the wall of the birth canal away from the baby's face. If you cannot complete this process, then try to place one fingertip into the infant's mouth and push away the birth canal wall with your other fingers.

3. Maintain the airway. Once you have created an airway for the baby, keep the airway open. **Do not pull on the baby.** Allow delivery to take place while you continue to support the baby's body and head.

4. If the head does not deliver in three minutes after you have created an airway, it is necessary to have the mother and infant transported to a medical facility immediately. Maintain the airway throughout *all* stages of care until higher-level EMS personnel relieve you. ■

Limb Presentation

The presentation of an arm or a single leg is not a breech birth. It is called a *limb presentation* and is an emergency requiring EMT or ALS personnel to transport the mother to a medical facility immediately. Ask dispatch to notify EMT or ALS responders of the emergency. Do *not* pull on the limb or try to place your gloved hand into the birth canal. Do *not* try to place the limb back into the vagina. Place the mother in the knee-chest position (Figure 12.20) to help reduce pressure on

remember

Call for immediate ALS assistance and transport for all limb presentations.

FIGURE 12.19
Create and maintain an airway for the baby during a breech birth.

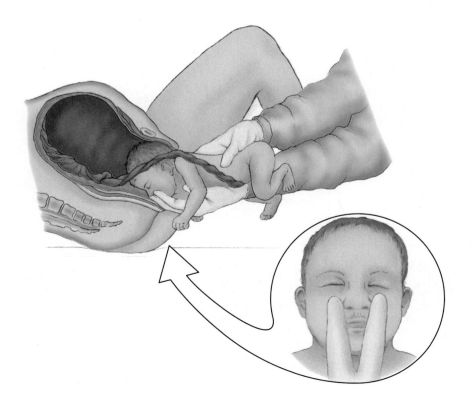

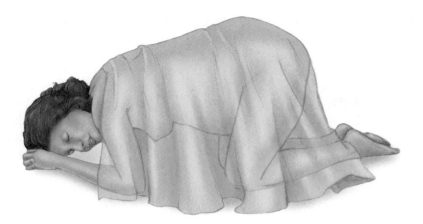

the fetus and the umbilical cord. Medical direction and protocols may instruct you to keep the mother in the typical delivery position. Follow your protocols.

Prolapsed Cord

First➤ When you examine the mother for crowning, you may find the umbilical cord protruding from the vaginal opening. When the umbilical cord delivers first, this is called a **prolapsed cord** and is common in a breech birth. Call for EMT or ALS personnel to transport the mother with a prolapsed cord to a medical facility immediately.

A prolapsed cord endangers the life of the baby. As the baby emerges through the vaginal opening, his head presses the umbilical cord against the vaginal wall, reducing or completely cutting off blood flow and oxygen. When oxygen flow through the cord is obstructed, the baby will try to breathe. But since the baby's face is pressed against the wall of the birth canal, the mouth and nose cannot take in air. To help the baby breathe, provide an airway, using the same methods described for breech birth. That is, place your fingers into the vaginal opening in front of the infant's face and make a "V." Do not try to push the cord back into the birth canal.

In addition, take the following steps. (Check with medical direction or your protocols to find out what First Responders are allowed to do.)

prolapsed cord a potential birth complication in which the umbilical cord presents through the vaginal opening before the baby's head. It is a birth complication if pressure from the baby's head compresses the cord during birth and cuts off oxygen and blood to the baby.

- Place the mother in a knee-chest position to reduce pressure on the cord.
- Try to maintain a pulse in the cord.
- Place wet dressings (use sterile water or saline if it is available) over the cord to keep it moist.
- Wrap the cord in a towel or dressings to keep it warm.
- Provide the mother with a high concentration of oxygen as soon as possible.
- Monitor vital signs and arrange for transport immediately. ■

NOTE: *The baby's chances for survival improve if you can keep the head from pressing on the umbilical cord and keep the cord pulsating. Check with your instructor to see if protocols allow you to insert several fingers into the mother's vagina and gently push up on the baby's head to keep pressure off the cord.*

Multiple Births

Multiple births are not necessarily abnormal. However, they do frequently involve premature delivery. Premature infants may not be fully developed and often have respiratory complications. If the mother is giving birth to more than one infant, she will have contractions begin again shortly after the birth of the first baby. These contractions may deliver the afterbirth of the first or another baby. If more than one baby is in the uterus, the mother's abdomen will remain rather large. Ask the mother if she has been told to expect twins (or more).

The procedures for assisting the mother remain the same. Normally, you will tie or clamp the cord of the first baby before the second baby is born, if the umbilical cord has stopped pulsating. Check with your instructor about the protocols in your area for caring for the cords in multiple baby births. Once the babies are delivered and they are breathing, assess each one, noting skin color (blue, dusky, pale), any deformities, strength of their cries, and whether they move on their own or just lie still. After a few minutes, note if there are any changes in these conditions. Perform resuscitation if necessary. Document the time of birth for each baby. Call for assistance as soon as possible.

Premature Births

Any baby weighing less than 5-1/2 pounds at birth is considered **premature**. Any baby born before the thirty-seventh week (prior to the ninth month) of pregnancy is considered premature. If the mother tells you the baby is early by more than two weeks, play it safe and consider the baby to be premature.

In addition to the procedures for normal births, you must take special steps to keep a premature baby warm. It is important to dry the baby. Wrap him in a blanket, sheet, towel, or aluminum foil (fold the edges of the foil to avoid cutting the baby). A blanket covered with foil is ideal. There are also commercial wraps available, which your unit may carry or your department may purchase. Cover the baby's head, but keep its face uncovered. Transfer the baby to a warm environment (90°F to 100°F), but do not place a heat source too close to the baby. Ventilate a premature baby who needs resuscitation using a mouth-to-mask technique or an appropriately sized bag-valve mask (see Appendix 2). Wipe or suction blood and mucus from the mouth and nose first before ventilating.

Stillborn Deliveries

Some infants are born dead and are called *stillborn*. Some die shortly after birth. Either event is very sad for the mother and father, family members, and care providers. Do not feel embarrassed to show your emotions, but be prepared to continue to act professionally and provide comfort to the mother, father, and other family members who are present.

If the infant shows no signs of life at birth (no attempts to breath and move) or goes into respiratory or cardiac arrest, provide the resuscitation measures described earlier in this chapter and in Chapter 8. Do *not* stop resuscitation until the baby regains respirations and a heartbeat, other emergency care providers relieve you, or you are too exhausted to continue.

There are cases in which a baby has died hours or longer before birth. Do not attempt to resuscitate a stillborn infant that has large blisters and a strong unpleasant odor. There may be other indications that the infant died earlier in the uterus such as a very soft head, swollen body parts, or obvious deformities.

OTHER EMERGENCIES

Trauma

Vital signs of a pregnant woman are usually different from a woman who is not pregnant. A pregnant woman's blood volume increases up to about 30% to 45%, a natural protection and preparation for the mother who will lose blood during delivery. Her heart rate increases by about 15 beats per minute, and her blood pressure falls 10-15 mmHg. Do not mistake the high pulse rate and low blood pressure

---

premature baby a baby that is born before the thirty-seventh week (prior to the ninth month) of pregnancy. Any baby with a birth weight of less than 5-1/2 pounds.

for signs of shock in the normal non-trauma pregnant woman. But in a trauma situation, the larger blood volume allows the mother's body to compensate for blood loss and may not show early signs of shock.

A pregnant woman can lose almost 40% of her maternal blood volume before she shows any signs of shock. In shock, the mother's body shunts blood away from the uterus first. Less blood to the uterus affects the fetus, causing harm well before the mother shows any signs. Blood loss may be internal and not obvious to the First Responder. Always suspect internal bleeding in any pregnant trauma patient, even if she seems to be initially unharmed and shows normal vital signs for a pregnant woman. Even if the mother is not injured, the fetus may be injured in an advanced pregnancy.

During the scene size up, look carefully at the environment, the patient, and the mechanism of injury. Try to determine what injuries might have been caused (Figure 12.21). Two common types of trauma that can cause significant harm to the mother and the fetus are blunt force and penetrating injuries:

- Blunt force injuries: common in falls, vehicle crashes, abuse, and assaults.

- Penetrating injuries: usually a result of gunshot wounds and stabbings or punctures from the debris of the auto wreckage.

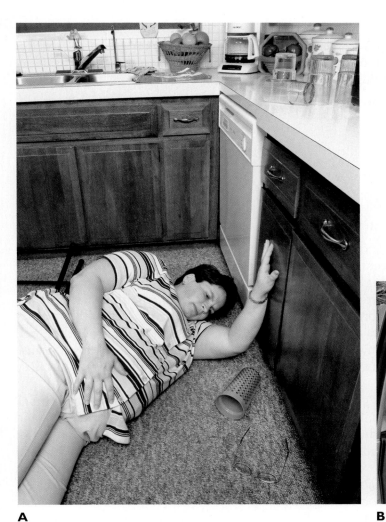

A

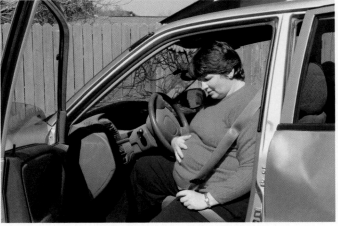

B

FIGURE 12.21

Look at the mechanism of injury and try to determine the possible injuries the mother may have received and the forces she was exposed to.

During the early months of pregnancy when the fetus is small, the fluids in the amniotic sac provide some protection from blunt force trauma. As the fetus grows, and especially in the last two months of pregnancy, blunt force trauma can cause more damage to the fetus. As a result, First Responders should provide direct care for the mother and indirect care for the fetus.

The greatest danger to both the mother and the baby is bleeding and shock. First ensure an airway and breathing and look for and control external bleeding. Provide a high concentration of oxygen as soon as possible and keep the patient warm but do not overheat her. The steps that prevent or care for shock will assist the fetus also. Arrange for immediate transport, and while waiting for EMT or ALS personnel to arrive, provide appropriate care based on the mechanism of injury, such as immobilization for possible spinal injuries, splinting for possible fractures, and dressing wounds.

In advanced pregnancies, the large fetus can press on the mother's inferior vena cava when she is lying on her back (supine) and restrict blood return to the heart, causing a condition called *supine hypotensive* (low blood pressure) *syndrome*. This condition greatly affects the fetus. If you immobilize an injured pregnant woman on a spine board, raise the right side of the board slightly and support it with rolled blankets or pillows. The weight of the fetus will shift to the left and off the vena cava, allowing better blood flow (venous return) to the heart.

Vaginal Bleeding

There are many reasons for excessive vaginal bleeding during pregnancy. First Responders must be aware of them and look carefully for the mechanism of injury that caused them, including the following:

- Blunt force and penetrating trauma.
- Intercourse.
- Sexual assault.
- Reproductive organ problems.
- Abnormal pregnancy.
- Placental tears and uterine rupture.

There are two types of placenta tears: *placenta previa* and *placenta abruptio*. In placenta previa the placenta lies low in the uterus and attaches itself over the opening of the cervix, meaning it would have to emerge before, or previous to, the fetus during birth. In this position, the placenta tears and bleeds when the cervix dilates during labor. Placenta abruptio can occur in a trauma situation when the force of the trauma abruptly tears the placenta partially or completely away from the wall of the uterus. The pregnant woman may have major internal blood loss because blood can be trapped between the placenta and the uterine wall. She may also lose blood vaginally.

The only indications you may have of internal blood loss and developing shock are changes in vital signs, feeling a hard uterus when examining the abdomen, and the mother's complaint that her abdomen is painful or tender. Get an initial set of baseline vital signs as soon as possible in your assessment and monitor the vital signs by retaking them every few minutes. Provide her with a high concentration of oxygen as soon as possible and maintain body temperature to help reduce the effects of shock. Arrange for immediate transport.

It is possible that the uterus will rupture in a rapid deceleration injury (vehicle crash) or with a direct compression injury (vehicle crash or blunt force injury). A ruptured uterus is almost always fatal to the fetus. The mother will bleed severely, and she will have a tender abdomen that is no longer large and evenly round but asymmetrical. When you palpate the abdomen, the mother complains of tenderness, and you may feel the head, arms, or legs of the fetus through the abdominal wall. The mother will quickly lose blood and go into shock. Provide a high concentration of oxygen and arrange for immediate transport.

The care for controlling vaginal bleeding includes the following:

- Place sanitary pads or bulky dressings over the vaginal opening.

- Replace pads or dressings as they become soaked.

- Do not place anything in the vagina.

- Save all blood-soaked pads and dressings. Place them in a biohazard bag for transport to the hospital and examination by physician.

Sexual Assault

Sexual assault or rape is always a psychologically and physically traumatic experience. The First Responder's professional manner, attitude, and emotional support are important steps in the care of the expectant mother who has been assaulted.

As the woman struggles or resists the attacker, and as the attacker uses force to make her submit, she can receive many types of injuries to the external soft tissues, the vaginal canal and the internal organs, and the musculoskeletal system. The fetus is also a victim in the assault. The injuries that the fetus receives may be direct from blows to the abdomen, or indirect as a result of injuries to the mother. The emotional trauma to the woman may be greater initially than the physical trauma.

You may have multiple roles to perform as a First Responder who is caring for a pregnant woman. You may have to provide care for injuries, including spinal immobilization, extremity splinting, and wound dressing. In sexual assault cases, you will need to provide emotional support and protect the patient from embarrassment from onlookers. Do not clean the vaginal area. Do not let the patient wash. Do not let her go to the bathroom. If she insists on cleaning herself and changing clothes, you cannot stop her. You should advise her that hospital personnel would be able to collect evidence from her that will help identify and convict the rapist. First Responders should collect clothing and any items that were used during the assault for examination and legal needs. Transport evidence in a paper container or wrap them in a towel. Do not place them in plastic.

For any emotional, violent, or traumatic injury and for complicated deliveries, provide care that will prevent or manage shock and arrange transport as soon as possible. Promote patient confidence by providing emotional support and physical comfort. Listen to your patient and talk to her throughout all procedures. You will find that some roles come easily. Other roles will take knowledge, practice, and skill.

Chapter Review

Begin caring for the pregnant mother by letting her know that you are a First Responder. Alert dispatch and gather all supplies and materials needed for delivery and for post-delivery care of the mother and baby.

Perform an initial and a focused assessment and determine if the mother is about to deliver. Ask if this is her first labor and how far apart the contractions are. Ask if she feels pressure or if she has the urge to move her bowels. Ask if her water has broken and if there was green or brownish-yellow discoloration (meconium staining). Ask if she feels the urge to push.

If you believe that birth may occur before the mother can be safely transported to the nearest hospital, provide the mother with as much privacy as possible. Position her on her back with her knees bent, feet flat, and legs spread apart. If this position makes her feel dizzy, position her slightly on her left side. Ensure your own protection by wearing gloves, mask, eye shield, and a gown. Remove any clothing obstructing your view of the vaginal opening. See if any part of the baby is visible or becomes visible **(crowning)** during contractions.

Assist the mother as she delivers her baby. It is normal if the skin between the vaginal and rectal openings **(perineum)** tears during delivery. Carefully support the baby's head as it is born. Spread your fingers flat around the baby's head. A slight, evenly distributed pressure will prevent an explosive birth. Provide support for the baby's entire body and head as birth proceeds.

If the umbilical cord is around the baby's neck, gently loosen the cord with your fingers and slip it over the baby's head. If the amniotic sac has not ruptured, puncture the sac and pull it away from the baby's mouth and nose.

For care of the newly born baby, clear the airway and be sure that he is breathing. If he is not breathing, encourage him to do so by rubbing his back or by snapping your index finger on the soles of his feet. For nonbreathing babies, provide ventilations at 40 to 60 breaths per minute. If using a bag-valve mask, only use one that is an appropriate size. After ventilating for 30 seconds, check the heart rate. If the heart rate is 100 beats per minute or greater, gradually reduce assisted ventilations. Gently rub the baby's back to maintain and improve his breathing and continue to provide oxygen. If the baby's respirations are inade-

quate or the heart rate is below 100 beats per minute, assist ventilations with a bag-valve mask. If the heart rate is less than 60 beats per minute, continue to assist ventilations and begin chest compressions. Perform CPR with either your fingertips or your thumbs with your hands encircling the chest. Continue resuscitation until the baby has spontaneous heart and lung actions.

Your local protocols may require you to tie or clamp the cord. Do not tie, clamp, or cut the cord until the baby is breathing on his own (unless you must start CPR).

Assist the mother as she delivers the afterbirth. Save all tissues for transport. Control vaginal bleeding by placing clean pads over the vaginal opening and massaging her abdomen from the pubic bone upward. Allow the mother to nurse her baby. Replace wet towels and sheets with clean, dry ones. Wipe clean the mother's face and hands.

Throughout the birth process, provide emotional support to the mother.

Be ready for complications during a delivery. Look for **meconium staining.** Provide an airway with your fingers in cases of **breech birth** and **prolapsed cord.** Maintain this airway until the baby is born or until you turn the mother over to more highly trained professionals. The EMS system should transport all mothers when there are emergencies that pose immediate life-threats to the baby (prolapsed umbilical cord or **limb presentation**). If there is severe bleeding before delivery, place pads at the vaginal opening, provide care for shock (hypoperfusion), and arrange for transport as soon as possible.

Expect a multiple birth if the abdomen is still large and contractions of the same intensity continue after a first baby is born. When possible, tie or clamp the umbilical cord of the first baby before the next baby is born.

Keep all babies warm. It is especially critical to keep premature babies warm. Be prepared to resuscitate premature babies.

In cases of a possible miscarriage, provide emotional support to the mother. Place pads at her vaginal opening if there is bleeding. Save all blood-soaked pads and any passed tissues and place them in a biohazard bag for transport and examination. Provide care for shock.

For stillborn infants, remain professional and provide emotional support to the mother, father, and other family members.

When the mother is involved in trauma, sexual assault, or is bleeding heavily from the vagina, care for injuries and provide emotional support. The greatest danger to both mother and baby is bleeding and shock. The pregnant mother's increased blood volume compensates for blood loss and masks the signs of shock. Provide a high concentration of oxygen and maintain body temperature. Transport as soon as possible.

IMPORTANT: *Avoid the risk of infection by taking appropriate BSI precautions when caring for patients. Wear all appropriate personal protective equipment including gloves, mask, eye shields, and gown to avoid contact with the patient's blood, body fluids, wastes, and mucous membranes. Don gloves and face protection before checking for crowning in a woman in active labor. Put on a gown to assist delivery.*

REMEMBER AND CONSIDER

✔ Does your response unit carry any supplies for assisting in childbirth?

Check your station or department and your unit or first responder kits. Find out where the supplies are kept. Do you have a commercial package or have company members created a special "jump bag" or OB kit for childbirth incidents? What would you put into a childbirth jump bag or kit? Find out how many childbirths your unit or personnel have responded to in this past year. Why do you think there are so few, or so many, in your area? Will obstetric patients go to the local hospital or to a specialized one? Are there separate birthing centers in your area? Do they handle only normal deliveries or complicated ones as well? Visit a birthing center and obtain additional information on childbirth and delivery.

INVESTIGATE...

✔ After you have checked for childbirth supplies, ask your supervisor or supply officer about the procedure for replacing used items. Many childbirth items, such as gauze pads and trauma dressings, are used for wound care and trauma management as well. Ask if it would be practical to keep childbirth items in a separate cabinet, jump bag, or kit. Offer to set up, stock, and monitor supplies and replace them as needed. When extra dressings are needed for trauma emergencies, the childbirth dressings will be used, and supplies that were set aside for childbirth may be overlooked when personnel replace items after an incident.

✔ Assisting childbirth in the field is rare, but First Responders must be ready for the event. If you have a training officer, ask if he or she is planning a drill or refresher class on childbirth. Find out what you can do to help prepare for or present the program. County and state training agencies will have films you can borrow. Health departments will have materials and information for handouts. Obstetricians from local hospitals will be interested in speaking to emergency personnel who will be responsible for assisting childbirth in the out-of-hospital situation.

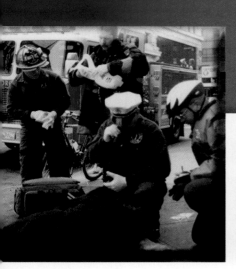
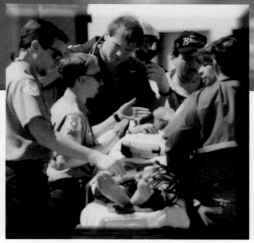
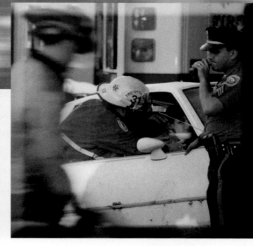

Infants and Children

This chapter introduces methods used in providing care for pediatric medical and trauma emergencies. It also takes into account the fact that children can be the First Responder's most difficult patients. They must be managed and cared for differently than adults, because of their age, physical and mental development, personalities, and experiences. Children respond well to familiar, normal routines and have difficulty handling strange situations and unfamiliar adults, including First Responders, who suddenly arrive in their environment to look at them and handle them. Seriously ill and injured children also provoke strong emotions. But through training and practice, First Responders can increase their professional confidence and manage the pediatric incident calmly and effectively. As a result, pediatric patients will find an empathetic care provider in the First Responder.

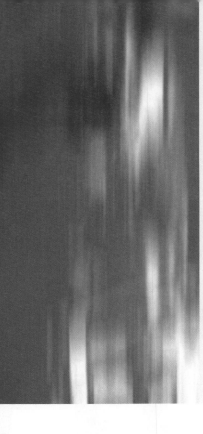

NATIONAL STANDARD OBJECTIVES

This chapter focuses on the objectives of Module 6, Lesson 6-2, of the U.S. DOT First Responder National Standard Curriculum and serves as an instructional aid to help you meet any specific objectives added to the course by your local EMS system.

By the end of this chapter, you will be able to (from cognitive or knowledge information):

6–2.1 Describe differences in anatomy and physiology of the infant, child, and adult patient. (pp. 461, 463–466)

6–2.2 Describe assessment of the infant or child. (pp. 466–470)

6–2.3 Indicate various causes of respiratory emergencies in infants and children. (pp. 471–474)

6–2.4 Summarize emergency medical care strategies for respiratory distress and respiratory failure/arrest in infants and children. (pp. 471–474)

6–2.5 List common causes of seizures in the infant and child patient. (pp. 474–475)

6–2.6 Describe management of seizures in the infant and child patient. (pp. 474–475)

6–2.7 Discuss emergency medical care of the infant and child trauma patient. (pp. 481–494)

6–2.8 Summarize the signs and symptoms of possible child abuse and neglect. (pp. 487–494)

6–2.9 Describe the medical-legal responsibilities in suspected child abuse. (pp. 490, 491, 492, 493, 494)

LEARNING TASKS

This chapter describes some of the many characteristics of children. The text and your instructor will help you understand how to handle children in many types of emergency situations. No emergency is routine, but with some experience you will become confident with what to do. With pediatric patients, though, you will find you may have to adjust your approach and care. As you read this chapter, think about and be able to:

✔ State the special problems that may arise when caring for the pediatric patient.
✔ Describe the changes in the approach to care when dealing with infants and children.

As children develop, their physical and emotional characters change. As they grow and get older, they also want to be treated differently, but may often regress when faced with a frightening emergency. Think about children you know and how they act in different situations. Then talk with classmates and members at your station about the response of children in different age groups and how to handle them. Be able to:

✔ List the age categories of infants and children.
✔ List some methods to use that will help in interacting with pediatric patients.

First Responder units may or may not carry oxygen. If your unit does, you will want to learn how to administer it. Your instructor will show you the equipment, demonstrate how to use it, and let you practice. Once you have learned how to operate the equipment, also be able to:

✔ Describe the methods and devices used for delivering oxygen to pediatric patients.

Children are afraid of strangers, and they can be most uncooperative when frightened by an emergency. Think about how children might respond, recall your

6–2.10 Recognize the need for First Responder debriefing following a difficult infant or child transport. (pp. 456, 494)

Feel comfortable enough to
(by changing attitudes, values, and beliefs):

6–2.11 Attend to the feelings of the family when dealing with an ill or injured infant or child. (pp. 460, 461, 470, 473, 478)

6–2.12 Understand the provider's own emotional response to caring for infants or children. (pp. 456, 490, 494)

6–2.13 Demonstrate a caring attitude towards infants and children with illness or injury who require emergency medical services. (pp. 456–457, 460–461, 462–463, 491)

6–2.14 Place the interests of the infant or child with an illness or injury as the foremost consideration when making any and all patient-care decisions. (pp. 456–457, 460–461, 462–463, 493)

6–2.15 Communicate with empathy to infants and children with an illness or injury, as well as with family members and friends of the patient. (pp. 460, 461, 470, 473, 478, 490–491, 492)

Show how to
(through psychomotor skills):

6–2.16 Demonstrate assessment of the infant and child. (pp. 466–470)

patient assessment steps, and discuss how you could approach children to gain their confidence. Be able to:

✔ List the steps for performing a scene size-up, initial assessment, focused history and physical exam, detailed physical exam, and ongoing assessment for infant and child patients. Highlight the steps that are unique to infants and children.

You will provide emergency care to infants and children that is similar to the care you would provide to an adult. Recall some emergency situations and be able to:

✔ List assessment and care concerns for the pediatric patient who has signs and symptoms of fever, hypothermia, vomiting and diarrhea, and suspected neglect and abuse.

✔ Describe the care you will provide to the patient in suspected child abuse situations.

✔ List the signs and symptoms of shock and describe emergency care.

✔ List the causes and signs of altered mental status.

✔ Describe the steps to take with an infant and his parents when managing a sudden infant death syndrome (SIDS) incident.

✔ Define shaken baby syndrome and describe its signs.

By the time you finish reading the chapter and working with your instructor and other classmates, you will feel comfortable with what you know. In class, you will begin to practice the skills you need to perform when responding to infant and child emergencies. Take every opportunity to practice in and out of class so you can:

✔ Demonstrate on an infant or child manikin the emergency care for trauma emergencies, including care for shock, burns, and spinal injuries.

✔ Demonstrate on an infant or child manikin the emergency care for medical emergencies, including airway obstruction, respiratory infection, fever, asthma, seizures, altered mental status, poisoning, near drowning, and sudden infant death syndrome (SIDS).

✔ Discuss how to work with the parents of children who are hooked up to technical medical equipment at home and need emergency care.

INTRODUCTION

Responding to a call for a child's illness or injury can be stressful for the First Responder. Some situations will make you feel sad or angry. You will not be able to express your emotions in front of the child or parent. When faced with the assessment and care of an infant or a child, you may at first feel that you do not know what to do or where to start. An anxious, fretful, or frightened child who cannot be comforted may further add to your stress level and reduce your confidence. Remember that many of the assessment and care techniques used for adults are the same for children, with some modifications. These modifications take into account the child's age, physical development, and emotional response.

After caring for the child and dealing with the parents, be aware of how you feel. Do not hesitate to talk with other care providers, support groups, or your family about your feelings. You will not have to go through the tough, stressful calls by yourself. Knowing that others have gone through the same emotions can help you become more comfortable with your own.

First Responders who are unsure of what to do in pediatric emergencies are likely to have a stronger emotional response during and after an incident than those who are prepared and confident in their actions. By training, practicing, and drilling to prepare for pediatric incidents, you will not only improve your confidence and decrease your stress but improve patient outcome as well.

Following are some methods that will help you understand and care for pediatric patients.

CHARACTERISTICS OF INFANTS AND CHILDREN

Everyone has some fear of the unknown. Since so many things are unknown to a child, it is easy to see why emergencies can be so frightening for them. A severe illness or injury is a new and unknown experience for children, and it is an experience that increases their anxiety, especially if parents are not there. For most children, security comes from their parents. Wanting parents may be a child's first priority, even above having you offer help, comfort, or relief of pain.

FIRST➤ When you are dealing with children, you need to gain their trust. You can attempt to calm and reassure them by using the following techniques:

- Approach them slowly, establish contact from a safe distance, and ask permission to get closer. Offering them something (a toy of their own or one you brought) may also help to prevent them from feeling threatened by your approach. (Many first response units carry teddy bears for their pediatric patients.)
- Let them know that someone will call their parents.
- Sit down with them so you are at their level. Standing makes you appear large and frightening.
- Let them see your face and expressions. You want to appear friendly, yet concerned and willing to listen. Speak directly to them. Speak clearly and slowly so that they can hear and understand you. Keep your voice gentle and calm even when you need to be firm. Try not to raise your voice or talk loudly to a

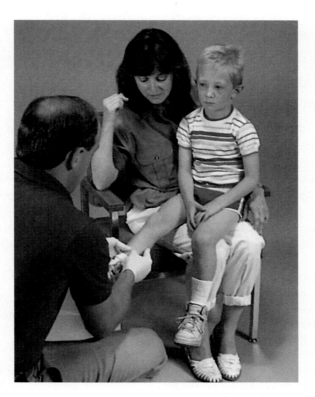

crying or screaming child. Some children are bashful or uncomfortable with strangers and may not look at you. Try to maintain eye contact (Figure 13.1).

- Pause frequently to find out if they understand what you have said or asked. Even if you communicate easily with your own children, never assume that other children understand you. Find out by asking questions.

- Quickly determine if there are any life-threatening problems and care for them immediately (Scan 13-1). If there are no immediate life threats, continue with patient assessment at a relaxed pace. Avoid moving children if possible. Movement may cause additional injury or, with certain medical problems, extreme responses. Children may be frightened by a rapid-pace exam and a stranger's questions. Alert young children may become frightened if you start your exam with their head and face. If children show fear as you reach out to touch them, begin the physical examination at the feet and slowly work your way up to the head, if they are not critically injured. While you are performing this toe-to-head assessment, you can look for the same signs of illness and injury as you do when assessing the adult patient. Take time, though, to consider special assessment needs based on the anatomy of the child (Figure 13.2).

- Always tell children what you are going to do before each step of the patient assessment. Do not try to explain the entire procedure at once. Explain one step, do it, then explain the next step.

- **Never lie to children.** Tell them if it will hurt when you are examining them. If children ask if they are sick or hurt, tell the truth; but reassure them by saying that you are there to help, and other people also will be helping. While you talk and work with them, smile. It carries a lot of weight with most children.

- Offer comfort to children by stroking their foreheads or holding their hands. Children will let you know if they do not want to be touched. Most children have learned from parents and teachers that they should not let strangers touch them. Special child safety programs make children aware of what kind of touching is allowable and what is a "good touch" or a "bad touch." Children

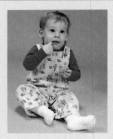

INFANTS

Birth to 1 Year

- Perform a scene size-up. In your initial assessment, get a general impression from a distance.
- Control your emotions and facial expressions to help reduce the child's fear.
- Protect the head and spine.
- Ensure an adequate airway. If needed, provide ventilations.
- Provide care to prevent shock. (A small amount of blood loss can cause shock.)

Establishing Responsiveness: The infant should move or cry when gently tapped or shaken. Is he alert, responsive to voice or to pain stimulus, or unresponsive?

Opening the Airway: Use slight head-tilt, chin-lift. (Use the jaw-thrust for possible spinal injury.)

Evaluating Breathing: If the infant is responsive but cyanotic, struggling to breathe, or has inadequate breathing, arrange for immediate transport. If the infant is unresponsive, look, listen, and feel for breathing. If there is no breathing, provide breaths.

Providing Breaths: Provide two ventilations while watching the chest rise. Ventilate with the mouth-to-mask technique, using an appropriate pediatric-size mask or a pediatric bag-valve mask. If there is evidence of airway obstruction, clear the airway.

Clearing the Airway

- Make certain that you have not overextended or under-extended the neck. Place a folded towel under shoulders to keep the head in a neutral position. If this does not open the airway, then . . .
- Place the infant over the length of your arm face down with the head lower than the trunk. Support the head with your hand placed around the jaw. Support your fore-arm by placing it on your thigh.
- Deliver five back blows between the shoulder blades with the heel of your free hand.
- Place your free arm on the infant's back and support the back of his head with that hand. Sandwich him between your arms and hands and turn him over. Support your arm on your thigh. Keep the head lower than the trunk and deliver five chest thrusts. If the airway remains ob-structed, but the patient is responsive, continue back blows and chest thrusts.
- If the airway remains obstructed, and the patient is unre-sponsive, wrap your fingers around the lower jaw, place your (gloved) thumb inside the mouth, and pull the mouth open to look for an obstruction.
- Do not attempt blind finger sweeps. You must see the ob-ject before you sweep the mouth with your little finger.
- Even if you did not see or dislodge an obstruction, give two breaths and repeat: reposition the head, attempt to ventilate, give back blows and chest thrusts, look for and remove visible obstructions, and attempt to ventilate again.

Continuing Rescue Breathing

- If patient is still not breathing but you gave two successful breaths, check for a brachial pulse (infant); or listen for

the heartbeat with your ear or a stethoscope over the chest or feel for a pulse at the base of the umbilical cord (newborn).

- If there is a pulse, but no breathing, continue to breathe giving 20 breaths a minute (one every 3 seconds) for the infant and 40 to 60 breaths a minute (one every 1 to 1-1/2 seconds) for the newborn. If there is no pulse, start CPR.

Performing CPR

- If the patient is unresponsive and not breathing, open the airway and look, listen, and feel for breathing. If there are no breaths, provide two initial breaths. (Assure the chest rises.) If there is no indication of obstruction, but the patient is unresponsive and is not breathing, check pulse.
- Check brachial pulse (infant) or listen for heartbeat with your ear or a stethoscope over the chest or feel the base of the umbilical cord (newborn). If there is no pulse and no breathing, start CPR. If you are alone, do CPR for one minute before calling dispatch.
- Start compressions. For the infant, the compression site is one finger-width below an imaginary line drawn across the nipples. Compress with the tips of two or three fin-gers 1/2 to 1 inch or approximately 1/3 to 1/2 the depth of the chest at a rate of at least 100 per minute. For the newborn, use overlapping or side-by-side thumbs and compress on the middle third of the sternum just below the nipple line. The remaining fingers encircle the chest and support the back. Compress 1/2 to 3/4 inch deep at a rate of at least 120 per minute.
- Deliver a ventilation once every five compressions for the infant and once every three compressions for the newborn.
- Check for a pulse after the first minute, then every few minutes.

Controlling Bleeding

- Use direct pressure as a primary method to control bleeding.
- If bleeding is not controlled, use elevation combined with direct pressure. If bleeding is still not controlled, use pres-sure points combined with elevation and direct pressure.
- A small amount of blood loss (25 milliliters) is serious. Care for shock.

continued...

Pediatric Emergencies—Initial Assessment and Basic Life Support

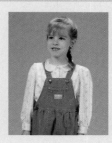

CHILDREN

1 to 8 Years

- Perform a scene size-up. In your initial assessment, get a general impression from a distance.
- Control your emotions and facial expressions to help reduce the child's fear.
- Protect the head and spine. A child's head is proportionately larger than her body.
- Ensure an adequate airway. If needed, provide ventilations as you watch for the chest to rise.
- Evaluate blood loss. Provide care to prevent shock. (A small amount of blood loss can cause shock.)

CAUTION: A child's size and weight may be more important than age when providing care.

Establishing Responsiveness: The child should move or cry when gently tapped or shaken.

Opening the Airway: Use slight head-tilt, chin-lift or jaw-thrust, as appropriate.

Evaluating Breathing: If the child is responsive but cyanotic or struggling and failing to breathe, arrange for immediate transport. If the child is in respiratory arrest, open the airway and look, listen, and feel for breathing. If there is no breathing, provide breaths.

Providing Breaths: Provide two ventilations while watching the chest rise. Ventilate with the mouth-to-mask technique, using an appropriate pediatric-size mask or a pediatric bag-valve mask. If there is evidence of airway obstruction, clear the airway.

Clearing the Airway

- Make certain that you have the proper head-tilt for an unresponsive child. Place a folded towel under shoulders to keep the head in a neutral position. If this does not open the airway, then . . .
- Rapidly deliver five abdominal thrusts for the unresponsive child.
- If the airway remains obstructed, and the patient is responsive, continue with abdominal thrusts.
- If the airway remains obstructed, and the child is unresponsive, place her on her back on a hard surface. Wrap your fingers around the lower jaw and pull the mouth open to look for an obstruction.
- Do not attempt blind finger sweeps. You must see the object before you sweep the mouth. Use your little finger.
- Even if you did not see or dislodge an obstruction, attempt to give two breaths and repeat: reposition the head, attempt to ventilate, provide abdominal thrusts, look for and remove visible obstructions, and attempt to ventilate again.

Continuing Rescue Breathing

- If patient is still not breathing but you gave two successful breaths, check for a carotid pulse.
- If there is a pulse, but no breathing, continue to provide breaths at a rate of 20 per minute. If there is no pulse, start CPR.

Performing CPR

- If the patient is unresponsive and not breathing, open the airway and look, listen, and feel for breathing. If there are no breaths, provide two initial breaths. (Assure the chest rises.) If there is no indication of obstruction, but the patient is unresponsive and is not breathing, check pulse.
- Check carotid pulse. If there is no pulse and no breathing, start CPR. Have someone call dispatch. If you are alone, do CPR for one minute before calling.
- Start compressions with the heel of one hand.
- Depress sternum 1 to 1-1/2 inches or approximately 1/3 to 1/2 the depth of the chest.
- Deliver compressions at a rate of 100 per minute.
- Deliver a ventilation once every five compressions.
- Check for a carotid pulse after the first minute, then every few minutes.

Controlling Bleeding

- Use direct pressure as a primary method to control bleeding.
- If bleeding is not controlled, use elevation combined with direct pressure. If bleeding is still not controlled, use pressure points combined with elevation and direct pressure.
- A blood loss of 1/2 liter (about one pint) is serious. Care for shock.

FIGURE 13.2
Special assessment considerations.

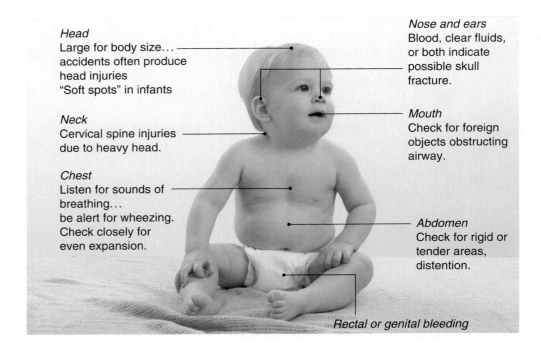

Head
Large for body size...
accidents often produce
head injuries
"Soft spots" in infants

Nose and ears
Blood, clear fluids,
or both indicate
possible skull
fracture.

Neck
Cervical spine injuries
due to heavy head.

Mouth
Check for foreign
objects obstructing
airway.

Chest
Listen for sounds of
breathing...
be alert for wheezing.
Check closely for
even expansion.

Abdomen
Check for rigid or
tender areas,
distention.

Rectal or genital bleeding

will show their acceptance of you by their reactions to your touch. Do not expect rapid acceptance. Use your smile and gentle words to provide comfort. ■

If the parents are present, do *not* direct all your conversation to them. Talk to the child. If you are at the scene of an accident in which the parents are also injured, let the child know that people are caring for their parents, too.

While assessing and caring for children, you will have to consider and work with the reactions of the parents or other adults who care for the child. Usually, the responses of a parent or guardian are positive and helpful even while they are concerned. Although sometimes parents will react with strong emotional responses that can hinder your care of the child. Both types of reactions are natural. Ask the anxious parent or guardian to help you with tasks, such as holding and reassuring the child, holding the dressing in place, holding the oxygen mask, or assisting with any other device you need to use in your care of the child. If this does not work to calm the parent, have a friend, neighbor, or other First Responder distract the parent with questions about the child's history or with getting the child's toy, favorite blanket, or clean clothes. Lastly, have someone gently and tactfully guide the parent away from the scene while you evaluate the child.

Some children who are seriously ill or injured are recuperating or being cared for at home while hooked up to medical equipment. These children may be on special monitors, have special tubes in their throats or abdomens, have intravenous drips containing medications, or be in special traction units. The parents have been trained by the child's doctors and nurses to operate the child's special equipment, but these children still have emergencies, and the parents will call EMS for help. You do not have to learn how to operate all the different types of special equipment, nor are you expected to. The parent will know how to manage the equipment. Your concern will be how to help the child, and the parent can likely guide you in that. However, some parents may hesitate, especially when EMS personnel arrive. Some may be nervous or unsure about working the equipment. Encourage them to go ahead and do what they have been trained to do and explain that they are more familiar with the equipment than you are. Ask the parents what they need you to do and how. Then help the parents do it.

Sometimes this special equipment malfunctions and, again, the parent may be anxious and unsure. Calm the parents and remind them that they have had training and you will do what you can to help as they give you instructions. If the parents still hesitate, ask them to contact the child's doctor or the medical supply company that provided the equipment. Most of these companies will have emergency contact numbers and staff on call 24 hours a day, 7 days a week to assist with equipment emergencies. After you and the parents have managed the child's emergency and the special equipment, call for EMT or ALS personnel to transport if necessary.

Take advantage of public education or public relations opportunities to encourage families to notify local emergency responders of children with special needs in the community. Arrangements can then be made to make sure the proper personnel and equipment are dispatched to them when emergencies occur.

AGE, SIZE, AND RESPONSE

FIRST➤ You will find that you instinctively treat infants and children differently from adults. You will know that an infant needs to be handled and cared for differently than a toddler, and that a toddler is spoken to and cared for differently than a school-age child or a teenager. In your training and with experience, you will become familiar with the age ranges, mental and physical development, personality, and experience levels of child patients so you can assess and care for them appropriately.

You already learned that for the purpose of performing CPR, pediatric patients are classified as newly born (immediately after birth), newborns (up to one month), infants (up to one year), and children (1 to 8 years). After that, CPR is performed on them the same as it is performed on an adult.

However, in general, when assessing and caring for pediatric patients, you must keep the following developmental categories in mind (Table 13-1):

- Infants—birth to 1 year.
- Toddlers—1 to 3 years.
- Preschool—3 to 6 years.
- School age (usually in elementary school)—6 to 12 years.
- Adolescent (usually in middle and high school)—12 to 18 years. ■

Each of these developmental stages requires a slightly different approach to assessment. However, there will be times when you are unable to determine the age of an infant or child. Some are large or small for their age, and parents may not be there to help you. You will have to estimate age based on the physical size, emotional responses, interaction with you, and language skills.

SPECIAL CONSIDERATIONS

You already realize that infants and children are not the same as adults in size, emotional maturity, and responses. You need to be aware that there are important anatomical differences as well. Because of these differences, your care will sometimes be somewhat different than it is for adults. Consider the following important differences and comparisons.

Head and Neck

A child's head is proportionately larger and heavier than her body. The body will catch up with the size of the head at about age 6. Because of the size and weight of the head, the child can be considered top heavy, and is likely to land head first in a

TABLE 13-1 DEVELOPMENTAL CHARACTERISTICS OF INFANTS AND CHILDREN

AGE GROUP	CHARACTERISTICS	ASSESSMENT AND CARE STRATEGIES
Newborns—birth to 1 month & infants— birth to 1 year	Infants do not like to be separated from their parents. They have minimal stranger anxiety. They are used to being undressed but like to feel warm, physically and emotionally. The younger infant follows movement with his or her eyes. The older infant is more active, developing a personality. They do not want to be "suffocated" by an oxygen mask.	Have the parent hold the infant while you examine him or her. Be sure to keep the infant warm. Also, warm your hands and stethoscope before touching the infant. It may be best to observe the infant's breathing from a distance, noting the rise and fall of the abdomen for normal breathing and the chest for respiratory distress, the level of activity, and the infant's color. Examine the heart and lungs first and the head last. This is perceived as less threatening and therefore less likely to cause crying. A pediatric nonrebreather mask may be held near the face to provide blow-by oxygen.
Toddlers— 1 to 3 years	Toddlers do not like to be touched or separated from their parents. They may believe that their illness is a punishment for being bad. Unlike infants, they do not like having their clothing removed. They frighten easily, over-react, have a fear of needles and pain. They may understand more than they communicate. They begin to assert their independence. They do not want to be "suffocated" by an oxygen mask.	Have a parent hold the child while you examine him. Assure the child that he was not bad. Remove an article of clothing, examine the toddler, and then replace the clothing. Examine in a toe-to-head approach to build confidence. (Touching the head first may be frightening.) Explain what you are going to do in terms he can understand. (Taking the blood pressure may be a "squeeze" or a "hug on the arm.") Offer the comfort of a favorite toy. Consider giving him a choice: "Do you want me to look at your belly first or your feet first?" A pediatric nonrebreather mask may be held near the face to provide blow-by oxygen.
Preschool— 3 to 6 years	Preschoolers do not like to be touched or separated from their parents. They are modest and do not like their clothing removed. They may believe that their illness is a punishment for being bad. They have a fear of blood, pain, and permanent injury. They are curious, communicative, and can be cooperative. They do not want to be "suffocated" by an oxygen mask.	Have a parent hold the child while you examine him. Respect the child's modesty. Remove an article of clothing, examine him, and then replace the clothing. Have a calm, confident, reassuring, respectful manner. Be sure to offer explanations about what you are doing. Allow the child the responsibility of giving the history. Explain as you examine. A pediatric nonrebreather mask may be held near the face to provide blow-by oxygen. Do not lie. Explain that what you do to help may hurt.

continues

TABLE 13-1 CONTINUED

AGE GROUP	CHARACTERISTICS	ASSESSMENT AND CARE STRATEGIES
School age—6 to 12 years	This age group cooperates but likes their opinions heard. They fear blood, pain, disfigurement, and permanent injury. They are modest and do not like their bodies exposed.	Allow the child the responsibility of giving the history. Explain as you examine. Present a confident, calm, respectful manner. Respect their modesty. Do not lie. Explain that what you do to help may hurt.
Adolescent—12 to 18 years	Adolescents want to be treated as adults. They generally feel that they are indestructible but may have fears of permanent injury and disfigurement. They vary in their emotional and physical development and may not be comfortable with their changing bodies.	Although they wish to be treated as adults, they may need as much support as children. Present a confident, calm, respectful manner. Be sure to explain what you are doing. Respect their modesty. You may consider assessing them away from their parents. Have the physical exam done by a First Responder of the same sex as the patient if possible. Do not lie. Explain that what you do to help may hurt.

sudden fall or stop. Common examples include falls from shopping carts and unrestrained children who are propelled head first through windshields in motor-vehicle collisions. Both of these incidents result in severe head injuries to pediatric patients. Be especially suspicious of a mechanism of injury (MOI) that suggests a possible fall from a height taller than the child.

Always handle the head of the newborn with caution because of the soft spots (fontanelles). The largest soft spot, the one on top of the head, does not close completely until about 18 months of age. This soft spot is flat when the infant is quiet, and you may see it pulsate with each heartbeat. If the soft spot is sunken, the child may have lost a lot of fluids (dehydration) because illness has caused inadequate fluid intake and/or diarrhea and vomiting. If the soft spot is bulging, it may indicate that there is increased pressure inside the skull. This can be due to brain swelling from trauma or from an illness such as meningitis. Since the fontanelles can also bulge when the infant is agitated and crying, they should be assessed when the infant is quiet. Again, consider the mechanism of injury or nature of the illness during your assessment and care.

In any head injury, look for blood and clear fluids leaking from the nose and ears, just as you would in adults.

When infants and small children suffer head injuries and also show signs of shock, suspect and assess for internal injuries as well. A head injury alone is seldom a cause of shock.

Airway and the Respiratory System

The airway and respiratory systems of the infant and child have not developed fully. The tongue is large relative to the size of the mouth and the airway is narrower than the adult airway and thus more easily obstructed. In addition, because the muscles in the neck are not fully developed, it may be difficult for a child to hold his head in an open-airway position when sick or injured.

When a child is lying on his back, the large head may cause the airway to flex forward and close. So place a towel that is folded flat under the child's shoulders to

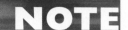

NOTE

Children are more vulnerable to spinal injuries than adults because of the larger, heavier head and the underdeveloped neck muscles and bone structure.

remember

Do not perform blind finger sweeps when trying to clear an airway obstruction.

FIGURE 13.3

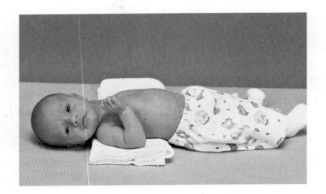

NOTE

Infants are obligate nose breathers. They will not automatically open the mouth when the nose is obstructed.

help keep the head in line with the body (a neutral position) and the airway open (Figure 13.3). For infants and small children, use a slight head-tilt.

There are some unique points to remember about children's breathing. Infants are obligate nasal breathers. That is, if the nose is obstructed, the infant will not immediately open his mouth to breathe as an adult would. Make sure the nostrils are clear of secretions so the patient can breathe freely. Remember that the child's windpipe (trachea) is also softer, more flexible, and narrower than an adult's windpipe, and it will obstruct easily. For this reason, you must be careful when opening the airway.

Chest and Abdomen

Since the diaphragm is the major breathing muscle for normal respirations in the infant and child, you will see more respiratory movement in the abdomen than in the chest. But the chest is more elastic, so when the child's breathing is labored or distressed, chest movement is obvious in all the muscles between the ribs and in the muscles above the sternum around the neck and shoulders. The use of these *accessory muscles* for breathing is important to note and indicates the child is in urgent need of medical care.

The child's less developed and more elastic chest may have an advantage over an adult's chest. In a crushing trauma, the bones of the child's chest may not break but they will flex. The disadvantage of this is that the more flexible chest offers less protection to the vital organs underneath—the heart and lungs. In your physical assessment, the mechanism of injury is important and will help you determine possible internal injury, especially if there is no obvious external injury. Some signs to look for are loss of symmetry (unequal appearance on both sides of the chest), unequal chest movement with breathing, and bruising over the neck and/or ribs.

Injury to the abdomen can result in tenderness, distention, and rigidity just as it can in adults. The abdominal muscles are not as well developed as they are in the adult and provide the child less protection. The abdominal organs (especially the liver and spleen) are large for the size of the cavity and are more susceptible to trauma. A child who has a blunt abdominal injury can bleed out within minutes. Injury that causes distention or swelling can restrict movement of the diaphragm muscle and make it difficult for the child to breathe.

Pelvis

The child can lose a large amount of blood into the pelvic cavity as a result of trauma to the pelvic girdle. If you suspect hip or pelvis injury, monitor vital signs for shock just as you would in the adult and arrange for transport to a medical facility as soon as possible. Check for bleeding or bloody discharge from the genital area. Do not rock the hips to check for instability.

Extremities

Assess for circulation, sensation, and motor function at the distal ends of all extremities. Assess circulation by checking the pulse and capillary refill. Capillary refill is checked by pressing briefly and gently on the hand, foot, forearm, or lower leg. You do not have to press the tiny nail bed. Pressing on the skin will push blood out of the area and cause it to briefly whiten (blanch) and then suddenly refill when pressure is released. Capillary refill time should be less than two seconds.

Injuries that cause soft-tissue swelling or bones to be displaced, bent, or splintered can restrict circulation. Always check both pulses and capillary refill in injured extremities. If First Responders perform splinting or other immobilization procedures, they must recheck the pulse after the splint is in place. EMT or ALS personnel will recheck it regularly en route to the hospital.

Adult bones may fracture in a trauma situation. Children's bones are less developed and more flexible and will bend and splinter before they break. Provide care for injury sites where there are signs and symptoms of painful, swollen, and deformed extremities, especially at any joint (fingers, wrists, elbows, ankles, knees, hips).

Children have growth plates at the ends of each long bone. A growth plate is developing tissue and the weakest area of a growing skeleton. A child who seriously injures a joint is likely to damage the growth plate, which determines the future length and shape of the mature bone. Growth-plate injuries may be the result of a fall, competitive sports (football), recreational activities (biking, skateboarding), and even from overuse (gymnastics, softball pitching). Pay special attention to a child who complains of pain or who has swelling or deformity in any joint.

Body Surface Area

Infants and children have a large amount of total surface area (skin) in proportion to total body mass. The large surface can easily lose heat and cause the pediatric patient to become chilled, or *hypothermic*, even in an environment in which an adult feels comfortable. It is important to keep infants and children covered and warm, especially if there is trauma and blood loss or illness and fluid loss.

Blood Volume

The smaller the patient, the less blood volume the patient has. The newborn may have slightly less than 12 ounces, or about a cup and a half of blood, and cannot afford to lose many drops. As children grow, their blood volume increases. By eight years old, they will have about two liters (roughly 1/2 gallon) of blood. Moderate blood loss in an adult may not concern you if it is easily controlled, but the same amount of blood loss in an infant or small child can be life-threatening.

Vital Signs

Pulse and respiratory rates vary with the size of the child. The smaller the child, the higher are the pulse and respiratory rates. Table 13-2 lists pulse and respiratory rates for infants and children.

Blood pressure also varies in children and depends on their sex, age, and height. Boys have slightly higher blood pressure than girls do. Taller children have higher blood pressure than shorter children. The following factors will also influence blood pressure readings:

- *Time of day.* Blood pressure fluctuates during waking hours and is lower during sleeping hours.

- *Child's physical activity.* Blood pressure is higher during and immediately after exercise or activity, such as running, playing ball, or jumping rope, and it is slower during inactive periods, such as reading, coloring, or watching television.

TABLE 13-2 PULSE AND RESPIRATORY RATES

AGE	AVERAGE PULSE RATE (PER MINUTE)	AVERAGE RESPIRATORY RATE (PER MINUTE)
Newborn (birth to 1 month)	120–160	30–50
Infant (1 month to 1 year)	80–140	25–30
Toddler (1 to 3 years)	80–130	20–30
Preschool (3 to 6 years)	80–120	20–30
School age (6 to 12 years)	70–110	15–30
Adolescent (over 12 to 18 years)	60–105	12–20

- *Child's emotional moods or feelings.* Blood pressure fluctuates when the child is afraid, angry, stressed, or happy.

- *Child's physical condition.* The blood pressure will rise or fall based on the type of illness or an injury.

If you are trained to take blood pressure, use the appropriate size cuff when you take a child's blood pressure. It should cover about one-half of the child's upper arm. Cuffs that are too small or too large may give inaccurate readings. Although there are so many factors that can affect a child's blood pressure, you can still determine an appropriate systolic range by using some simple calculations:

- To determine the upper limit of a child's systolic blood pressure, multiply the child's age in years by 2 and add 90 (age $\times$ 2 + 90 = upper limit of systolic blood pressure).

- To determine the lower limit of a child's systolic blood pressure, multiply the child's age in years by two and add 70 (age $\times$ 2 + 70 = lower limit of systolic blood pressure).

It is not necessary to measure a blood pressure on a child under the age of three in the prehospital setting.

ASSESSMENT OF INFANTS AND CHILDREN

You may wish to review Chapter 7, "Patient Assessment," at this time.

SCENE SIZE-UP

FIRST➤ Size up the scene involving a pediatric patient just as you would a scene involving an adult, but approach slowly so you do not frighten the child. Determine scene safety and the number of patients involved in the emergency. Determine the mechanism of injury or the nature of illness. Prepare for patient care by putting on appropriate personal protective equipment. If you think you may need additional resources, call for them immediately. ■

INITIAL ASSESSMENT

General Impression

FIRST➤ To get a general impression, look at the child and the environment as you approach. Quickly gather critical information that will help you decide whether to hurry or take your time. From a short distance or from across a room, you can see if the child is alert, struggling to breathe, crying, quiet and listless, or unresponsive to your approach. Is the skin pale, bluish, or flushed? How is the child interacting with the environment, with those around him, and to you as you approach? What is the child's body position? From these clues, you can get a general impression of the child's status. In children, the general impression is an important indicator of the severity of illness.

Once you reach the child, you can quickly determine mental status using the AVPU scale. Is the child alert? Is he responsive to your voice or only to a painful stimulus like squeezing his shoulder? Or is he unresponsive? Is he oriented to person, place, and time? An infant or a very young child is not able to answer questions about his name, where he is, or what day it is; however, parents or caregivers can explain if the child's actions are as they would normally expect them to be.

Next, quickly assess the child's ABCs. You may assume that the crying child has an airway, breathing, and circulation. For the quiet or unresponsive child, check the airway. Is it open? Check breathing. Is the child breathing normally or with effort? What is the rate? Is chest expansion present and equal? Are there noises like grunting or a high-pitched sound (stridor) associated with the child's respiratory efforts? Is the skin blue (cyanotic), indicating low oxygen levels? Check circulation. Is the pulse strong and regular? Is there any bleeding? For all children, you will want to find out: Is the skin warm and dry, indicating normal circulation? Or is it cool and clammy, suggesting blood loss and shock? What skin areas are most accessible for you to determine cool and clammy skin? Is capillary refill time less than two seconds? Care for the life-threatening conditions that affect airway, breathing, and circulation first. Remember that the unresponsive child needs immediate care.

When you determine priority of transport, you have a high-priority patient if the infant or child:

- Gives a poor general impression.
- Has an altered mental status.
- Has an airway problem.
- Is in respiratory arrest, or has inadequate breathing or respiratory distress.
- Has a possibility of developing shock.
- Has evidence of uncontrolled bleeding that may soon result in shock. ■

Managing the Airway

The airway is your first concern in the care of any patient. Always ensure that the airway is open and clear and that the patient is breathing adequately or is receiving appropriate ventilations and supplemental oxygen when necessary. (You may wish to review airway care techniques for infants and children in Chapter 6 at this time.)

Opening the Airway

FIRST▶ When a child lies on his back, the tongue will fall to the back of the throat as it does in adults. Remember, though, that in an infant or child the tongue is larger and can more easily obstruct the airway. Also, when lying on the back, the larger head of the infant may cause the head to flex or bend too far forward and close off the airway. In small children, if you are not careful when opening the airway, you may cause hyperextension or bend the head too far back, which also can close off the airway. You must be sure to align the head and neck or place it in a neutral position so that the airway is open. As noted earlier in this chapter, you can

remember

Never perform a blind finger sweep on an infant or a child and never perform abdominal thrusts on an infant.

NOTE

An infant's tongue can easily obstruct the airway. So can an hyperflexed or hyperextended head.

easily position the infant or small child correctly by placing a towel under the shoulders. Check for breathing before repositioning the head. Then, if necessary, perform a slight head-tilt or a jaw-thrust maneuver (for trauma) to assess breathing and provide ventilations. ■

Clearing and Maintaining the Airway　If air does not enter easily or the chest does not rise when providing artificial ventilation, reposition the head and try again. If you still have no success in ventilating the patient, give back blows and chest thrusts on an infant (younger than one year of age) and abdominal thrusts for children over one year. Then check the mouth to see if there is an obstruction. If you see one, sweep the mouth with the little finger of your gloved hand. Do not perform blind finger sweeps.

If there are fluids in the airway, clear them by sweeping the mouth with a gauze pad or by suctioning. Check with your instructor to see if First Responders are allowed to use suctioning equipment in your area. If so, your instructor will provide you with training. You also may be able to use nasopharyngeal and oropharyngeal airways in the infant and child patient. Again, your instructor will let you know and give you appropriate training.

Providing Oxygen　In some jurisdictions, and for some EMS agencies, training for First Responders in oxygen delivery is optional. If you are allowed to provide oxygen to patients, your instructor will have the appropriate equipment and train you how and when to use it with pediatric patients.

The oxygen requirement for children is twice that of adults. Children must receive a high concentration of oxygen when they are in respiratory distress, have inadequate respirations, or have blood loss that can result in shock. A low oxygen level (hypoxia) causes serious physical reactions in children. It can affect the heart rate, slowing the pulse and reducing oxygen circulating to tissues. This in turn affects the brain, decreasing oxygen to cells and causing altered mental status and tissue death. Always follow the rule: "If they are blue, give O_2."

Providing oxygen may be a vital part of the emergency care procedures used in caring for children. However, it may be difficult to deliver in the prehospital setting. Many adults are not comfortable wearing an oxygen mask because it feels confining and suffocating. Children also will fear having a mask placed over the face, and the flow of oxygen may even cause children to hold their breath. The First Responder can still provide enriched oxygen to children who need it by using a *blow-by technique.*

To perform the blow-by technique, hold, or have the parent hold the oxygen tubing or the pediatric nonrebreather mask about two inches from the child's face. The oxygen will enrich the area in front of the face as it blows by and the child inhales (Figure 13.4). Oxygen tubing can be plugged into the bottom of a colorful paper cup and provide oxygen effectively. The advantage to this method is that the child will likely be curious about the cup and hold it to his face to examine it or try to drink from it. At the same time the child is receiving oxygen, he will also calm down because he has something of interest to keep his attention. You have provided a toy and gained confidence so your exam can proceed more smoothly. You may also use a paper cup for blow-by oxygen. Do not use a styrofoam cup, because it will crumble and particles can blow into the child's face, eyes, and airway.

If the patient is not breathing, provide artificial ventilation. For the newborn, provide it at a rate of 40 to 60 breaths per minute. For both the infant and child under eight years old, provide 20 breaths per minute (once every 3 seconds) using a pediatric-size pocket face mask or a bag-valve-mask ventilator of the correct size. Remember the following steps when ventilating:

remember

Use a paper cup. A styrofoam cup will crumble and particles can blow into the child's face, eyes, and airway.

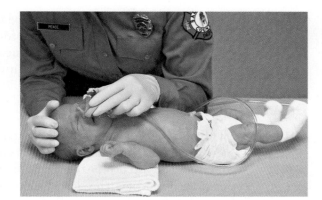

FIGURE 13.4
You can deliver oxygen by using the blow-by method.

- Breathe less forcefully through the pocket face mask. Watch for the chest to rise. Ventilate slowly so as not to cause stomach distention.

- Excessive force is not needed with the bag-valve-mask ventilator. Watch for the chest to rise.

- Use a properly sized face mask to get a good mask-to-face seal.

- Do *not* use flow-restricted, oxygen-powered ventilation devices.

- If ventilations are not successful, perform the procedures for clearing an obstructed airway. Then try to ventilate again.

FOCUSED HISTORY AND PHYSICAL EXAM

FIRST➤ After completing your initial assessment, focus on getting a history and conducting a physical exam. These steps may be done at the scene with the responsive patient and while you are waiting for the EMT or ALS personnel to arrive, or they may be done while en route to the hospital. Normally, infants or very young children will not respond to your questions, but children older than two or three years will be able to answer questions that require a yes-or-no answer, and they can tell you or point to where it hurts. Otherwise, parents or other responsible adults, such as baby-sitters or teachers, will have to give you information about the child's history and how he became sick or hurt.

While you are getting a general impression of the child, decide if he is seriously injured or sick. For any child who is critically injured or sick, perform a rapid assessment, as you would do for an adult:

- *Rapid trauma assessment (patient with significant MOI)*—check ABCs first, with manual in-line stabilization of the head and spine; inspect and palpate each body area; get baseline vital signs; and, if possible, get a history.

- *Rapid physical exam (unresponsive patient)*—perform any medical interventions, such as open and clear the airway, ventilate, start CPR; inspect and palpate each body area; get a history or as much information as possible about the events leading to the illness; get baseline vital signs.

If you decide from your general impression that the child is responding or acting normally, then perform the appropriate focused assessment:

- *Focused history and physical exam (trauma patient with no significant MOI)*—find out the chief complaint, or what hurts; inspect and palpate the area; get baseline vital signs; get a history that focuses on events that caused the injury and the injury itself.

- *Focused history and physical exam (responsive medical patient)*—find out the chief complaint, or the nature of illness; get a history of the events leading up to the illness and the illness itself; focus your physical exam on the area of complaint, or inspect and palpate the part of the body involved; get baseline vital signs. ■

DETAILED PHYSICAL EXAM

FIRST➤ Now that you have completed a focused assessment, you may have time to perform a more detailed physical exam. This exam will be very similar to what you do for the adult, except it is performed in reverse order (toe to head) when you examine the alert but frightened or crying infant or young child. This will give the child an opportunity to get used to you and your touch if he has not done so during the short focused assessment.

In a medical situation, you can examine the child in more detail from toe to head, while he is in the parent's lap or being held by someone else he knows well. In a trauma situation with no significant MOI, you can again let the parent or other known adult help comfort the child while you begin your detailed toe-to-head physical exam and assess for DCAP-BTLS, instability, and crepitis (grating noise or sensation).

Always explain to the child and parent what you are doing and make sure that both understand. Most young children are used to being dressed and undressed and examined by their doctors and will not be embarrassed. As they get older, children are more modest and have learned that strangers should not touch them. Adolescents are concerned about body changes and wonder if they are normal. Remove or rearrange only the necessary clothing during your exam. Then replace it when you have examined that part of the body.

Trauma patients with a significant MOI or unresponsive medical patients who require a rapid assessment are usually unresponsive or too critically injured or ill to know or care where you start your assessment. Stabilize the head and neck before you reposition the head to assess the ABCs in a trauma case, and then follow the steps described above. ■

ONGOING ASSESSMENT

FIRST➤ You are never finished with your patient until he has been turned over to an equal or higher level of medical care. This means that when you finish your detailed physical exam, you will start again. This is called the ongoing assessment, and it will continue until EMT or ALS personnel arrive. The status of a child can change rapidly and frequently, so you will need to reassess mental status, maintain airway, monitor breathing, check pulse, and re-evaluate skin color, temperature, and condition. Take and record vital signs every 5 minutes for unstable patients and every 15 minutes for stable patients. Continue to monitor the effects of interventions, provide appropriate care, and give emotional support. ■

MANAGING SPECIFIC MEDICAL EMERGENCIES

Many of the specific medical emergencies listed here have been described in detail in other chapters. Much of the care you will provide to infants and children is similar to what you would provide to adults.

RESPIRATORY EMERGENCIES

First Responders do not usually receive the in-depth training for determining different respiratory illnesses and causes of airway and breathing problems in pediatric patients. This section will list some common causes, cover general signs and symptoms, and describe management of respiratory emergencies in pediatric patients.

Guidelines for the assessment and emergency care of a pediatric patient with any respiratory emergency are summarized in Figure 13.5. It is important to note that the most common cause of cardiac arrest in infants and children is respiratory arrest. Identifying and caring for a respiratory problem early can minimize the chances of cardiac arrest.

Airway Obstruction

You may wish to review the signs and symptoms and the management of partial and complete airway obstruction for pediatric patients in Chapter 6. Continue to review and practice them during and after your training. This will enable you to act quickly to assure an open airway and adequate breathing for all patients. Since the steps of relieving an obstructed airway in infants are different than for adults, practice the steps of back blows and chest thrusts frequently so that you can perform them quickly and effectively. Remember that the unresponsive child needs immediate care.

Difficulty Breathing

There are many types of airway and respiratory infections and conditions that cause airway and breathing problems. A simple cold can plug the nose and make breathing difficult, but the nose can be easily cleared by blowing or suctioning. A respiratory infection can cause swelling of the respiratory tract or blocking by mucous secretions, making it difficult to breathe. Another respiratory problem that occurs in some infants involves periods of time when they will stop breathing and then start up again on their own. This period of interrupted breathing is known as **apnea**. In almost all cases, apnea occurs while sleeping. For this reason it is called *sleep apnea*. Some cases of sleep apnea are related to airway obstruction, while others are associated with failure in the central nervous system to stimulate respiration during sleep. The close relationship between apnea and sudden infant death syndrome is still under study.

apnea (ap-ne-ah) absence of breathing.

Respiratory Infections

Two common respiratory infections in infants and children include croup and epiglottitis. Any infant or child with noisy respiration and a hoarse cough may have croup. **Croup** is an infection caused by a virus and affects the larynx (voice box), trachea, and bronchi. It usually causes the tissues in the upper airway to become swollen, which restricts airflow. In **epiglottitis**, the epiglottis (the flap that closes over the trachea while swallowing) becomes inflamed. Epiglottitis can have a sudden onset in what seemed to be an otherwise healthy child. Suspect this respiratory emergency if the child develops a rapid fever, has cold-like symptoms, has difficulty swallowing, and is drooling. Children with epiglottitis will also sit upright in a *tripod position* (leaning forward with arms braced on the edge of the bed or chair) with the chin thrust out and the mouth wide open. You will notice that they will use the muscles in their upper chest and those around their shoulders and neck to breathe. This effort to breathe is very tiring for the child. The First Responder must act quickly. Though rare, epiglottitis is considered life-threatening.

Because it may be difficult to determine what type of respiratory emergency an infant or a child is having, consider any airway problem or breathing difficulty an

croup (KROOP) acute respiratory condition found in infants and children, which is characterized by a barking type of cough or stridor.

epiglottitis (ep-i-glot-I-tis) swelling of the epiglottis that may be caused by a bacterial infection. It can obstruct the airway and is potentially life-threatening.

Pediatric Respiratory Emergencies

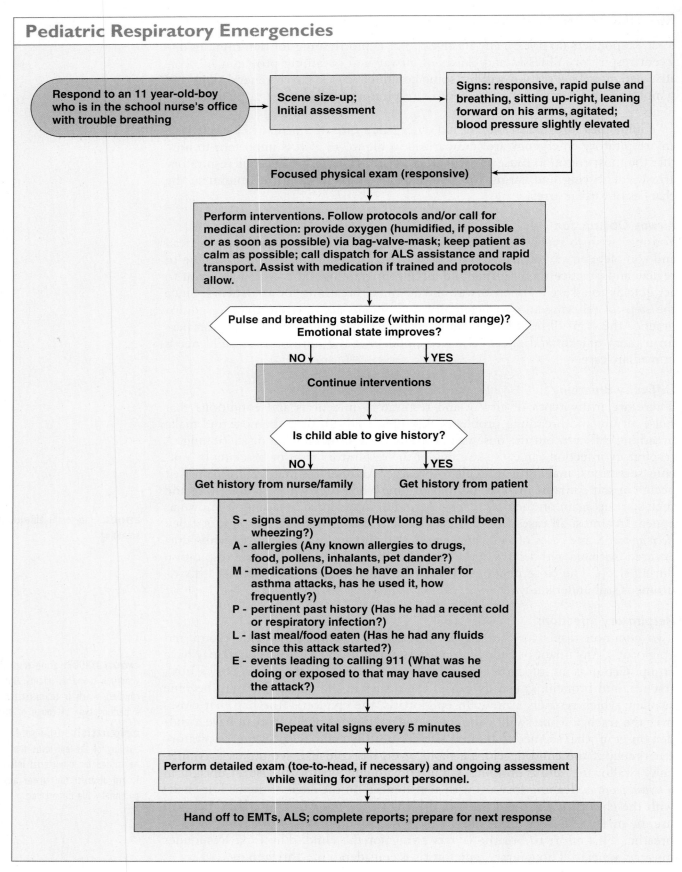

Respond to an 11 year-old-boy who is in the school nurse's office with trouble breathing

Scene size-up; Initial assessment

Signs: responsive, rapid pulse and breathing, sitting up-right, leaning forward on his arms, agitated; blood pressure slightly elevated

Focused physical exam (responsive)

Perform interventions. Follow protocols and/or call for medical direction: provide oxygen (humidified, if possible or as soon as possible) via bag-valve-mask; keep patient as calm as possible; call dispatch for ALS assistance and rapid transport. Assist with medication if trained and protocols allow.

Pulse and breathing stabilize (within normal range)? Emotional state improves?

NO   YES

Continue interventions

Is child able to give history?

NO   YES

Get history from nurse/family   Get history from patient

S - signs and symptoms (How long has child been wheezing?)
A - allergies (Any known allergies to drugs, food, pollens, inhalants, pet dander?)
M - medications (Does he have an inhaler for asthma attacks, has he used it, how frequently?)
P - pertinent past history (Has he had a recent cold or respiratory infection?)
L - last meal/food eaten (Has he had any fluids since this attack started?)
E - events leading to calling 911 (What was he doing or exposed to that may have caused the attack?)

Repeat vital signs every 5 minutes

Perform detailed exam (toe-to-head, if necessary) and ongoing assessment while waiting for transport personnel.

Hand off to EMTs, ALS; complete reports; prepare for next response

FIGURE 13.5

urgent emergency and call for ALS transport immediately. Provide oxygen as soon as possible using a blow-by technique if you cannot get the child to accept a face mask or a nasal cannula. *Do not place anything in the mouth, such as a tongue depressor, in an attempt to examine the airway.* Probing the mouth can cause spasms that will further close the airway. Avoid any actions that might agitate or stimulate the child.

FIRST➤ Signs and symptoms of respiratory distress include the following:

● Wheezing or a high-pitched harsh noise, or grunting.
● Exhaling with effort.
● Breathing that is faster or slower than normal is inadequate and requires assisted ventilations and oxygen.
● Straining to use (retraction of) the chest muscles, especially around the neck and shoulders.
● Child is sitting up and supporting himself in a tripod position.
● Drooling.
● Nasal flaring.
● Cyanosis (late sign).
● Capillary refill of more than two seconds (late sign).
● Slow heart rate (late sign).
● Altered mental status (late sign). ■

Asthma is also a respiratory condition common to children. It can become life-threatening if left untreated. Most children who have asthma use a medication or inhaler prescribed by their doctors. Parents or caregivers call for assistance for a child with asthma if the signs and symptoms are new and unfamiliar, do not respond to at-home care, or the child is not responding to the usual prescribed treatment. Signs and symptoms of asthma occur when the small airways in the lungs go into spasm and constrict, or become too narrow for air to pass through. Something the child eats or breathes or some unusual excitement may trigger the attack.

FIRST➤ Signs and symptoms of asthma include:

● Loud wheezing and breath sounds in a mild attack, becoming less audible as the attack worsens.
● Shortness of breath.
● Obvious respiratory distress with easy inhalation and forced expiration.
● Cough. A non-productive cough (one that does not produce sputum), with or without wheezing and a slow pulse rate, called *bradycardia* (bray-de-KAR-de-ah), is a sign of severe distress.
● Faster than normal breathing rate.
● Increased heart rate; faster, weaker pulse.
● Sleepiness or slowed response.
● Bluish (cyanotic) tint to the skin, especially around the lips and eyes. ■

FIRST➤ Provide emergency care to the pediatric patient who has difficulty breathing and the above signs and symptoms by following these steps:

1. Act calmly and with assurance, which will help calm and reassure the child and the parents or caregiver. For mild distress, the child will be agitated. For severe distress, the child will be exhausted and unable or unwilling to move. Signs of sleepiness and slow response mean low oxygen levels.

2. Place the child in a sitting position. The child will likely have taken a position of comfort that makes it easy for him to breathe, usually a tripod position, leaning forward and bracing himself on his forearms.

3. Administer humidified oxygen (follow local protocols). Ask the child to breathe in normally but to blow out air forcefully, as if blowing out the candles on a birthday cake or blowing up a balloon. Show the child how and breathe with him.

4. If you are allowed to assist in giving medications, help the parents or caregiver administer the child's medication. Check local protocols and always call for medical direction before assisting a patient with medications (see Appendix 3).

5. Have the parents or caregiver contact the child's physician.

6. Arrange for transport by EMT or ALS personnel. If the signs and symptoms are not relieved with your care and the child continues to worsen, call for ALS assistance immediately. A severe and ongoing asthma attack that is not relieved by medication and oxygen may be *status asthmaticus*, a very serious and life-threatening condition. ■

WARNING: *First Responders should consider all respiratory disorders in children serious and take action immediately. Respiratory distress and low oxygen levels in children are the primary causes of cardiac arrest not related to trauma. In cases of cardiac arrest, call for ALS support immediately. For respiratory distress, provide oxygen by a pediatric-sized nonrebreather mask (Figure 13.6) or by using the blow-by technique. For severe distress and respiratory arrest, provide assisted ventilations with a pediatric-sized bag-valve-mask ventilator and supplemental oxygen and call for ALS support (Figure 13.7).*

Always allow the child to assume a comfortable position. The alert child will naturally find the position in which it is easiest to breathe. Remember, if you are not trained to use oxygen or do not carry it, call for ALS support at the first sign of respiratory distress in children.

SEIZURES

FIRST➤ A seizure will cause a sudden change in sensation, behavior, or movement. The more severe forms of seizure cause violent muscle contractions called *convulsions*. Seizures may be the result of high fever, epilepsy, infections, poisoning, low blood sugar (hypoglycemia), or head injury. They may also occur when the brain does not receive enough oxygen because of inadequate blood circulation (shock) or inadequate oxygen in

FIGURE 13.6
For respiratory distress, provide oxygen with a correctly sized pediatric nonrebreather mask placed on the child or use the blow-by method.

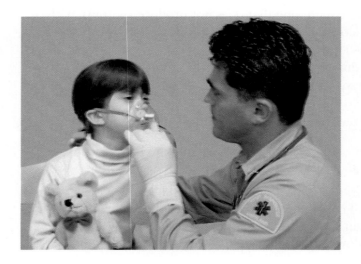

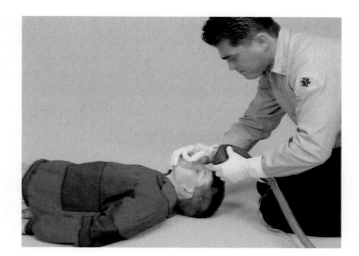

the blood (hypoxia). In some cases, there is no known cause. Many children suffer seizures, but they are rarely life-threatening. Seizures caused by fever (febrile seizures) should be taken seriously. If a child is having prolonged or multiple seizures and has an altered mental status, consider these conditions as a life-threatening emergency and call for ALS support immediately.

In many cases, a patient's seizures stop before EMS arrives. After a seizure, it is normal for children to be either lethargic (drowsy) and difficult to arouse or agitated and combative. Look for signs of illness or injury and question the child or family about symptoms. Also get the following information. Ask:

- Has the child had prior seizures? How long did they last? What part of the body was affected?
- Has the child had a fever?
- Has the child had an injury or fall in which the head may have been struck?
- Is the child taking any medications, specifically medication for seizures?
- Did the child's skin (nail beds and mucous membranes) change from its normal color to bluish or grayish, indicating low oxygen (hypoxia)?

Any child who has had a seizure must have a medical evaluation. Arrange for transport as soon as possible. In the meantime, provide the following emergency care steps:

1. Maintain an open airway and insert nothing in the mouth.
2. Look for evidence of injury suffered during the seizure.
3. If you do not suspect spinal injury, position the child on his side.
4. Be alert for vomiting.
5. Provide oxygen or assisted ventilations with supplemental oxygen, if allowed to do so.
6. Monitor breathing and altered mental status. ■

ALTERED MENTAL STATUS

Any medical or trauma emergency that affects the brain can cause an altered mental status. Examples include low blood sugar (hypoglycemia), poisoning, infection, head injury, decreased oxygen levels, shock, or the period after a seizure. As you assess the child, note the mechanism of injury or nature of illness, which will give clues to causes of the child's mental status. Look for signs of poisoning (ingested, inhaled, or absorbed) and ask family members or teachers if there is a history of diabetes or seizure disorder. Take and monitor vital signs, which can indicate shock as a cause. While observing and examining the child, you may notice signs of sleepiness, confusion, agitation, or listlessness.

As you gather information, perform the following emergency care steps:

1. Maintain an open airway, but protect the spine in cases of trauma. If necessary, ventilate the patient.

2. Provide oxygen as soon as possible by nonrebreather mask, or assist ventilations with a bag-valve-mask ventilator and supplemental oxygen.

3. Place the patient in the recovery position if there is no indication of spinal injury. Care for shock.

4. Arrange to transport as soon as possible.

SHOCK

Common causes of shock in infants and children include losing large amounts of fluid from diarrhea and vomiting, blood loss, and abdominal injuries and other trauma. Shock from fluid loss occurs quickly in infants and is a serious emergency; call for ALS support immediately. Though not as common, shock can also be caused by allergic reactions, poisoning and, rarely, by cardiac-related problems.

The child's body can compensate for shock for a long time, but the body's compensating mechanisms can suddenly fail. This failure is called *decompensated shock*. It occurs when the body can no longer function or compensate for low blood volume or lack of perfusion of oxygenated blood to the brain. As a result, the child has an altered mental status and the blood pressure drops (hypotension). When a child goes into the decompensated shock stage, signs and symptoms of shock can develop rapidly.

NOTE: *In the adult, shock typically develops more gradually, and the signs tend to be easier to recognize. In the child, you must suspect and anticipate shock and begin caring for it immediately, even before you see definite signs of it.*

FIRST➤ Signs and symptoms of shock include (Figure 13.8):

- Rapid heart and respiratory rate. (Both heart rate and respiratory rate will reflect the course of shock.)
- Weak or absent pulse.

FIGURE 13.8
Signs of shock in an infant or a child.

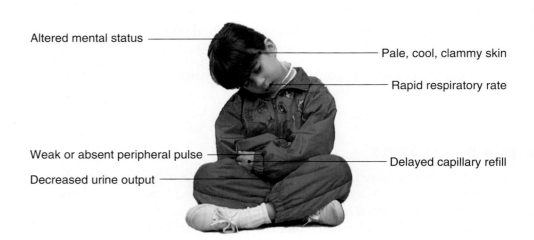

Altered mental status

Pale, cool, clammy skin

Rapid respiratory rate

Weak or absent peripheral pulse

Decreased urine output

Delayed capillary refill

- Delayed capillary refill.
- Decreased urine output (information from parents), which indicates dehydration.
- Altered mental status.
- Pale, cool, clammy skin.
- Sunken fontanelles.

Provide the following care in your management of the sick or injured infant or child who has evidence of shock (Figure 13.9):

1. Assure an open airway, but protect the spine in cases of trauma. Provide ventilations, if necessary.

2. Provide oxygen by nonrebreather mask or assist ventilations by bag-valve-mask ventilator with supplemental oxygen as per local protocols.

3. Control any bleeding and dress wounds.

4. Elevate the legs if there is no trauma or suspected spinal injury.

5. Maintain body warmth but do not overheat.

6. Arrange to transport as soon as possible.

7. While waiting for EMT personnel to arrive or while en route, continue to monitor airway, breathing, and vital signs and continue any care. ■

SUDDEN INFANT DEATH SYNDROME (SIDS)

In the U.S., sudden infant death syndrome (SIDS) claims thousands of infants each year. It is the sudden unexplained death during sleep of an apparently healthy baby in the first year of life—even a baby who is receiving proper care and has just

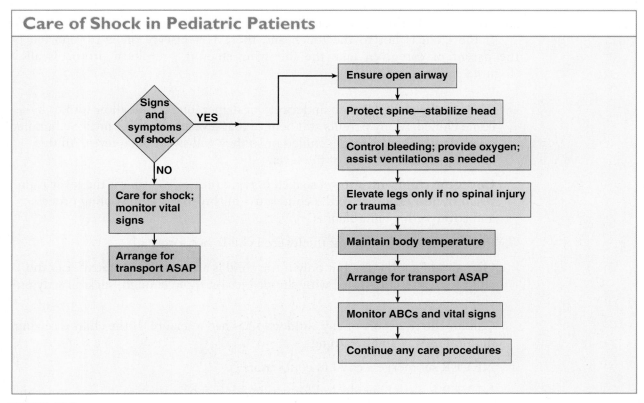

Care of Shock in Pediatric Patients

FIGURE 13.9

passed a physical exam. Possible causes and theories are still being investigated. It is known that SIDS is not caused by external methods of suffocation, by vomiting, or by choking.

When First Responders arrive, they may see distraught parents with their infant in respiratory and cardiac arrest during the scene size-up. Since First Responders cannot diagnose SIDS, you must immediately start emergency care as you would for any patient in arrest. Provide resuscitation and arrange transport to the hospital. Assure the parents that everything is being done for the baby. Normally, First Responders will not begin resuscitation if there is obvious rigor mortis (stiffening of the body) or if blood has pooled (lividity) along whatever side the child was lying on. Check with your instructor to find out what your protocols require for this situation. In either case, be sure to provide emotional support to the parents.

FEVER

The body's normal response to many childhood diseases and infections is a high temperature or fever. But the rise in body temperature may also be caused by heat exposure, by a non-infectious disease problem, and even by childhood immunization shots. The parents probably monitored their child's temperature and can report the temperature readings taken before you arrived. Try to find out how high the fever is and how rapidly it rose. Increased temperature is not necessarily what causes a seizure, but a rapid rise in body temperature can cause one.

A fever with a rash, long bouts of diarrhea and vomiting, little intake of fluids, or one that rose rapidly with or without seizure are all indications that a potentially serious medical condition may be present. Call for EMT or ALS transport as soon as possible.

It is not necessary to try to take a temperature. If the skin feels very warm to touch, report this finding along with skin color and condition. A child with a high fever will likely be flushed and dry. A mild fever may quickly elevate to a high fever and become a life-threatening problem.

If the child is hot to the touch and there is a history of fever reported by the parent or caregiver, take the following steps if your local protocols allow (Figure 13.10):

- Undress the child down to underwear or diaper, but do not allow him to become chilled. Many parents still believe that feverish children must be bundled up so they will not become chilled or so they will sweat out a fever. All this clothing retains the heat of the fever.

- Cover the child with a towel soaked in tepid (not cold) water if the fever is the result of heat exposure. If the child starts to shiver, stop the cooling process and cover with a light blanket.

- Place damp, cool cloths on the fevered child's hot forehead.

- Give sips of cool water, but only if the child is alert and cooperative. Let the child suck on a cloth filled with chipped ice or, if old enough, suck directly on chipped ice.

- Call for the transport of any child who has had a seizure. If the child is seizing, monitor airway and breathing.

- NEVER submerge a child in cold water.

- NEVER use rubbing alcohol for cooling. It can be absorbed in toxic amounts through the child's skin.

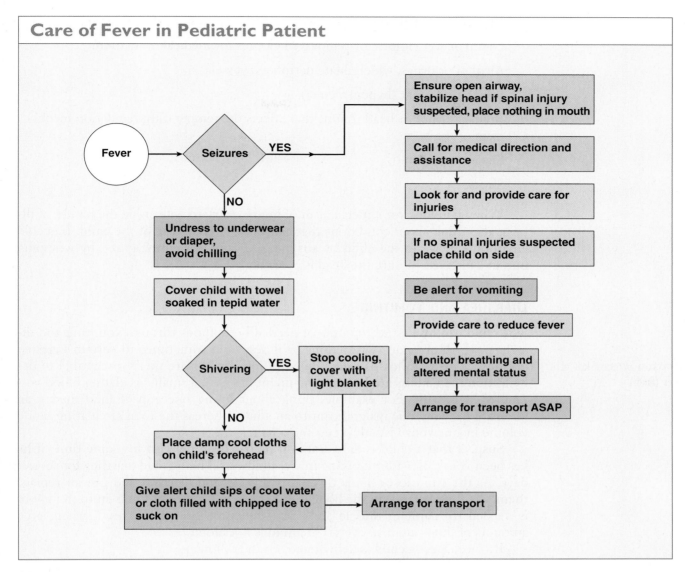

Care of Fever in Pediatric Patient

Fever → **Seizures** —YES→ Ensure open airway, stabilize head if spinal injury suspected, place nothing in mouth → Call for medical direction and assistance → Look for and provide care for injuries → If no spinal injuries suspected place child on side → Be alert for vomiting → Provide care to reduce fever → Monitor breathing and altered mental status → Arrange for transport ASAP

Seizures —NO→ Undress to underwear or diaper, avoid chilling → Cover child with towel soaked in tepid water → **Shivering**

Shivering —YES→ Stop cooling, cover with light blanket → Place damp cool cloths on child's forehead

Shivering —NO→ Place damp cool cloths on child's forehead → Give alert child sips of cool water or cloth filled with chipped ice to suck on → Arrange for transport

FIGURE 13.10

Be cautious about cooling a fevered child. You can cause hypothermia or reduced body temperature. Wet towels and sheets cool rapidly and become cold, which causes the child to shiver and become chilled.

HYPOTHERMIA

Children lose a lot of body heat through their heads. The surface area of the child's head is proportionately larger than the rest of the body. The large head radiates and loses heat when it is uncovered. When the head is exposed, the body will make every effort to keep the brain warm and functioning, so it sends heat from other parts of the body to the head. Since the child cannot conserve heat well, it will not take long to use up any reserves and develop hypothermia. Keep the head covered to prevent heat loss when caring for infants and children in cool environments.

Children's bodies are unable to regulate temperatures as well as adult bodies can, even in normal room temperatures (68°F). Most children do not have much fat stored under their skin and cannot conserve heat. They can become chilled through the environment, injury, or illness, including:

- Exposure to cool weather and water.
- Damp or wet clothes, or removal of clothes for medical evaluation.
- Alcohol or drugs, which dilate peripheral vessels.
- Low blood sugar (hypoglycemia).
- Brain disorder or head trauma that affects the temperature regulation mechanism of the body.
- Severe infection.
- Shock.

When you look for a mechanism of injury or try to determine the nature of illness, also think about conditions that can cause overcooling of the child. In a cold environment, warm the child by stripping off any wet clothing and by wrapping him in a blanket. Be sure the head is covered.

DIARRHEA AND VOMITING

dehydration excessive loss of body water (fluids).

The child can lose large amounts of needed body fluids through vomiting and diarrhea, which are normal reactions to illness (and sometimes to certain ingested poisons). This fluid loss is called **dehydration**. Infants are more susceptible to dehydration than adults are because the infant has such a small circulating blood volume to start with. For example, think about losing one cup of fluid during an illness. This would be insignificant to an adult, whereas the total circulating blood volume in a newborn is only a cup and a half.

Suspect that a child is dehydrated if he has been feverish for some time, if he has been vomiting without taking in any fluids, or if he has had diarrhea for several days. As the child loses fluids through vomiting and diarrhea and cannot replace them, the fluid balance in the body is disturbed. A balance of fluids-in to fluids-out is needed to maintain muscle and organ function. Shock can result when large amounts of fluids are lost, even if the fluid is not blood.

If you suspect a child is dehydrated, do the following:

1. Monitor the airway.
2. Position the child so the airway will not be obstructed if the child vomits. Elevating the legs may help if the patient is showing signs of shock.
3. Monitor respirations and administer blow-by oxygen as per local protocols.
4. Check vital signs. If they indicate shock, arrange to transport immediately.
5. If protocols permit and the child is alert, allow him to sip water or suck on chipped ice.
6. If possible, save some vomitus for hospital personnel to examine.

POISONING

Part of a child's learning experience includes exploring and tasting things. This can sometimes lead to exposure to or ingestion of poisonous substances. Poisons can affect any or all of the body's systems and can rapidly threaten the life of a child. Much of your assessment and care will be the same as for an adult. Know your local protocols for contacting medical direction or a poison control center if there is any indication or suspicion that a child has been exposed to a poison. Be aware that some poisons may be considered hazardous materials, which will require response by specialized personnel trained to handle them. The hazmat team will perform decontamination procedures.

NEAR-DROWNING

The child who has been submerged in water may still be alive or clinically dead (no breathing and no heartbeat), but not biologically dead (brain cells are still alive). Many patients have been revived after over 30 minutes of submersion in cold water. Children have been successfully revived more often than adults in these situations. When caring for a possible near-drowning patient:

1. Make sure the airway is clear and free of fluids.

2. Provide artificial ventilations or CPR as necessary.

3. Protect the spine in cases where the near-drowning was the result of a diving or boating incident.

4. Get the patient to a warm and dry environment away from wind to prevent or care for hypothermia. Remove wet clothing.

5. Place the child in the recovery position to prevent aspiration. Administer high-concentration oxygen (as per local protocols).

6. Obtain a baseline set of vital signs.

7. Arrange to transport all near-drowning patients, even if they have recovered and are breathing on their own. It is possible that they will deteriorate hours after they have recovered.

MANAGING TRAUMA EMERGENCIES

GENERAL CARE OF THE CHILD TRAUMA PATIENT

Because of their size, curiosity, and lack of fear due to their inexperience, infants and children are frequent victims of trauma. It is the number-one cause of death in people 1–18 years of age—as a result of motor-vehicle crashes, drowning, burns, firearms, falls, blunt and penetrating trauma, abuse, entrapment, crushing, and various other mechanisms of injury (Figure 13.11).

When performing a physical exam on a stable, responsive child you can reverse your assessment order and do a toe-to-head physical exam. For unresponsive or unstable patients, perform the head-to-toe assessment, focus on the ABCs, and determine priority of transport.

When managing injuries in children, keep in mind that their larger head size and weight will make them more prone to head and neck trauma in motor-vehicle collisions, especially if unrestrained. This is also true of bicycle mishaps if children are not wearing helmets, in mishaps in which they are struck, in swimming and diving mishaps, and in sports mishaps. Suspect abdominal and pelvic injuries in vehicle crashes in which the child is restrained, and extremity injuries in falls of three times their height or greater.

FIRST➤ General emergency care steps for the infant or child trauma patient include the following (Figure 13.12):

1. Ensure an open airway. Manually stabilize the head and neck. Use a jaw-thrust maneuver to open the airway and protect the spine. Place a folded towel under the shoulders to maintain a neutral position for the airway and alignment of the head.

FIGURE 13.11
Look for the mechanism of injury.

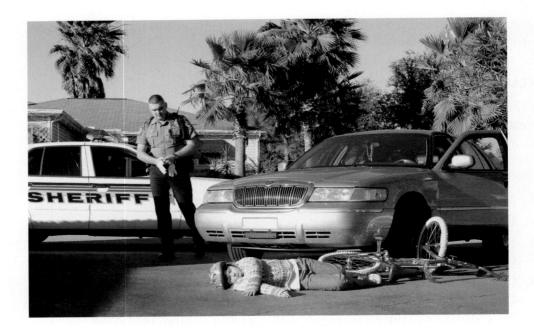

2. Make sure the airway is clear. Suction, if local protocols allow. If necessary, provide ventilations.

3. Provide oxygen by nonrebreather mask or assist ventilations with a bag-valve-mask ventilator with supplemental oxygen as per local protocols.

4. Control bleeding by applying appropriate dressings.

5. Stabilize painful, swollen, deformed injuries to extremities.

6. Maintain manual stabilization of the patient's head and neck until EMT or ALS personnel arrive.

7. Arrange for transport as soon as possible.

8. While waiting for the EMTs to arrive or while en route, perform your detailed and ongoing assessments. ■

For a summary of the assessment and emergency care of pediatric patients with specific musculoskeletal injuries, see Figure 13.13. For assessment and care of bleeding, shock, and specific soft-tissue injuries, see Figure 13.14.

SAFETY SEATS

Too many safety seats are not installed correctly, and children often are not secured properly by the safety straps and harnesses. Any movement of the seat or the child can throw both forward in a crash. As a result, the child receives internal injuries, which emergency care providers may not be able to initially detect. Usually, the child's body will compensate for these internal injuries and bleeding, which can lull the rescuers into thinking the child is unharmed and stable.

Based on crash-result studies over recent years, it has been determined that removing children from their safety seats and immobilizing them on spine boards is the best procedure for children involved in vehicle crashes. The National Safe Kids Campaign is working to promote this change based on crash studies (Table 13-3).

Any vehicle crash should lead you to suspect that the child has been injured, even if you do not see any damage to the safety seat. Carefully extricate the child from the safety seat and place him on a spinal immobilization device, if local proto-

Pediatric Trauma—Standard Protocol

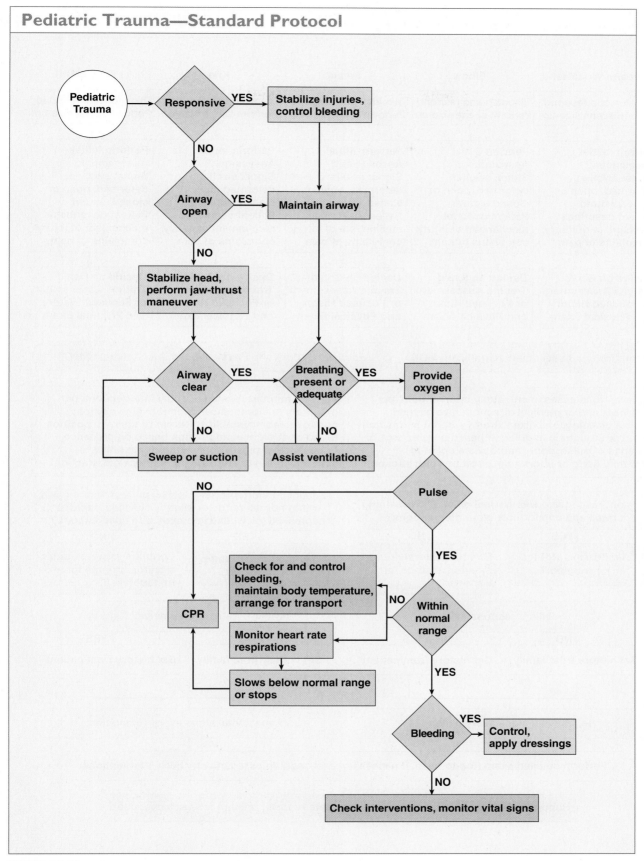

FIGURE 13.12

Pediatric Musculoskeletal Emergencies

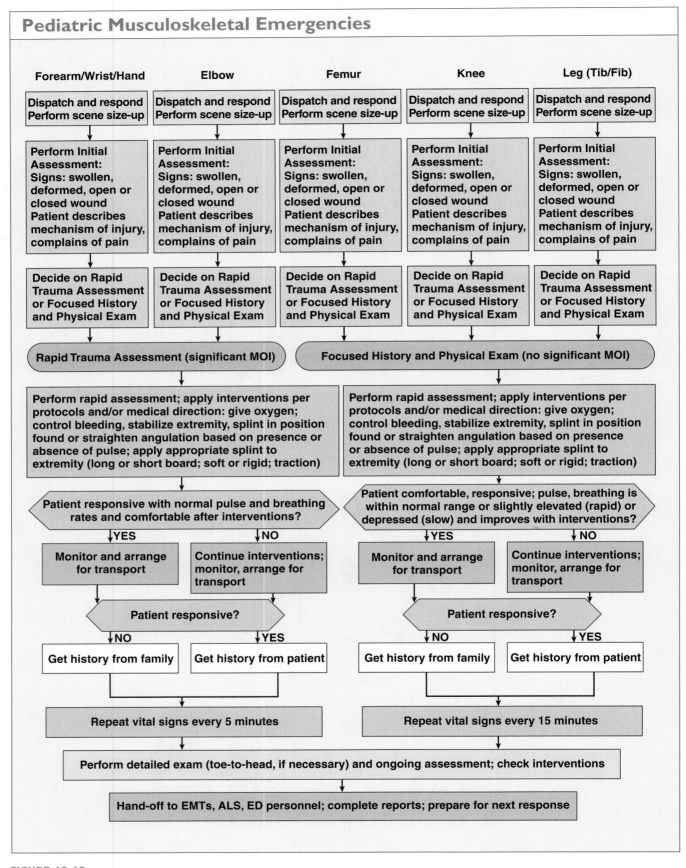

FIGURE 13.13

Pediatric Bleeding, Shock, and Soft-Tissue Injuries

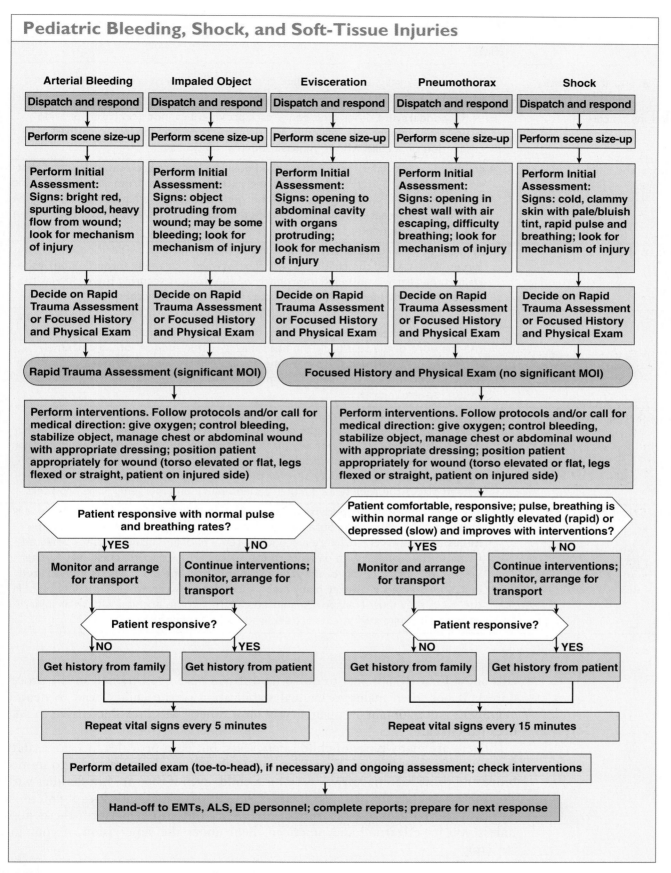

FIGURE 13.14

TABLE 13-3 CHILD SAFETY SEATS

ISSUES	FACTS
Installation and child security	Too many safety seats are not installed correctly, and children are often not secured properly by the safety straps and harnesses.
Restrictions on care	First Responders and other emergency care providers cannot adequately provide airway management care, maintain an open airway, or provide bag-valve-mask resuscitation on a child who is immobilized in a safety seat.
Position of the child	A child's torso in a safety seat is in a flexed position because the seat is designed that way. Spinal immobilization straightens and extends the spine from the cervical spine (the neck) to the sacrum (the part of the spine between the hip bones). Leaving the child in a safety seat continues to stretch the spine in a curved position rather than in a straight, extended position.
Injuries to the child	If an infant or small child of any age is riding in the forward-facing position, the crash forces likely caused the child's body to flex forward extremely (hyperflexion), especially if the seat was installed improperly or the harness securing the child was too loose. This sudden forward flexion causes injury to the cervical spine.
Protection for the child	Children up to age 4 and up to 40 pounds may be too large for their child safety seat to support the head and protect them properly. If the child's head extends above the top edge of the seat back, the head may hyperextend (be forced extremely backward) in a crash. At the same time, the body is thrust forward. All this sudden and extreme motion stretches the ligaments and muscles of the spinal column, causing severe injuries.
Car seat damage and stability	The safety seat involved in a vehicle crash (especially an improperly installed one) is likely to be damaged, though the damage may not be noticed even on close inspection. A damaged seat will not adequately immobilize and support the child. Further, manufacturers state that child safety seats are not designed to be used as immobilizing devices. Using the safety seat for purposes other than the manufacturer intended places the liability for further patient injury on emergency care providers.
Transport considerations	Safety seats cannot be properly secured in the ambulance. Further, if the ambulance is involved in a collision en route to the hospital, the safety seat cannot endure the forces of another crash. There are enough reports of ambulance crashes while en route to the hospital with patients to cause concern. A second crash may further weaken the effectiveness of the safety seat and leave the child, who is immobilized in it, unprotected. However, many ambulances are now carrying child safety seats in the event they must transport uninjured children to the hospital with their injured parents. The child safety seats are secured in the captain's chair.

cols allow First Responders to do so (and if you have been trained in the procedures). If not, then maintain manual stabilization of the child's head in neutral alignment and maintain an open airway until other EMS providers arrive to take over patient care.

There are many types of child safety seats, but each provides the same safety functions if properly used. First Responders should not hesitate to act to immobilize and provide initial airway care for a child, even if they are not familiar with the safety seat they find at a crash site. Use the following guidelines if you must extricate an infant or a child from a safety seat, but do not perform these steps unless you have learned and practiced them under the supervision of your instructor:

- Do a quick visual inspection of the vehicle interior: Did the crash force the safety seat from its position, even slightly? Was the safety seat in the rear or front vehicle seat? Was the safety seat a rear-facing or forward-facing seat? Is there structural damage to the seat?

- Throughout the assessment and immobilization process, be sure that someone maintains manual stabilization of the infant's or the child's head.

- Assess the patient for airway, breathing, and circulation. Assess for injuries.

- If the safety seat has a protection plate over the patient's chest, remove it (cut the straps securing it, if necessary) in order to assess the chest area and provide care, such as lung assessment and bleeding control. (Before performing chest compressions, remove the infant onto an immobilization device.)

- As you assess the patient, check for loose straps, which would have provided little protection. Extricate the child onto an immobilization device, which can then be secured to the ambulance stretcher (Scan 13-2).

PNEUMATIC ANTI-SHOCK GARMENTS

Pneumatic anti-shock garments (PASGs) are rarely used for pediatric patients. They are only used for certain injuries. Check with your instructor to see if your jurisdiction allows First Responders to become trained in using them for stabilizing pelvic injuries in pediatric patients. If so, your instructor will provide you with the equipment and training. When using a PASG for a pediatric patient, it is critical that it fit the patient so it does not compromise respirations. Check your local protocols.

BURNS

Burns in infants and children are assessed somewhat differently than for adults because of the child's larger surface area, larger heads, and smaller extremities. In the rule of nines, for example, the percentage of body surface area assigned is slightly different: 18% to the head and neck, 18% to the chest and abdomen, 9% to each arm, 18% to the entire back, 14% for each leg, and 1% to the genital area. If you find it is difficult to do the estimations with accuracy while you are trying to quickly care for and stabilize the patient, do not worry about precision. The safest procedure is to estimate quickly and overestimate rather than underestimate the body surface area burned. The younger the child, the more important it is that he is seen in a burn center because of concerns about abuse and long-term morbidity.

Carefully and quickly care for the burned area with dry, sterile, and non-adherent dressings or sheets. Dry dressings will keep air and foreign materials or dirt off the burn and will help keep the child warm, which will help in preventing shock. Moist dressings may chill the child and could speed the shock response. Follow local protocols for burn management. Arrange to transport the burned child as quickly as possible. Check local protocols for determining the type of cases (degree of severity, respiratory burns) that should be transported to a burn center. Burns are excruciatingly painful, and children are likely to be frantic. Rapid transport is important for obtaining pain relief for the child as well as for care of the burns.

SUSPECTED NEGLECT AND ABUSE

The news media have been reporting more stories of child neglect and abuse in recent years. These events are not something new. Rather, they have always existed but are now more recognized and reported. A case of child abuse or neglect is one of the most difficult emergency situations for the First Responder to handle. It is

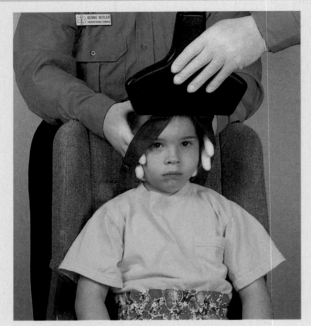

1. Rescuer #1 stabilizes car seat in upright position and applies manual head/neck stabilization. Rescuer #2 prepares equipment, then loosens or cuts the seat straps and raises the front guard.

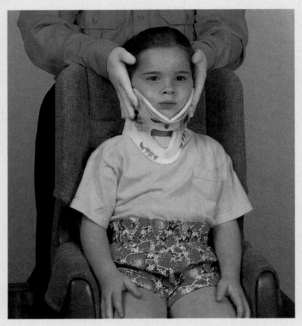

2. Cervical collar is applied to patient as Rescuer #1 maintains manual stabilization of the head and neck.

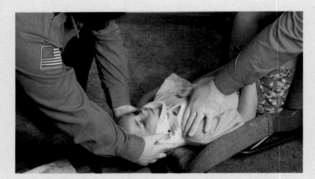

3. As Rescuer #1 maintains manual head/neck stabilization, Rescuer #2 places child safety seat on center of backboard and slowly tilts it into supine position. Both rescuers are careful not to let the child slide out of the chair. For the child with a large head, place a towel under area where the shoulders will eventually be placed on the board to prevent head from tilting forward.

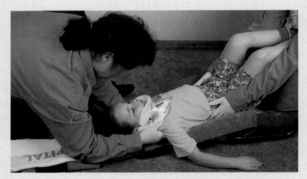

4a. Rescuer #1 maintains manual head/neck stabilization and calls for a coordinated long axis move onto the backboard.

continued...

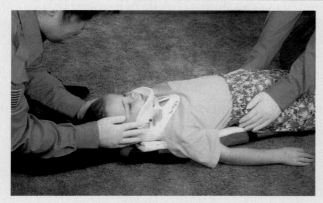

4b. Rescuer #1 maintains manual head/neck stabilization as the move onto board is completed, with the child's shoulders over the folded towel.

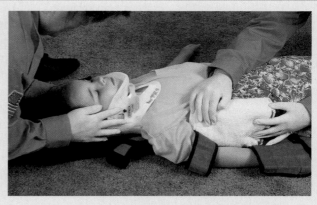

5. Rescuer #1 maintains manual head/neck stabilization. Rescuer #2 places rolled towels or blankets on both sides of the patient.

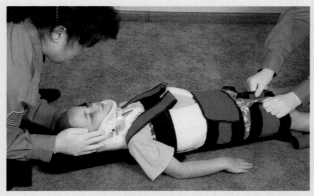

6. Rescuer #1 maintains manual head/neck stabilization. Rescuer #2 straps or tapes patient to board at level of upper chest, pelvis, and lower legs. Do not strap across abdomen.

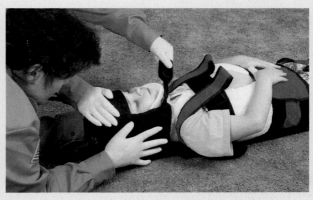

7. Rescuer #1 maintains manual head/neck stabilization as Rescuer #2 places rolled towels on both sides of head, then tapes head securely in place across forehead and maxilla (jaw bone) or cervical collar. Do not tape across chin to avoid putting pressure on neck.

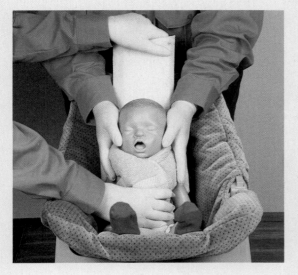

The infant procedure is exactly the same as for a child, except that an arm board is inserted behind the infant in step 2. If the infant is very small, the arm board may actually be used as the spine board.

normal to experience some very strong emotions that you must control in order to assess and care for the child. After the call, it is important to talk out your feelings with those who can offer support and understanding. Remember to maintain patient confidentiality. You cannot name the child or family to anyone but medical or juvenile authorities or the police.

You must collect information, perform your assessments, and provide care without making a judgment or expressing your suspicion, distaste, or disbelief. Keep in mind that the abuser also needs help. Remember that your suspicions may be unfounded and that not every injury or sign of possible abuse to a child is the result of actual abuse. It is not your place to accuse the parents or caregiver, because they may not even be the abuser. You will need to check for patterns in responses and reports to confirm your suspicions. Report your concerns and impressions to EMT or ALS personnel, medical direction, or to social services, the health department, or the police as required by local protocols. In most jurisdictions, there is a legal obligation to report suspected child abuse. Be aware of your local laws and protocols regarding reporting abuse.

FIRST> There are several different forms of child abuse, and they frequently occur in combination (Figure 13.15):

- Psychological abuse.
- Neglect.
- Sexual abuse.
- Physical abuse. ■

Psychological Abuse

It may be rare that First Responders are called to care for a patient who has been psychologically abused, because there is no physical injury. However, there may be emotional signs and symptoms that may be difficult to assess unless you know the patient. **Psychological abuse** includes emotional or verbal abuse that seriously affects the child's positive emotional development, well-being, and self-esteem. Children exposed to psychological abuse may feel rejected, degraded, or terrified. They may be forced into isolation with limited freedom or contact with others. They may be exploited or corrupted and forced to accept the beliefs of another, such as a cult or gang leader. Verbal abuse that affects emotional well-being and self-esteem and causes feelings of rejection or degradation in children includes phrases such as, "You're stupid," "You are no good," "You are not like your sister," "I wish you were never born," or "I hate you." Some parents isolate their children, locking them in

psychological abuse
persistent emotional or verbal abuse that affects a child's positive emotional development, self-esteem, and emotional well-being.

FIGURE 13.15
Example of injuries caused by abuse and neglect.

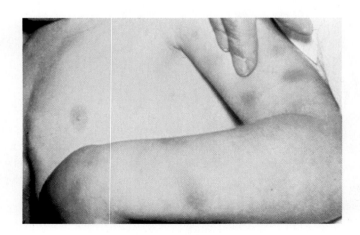

closets or not letting them attend school. Cult and gang leaders often exploit the emotions of vulnerable teenagers, making them believe that the cult loves them or the gang gives them power and freedom and their parents do not.

Though psychological abuse can occur alone, victims often suffer other forms of abuse with it, such as sexual and physical abuse. The victims of psychological abuse, as well as other forms of abuse, are those with the least power and resources—children and women. Possible signs of psychological abuse include the following:

- Depression.
- Withdrawal.
- Extreme anxiety.
- Low self-esteem.
- Feelings of shame and guilt.
- Fear.
- Lack of normal social skills because of isolation.
- Avoidance of eye contact.
- Extreme passiveness or compliance.
- History or indications of self-harm.
- Substance abuse.
- Increased tension or anxiety when the abuser is present.

Provide care and emotional support by listening to and believing what the child tells you and expressing your understanding. Let the child know that there are people who will help and that you can get help. Arrange to have the child transported to get him away from the abuser if necessary. Be sure to report your findings to the transport personnel, and to social services, the health department, or the police as required by your protocols.

Neglect

Emergency responses are usually for the obvious traumas that occur in physical and sexual abuse, not for neglect. However, long-term **neglect** may result in physical deterioration and injury or medical problems. Child neglect occurs when parents or caregivers do not provide for any or all of the following basic needs of the child:

- Food and water.
- Appropriate shelter and clothing.
- Medical care.
- Education.

neglect failure of the parents or caregivers to provide for the child's basic physical, social, emotional, medical, and/or medical needs.

On arrival, your scene size-up may reveal obvious signs of neglect, such as a child who is dressed inappropriately for the weather, a child who is lean, lethargic, and has signs of dehydration, or an environment with unclean living conditions, particularly where the child sleeps or is confined. Consider also the circumstances of the family: they may not be able to financially afford to provide for the basic needs of the child or even themselves, and the entire family may need help from social services. Provide appropriate care for the child's illness or injuries and arrange to transport. Follow your protocols for reporting your concerns.

Sexual Abuse

sexual abuse physical sexual contact with or exposure to children and sexual exploitation of children by exposing, displaying, or photographing them for sexual purposes or with sexual intent.

There are many forms of child **sexual abuse**, including physical sexual contact or exposure and sexual exploitation by displaying or photographing children for sexual purposes or with sexual intent. First Responders usually receive a call for sexual abuse if the child is injured or showing signs of a sexually related medical condition. A child can be the victim of sexual abuse from a parent or other relative and sometimes from a neighbor, teacher, or other trusted individual. Do not expect the abuser to admit that sexual abuse is the reason for the call. Many excuses and reasons are given for the child who has genital injuries or who has signs and symptoms of sexually transmitted diseases. Continue to act professionally and control your emotions. When providing care, avoid embarrassing the child or making him feel guilty. Let the child know that you and the people at the hospital will help. Some signs of sexual abuse include:

- Obvious injuries to the genital area, including burns, cuts, bruises, abrasions.

- Rashes or sores around the genitals, discharges (such as seminal fluid), bleeding from the genital openings or on underclothing.

- Information from the child that he was exposed, touched, or assaulted.

FIRST➤ Be sure to report your suspicions and findings to EMT or ALS personnel or to the appropriate agency as per local protocols. Use these emergency care steps:

1. Dress wounds and provide other appropriate care for injuries.

2. Save any evidence of sexual abuse, such as soiled or stained clothing. Do not let the child use the bathroom to urinate or defecate. If the child must go to the bathroom, try to collect it in a container for hospital examination. Do not let the child drink any fluids or eat anything. Do not wash the child or let the parent wash the child or change clothes. (The parent may insist on washing the child and changing his clothing; the child may insist that he must use the bathroom. Be aware that you cannot prevent them from doing so.)

3. Minimize embarrassment by covering the child with a blanket if necessary.

4. Arrange for transport as soon as possible.

5. Provide emotional support and reassurance. Remember, you are still caring for a child. Try to engage him with toys or age-appropriate conversation or games. ■

Physical Abuse

physical abuse inflicting any type of physical injury or performing any physical act that harms or disfigures the child.

Any form of violent, harmful contact with a child or any disfiguring act performed on the child is **physical abuse**, no matter what the intent of the adult. Some of the indications of physical abuse include the following:

- Outline of marks or bruises that are the size or shape of the object used to strike the child, such as the hand, a belt, strap, rope, or cord.

- Areas of swelling, black eyes, loose or missing teeth, split lips.

- Lacerations, incisions, abrasions.

- Any unexplained bruises, broken bones, or burn marks.

- Broken bones, signs of injuries healing incorrectly (misshaped limbs), or a history of numerous broken bones.

- Head injuries or indications of closed head injuries that could be the result of violent shaking (bulging fontanelles, unresponsiveness), especially in infants and small children.

- Bruises—old and new—in various stages of healing.

- Abdominal injuries with signs of bruising, distention, rigidity, or tenderness that could be the result of punching or kicking.

- Genitalia injuries with lacerations, avulsions, or bleeding.

- Bite marks showing the pattern and size of an adult mouth.

- Burn marks or patterns caused by cigarettes, hot irons, stove burners; water burns or scalding marks on the legs, such as stocking burns from dipping in hot water or a hand mark on the buttocks where the child's skin was protected from immersion. The creases at the knees and thighs are also protected when the child flexes his legs while being dipped in hot water.

The child's relationship with the parents or a parent's attitude toward the child or the situation may be a clue to abuse. However, these will not always be reliable indicators of the family relationship. Look for the following:

- Story of how the injury occurred that does not match the injury found.

- Child who seems afraid to say how the injury happened.

- Child who is obviously afraid of a parent or other person at the scene.

- Child who seems to expect no comfort from the parent.

- Child who has no apparent reaction to pain.

- Parent who does not wish to leave you alone with the child.

- Parents who tell conflicting stories or change explanations.

- Parent who blames the child for being clumsy or accident-prone.

- Parent who seems inappropriately concerned or unconcerned.

- Parent who is angry and is having trouble controlling it.

- One parent who appears depressed or withdrawn while the other parent is expressing anger or giving explanations.

- Any signs of alcohol or drug abuse.

- Any expression of suicide or seeking mercy for their children.

- Parent who is reluctant to give the child's history or to permit transport or who refuses to go to the nearest hospital.

You must be the child's advocate and convince the parents that the child needs to be seen by a physician because of "the difficulty of determining the seriousness of injuries in the field." Do not accuse anyone of any wrongdoing.

You may respond to a call for an injured child and have no idea that the injury is related to abuse. You may observe that the child and parents relate well and that there is a strong bond among them. There are still abuse indications that will make you suspicious over time. Be alert for:

- Repeated responses for the same child or children in the same house.

- Signs of past injuries during your assessment.

- Signs of poorly healing wounds.

- Signs of burns that are fresh or in various stages of healing.

- Many types of injuries on numerous parts of the body.

Obvious abuse situations can trigger strong emotions in you. Most people feel it is their duty to protect young children. Your first reactions to an abuse situation may be anger and disgust. However, you should not display these feelings while caring for the child or dealing with the parents or other caregivers. Providing necessary care for the child's injuries, clearly documenting objective findings, and alerting the proper authorities of your suspicions are appropriate actions. If you suspect abuse and the parent or caregiver will not allow the child to be transported, call for law enforcement assistance. Keep in mind that you may also need to get help in dealing with the aftereffects of dealing with child-abuse cases. Consider contacting your critical incident stress management (CISM) team.

Shaken Baby Syndrome

Another type of abuse is shaken baby syndrome. It is a group of signs and symptoms that usually occur in children younger than two years old but may be seen in children up to five years. The syndrome results from the trauma caused by an angry or an extremely frustrated parent or caregiver who shakes the baby as a punishment or as an attempt to quiet him. The intent, usually, is not to harm the baby. Rarely, the syndrome may be caused accidentally by tossing the baby in the air or jogging with the baby in a backpack. It is not a result of gentle bouncing.

Infants and children have large heavy heads, weak and not fully developed neck muscles, and space between the brain and the skull to allow for growth. The skull is also soft and pliable and not yet strong enough to absorb much force. During violent shaking, the brain will rebound against the inside of the skull and bruise, swell, and bleed, which causes increased pressure. Shaking also can cause injury to the neck and spine and to the eyes, causing loss of vision.

If you are called to the scene of a sick or injured child, ask the parent or caregiver questions to obtain a history. Look for signs and symptoms of illness or injury in your assessment. A shaken baby may have no obvious signs of trauma, such as bruising, bleeding, or swelling. The history and some of the signs and symptoms of shaken baby syndrome may include the following, but they may also be indications of other illnesses:

- Change in behavior.
- Irritability.
- Lethargy or sleepiness.
- Decreased alertness.
- Unresponsiveness.
- Pale or bluish (cyanotic) skin.
- Vomiting.
- Convulsions (seizures).
- Not eating normally.
- Not breathing.

Shaken baby syndrome is a serious emergency. Call for ALS support immediately for any child with the above signs and symptoms. While waiting for them to arrive, ensure that the baby has an airway, is breathing, and has a pulse. Perform rescue breathing or CPR as needed and provide oxygen, if you are trained and allowed to do so. If the child is vomiting, protect and clear the airway. Be sure to turn the infant as a unit, keeping the head in line with the body. If the infant is having seizures, protect him from further injury.

Chapter Review

Assessment and emergency care of infants and children is basically the same as for adults. However, you must consider the special characteristics of the pediatric patient's anatomy, physiology, and emotional responses when assessing and caring for them. For example, to help keep an infant or a child calm, reverse the order of the physical assessment. Begin at the toes and work toward the head. Infants and children may also be examined while sitting on a parent's lap.

One example of a child's different anatomy compared to that of an adult's is the head. In infants and children, the head is larger and heavier in proportion to the rest of the body. Be suspicious of mechanisms of injury that have the potential to cause head and spine injury. Also, carefully handle the head of an infant up to 18 months; do not apply any pressure to the soft spots (fontanelles).

Infants breathe through the nose. If it is obstructed, they may not immediately open their mouths to breathe. Be sure to clear the nostrils of secretions. Remember also that because the tongue is larger in an infant and a child, it can cause airway obstruction. When managing the airway of an infant, make sure the large head is in a neutral position, neither hyperflexed nor hyperextended. Place a folded towel under the infant's or the child's shoulders to maintain the spine and the airway in neutral alignment.

Care for respiratory distress in infants and children immediately. For respiratory distress, provide oxygen with a pediatric-size nonrebreather mask or by using the blow-by technique. For severe distress and respiratory arrest, provide assisted ventilations with the appropriate device, such as a pocket face mask or pediatric bag-valve-mask ventilator and supplemental oxygen. Do not place anything in the mouth of the infant or child unless you see an obstruction. Arrange for transport immediately.

Children tolerate high fevers better than adults do, but a fever that rises rapidly can cause seizures. Arrange to transport the feverish child as soon as possible. Also arrange to transport the child who is vomiting and has diarrhea.

The surface area of a child's body is large in proportion to weight. This makes infants and children more vulnerable to hypothermia. Covering the patient, especially the head, will help maintain warmth.

Care for shock early. In an infant or child, signs and symptoms of shock mean it has progressed and is in the late stages. If you suspect that shock may result from the mechanism of injury or nature of illness, provide emergency care immediately.

Because of their size, curiosity, and a lack of fear due to their inexperience, infants and children are frequent victims of trauma. When assessing and providing emergency care, keep in mind that their larger head size and weight make pediatric patients more prone to head and neck trauma. In addition, be calm, professional, and discreet about suspicions of abuse or neglect in the presence of caregivers. Be an advocate for the child and remember your obligation to report any suspicions to the proper authorities.

Children are curious and daring, and they like to have fun. Sometimes they get into fights or into situations in which they get hurt. Many result in bumps and scrapes that are easy for a parent to care for, but sometimes an illness or injury is serious enough, or frightening enough to the child or parent, that EMS is needed.

✔ What are some of the types of injuries you expect to see in certain age groups?

✔ What can you do to help calm a crying and frightened child?

✔ Think about the many activities that children are involved in today. How do they compare with what you did as a child? Do children have more opportunities, freedom, and choices of activities today? Do these activities bring a higher potential for illness or injury?

✔ Find out how many pediatric calls your department or agency had this past year and what types they were. Were there more responses to illnesses or to injuries?

With this information, you can get an idea of where you will want to concentrate your learning and practice. Many emergency responders are nervous about caring for children. It may be because they have little experience with children who are healthy and much less experience with those who are seriously ill or injured. It may also be because children appear small and helpless, and care providers are often afraid of causing more pain while trying to help. Many chil-dren are afraid of strangers, and the care provider will find it hard to communicate with them, which may make you uncomfortable. As a result, you may not know what to do. This is normal, but you cannot allow it to interfere with your ability to care for these patients. If you never have the opportunity to work with or be around children, it is, of course, more diffi-cult to work with them in an emergency. If you have the time to work with children as a baby-sitter, coach, camp counselor, or tutor, you will learn more about their personalities and feel more comfortable working with any child.

INVESTIGATE...

✔ Locate the schools and day-care centers in your area.

Find out if the schools have health rooms and school nurses. Are the nurses on duty every day? What does the school or day-care center do when a child is taken seriously ill or is injured? Are parents or is EMS called first? Will you be able to provide care for or transport a child without a parent present? (You may wish to review legal and consent issues in Chapter 2.) Ask other EMS providers to tell you about their experiences.

✔ Locate the ball fields, parks, and playgrounds in your area.

During what seasons are these areas the most pop-ulated by children? What sports do they play, who su-pervises them, and what policies are followed if a child is hurt at an organized game? What injuries would you expect to find at a baseball or softball game; at a field- or ice-hockey game; at a soccer, basketball, or football game? Are the coaches trained in providing care for sports injuries? If the parents are not at the game, how can they be contacted? Will you care for the child without consent?

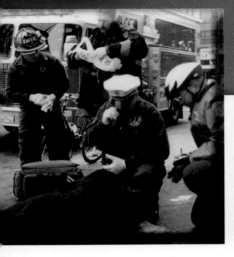
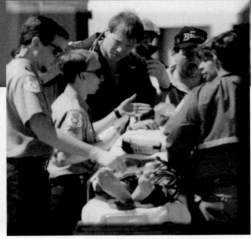
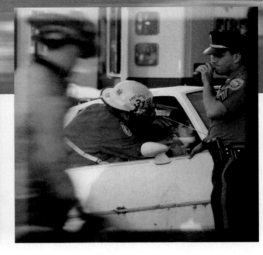

Gaining Access and Hazards on Scene

CHAPTER

14

First Responders are one part of an EMS system that functions and responds 24 hours a day every day of the year. These operations include many services involving a wide range of skills. First Responders provide basic services such as responding to minor illnesses and injuries. First Responders are also prepared for more serious medical and trauma incidents. They help EMT and ALS personnel in monitoring and providing care for critically injured patients at vehicle crashes, building fires and other hazardous scenes, and multiple-casualty incidents. Learning what steps to take, what care to provide, what assistance to give, and performing these tasks in cooperation with other personnel and services in the system are all part of EMS operations.

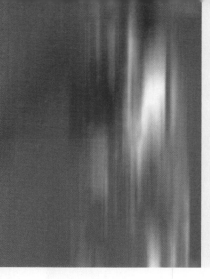

NATIONAL STANDARD OBJECTIVES

This chapter focuses on the objectives of Module 7, Lesson 7–1, of the U.S. DOT's First Responder National Standard Curriculum and serves as an instructional aid to help you meet any specific objectives added to the course by your local EMS system.

By the end of this chapter, you will be able to (from cognitive or knowledge information):

7–1.1 Discuss the medical and nonmedical equipment needed to respond to a call. (pp. 500–501)

7–1.2 List the phases of an out-of-hospital call. (pp. 499–502)

7–1.3 Discuss the role of the First Responder in extrication. (pp. 503–513)

7–1.4 List various methods of gaining access to the patient. (pp. 503–513)

LEARNING TASKS

This chapter explains the operations of the EMS system and how all system services and personnel coordinate their activities to rescue and provide care in critical or disaster situations. As you work through this chapter to meet the above objectives, there is some additional information that will be essential to consider and act upon at the scene of certain critical incidents.

One of the most common critical incidents for a First Responder may be a motor-vehicle collision, especially if you are a police officer. You should be able to:

✔ State what elements you must evaluate at the scene of a motor-vehicle collision or incidents involving multiple vehicles.

✔ Describe safety steps to take at a motor-vehicle collision scene before you gain access to patients.

✔ Describe how to stabilize a vehicle that is on its side.

✔ State how you would gain access to patients who are in a stabilized vehicle that is on its side.

✔ State how you would free patients pinned in a vehicle.

If your training agency provides old vehicles for practicing extrication skills, your instructor will teach you how to use simple tools to gain access to the patient. If so, you should be able to:

✔ Demonstrate the steps of evaluating and making the scene safe.

✔ Demonstrate how to stabilize an upright vehicle.

✔ Demonstrate how to stabilize an overturned vehicle.

✔ Demonstrate how to gain access to patients in vehicles, using simple tools.

Many First Responders are firefighters who often discover, report, or arrive first at structure fires. Firefighters wearing appropriate protective gear may be assigned to find victims in the building and to care for patients brought from a building. You should be able to:

✔ Describe the basic ways to gain access to patients found in a variety of structures.

✔ Identify those hazards that are unique to a fire scene.

✔ State what you should do if electrical or gas hazards exist at the scene.

Hazardous-materials training is a separate and special program. Many jurisdictions require all emergency services personnel to complete the awareness level of hazardous-materials training before they may respond on any emergency call. For any emergency incident involving possible hazardous materials, you should be able to:

✔ State how to recognize a possible hazardous-materials incident.
✔ Describe First Responder duties at hazardous-materials incidents.
✔ List the types of information that must be gathered from and reported on a hazardous-materials scene.

SAFETY

Your first consideration at any emergency scene is your own safety. To ensure your safety, follow standard operating procedures (SOPs) or standard operating guidelines (SOGs), limit your actions to your training level, and use the proper equipment and the required number of trained persons for any task (Figure 14.1).

There are always risks, but EMS personnel must minimize the risks and learn what risks they can control before acting. For example, you have no control over the chance that a drunk driver could crash into you as you provide care at the scene of a traffic collision. But by using proper warning devices to divert traffic (for example, flares) and by positioning your own vehicle or response unit at a proper distance from the scene, you can minimize your risks of being injured by passing cars (Figure 14.2). At any emergency scene, you must always:

> **NOTE**
>
> When you are restricted to following SOPs or SOGs, you must follow a procedure, which may not fit every variable encountered on an incident. However, a guideline provides some leeway for decision-making for trained and experienced EMS providers.

1. *Evaluate the scene.* Before you approach the patient, make certain that you will be in no danger while you work on the patient. If there is a hazard, make sure you can control it before you approach. If you cannot control a hazard, wait for assistance.

2. *Wear proper protective gear.* Use the gear that is appropriate for the situation and that you are certified or qualified to wear. Examples include firefighting turn-out gear, hazmat suit, reflective vest, eye protection, gloves.

3. *Do only what you have been trained to do.* Legally and ethically, you are limited by your level of training. If you attempt to act beyond your level of training, you may risk injury to yourself, cause harm to the patient, or add to the extent of the incident.

4. *Call dispatch for the appropriate assistance.* Describe the incident so that the needed personnel and equipment may respond as soon as possible.

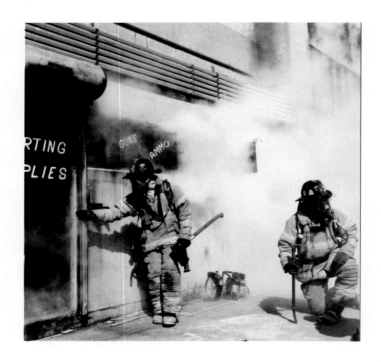

FIGURE 14.1
Ensure your own safety first at all emergency scenes.

PREPARING FOR THE CALL

First Responder responsibilities at motor-vehicle collisions will vary depending on the type of agency, jurisdiction requirements, regulations, and standard operating procedures (SOPs) or standard operating guidelines (SOGs). You must be prepared to perform First Responder duties on any emergency call (Figure 14.3).

All EMS responses progress through several phases. These phases may differ slightly depending on the level of care you provide. For First Responders, the phases of an emergency call include:

Phase 1 *Preparation:* Being prepared means having the proper training, tools, equipment, and personnel.

FIGURE 14.2
Make the scene safe before approaching.

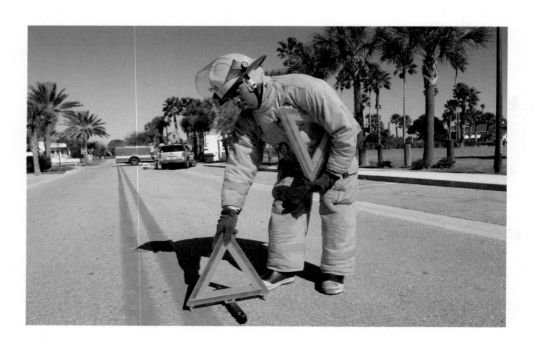

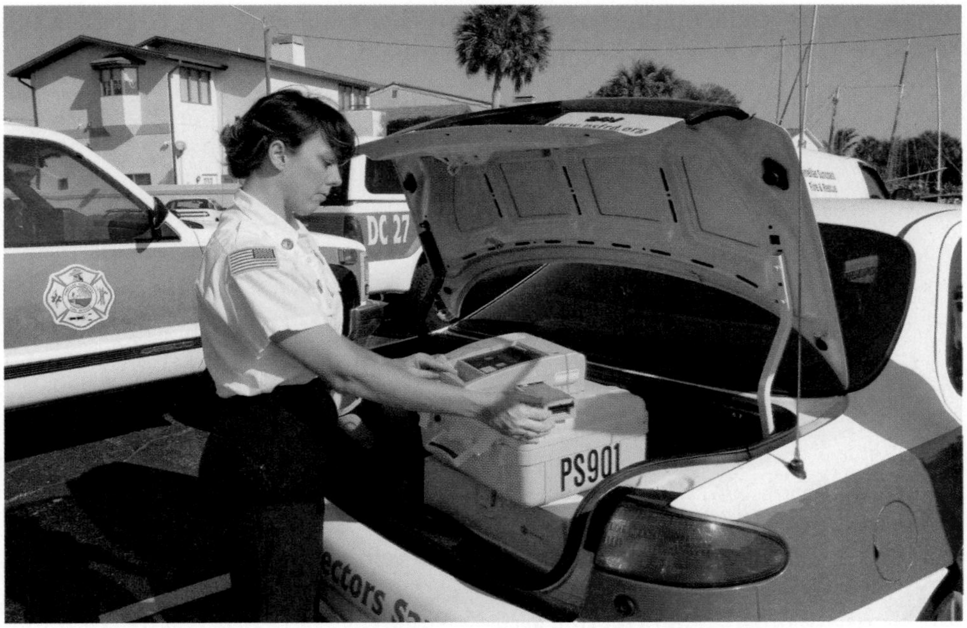

FIGURE 14.3
Always be prepared to perform your duties on any incident.

- *Medical supplies*—Make sure your unit is stocked with medical supplies such as BSI equipment, airways, suctioning equipment, artificial ventilation devices (pocket face masks, bag-valve-masks), and basic wound-care supplies (dressings, bandages).

- *Non-medical supplies*—Check for other necessary items such as personal safety equipment (helmets), flares, flashlights, fire extinguisher, blanket, simple tools (screwdrivers, hammer, spring-loaded punch), and area maps.

- *Equipment and supplies*—Be sure to check that all special equipment is on your unit and operating properly, that any malfunctioning equipment is replaced or repaired, and that all supplies are restocked. Check the engine compartment and fluid levels of your vehicle (fuel, oil, transmission, windshield washer). It is also important to check the emergency equipment, including flashing lights, sirens, and radios, at the beginning of every shift or on a daily basis.

- *Personnel*—Assure that the appropriate number of personnel are on duty and will be able to respond with you or can be dispatched to assist you if necessary.

Phase 2 *Dispatch:* Be familiar with your dispatch or communications system and what procedures you follow when dispatched. Note any information the dispatcher gives you about the call.

- Most dispatch systems have a central dispatch or communications center with 24-hour access.

- Dispatch centers are staffed with personnel especially trained to dispatch the most appropriate units. Many dispatch centers are training their personnel in Emergency Medical Dispatch programs so they may provide patient-care instructions to the caller over the telephone while EMS personnel are responding. All dispatchers are trained to gather as much information from the caller as possible and relay that information to responding units. Information such as the nature of the call, the location of the incident and/or the patient, the number of patients and the severity of illness or injury, as well as any other special problems that responders might encounter at the scene is all important and must be relayed to responding personnel.

Phase 3 *En route to the scene:* First Responder duties continue while en route to an emergency and include more than finding the location on the map.

- First, fasten your seatbelt and be sure you have personal protective equipment ready.

- Contact dispatch and let them know you are en route.

- Be sure you have the essential information on the call, such as location, potential hazards, and number of patients. Do not hesitate to check back with the dispatcher if you need more information.

Phase 4 *Arrival at the scene:* When arriving at the scene be extra alert and approach cautiously. Look for hazards. Position your response unit where you have access to it but where it will not interfere with traffic flow. Activate emergency lights or flashers. Always keep your eye on traffic. Do not become a victim.

- Notify the dispatcher of your arrival. Since dispatchers can only communicate what they are given from the emergency caller, you may have to provide additional information once you arrive on scene, such as the following: actual location of the incident if it is different from what was given on dispatch; type of incident; need for additional resources (engine company, helicopter medevac, rescue squad); number of victims or an estimate if there are many; where and by which unit the patient is being transported; and appropriate patient information. Many EMS agencies are now using cellular phones as a backup to radio communications.

- Size up the scene to assure that it is safe and contains no hazards. Put on your personal protective equipment. Don reflective vests. If you wear dark clothing, other drivers may not see you. As you approach, look for the mechanism of injury in trauma scenes or determine if it is a medical emergency. Always stabilize vehicles before entering them or attempting to extricate any patients. Determine if it is a multiple-casualty incident and, if so, determine the approximate number of patients. Evaluate patients quickly to determine if they are high or low priority. Do you need to move patients immediately? Can it be done safely? Will you need more assistance? Let the dispatcher know what additional resources you are going to need as soon as possible.

Phase 5 *Transferring patients:* First Responders will help lift, carry, and load patients on appropriate devices.

- Assist in preparing the patient for transport.

- Assist in lifting and moving patients, using appropriate lifting and moving procedures.

Phase 6 *After the emergency:* The phases of emergency calls are cyclic. Once a call is finished, you will prepare for the next call.

- Clean and disinfect equipment, restock the unit with supplies, and refuel the unit.

- Complete paperwork and file reports. Participate in debriefing.

- Notify the dispatcher that you are back in service.

make scene safe.

MOTOR-VEHICLE COLLISIONS

Once you ensure your own safety, your main duty at the scene of an emergency is to provide patient care. At the scene of a motor-vehicle collision, however, you may have other duties to perform before you can reach the patients to provide this care

Your responsibilities at the scene may include:

- Making the scene safe, assuring that no one else is hurt as they approach.

- Evaluating the situation and calling the dispatcher for appropriate help.

- Gaining access to patients.

- Freeing trapped patients.

- Evaluating patients and providing emergency care.

- Moving patients who are in danger from fire, explosion, and other hazards.

- Determining which patients may be moved so that you can reach and provide care for another more critically injured patient.

Many First Responders are injured when they attempt to help vehicle-collision victims. Usually, the First Responders are struck by another vehicle when they did not take initial steps to make the scene safe. Your first step is to secure an area around the scene so you can work safely.

FIRST➤ Law enforcement officers and firefighters must follow their department's SOPs or SOGs on vehicle collisions. However, if you are a First Responder without a special course in collision-scene procedures, use the items listed here as guidelines or follow your local protocols. Since each collision scene is unique, you will need to proceed with caution, carefully observe the scene, and decide what actions to take to control it.

1. Pull your vehicle completely off the road at least 50 feet from the scene. Turn on your vehicle's emergency flashers. You may want to use your headlights to light up the scene. If so, be sure to angle your vehicle so that it does not blind oncoming drivers.

2. Make certain that you have parked in a safe location. Look for fuel spills and fire. If you are downhill from the scene, fuel may run in your direction. Check the wind direction. Will the wind carry smoke or fire to where you have parked?

3. If your jurisdiction or agency has SOPs or SOGs for positioning your unit and using warning lights, follow those guidelines. If you turn off the unit, you cannot leave your warning lights on.

4. Set out emergency warning devices, such as flashing lights or flares, to warn others (Scan 14.1). On high-speed roads, place one of these devices at least 250 feet from the scene. On low-speed roads, set one of these devices at least 100 feet from the scene. Add at least 25 feet to these measurements if the scene is on a curved road.

← FLARES/CONES →

5. As you approach, check the scene again for safety. Is there fire, leaking fuel or gases, unstable vehicles, or downed electrical wires? If any of these conditions are present, make certain someone phones or radios for help. If a power line is down, get the nearest pole number so you may request that power be turned

Warning Devices

FLARES

To ignite a flare, remove the small outer cap to expose the striker surface. Then remove the large plastic cap and hold it against the fuse on the end of the flare. Be sure to keep both caps as they will be used to keep the flare from rolling off the roadway once placed in position. Swipe the flare firmly against the striker in a downward motion to ignite it. This may take several attempts, much like striking a match. Once the flare has ignited, replace both plastic caps on the back end of the flare and place it on the road surface.

IMPORTANT: When carrying a lighted flare, always keep it pointing towards the ground and to one side to avoid being hit by burning sulfur. Watch out for spilled or leaking fuel, dry grass, and debris on the road surface. Remember that leaking fuel will flow downhill.

EMERGENCY FLASHERS

Use your vehicle's emergency flashers and set up emergency warning devices approved for highway use. For low visibility and night use, you must use flashing lights or flares.

CONES AND REFLECTORS

Set up cones or reflectors in a graduated line from the shoulder to the corner of your vehicle.

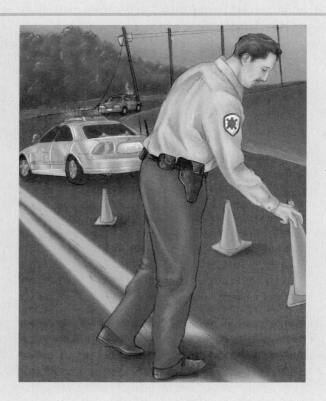

off. You may need the fire department and rescue squad at the scene. Some jurisdictions automatically dispatch these units for motor-vehicle collisions.

6. As you approach, observe the scene for clues. How many potential patients can you see? Could someone have been thrown from a vehicle? Could someone have walked away from the scene? Do you see signs indicating that children were in the vehicle (bottles, toys, school books, car seats)? Are there signs that a pedestrian or bike rider was involved? Have someone alert the dispatcher and report the number of possible patients.

7. If the scene is safe, stabilize the vehicle by chocking the wheels, gain access to the patients, do your assessments, and begin care on those who appear to be most critical. ■

Do not approach or attempt to gain access to patients if the scene is too dangerous. If you cannot control traffic, if electric lines are down, if there is fire at the scene, or if there are fuel or hazardous-materials spills, you are in danger. Call the dispatcher for additional resources for any of these conditions. If you are not trained to deal with fires, electricity, or hazardous materials, protect yourself and stay uphill and upwind from any spills.

FIRST➤ A First Responder's first priority is personal safety. Your primary duty is to provide patient care at a safe scene. Do only what you have been trained to do. ■

UPRIGHT VEHICLE

In most traffic collisions, the vehicles involved remain upright and are generally safer to approach than overturned vehicles. Even though the vehicles appear to be stable, with little chance of rolling or sliding away from the at-rest position, it is still necessary to take the safety precaution of stabilizing the vehicle.

Always evaluate vehicle stability when you assess the scene. As you look for traffic hazards, electrical hazards, spilled fuel, and fire, also see if there is any chance that the vehicle(s) may roll away or flip over. Make sure vehicles are in "park" and the ignition is turned off, if you have immediate access. You may find the following situations:

- *Hills or slight inclines*—The vehicle may have come to rest on a surface that slants enough to allow forward or backward roll. To keep the vehicle from rolling, place wheel chocks, spare tires, logs, rocks, or similar objects under one or more wheels (Figure 14.4).

- *Slippery surfaces*—Ice, snow, or oil can produce a slippery road surface. If available, sprinkle dirt, sand, ashes, or kitty litter, or place newspapers around the wheels and chock the wheels to reduce the chances of slipping.

- *Tilted vehicle*—Even upright vehicles may be tilted to one side by their position or by the terrain. Do not work beneath a tilted vehicle or on the downhill side of one. Chocking the wheels may prevent the vehicle from tilting over, but tying the vehicle in place is safer. If strong rope is available, tie lines to the frame of the car (not the bumper) in front and back or to both sides, then secure the lines to large trees or poles, guardrails, or heavier stable vehicles while waiting for fire-department units to arrive.

- *Stacked vehicles*—Part of one vehicle may be resting on top of another vehicle. There are several ways to stabilize them: chock the wheels of both vehicles; insert tires, lumber, blocks, or similar sturdy items between the road surface and the vehicles; use line or rope to tie and secure both vehicles.

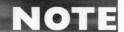
air bag can go off later.

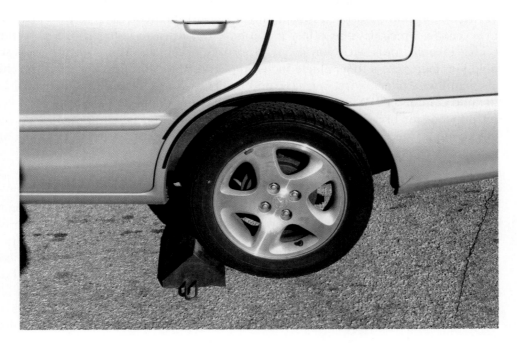

FIGURE 14.4
Stabilize the vehicle before beginning patient care.

FIRST Never try to enter or work around a vehicle until you are certain that it is stable.

Once you stabilize the vehicle, there are two access methods to use for reaching a patient: simple access and complex access. **Simple access** does not require equipment; **complex access** requires tools and special equipment, which also requires additional training. In most cases, you will approach an upright, stable vehicle and reach the patient by simple access. If the doors and windows are closed, there are four ways to gain access to the patients:

- *Open the doors.* Many people drive without locking the doors. However, many new models automatically lock once they reach a speed of five miles per hour. Some lock when the driver puts the transmission in "drive." Check all the doors, including side and rear doors on vans and hatchbacks before trying another entry method. If all doors are locked, one of the occupants may be able to unlock a door. Try before you pry.
- *Enter through a window.* If doors are locked or jammed, gain access through a window. The patient may be able to roll down a window; if not, you will have to break a window. When you begin using tools to access patients, the process becomes more complex.
- *Pry open the doors.* The doors on most cars made before 1967 can be pried open with a pry bar or jack handle. This method will not work for most cars made after 1967, when it *does* work, the method is very time consuming. Prying open doors is not considered a First Responder skill. Access through windows is usually more practical.
- *Cut through the metal.* The only other access when entry through doors and windows is not possible is cutting through vehicle roofs, trunks, and doors. This entry method takes special tools that First Responders do not usually carry unless they are also members of the fire department. If you cannot gain access through a door or window, it may be possible to cut around the lock of a door using a sharp tool (chisel or strong screwdriver) and a hammer. ■

Your instructor will teach you how to use these entry methods if they are First Responders skills in your jurisdiction.

Keep in mind that speed is sometimes crucial when you need to reach patients in a vehicle. Precious time is lost if you have to return to your vehicle to retrieve tools. Take all tools with you as you approach a vehicle. Many simple tools will help you gain access to a vehicle including slotted and Phillips screwdrivers, chisels, hammers, pliers, wire, washers, and pry bars. Some First Responder tool kits include commercial "Slim Jims" used for unlocking doors and spring-loaded center punches for breaking glass. Access with tools and special equipment is considered complex because it takes time, planning, and sometimes special training; and it requires taking additional safety precautions to protect the patient.

Unlocking Vehicle Doors

Special commercial tools for unlocking doors may be part of your First Responder kit. You might be able to unlock doors of older vehicles by slipping a commercial tool known as a "Slim Jim" between the window and the door. You also might be able to pry open the window with a wood wedge or pry bar and slip a wire coat hanger inside the window (Scan 14.2). Opening newer locks using these methods might be impossible, depending on the manufacturer. Some cars have a dead bolt system that cannot be unlocked with special tools. These types of locks are designed to unlock on impact and allow rescuers to gain access. If you cannot unlock or open a door, gain access through a window.

Unlocking Vehicle Doors

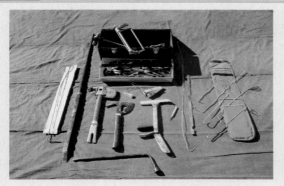

Various tools can be used to help unlock vehicle doors in older vehicles (check model years):

- Wire hook.
- Straight wire.
- Slim-Jim (or similar device).
- Screwdriver.
- Flat pry bar.

An oil dipstick or a keyhole saw may be used to help force up a locking button.

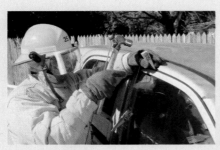

1. Framed windows. Pry the frame away from the vehicle body with a wood wedge and insert a wire hook.

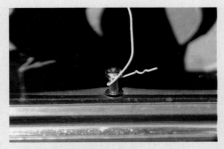

3. For flat-top locks, use a hooked wire. Snag the locking button and pull upward.

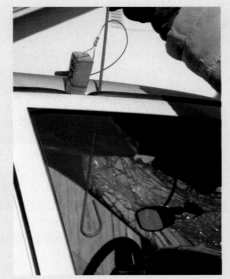

2. Or use a wooden wedge to pry away the frame before inserting the wire hook.

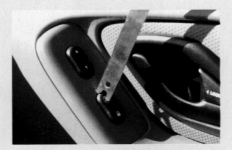

4. For rocker or push-button locks on the door panel or on the armrest, use a straight wire and press the lock open.

Before you attempt to unlock a door, confirm that all doors are indeed locked and windows are up, preventing access any other way, or have an occupant on the inside unlock it. Check the doors for damage. A severely damaged door may not open easily even if you do unlock it. If all of the doors are damaged, be prepared to break glass and gain access through the window. Look in the windows to see if the car has buttons in the armrest. It will not be easy to unlock doors with this type of locking device. Vehicles with electric locks and windows cannot be unlocked if the battery is disabled.

Gaining Access Through Vehicle Windows

To gain rapid access to patients who are unresponsive or unable when the doors are locked, use a spring-loaded center punch on the rear or side windows (Figures 14.5 and 14.6). A heavy hammer may work, but it requires that you aim carefully and strike forcefully (possibly several times), which may shatter and spray glass. Always wear protective equipment, especially goggles and gloves, when breaking glass.

At the scene of a collision, most people consider breaking the windshield of a vehicle first if they cannot gain access through the doors. However, this is the wrong approach. Windshields are made of laminated safety glass, which has great strength. Even when shattered, the glass will still cling to an inner plastic layer. All cars have laminated safety glass windshields. Many foreign cars have this type of glass in all windows of a vehicle. If it is necessary to remove windshields, First Responders should leave that task to personnel trained in this rescue technique.

Rear and side windows are usually made of tempered safety glass. When this glass is broken, there is no plastic layer to hold the pieces. Tempered safety glass will not shatter into sharp pieces or shards. Instead, this glass will shatter into small rounded pieces and will often drop straight down into the vehicle, if you break it in a corner with a spring-loaded center punch. The small glass pieces can cut, but the cuts are usually minor.

If you must use a hammer, do not bash the center of the glass with it, or you will send pieces throughout the entire passenger compartment.

remember

Wear gloves and have protection for your eyes.

FIGURE 14.5

Use a spring-loaded center punch to break windows.

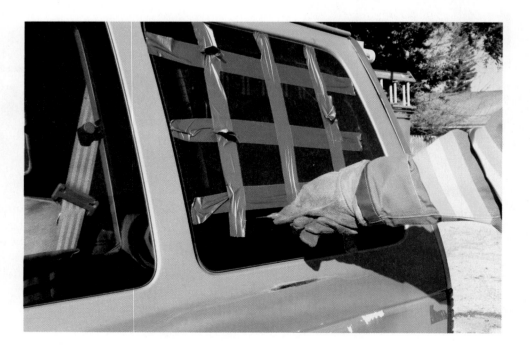

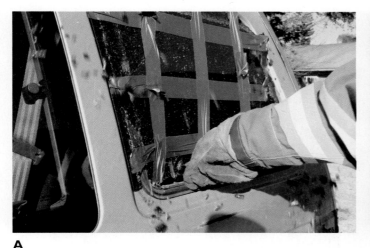
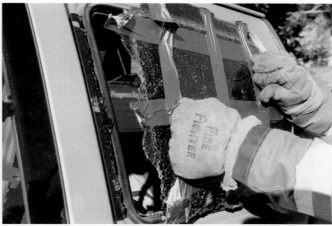

A **B**

FIGURE 14.6
Protect yourself when breaking and removing glass.

FIRST➤ When gaining access through a vehicle window, you should:

1. Make certain the vehicle is stable. If possible, have the driver turn off the ignition.

2. Confirm that all doors and windows are locked and secure.

3. Protect yourself by wearing gloves and eye protection.

4. If possible, select a window that is away from the patient. Place one gloved hand flat against the window, resting the heel of your hand on the corner of door. Place the spring-loaded center punch between two fingers in one of the lower corners of the window, as close to the door as possible. Press the center punch with your other hand. When the window breaks, the hand pressing the center punch will not go through the window.

5. After breaking the window, reach in and try to open the door. You may only have to unlock the door to open it. Often, jammed doors that will not open from the outside will open from the inside.

6. Turn off the vehicle ignition, place the transmission in "park," and set the parking brake. ■

OVERTURNED VEHICLE

Do not try to right an overturned vehicle. Even if you have enough help to turn the vehicle upright, moving it can cause further injury to the occupants. Stabilize the overturned vehicle while waiting for fire department units and before you try to reach the occupants. Always look for fuel spills, battery acid, and other chemical hazards around an overturned vehicle.

VEHICLE ON ITS SIDE

FIRST➤ If you find a vehicle on its side and have some simple equipment, take the following precautions to stabilize it. You should (Figure 14.7):

1. Stabilize the vehicle with items such as tires, blocks, lumber, wheel chocks, cribbing, rocks, or similar available materials. Place these items between the road surface and the roofline. Also place stabilizing items between the road surface and the lower wheels if the wheels are not resting on the road surface.

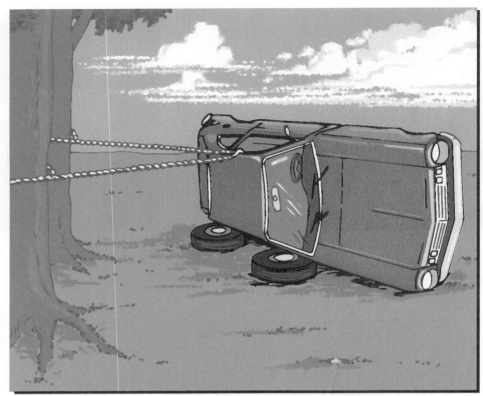

2. If the vehicle is still unstable, use strong rope or line to tie the vehicle to secure objects.

3. Attempt to gain access to occupants of the vehicle. Entry through a door is very dangerous since the door may be seven feet or more off the ground and your weight will move the vehicle as you climb on it. It will also be difficult to open the door with the vehicle on its side. Your first and more sensible entry point will be through a window. The rear window is the best approach to take. Never attempt access to a damaged interior through broken glass without adequate protective clothing and equipment.

4. If you open a door, tie it securely open. Do not use a prop. Props can slip or be knocked away, causing the door to slam on you or the occupants. ■

PATIENTS PINNED BENEATH VEHICLES

When a patient is pinned beneath a vehicle, call for a rescue squad immediately. Never place yourself in danger by reaching or crawling into the area where the patient is pinned. If it appears that the scene is too dangerous, First Responders can perform certain procedures to move the vehicle and free the patient, but this is often risky. Follow your department's SOPs or SOGs in these situations.

A jack or pry bar and blocks can be used to raise a vehicle, which will enable rescuers to move the patient from beneath the vehicle. When lifting one side of the vehicle off the patient, be sure you are not causing the other side of the vehicle to press on another part of the patient, for example his legs. With enough help, you may be able to lift the vehicle off the patient. In any attempt to raise a vehicle off a pinned patient, others must shore up the vehicle as you raise it so that it will not slip or fall back onto the rescuers or the patient. Use blocks, tires, lumber, or similar sturdy items at the scene. Do not attempt to enter the space to remove the victim until the entire vehicle is stable.

PATIENTS TRAPPED IN WRECKAGE

You may find patients with their arms, legs, or heads protruding through the window. Before trying to free them, you should:

1. Use blankets to shield any patients who are still in the vehicle, while other rescuers continue to open the vehicle to provide better access and extrication (Figure 14.8).

2. Use pliers, hammer claws, or a knife to carefully break or fold away glass around the patient's extremity.

FIRST➤ When patients are trapped inside crushed vehicles, you must wait for special power tools and skilled rescue personnel. Trained personnel can quickly and easily free or disentangle patients from the wreck.

First Responders working on vehicles with occupants pinned inside will often be able to free some patients:

- Simply remove wreckage from on top of and around the patient.
- Carefully move a seat forward or backward.
- Carefully lift out a back seat.
- Remove a patient's shoe to free a foot, or cut away clothing caught on wreckage.
- Cut seat belts. Be sure to properly support the patient during the cutting and after the tension has been released.

NOTE: *In general, cervical-spine immobilization should be applied by qualified personnel prior to performing maneuvers that will cause the patient to move.*

- Check air bag deployment. Follow manufacturer and agency guidelines for working around vehicles with deployed and undeployed airbags. Check the steering wheel beneath the deployed airbag for damage indicating that the patient might have struck it. Airbags may also activate in the front seat passenger area, and some more recent models have side air curtains. ■

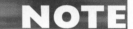

Powders used to lubricate an airbag may irritate the skin. Be sure to wear personal protective equipment when working around vehicles with deployed airbags.

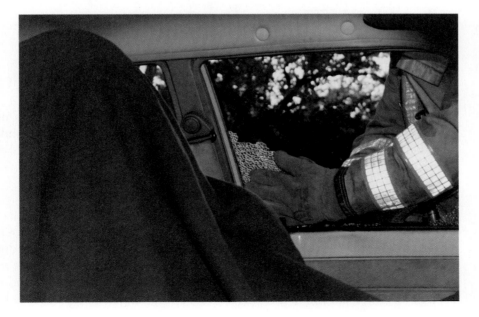

FIGURE 14.8
Cover the patient with a blanket to protect him from injury while removing glass.

In any attempt to free patients from vehicles, you must consider the immediate need for quick access. If immediate access and patient movement is necessary to save a life, make every attempt to reach the patient. If the patient's life is not at risk but immediate movement will cause further injury, then leave the patient in place until more highly trained personnel respond to the scene.

During the wait, talk to the patient to offer reassurance and explain why you are taking precautions. While you are talking to the patient, begin your initial patient assessment steps and provide oxygen while another First Responder stabilizes the head. If you must move the patient before more advanced care personnel arrive, make every attempt to maintain stabilization of the patient's spine during the move. Once EMTs and other EMS personnel arrive, report your patient assessment findings and provide them with any assistance they need, such as taking vital signs, controlling bleeding, gathering special equipment, or loading and lifting the patient.

BUILDINGS

FIRST RESPONDER RESPONSIBILITIES

Gaining access to a patient in a locked building may require special skills and tools outside the range of First Responder duties. There are many types of gates, doors, windows, and locks that restrict access to buildings. In addition to access problems, older buildings may have many hidden and unsuspected dangers; security devices will present special barriers, and guard dogs will limit or halt your actions until they are contained

First Responders are not expected to know how to open or destroy locks or have all the tools needed for the variety of windows, doors, and gates found in buildings. Unless you are trained in fire and rescue operations, you are not expected to know how to enter and make your way safely around an empty or abandoned building.

FIRST➤ Follow the guidelines below for gaining access to patients inside any type of building (homes, offices, stores, schools). You will be expected to:

- Request additional resources if necessary.
- Try opening and entering through open doors or windows first.
- Look for a key under mats or in mailboxes.
- Ask bystanders and neighbors if they have a key.
- Break glass to unlock doors or windows.

Follow your department's SOPs or SOGs regarding notification of local law enforcement prior to and following any forcible entry. ■

If you know or see that someone inside needs immediate care, do not try to gain access before calling for help. Your efforts to gain entry may fail, and you will need help as soon as possible. Call the dispatcher and request additional resources immediately.

ENTERING BUILDINGS

While waiting for help, try different entry points. Try to open a door. If the door is locked, try opening a few low windows on your way to finding a second door. If the second door is locked, break the glass in a window or a door and enter as quickly but as safely as possible. Do not attempt to break through doors or windows made of large sheets of tempered glass. Some newer buildings and homes may have been

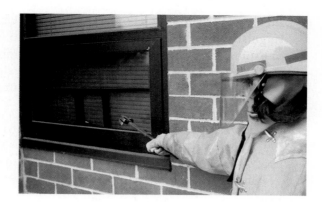

constructed with Lexan® resin (a type of plastic) or a special type of laminated glass that is designed to resist the forces of hurricanes and the debris carried by high winds. These materials are extremely difficult to break, and can bounce a hammer back into your face. Do not try climbing up walls or posts to reach a high window. Do not try to gain access to a window by walking across roofs. Call and wait for special rescue personnel who will have the appropriate equipment.

FIRST➤ When attempting to break a glass window, you should:

1. Make certain that the patient is not lying near the other side of the glass.

2. Use a hammer or similar blunt object to strike the glass near one of its edges (Figure 14.9). A nightstick or an aluminum aircraft flashlight will break most window glass. If you do not have tools, use a rock or a similar solid object to strike the glass.

3. Carefully clear all glass from the frame and reach in to unlock the door or window.

4. Make certain that you are stepping onto a safe floor. Be sure that you do not have an unusual drop when entering. Take a moment to visually inspect the floor for damage or poke the floor for signs of weakness. ■

HAZARDS

FIRE

Television and movies have led people to believe that they should enter burning buildings or run up to burning vehicles in order to save victims. This is a dangerous tactic. Those in the fire service are highly trained to do their jobs. They are given special equipment and use special strategies to fight fires, which minimizes the risks to their safety. Firefighting requires special training, protective clothing, the right equipment, and usually more than one firefighter.

If you are a member of the fire service, follow SOPs or SOGs for rescuing victims from vehicle and structure fires. If you are in law enforcement and have special training in rescuing victims from vehicle and structure fires, do only what you have been trained to do. If you are a First Responder without firefighting training, do not risk your life to approach a fire and provide care.

Motor-vehicle collisions do not usually produce fire, and most emergency calls to buildings do not involve fire. However, these events do occur, and you must be prepared to protect yourself. Your own safety is the first priority. First Responders with no training or little experience at fighting fires must follow the rules listed below to ensure their safety:

- Never approach a vehicle that is in flames. Using blankets, sand, or a fire extinguisher is appropriate if you know how to evaluate the fire and the danger of explosion and if you have protective clothing and know how to attack a fire. If you do not have the proper training to perform these tasks and do not have the necessary protection, stay clear. Make sure that the dispatcher knows there is a fire.

- Never attempt to enter a building that is obviously on fire or has smoke showing. Even a small fire can spread toxic fumes throughout the structure. If you enter, look and smell for signs of fire. Remember that fire could be hidden within the walls, floors, and ceilings.

- Never enter a smoky room or building or go through an area of dense smoke.

- Never attempt to enter a closed building or room giving off grayish yellow smoke. Opening a door to this building or room will cause a *back draft*, which is a condition that immediately increases the intensity of the fire and can cause an explosion due to the sudden increase in oxygen supply.

- Do not work by yourself or enter a building unless others know that you are doing so. If you are injured or trapped, you are an unknown victim who may not be rescued until it is too late.

- Always feel the top of a door before opening it (Figure 14.10). If it is hot, do not open it. (Note: Doorknobs and handles may also be hot.) If the door is cool, open it slowly and cautiously and avoid standing in its path as you open it.

- Never use the elevator if there is a possibility of a fire in a building. The elevator shaft can act as a flue and pull flames, hot toxic gases, and smoke into the shaft. Also, the fire can cause an electrical failure, which could trap you in the elevator. Some elevators have heat-activated call buttons. The elevator may take you to the fire floor, open, and expose you to lethal heat or toxic gases.

- If you find yourself in smoke, stay close to the floor and crawl to safety (Figure 14.11). If possible, cover your mouth and nose with a damp cloth.

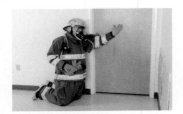

FIGURE 14.10
If a door is hot, do not open it.

GAS

If you notice the odor of natural gas at any scene, move patients away from the area, keep bystanders away from the scene, and alert dispatch, so that other services can be activated, and request that gas in the area be shut off or diverted.

FIGURE 14.11
If trapped by fire or smoke, stay low and crawl to safety.

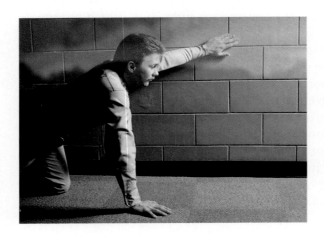

FIRST➤ The smell of natural gas in a building is a signal for immediate action. Evacuate the building and call dispatch to report the odor of gas. If the gas is coming from a bottled source, do not try to turn off this source unless you have experience with this type of gas system. You can vent the area by opening windows and doors as you leave. Do not enter an area to rescue a patient. You must wear a self-contained breathing apparatus (SCBA) and be trained to handle such emergencies. Remember that there is always a danger of fire or explosion from simple acts such as turning on or off a light switch, or even from the spark of an appliance turning on. Play it safe and request the help you will need. ■

warning

If you suspect a gas leak, do not turn lights on or off, do not use the doorbell, do not use any electrical equipment (including portable radios and flashlights), and do not use any open-flame products, such as matches or flares.

ELECTRICAL WIRES AND ABOVE-GROUND TRANSFORMERS

FIRST➤ If electrical wires are down at a scene and block your pathway to a patient, or if they are lying across a car, do not attempt a rescue. As you approach a scene with downed wires, position your vehicle at least a pole away from the downed wires. If the power is restored, the wires can whip and arc in a circle as wide as their free length, which can be to the next pole (Figure 14.12).

Never assume that power lines are dead or that a dead line will stay dead. Consider all downed lines as live. Do not be fooled by the fact that lights are out in the surrounding area. Even if lights are off all around you, the wire blocking your path may be live or could be re-energized as you pass by. Call or have someone alert dispatch to call the power company and request that the power is turned off. Even if you believe the power has been turned off, it is still best to wait for trained rescue personnel to arrive.

Many newer communities have underground electrical wires with access through an above-ground splice box or transformer. These above-ground transformer boxes are usually green, mounted on concrete pads, and often hidden by shrubbery (Figure 14.13). It may not be safe to approach a vehicle that has collided with an above-ground transformer box. Alert dispatch immediately and ask for special rescue assistance

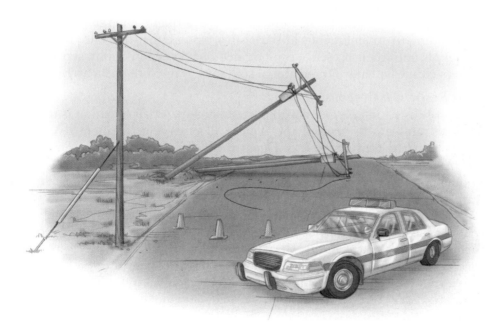

FIGURE 14.12
Place your vehicle at least a pole away from the pole with downed wires.

FIGURE 14.13
Pad-mounted transformer.

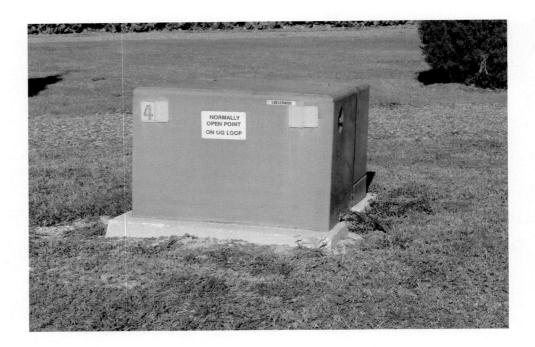

If patients are in a car that is touching a downed wire or is near one or has crashed into an above-ground transformer, tell them to stay in the vehicle and avoid touching any metal parts. If the patients have to leave the vehicle because of fire or other danger, you must tell them to jump clear of the car without touching it and the ground at the same time. If they touch both simultaneously, they will complete a circuit and may be electrocuted. ■

HAZARDOUS MATERIALS

There may be hazardous chemicals and other materials at the scene of an emergency. If so, do not attempt a rescue or perform patient care. No responders should enter a hazardous-materials area unless they are trained to do so.

The possibility of hazardous-materials incidents exists at every industrial site and every farm, truck, train, ship, barge, and airplane emergency incident. When responding to an emergency at these sites, assume that there are unsafe hazardous materials until their presence can be ruled out. When in doubt, stay clear and keep others clear of a hazardous-material spill until trained rescuers arrive.

First Responder Responsibilities

Your role as a First Responder in a hazardous-materials situation is to first protect yourself and others around the scene. All emergency response vehicles should carry a current copy of the U.S. Department of Transportation's *Hazardous Materials: Emergency Response Guidebook*. At a hazardous-materials incident, refer to the guidebook for information on the chemical or substance and the perimeter of the safe area.

You may have to set up safety zones. Set up a hot (danger) zone and keep all people out of this area. Set up a cold (safe) zone, which should be on the same level as and upwind from the hazardous-materials incident. Be aware that below-grade areas, such as ditches, trenches, and basements, will often have low-oxygen environments. Many gases are heavier than oxygen and will settle in low areas. The safe zone must not be downhill or downwind from the scene or on a high point that may be exposed to vapors if the wind shifts. Avoid low spots, streams, drainage fields, sewers, and sewer openings where spills may flow and fumes may collect.

Contact dispatch immediately with a description of the incident so you can get the appropriate help on the way. Advise the dispatcher of your position and stay on the line until you are told to disconnect. Ask and wait for information about the danger of the materials and for directions as to what you should do until the hazardous-material (hazmat) teams arrive. Make certain you give your name and call-back number.

If, for some reason, you cannot contact the dispatcher, call one of the following:

- CHEM-TEL on its 24-hour toll-free number at 800-255-3924 (for the United States and Canada). For calls originating from other areas, call 813-070-0626.

- CHEMTREC on its 24-hour toll-free number at 800-424-9300 (for the United States and Canada). For calls originating from other areas, call 703-527-3887.

When possible, provide the following information:

- Nature and location of the problem, an estimate of when the spill occurred, and if there are other possible hazardous materials near the scene.

- Type of material (gas, liquid, dry chemical, or a radioactive solid, liquid, or gas) and an estimate of how much material is at the scene.

- Name or identification number of the material. Look for labels or placards that are visible from your safe point. Use binoculars to help in reading this information.

- Name of the shipper or manufacturer. From a safe point or with binoculars, look for names on railroad cars, trucks, or containers. Ask bystanders, drivers, or railroad or factory personnel.

- Type of container. Is the material in a rail car or a truck? Is it in open storage, covered storage, or housed storage? Is the container still intact, or is liquid leaking, gas escaping, or a powder spilled? Report if the material is stable or if it is flaming, vaporizing, or blowing into the air.

- Weather conditions. Rain and wind are major concerns because they will carry hazardous materials to and contaminate other locations.

- Estimate of how many possible patients there are both in the hot zone (closest to the spill) and around the hot zone (in circles farther from the spill).

- Other significant problems at the scene such as fire, crowds, and traffic.

You may not be able to obtain and report most of this information, but any information you can provide is important to the responding units.

A major source of information at a hazardous-materials scene is the standard materials placard required by the U.S. Department of Transportation (Figure 14.14). This placard is on the vehicle, tank, or railroad car. The numbers, symbols, and colors provide information about the material in the container. Be aware that vehicles transporting hazardous materials insert placards into brackets. These placards may be made of metal or plastic and are hinged so they may be flipped to indicate a different cargo. During transportation or the incident, the placard may flip and show a different material. If possible, check with the driver, who must have a

FIGURE 14.14
Hazardous-materials placard.

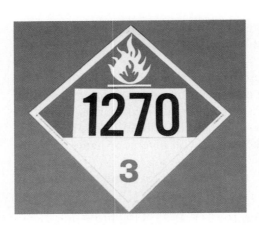

Material Safety Data Sheet (MSDS) on each hazardous material carried, to determine that the placard is correct. Some hazardous-materials transporters use placard stickers, which can be peeled off when the load is delivered. The driver applies another sticker for a different load of hazardous materials.

Refer to the U.S. DOT's *Hazardous Materials: Emergency Response Guidebook*. You may also want to become familiar with the information from the National Fire Protection Association (NFPA) "Standard 473 Competencies for EMS Personnel Responding to Hazardous Materials Incidents."

Managing Patients

All contaminated victims must remain in the hot zone until the hazmat team decontaminates them and brings them to the cold zone for care by EMS personnel. If a victim of a hazardous-materials incident leaves the hot zone, you must first protect yourself from exposure. Victims may have chemicals on their bodies and clothing that could be harmful to you. DO NOT attempt to care for these patients unless you have the proper protection. Initial care includes flushing with water any contaminated areas, such as the skin, clothing, and eyes for at least 20 minutes, unless the material is dry lime. (Brush away excess dry lime first, then flush.) Remove contaminated clothing and jewelry as you flush the patient with water. Once the patient is flushed, use blankets to protect him from the environment and to maintain body temperature.

Victims may be able to wash themselves or you may wash the victim. Use a small diameter hose and make sure the victim stands in a large tub, small wading pool, or similar collection container so the contaminated rinse water does not run off into nearby sewers or streams. Perform wash operations uphill and upwind from the site if possible. Do not place yourself at risk. If it is necessary to provide artificial ventilations, use an appropriate barrier device. Use resuscitation devices with one-way valves so contaminants do not blow back into your mouth or face.

The best thing for you to do at a hazardous-materials incident is to request the appropriate resources (Figure 14.15) and remain in the cold zone until the patient can be safely treated.

Radiation Incidents

FIRST➤ Stay clear of collisions involving radioactive materials. Your first duty is to protect yourself from exposure. Your next step should be to request the appropriate resources from a safe area away from the scene.

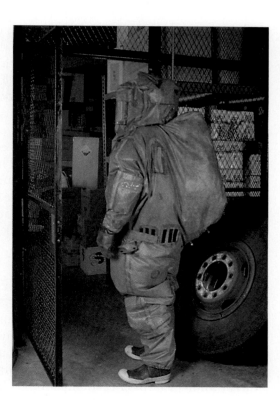

FIGURE 14.15
Special training and equipment, such as this fully encapsulated suit, are required at a hazardous-materials incident.

Look for radiation hazard labels (Figure 14.16). Stay upwind from any containers having these labels. Follow the same basic rules as you would when dealing with any hazardous material. The greater the distance you are from the source and the more objects that appropriately shield you from the source (concrete, thick steel, earth banks, heavy vehicles), the safer you will be.

When you are dispatched to hazardous-materials and radiation incidents, position your vehicle at a safe distance. Do not approach the scene unless you are specially trained to do so and are wearing the appropriate protective equipment (turnout coat, pants, boots, gloves, Nomex hood, helmet). Your protective equipment will provide some protection from most types of radiation, but be aware that it does not protect you enough to work close to a high-level radiation source for any period of time. ■

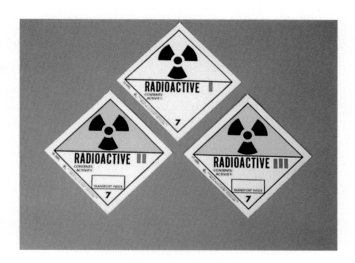

FIGURE 14.16
Radiation hazard labels.

Patients may be exposed to radiation, contaminated by it, or both. A patient who is exposed (not contaminated) was in the presence of radioactive material, but the material did not actually touch his clothing or body. Exposure to radiation may be harmful to the patient, but he is not radioactive and cannot pass on the exposure to you. However, the actual source of the radiation can be harmful to you. If the patient is still in the area of the radiation source, you must wait until the hazmat team brings him to the safe area.

Patients are contaminated when they come in contact with radiation sources, which may be gases, liquids, or particles. The radioactive materials may be on a patient's clothes, skin, or hair and will contaminate you when you touch the patient during assessment or care. The hazmat team will have to decontaminate the patient before you can provide care. Do not attempt to clean or care for radiation patients until they are in a safe area and are decontaminated.

HELICOPTER OPERATIONS/AIR MEDICAL TRANSPORT

Most EMS systems use helicopters to transport critically ill or injured patients to specialty referral centers—such as trauma, burn, and pediatric centers—or to evacuate patients from hard-to-reach or hazardous areas. Your instructor will tell you the circumstances that usually require a helicopter, often referred to as a *medevac unit*, or *medical evacuation unit*. Check your local protocols for medevac procedures and contact on-line medical direction about patients who may need a medevac.

Generally, for helicopter transport, take the following steps:

1. Request the helicopter . . .
   — If the patient needs to be transported to a specialty center that is more than a reasonable distance or drive time from the incident and air transport will save time over ground transport.
   — If the patient is a high-priority one who is trapped and extrication time will be prolonged.
   — If the patient is in a remote area that cannot be reached by ground units or if ambulance access is blocked.

2. Consider these factors prior to requesting a medevac helicopter . . .
   — Extended ground transport time.
   — Shock.
   — Chest abdominal, or pelvic trauma with respiratory distress or shock.
   — Serious mechanism of injury with altered vital signs or altered mental status.
   — Penetrating injuries to any body cavity.
   — Carbon monoxide poisoning.
   — Heart attack.
   — Amputation of limbs.

3. Provide information to the helicopter . . .
   — Your name, agency name, call-back number or radio frequency.
   — Nature of the incident.

— Exact location of the incident with landmarks and crossroads where possible, or latitudes and longitudes where known and appropriate.

— Exact location of the landing zone.

4. Set up the landing zone . . .

— Select a flat area that is clear of obstructions, such as utility poles and wires, radio towers, trees and shrubs. For day landings, the area should be at least 60 by 60 feet; for night landings, 100 by 100 feet. For large helicopters, double the landing area. (Check with your jurisdiction, as different aircraft have different landing requirements.) Pick up loose items that might blow into bystanders or into the helicopter's rotor blades.

— The landing area should be at least 50 feet away from the incident so rescuers are not hampered by noise and rotor wash. If necessary, the patient may be packaged and placed in the ambulance and transported to the helicopter landing site.

— If the landing area must be a highway, stop traffic in both directions, even if the helicopter will land only on one side of the highway.

— Warn the helicopter crew of nearby obstructions, such as utility lines, radio towers, antennas, and trees.

— Mark the corner of the landing area with high-visibility objects: iridescent flags or tape by day; lights at night; flares for either day or night, if there is no danger of fire. Never shine lights up to the helicopter at night. Bright lights directed toward the pilot take away his night vision, and make it more difficult for the pilot to see.

— Keep rescue crews and bystanders at least 200 feet away while the helicopter is landing.

— Do not approach the helicopter until the pilot signals you. Never approach from behind the helicopter where the pilot cannot see you and where the tail rotor is located. Always cross in front of the helicopter.

— Approach the aircraft in a crouch to avoid being struck by the dipping rotor blades. If the helicopter has to land on an incline, approach only from the downhill side.

— Remove loose items such as hats and scarves when approaching the helicopter so nothing will blow into the rotor blades.

Chapter Review

SUMMARY

As a First Responder, your first priority is your own safety, and your first duty is patient care. Before approaching a patient, make sure the scene is safe. Begin evaluating the scene as you approach. Evaluate for hazards, such as traffic, fire, downed electrical lines, hazardous materials, and unstable vehicles. Also size up the scene for ejected patients and for those who are standing or walking.

Always make certain that an upright vehicle will not roll. Stabilize vehicles that are on inclines or slippery surfaces. If one vehicle is stacked on another or on its side, stabilize both before trying to reach patients. Do not attempt to provide patient care in or around unstabilized vehicles or try to right overturned vehicles.

Gain access to patients in a stabilized vehicle by trying doors first. If door access is not possible, attempt to gain access through a rear or side window. Break glass only after stabilizing the vehicle. Wear gloves and eye protection, or cover the glass and your face before breaking it. Break a window that is farthest from the patient.

Remove patients from vehicles only when there is danger or if life-saving care is required. First Responders may not have the skills or tools to remove patients trapped under a vehicle. If you must free a pinned patient, use a jack or pry bars to lift the vehicle and, while lifting, place blocks to stabilize and shore up the vehicle.

When caring for a patient with a body part protruding through a window, cover the body part first. Then break or fold the glass away before moving the patient.

Patients who are jammed or trapped in wreckage often can be freed by removing wreckage from around them, adjusting or removing seats, removing shoes, or cutting away clothing or seat belts.

The initial routes for gaining access to patients in buildings are doors, then windows. If you must break glass, protect yourself with gloves and goggles or cover the glass and your face. Be sure the patient is safe from flying glass and that you are stepping onto a safe floor.

At the scene of a fire, do not approach a burning vehicle or building unless you have the proper equipment and have been trained to assess the hazards and fight the fire. Do not enter a building that may be on fire. Do not try to go through smoke or potentially toxic gases. Do not attempt to enter a building or room that has any smoke coming from doors, windows, or vents. Do not open a door if it is hot. If caught in a burning building, stay low and crawl to safety.

Only trained personnel should shut off gas or electricity. If you smell natural gas, do not approach, but do alert dispatch. If there are electrical hazards, do not attempt a rescue. If electrical wires are touching a vehicle, have passengers stay in the vehicle and instruct them to avoid touching any metal objects inside the vehicle. If they must get out, warn them to jump clear without touching the vehicle and the ground at the same time.

If the scene contains hazardous or radioactive materials, stay in a safe area and request the appropriate resources. Provide the dispatcher with essential information.

Medevac helicopters are becoming a common sight in many EMS systems. It is important for First Responders to know the capabilities of these vital resources and the specific requirements for setting up a landing zone for both day and night operations.

✔ If you came upon a situation in which a person was trapped in a vehicle or a building, what would you do first? Remember that the first thing to consider is your own personal safety. Are you equipped to handle a rescue on your own? If not, what kind of help is available for different types of rescue situations?

Check with your department and find out what emergency support personnel and equipment are available to be sent to assist First Responders for emergencies where people are trapped.

✔ What tools do you carry in your vehicle or on your unit? Are they simple tools that typically do not need a special training class to show you how to use them? Or are the tools more mechanical with special attachments that require training in order to use them properly? Regardless of the type of tool, will you know what to do with it when you need it to free a person from an entrapment situation?

Even simple tools are useless unless you know what to do with them or how to apply them effectively and safely in certain situations. If you have never actually removed a windshield with a putty knife, glazier's tool, or screwdriver, find out if your department can get an old junked vehicle to practice on. Work under the guidance and instruction of someone who has had training or experience in auto extrication so that you can learn the appropriate techniques in a safe environment.

Many response areas include a variety of building types in their residential, commercial, and industrial neighborhoods.

✔ Orient yourself and other department personnel to the different types of buildings in your response area by examining various neighborhoods and noting the type of construction, what the normal entry points are, and what other entry points there may be. Consider how you would enter different buildings if you could not gain access to trapped victims by the normal entry point.

Firefighters work with local businesses and industries to preplan their fire attack and rescue operations in the event of a fire or other disaster. First Responders should do the same.

✔ Check with personnel at schools, stores, businesses, warehouses, and other commercial properties to find out where their first-aid room is, what medical personnel may be on duty and when, what is the closest access point to work areas, first-aid rooms, and offices or classrooms. Find out which areas will be difficult to access if there is an emergency and what hazards may hinder your care of any personnel or students.

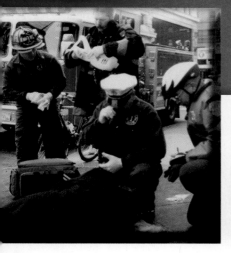
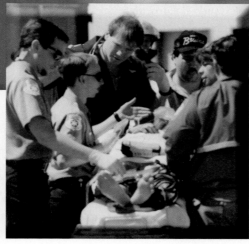
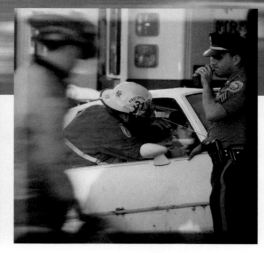

Multiple-Casualty Incidents, Triage, and the Incident Management System

The chapter discusses the role of the EMS system and that of the First Responder in emergencies involving multiple victims. Multiple-casualty incidents can be caused by anything, including vehicle collisions, hurricanes, and terrorist events such as those on September 11, 2001.

NATIONAL STANDARD OBJECTIVES

This chapter focuses on the objectives of Module 7, Lesson 7-1, of the U.S. DOT's First Responder National Standard Curriculum and serves as an instructional aid to help you meet any specific objectives added to the course by your local EMS system.

By the end of this chapter, you will be able to (from cognitive or knowledge information):

7–1.8 Describe the criteria for a multiple-casualty situation. (p. 526)

LEARNING TASKS

Although relatively uncommon, multiple-casualty incidents, whether caused by nature or by human beings, are a fact of life and will remain a part of our world. It is necessary for First Responders to understand their role in such an incident and the overall structure of an Incident Management System. You should be able to:

✔ Define multiple-casualty incident (MCI).
✔ Describe the First Responders role at the scene of an MCI.
✔ Define Incident Management System (IMS).
✔ Describe the basic structure of an IMS.

When an emergency involves multiple patients and the available resources cannot care for all patients at one time, a method must be used to identify those patients most in need of immediate care. This process is called *triage*. After you learn about multiple-casualty incidents and how to triage, you should be able to:

✔ Define triage.
✔ Discuss the First Responders role in the triage process.
✔ List the major steps of the triage process.
✔ Discuss how you might triage a simulated multiple-casualty incident.
✔ List the START triage criteria for assessing patients in a multiple-casualty incident.

MULTIPLE-CASUALTY INCIDENTS (MCIs)

If taken literally, the definition of a multiple-casualty incident (MCI) is any emergency with more than one victim (Figure 15.1). While MCIs do indeed involve more than one victim, a more realistic definition is: any emergency that involves multiple victims and overwhelms the first responding units. Most fire departments, rescue squads, and ambulances are prepared and capable of managing a scene with more than one patient. However, can they manage a scene with three or four? How about five or six? What if the victims are all critical and need immediate transport?

In most cases, it is up to the first emergency personnel on the scene to make a judgment call and declare an MCI. If they feel that they can manage the number of patients with the immediately available resources, then an MCI may not be declared. If they cannot manage the number of patients, then an MCI is declared and an Incident Management System is put into action.

INCIDENT MANAGEMENT SYSTEM (IMS)

The Incident Management System (IMS), also called an *Incident Command System (ICS)*, is a model tool for the command, control, and coordination of resources at the scene of a large scale emergency involving multiple agencies. It consists of procedures for organizing personnel, facilities, equipment, and communications.

The first formal Incident Management Systems were formed as a result of a mandate from Congress to analyze the aftermath of a devastating series of wildfires in southern California back in the early 1970s. Since that time, EMS, fire, and police agencies all across the nation continue to develop and implement such plans.

Most Incident Management Systems are based on well established management principles of planning, directing, organization, coordination, communication, delegation, and evaluation. They must be flexible enough to accommodate a single agency/single jurisdiction emergency as well as multi-agency/multi-jurisdictional events. Most Incident Management Systems employ a top-down modular structure that can be scaled to any size event. Some of the modules that might be included in a typical IMS are as follows:

- Command.
- Operations.
- Planning.
- Logistics.
- Finance.

It is easy to imagine how chaos can occur when so many different agencies and departments respond to a single large-scale emergency. Designing and implementing an organized approach to such an event will ensure a more positive outcome

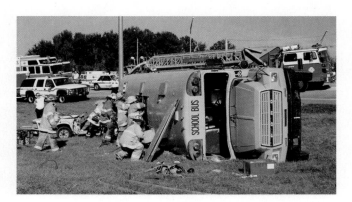

FIGURE 15.1
Plenty of resources have been called to the scene of this school bus wreck.

FIGURE 15.2
The incident manager delegates duties to the various sector officers.

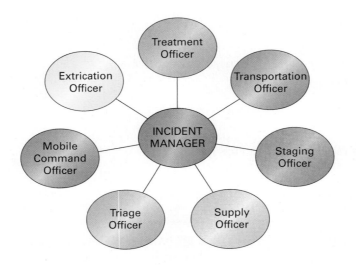

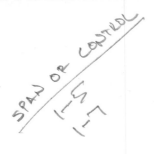

for both the rescuers and the victims. See Figure 15.2 for an example of the EMS portion of a large Incident Management System.

TRIAGE

triage a method of sorting patients for care and transport based on the severity of their injuries or illnesses.

When there are many victims at an emergency, it is nearly impossible to provide care to all those who need it when they need it. So a system called **triage** has been developed to help identify those victims who are most in need of immediate care. Triage is a process for sorting injured people into groups based on their need for or likely benefit from immediate medical care. Triage is used in hospital emergency departments, on battlefields, and at emergencies when there are multiple victims and limited medical resources (Figure 15.3).

PRIORITIES

FIRST> Triage is a process of sorting a number of patients into categories and ordering their medical care and transport based on the severity of their injuries and medical conditions. This process is used at the scene of mul-

FIGURE 15.3
At the scene of a multiple-casualty incident, triage is the system used to identify victims who are most in need of immediate medical care.

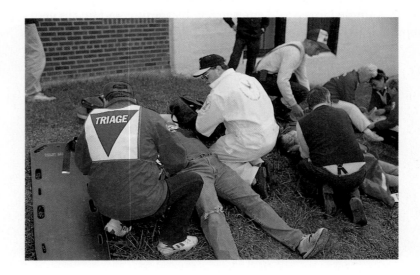

tiple-casualty incidents. When there are more victims than there are rescuers, the process of triaging helps to ensure that the most critical but still salvageable patients are cared for first. ■

For many MCIs, there may be a delay before additional help is on scene. If the emergency is large enough or in a remote area, an hour or more may pass before there are enough rescuers present to render care for all the patients. So triage is also used to determine the order of transport for patients. Patients who appear to have serious medical- or trauma-related problems—such as heart attack, shock, major injuries, and heat stroke—must be transported quickly, while patients with minor injuries or illnesses are transported later.

Since First Responders are first on the scene, they must be able to triage patients and initiate care. When additional EMS personnel arrive, First Responders pass on information, continue to help complete the triage process, and help provide care to the worst patients first. You cannot begin to provide care to patients randomly. You must begin caring for those people who have the highest priority based on their condition. You will need to make brief notes on each patient while you are performing triage.

Some jurisdictions have their First Responders use triage tags for patient information (Figure 15.4). Even if you do not carry these tags, you should be familiar with them in case you are called on to help when others are using triage tags. Use one triage tag per patient and leave the tag attached to the patient so that others arriving at the scene can have immediate access to information. Do not delay the triage process in order to make elaborate notes.

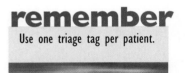

remember
Use one triage tag per patient.

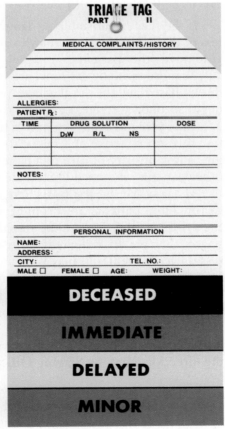

FIGURE 15.4
The METTAG, shown front and back, is an example of a standard triage tag.

The typical triage process includes both an initial and secondary step. The initial step does not allow for you to stop and provide interventions for each person in need of care. The purpose of an initial triage is to assess the patient's condition, determine the urgency of the patient's condition, and assign a treatment priority.

To begin the triage process, perform an initial triage assessment. Depending on what is found during this initial assessment, patients will be placed into one of four categories. The categories are as follows:

- Priority 1—Immediate.

- Priority 2—Delayed.

- Priority 3—Minor.

- Priority 4—Deceased.

The initial assessment includes the following elements:

Check responsiveness. If the patient is unresponsive, check for breathing and pulse. If there is no breathing or no pulse, do not provide care; tag the patient "Priority 4" and move on to the next patient.

Check the airway. If it is not open, open it. If the patient responds or begins to breathe on his own, tag the patient "Priority 1" and move on to the next patient.

Check pulse. If you feel a pulse, check for severe bleeding. If there is severe bleeding, quickly apply a pressure dressing, tag the patient "Priority 1," and move on to the next patient.

If the scene is unstable or dangerous in any way, begin to move people regardless of their injuries. Patients who are able to move and walk on their own can help you move other patients.

As more trained personnel arrive, they will take assigned positions and perform duties based on the local triage protocols. Those assigned to provide care will begin secondary triage, or caring for the patients who have been tagged "Priority 1," while you and others complete the initial triage of all patients. Even when additional rescuers arrive and begin to sort patients into treatment groups, they may give a low priority of care to a patient in cardiac arrest because there are too many other patients who need immediate life-saving care.

At many MCIs, secondary triage begins when a triage officer sets up a triage sector. Here patients are brought and separated into treatment groups based on the priority given them in the initial triage. As rescuers move patients to the triage sector, they are re-evaluated and re-categorized if necessary. The triage officer assesses each patient and may upgrade to a higher priority, allow the patient's status to remain the same, or downgrade to a lower one. Once patients are re-assessed in the triage sector, they are then sent to treatment sectors.

If you are dispatched and respond to an MCI already operating under the direction of an Incident Commander, report to the Staging Officer if there is one, or to the command post. Identify yourself and your level of training, and then follow the directions that the Staging Officer or Incident Commander gives you.

FIRST➤ There are several triage systems. Each uses slightly different criteria for classifying patients. Use the specific triage system and classifications that your jurisdiction has adopted. ■

---

note

When caring for victims who have been triaged, begin with the highest priority (most critically injured with a chance at survival).

---

remember

Victims in cardiac arrest or who present with a fatal injury are not given immediate treatment so that enough personnel may be available to care for those with life-threatening, but survivable, injuries.

[handwritten margin notes: Respirations — over 30 immediate. Profusion — radial pulse, cap refill. Mental Status.]

The following is an example of a typical four-category triage system:

- **Priority 1** (immediate; red tag)—treatable life-threatening illness or injuries.
  - Airway and breathing problems.
  - Severe or uncontrolled bleeding.
  - Altered mental status.
  - Severe medical problems.
  - Shock.
  - Critical burns.

- **Priority 2** (delayed; yellow tag)—serious but not life-threatening illness or injuries.
  - Burns without airway problems.
  - Multiple injuries or injuries to major bones.
  - Back injuries with or without spinal-cord damage.

- **Priority 3** (minor, green tag)—"walking wounded."
  - Minor musculoskeletal injuries (pain or stiffness, but able to move normally).
  - Minor soft-tissue injuries (minor lacerations, bruises). In three-category triage systems, those who are dead or fatally injured are also included as low priority and placed in Priority 3.

- **Priority 4** (deceased; gray or black tag)—dead or fatally injured.
  - Open head injury with exposed brain matter.
  - Cardiac arrest.
  - Severed trunk.
  - Decapitation.
  - Incineration.

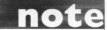

Victims who can walk should be directed to a specific location away from the immediate emergency scene.

NOTE: *Instead of a "deceased" category, your system may use a "probable death" category, which includes obvious death, mortal wounds, and all injuries where death is considered to be certain under the conditions in which the rescue is taking place.*

Many factors can change the patient's priority during the triage process. These factors include the type of incident, location, how quickly the patient can be assessed, weather conditions, number of patients, types of injuries, number of rescuers, availability of high-level trauma services, and limitations of the EMS system. A significant factor that affects the triage process is the fact that patients do not always maintain their initial condition or triage status. Their conditions change. During the secondary triage, a patient's status may need to be upgraded or downgraded.

You also will have to modify care procedures if you are trying to manage a large number of patients. For example, you may initially classify an unresponsive patient as Priority 1. Then sometime later that patient becomes responsive and may be reclassified as a Priority 2 or 3 due to their improved condition. The opposite may also be true. That is, a patient who is initially classified as Priority 3 may be re-classified as a Priority 1 when he becomes unresponsive.

FIRST▶ It is important to understand that patients will constantly be re-assessed as time and resources permit. ■

START TRIAGE SYSTEM

One variation of a triage system that is common in fire departments and EMS is the **START triage system** developed by the Newport Beach, California, Fire and Marine Department and Hoag Hospital. The letters START stand for Simple Triage and Rapid Treatment. START is based on the rapid assessment patients using the following three criteria: respirations, perfusion, and mental status (RPM).

Patients are classified into one of four categories—immediate, delayed, minor, and deceased—based on the RPM assessment (Figure 15.5).

Initial Triage

The first rescuers on the scene begin the triage process and quickly identify and separate those patients who are probably the least injured. They are initially classified as "minor." This is accomplished by directing all the walking wounded to a specific location away from the immediate emergency scene. By responding to the direction to move, patients who are able will move and therefore self triage into the "minor" category, at least initially. It is important not to send these patients too far away as some of them may be able to assist with the care of more injured patients.

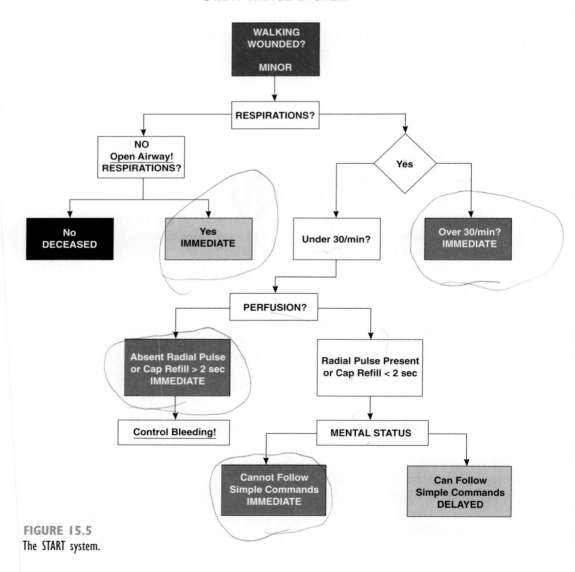

START TRIAGE SYSTEM

FIGURE 15.5
The START system.

TABLE 15-1 START TRIAGE SYSTEM

	IMMEDIATE	DELAYED	MINOR	DECEASED
Respirations	> 30 per minute	< 30 per minute	< 30 per minute	Absent
Perfusion	Capillary refill > 2 seconds or radial pulse absent	Capillary refill < 2 seconds or radial pulse present	Capillary refill < 2 seconds or radial pulse present	Absent
Mental status	Unable to follow commands	Able to follow commands	Able to follow commands	Absent

Once the walking wounded have exited the scene, the next step will be to begin triaging the remaining patients. START triage recommends you to "start where you stand." That is, begin assessing the patients closest to you and work your way out to all of the patients (Table 15-1).

- *Check respirations.* Each remaining patient is assessed for the presence of respirations. Open the airway and check for breathing. If the patient takes a breath, he is tagged "immediate." If he is not breathing, he is non-salvageable and is tagged "deceased." Responsive patients with respirations less than 30 per minute are assessed for perfusion status.

  – No respirations: dead/non-salvageable (black or gray tag).

  – Respirations above 30 per minute: immediate (red tag). No further assessment needed.

  – Respirations below 30 per minute: assess perfusion.

  All respiratory rates are estimates based on quick observation. It is not necessary to take actual rates during the triage process.

NOTE: *Patients who were identified as ambulatory can assist in keeping the airway open for an unresponsive patient. If other patients cannot help, use items on the scene to position the head and maintain the airway.*

- *Assess perfusion.* Check the breathing patient's radial pulse. The presence of a radial pulse indicates a systolic blood pressure of at least 80 mmHg. Any patient with a radial pulse is assumed to have adequate perfusion. Therefore, assessment of mental status is the next step before categorizing the patient. Any patient without a radial pulse is assumed to have inadequate perfusion and is tagged "immediate."

  Some triage systems use capillary refill to assess perfusion. However, it is often unreliable because of many variables, such as age, sex, and environment. If your protocols require that you check capillary refill, the following criteria will guide you: If capillary refill is greater than two seconds or the radial pulse is absent, categorize the patient as "immediate" and move on to the next patient. If capillary refill is less than two seconds and the patient has a radial pulse continue to assess mental status.

  During the perfusion assessment, if you find major bleeding, do what you can to attempt to control the bleeding. Have the patient or one of the walking wounded hold direct pressure over the wound. Elevate the legs of any patient with no radial pulse and keep him in this position.

- *Mental status.* The final step in the START triage process requires assessment of the patient's mental status. This is accomplished by determining if they can follow simple commands, for example, open or close the eyes or squeeze your fingers. If the patient is able to follow simple commands they are categorized "delayed" and you will then move on to the next patient. If the patient is unable to follow simple commands they are categorized "immediate" and you will then move on to the next patient.

NOTE: *When working with the START triage process, it is good to know that all unresponsive breathing patients are automatically categorized as "immediate."*

JumpSTART Pediatric MCI Triage System

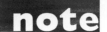

If a victim appears to be a young adult, use the START triage system. If he appears to be a small child, use JumpSTART.

The START triage system works well for rapidly assessing adults, but rescuers need to use different criteria to assess pediatric patients in multiple-casualty incidents. Using the START system, a respiratory rate of less than 30 breaths per minute in adults is a good sign, while a rate faster than 30 breaths a minute indicates a problem. Small children, especially crying infants, will normally have a respiratory rate greater than 30 breaths a minute. A child with a respiratory rate of 8 breaths a minute would be categorized "delayed" using the START system, when actually he is in respiratory failure and should be categorized "immediate."

There are similar assessment problems when checking circulation in children. Adults usually have circulatory failure followed by respiratory arrest. Children have respiratory failure followed by circulatory failure, meaning that a non-breathing child could still have a pulse. But the START system would categorize the child with no respirations as "deceased." START also uses capillary refill as an assessment tool, and it can be a useful assessment for children in normal environments. However, the reliability of capillary refill as an assessment tool varies with age, sex, and the environment, and measuring it requires good lighting. The JumpSTART system does not recommend using capillary refill for assessing perfusion.

When checking mental status in children, there is a broad range of responses possible, depending on the child's age. Infants will not be able to obey commands; small children do not have the developmental ability to respond appropriately to commands. However, rescuers can check for signs of mental status using the AVPU scale (alert, responsive to voice, responsive to pain, or unresponsive).

To meet the needs of children involved in MCIs, Dr. Lou Romig, Medical Director for the South Florida Regional Disaster Medical Assistance Team, developed a special triage system for pediatric patients, the JumpSTART Pediatric MCI Triage system (Figure 15.6). JumpSTART can be used on children from 12 months to 8 years of age, although rescuers can use it on older children as well. The age ranges were determined by several criteria:

- Children from 12 to 18 months are beginning to walk and can be sorted as "walking wounded," or ambulatory patients.

- Children over 8 years of age have airway anatomy and physiology similar to that of an adult.

Dr. Romig suggests that if the patient looks like a young adult, use START; if the patient looks like a child, use JumpSTART.

The assessment categories for the JumpSTART system are the same as for the START system: respirations, perfusion (peripheral pulses), and mental status (AVPU).

JumpSTART Steps
1. Move all children who are able to walk to an area set aside for minor injuries. There, rescuers will perform a secondary triage, including respirations, pulse,

for kids

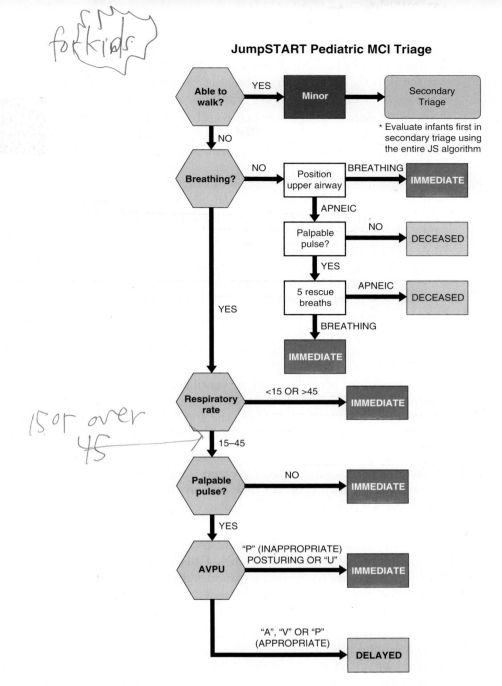

JumpSTART Pediatric MCI Triage

FIGURE 15.6
The JumpSTART Pediatric MCI Triage system. *(Copyright 2002 Lou Romig, MD, FAAP, FACEP)*

15 or over 45

and mental status. Infants who are not yet walking are assessed during initial triage, using the JumpSTART steps, or in the secondary triage area, if someone carries them there. Infants and children who are ambulatory (able to walk), have respirations, perfusion, and appropriate mental status, and have no significant external injury are categorized as "minor."

On an MCI, it is possible to have a child with special health care needs. These children may not be ambulatory and may also have chronic respiratory problems and elevated respiratory rates. Assess these special-needs children the same as you would infants. It may also be difficult to assess mental status because of the child's special health care or developmental status. Look for the child's parent or caregiver to get information if this person is present and uninjured.

2. **a.** Assess non-ambulatory children for the presence or absence of spontaneous breathing. If there is breathing, assess the respiratory rate (see Step 3).

Open the airway of any child who is not breathing or who is not breathing for more than 10 seconds. Clear a foreign body airway obstruction *only* if you see it. If the child begins to breathe spontaneously with an open airway, categorize the child as immediate, and move on to the next patient.

b. If the child does not begin spontaneous breathing when you open the airway, palpate for a peripheral pulse (radial, brachial, or pedal). If there is no peripheral pulse, categorize the patient as deceased, and move on to the next patient.

c. If the child does not begin spontaneous breathing when you open the airway, and the child has a pulse, ventilate the patient five times using an appropriate barrier device. Giving breaths is considered the "jumpstart" part of the pediatric triage system. Children may stop breathing or have a period of not breathing (apnea) but still maintain a pulse. The START system would categorize the non-breathing child as "deceased," but the Jump-START system modifies the process to include a pulse check for the non-breathing child and five ventilations if there is a pulse. The ventilation is meant to jumpstart the child's breathing.

However, if ventilations *do not* trigger spontaneous respirations, categorize the child as "deceased" and move on to the next patient. If the child begins to breathe spontaneously, categorize the child as "immediate" and move on without providing further ventilations. It is possible that the child may not be breathing when another rescuer arrives to begin secondary triage. This rescuer will determine the appropriate intervention based on the number of patients and the number of rescue personnel.

3. In this step, all patients have spontaneous respirations. If the respiratory rate is 15–45 breaths per minute, proceed to Step 4 and assess perfusion. If the respiratory rate is less than 15 (slower than one breath every four seconds) or faster than 45 breaths a minute or very irregular, categorize the child as "immediate" and move on.

4. In this step, all patients have adequate respirations. Assess perfusion by palpating peripheral pulses on uninjured limbs. Check peripheral pulses rather than capillary refill because of the many variables that affect accuracy. If the child has palpable peripheral pulses, assess mental status (Step 5). If there are no peripheral pulses, categorize the patient as immediate, and move on.

5. In this step, all patients have adequate ABCs. Check the child's mental status by using a rapid AVPU assessment. Keep in mind that the developmental age of the child will affect results. If the child is alert, responds to your voice, or responds appropriately to pain (localizes the pain, or knows where you are pressing or grasping, and withdraws or pushes you away), categorize the patient as "delayed." If the child does not respond to your voice and responds inappropriately to pain (makes a noise, moves sporadically, or does not localize the pain), shows "posturing" (decorticate, with arms curled onto the chest toward the midline of the body; or decerebrate, with arms stiff at their sides and hands flexed away from the body), or is unresponsive, categorize as "immediate," and move on.

PATIENT ASSESSMENT

It is critical to consider the mechanism of injury and the findings from the initial and focused assessments when you determine order of care for multiple-casualty incidents. Vital signs and significant signs of injury will help you determine priority and care. Relate patient signs to possible injuries or illness (Figure 15.7).

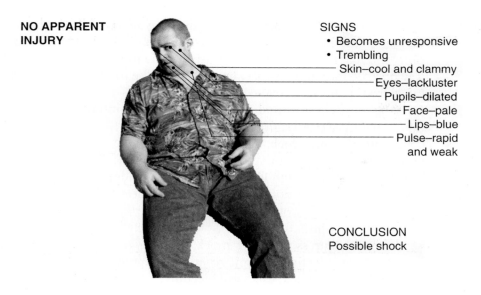

NO APPARENT INJURY

SIGNS
- Becomes unresponsive
- Trembling
- Skin–cool and clammy
- Eyes–lackluster
- Pupils–dilated
- Face–pale
- Lips–blue
- Pulse–rapid and weak

CONCLUSION
Possible shock

FIGURE 15.7
First Responders must be able to relate signs to specific illnesses and injuries.

NO APPARENT INJURY

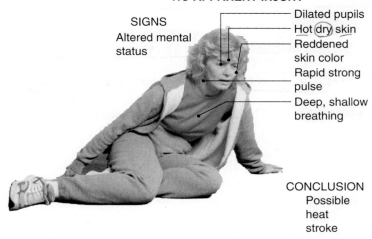
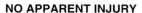

SIGNS
Altered mental status

- Dilated pupils
- Hot dry skin
- Reddened skin color
- Rapid strong pulse
- Deep, shallow breathing

CONCLUSION
Possible heat stroke

FIRST➤ As a First Responder, you must be able to apply the following information to the assessment and care of patients:

- Pulse (vital sign).
  - *Rapid, strong:* fear, overexertion, heat stroke and advanced heat exhaustion, high blood pressure, early stages of internal bleeding.
  - *Rapid, weak:* shock, blood loss, developing heat exhaustion, diabetic coma, falling blood pressure.
  - *Slow, strong:* stroke, possible skull fracture.
  - *No pulse:* carotid = cardiac arrest; distal = injury to the extremity (usually a possible fracture or dislocation) or shock with low blood pressure.
- Respiration (vital sign).
  - *Rapid, shallow:* shock, heart problems, heat exhaustion, insulin shock, congestive heart failure.
  - *Deep, grapsing, labored:* airway obstruction, congestive heart failure, heart problems, lung disease, lung injury from excessive heat, chest injuries, diabetic coma.
  - *Snoring:* stroke, possible fractured skull, drug or alcohol abuse, airway obstruction.
  - *Stridor:* high-pitched sounds on inspiration.

- *Crowing:* abnormal breathing sound indicating airway obstruction.
- *Gurgling:* liquid in the airway—for example, vomitus, blood, or normal secretions and inability to clear them—usually due to impaired mental status; airway obstruction; lung disease; lung damage due to excessive heat; fluids in lungs from pulmonary edema.
- *Coughing blood:* chest wound, possible rib fracture, internal injuries.

● Skin temperature (vital sign).
- *Cool, moist (clammy):* shock, heat exhaustion.
- *Cool, dry:* exposure to cold.
- *Hot, dry:* heat stroke, high fever, chemical (pesticide) exposure.
- *Hot, moist:* heat exhaustion or heat stroke (but heat stroke may be either sweaty or dry), infectious disease.

● Skin color (vital sign).
- *Red:* high blood pressure, heart attack, heat stroke, diabetic coma, minor burn, fever or infection, allergic reaction (anaphylaxis).
- *Pale:* shock, heart attack, excessive bleeding, heat exhaustion, fright, insulin shock.
- *Blue (cyanosis):* heart failure, airway obstruction, lung disease, certain poisonings, shock.

● Pupils (vital sign).
- *Dilated, unresponsive to light:* cardiac arrest, unresponsiveness, shock, bleeding, heat stroke, drugs (LSD, uppers).
- *Constricted:* damage to the central nervous system, drugs (heroin, morphine, codeine).
- *Unequal:* stroke, head injury—only useful in setting of profoundly altered mental status.

● Mental status.
- *Confusion:* fright, anxiety, illness, minor head injury, alcohol or drug abuse, mental illness, shock, epilepsy, hypoxia.
- *Stupor:* head injury, alcohol or drug abuse, stroke.
- *Altered mental status:* head injury, fainting, epilepsy.
- *Unresponsiveness:* stroke, allergy shock, head injury, poisoning, drug or alcohol abuse, diabetic coma, heat stroke or advanced heat exhaustion, shock, heart attack.

● Paralysis or loss of sensation.
- *One side of body:* stroke, head injury.
- *Arms only:* spinal injury in neck.
- *Legs only:* spinal injury along back.
- *Arms and legs:* spinal injury in neck and possibly along back.
- *No pain, obvious injury:* spinal-cord or brain damage, shock, anxiety, drug or alcohol abuse. ■

You have learned about the significance of the injuries and how to provide care for patients with these signs and symptoms throughout your First Responder course. When you are faced with multiple casualties at critical incidents, also be aware of your mental and physical stress levels. Critical incident stress debriefing (CISD) sessions or other qualified psychological support should be available after a disaster or unusual emergency to address the needs of rescuers who may have been influenced by the scene and the stress generated in providing emergency care.

Chapter Review

SUMMARY

While relatively rare multiple-casualty incidents (MCIs) can easily overwhelm the first responding units at the scene. It is up to those first units to quickly request additional resources and begin to establish command over the incident.

An **incident management system,** or incident command system, is a tool used to manage overall control of large scenes involving many resources and multiple agencies.

Triage is the sorting of patients based on the severity of their injuries and/or illnesses. The goal of triage is to save as many patients using the available resources. Triage systems vary by jurisdiction, but generally use a three- or four-category system. Typical categories include **immediate** for the most critical but salvageable patients, **delayed** for those less critical but still in need of care, **minor** for those who are generally ambulatory at the scene, and **deceased** for those who show no signs of life.

One variation of a triage system is the **START system**—a Simple Triage and Rapid Treatment program that uses respirations, perfusion, and mental status assessments to categorize patients into one of four treatment categories.

A variation of the START triage system designed specifically for pediatric patients is called the JumpSTART system, which takes into account the unique needs and presentation of pediatric patients.

Patient assessment is an important part of MCIs, because patients will need continued care following the initial triage process. Taking multiple vital signs and other key signs will help to determine the seriousness of the patient's injuries and to determine if they are getting worse or remaining stable. MCI patients must be continuously assessed by field personnel until they reach a destination hospital.

REMEMBER AND CONSIDER

Any emergency that involves multiple victims and overwhelms the responders who arrive first on scene qualifies as an MCI. It is important to bring order to chaos; therefore, use the procedures within the Incident Management System to organize responding personnel and equipment. If you respond to an MCI, report to the Staging Officer or command post to receive instructions. Do not enter a declared MCI scene without being aware of and understanding potential life-threatening hazards or where you can have the greatest impact.

Victims at an MCI must be initially triaged to determine treatment priority. Care will be provided by other emergency personnel in an order that benefits the most critically injured first. Additional triage assessments will follow and may result in documented changes in a patient's medical condition.

✔ It can be difficult to avoid providing immediate care to MCI victims. However, initial triage is necessary to determine how the greatest good can be provided for the greatest number of patients. By performing this task without distraction, more lives may potentially be saved.

Two popular triage systems—START and JumpSTART—address the differences between acceptable pulse and respiratory values and mental status assessment. Understanding these variations will help your patient assessment skills in other areas of emergency medical care.

Check your First Responder vehicle for triage tags. Take the time to understand the definition and values assigned to each tag. Ask an experienced rescuer to explain your agency's Incident Management System.

✔ Does your agency carry on-scene identifiers such as vests, tarps, or cones? Where are they located?

✔ Who in your department is best suited or appointed for leadership at an MCI?

Ask if you can participate in a table-top MCI exercise. This exercise will allow you to experience a multiple-casualty response in a controlled setting, permit a global view of the incident, and perhaps give you an opportunity to sample various leadership roles.

✔ How often does the local EMS system perform a drill to test the system?

Many times the people coordinating such drills need volunteers to help serve as victims for the event. This would be a great opportunity to see how the system functions from the perspective of a patient. Contact your local EMS agency or fire department to inquire about helping with their next drill.

Appendix I

Determining Blood Pressure

Note: This Appendix is based on materials presented and followed by the American Heart Association (AHA). Keep track of AHA updates and adjust your techniques as changes are made. It is recommended that you follow the AHA guidelines for determining blood pressure unless your state EMS system or local protocols recommend a different method.

In some localities, particularly those in which First Responders work in isolated areas, a special training program for learning to assess blood pressure is included in the standard First Responder course. If this is not part of your course, do not try to train yourself in the use of the blood pressure cuff. Do only what you have been trained to do in your program.

WHAT IS BLOOD PRESSURE?

Blood pressure is a vital sign. It is the measurement of the pressure of blood against the walls of the arteries. A blood pressure reading that is significantly above or below the normal range for a patient can be valuable in determining what may be wrong with the patient (for example, shock). Repeated blood pressure measurements also help you monitor the patient's condition and check the patient's stability as you wait for the EMTs to arrive.

Blood pressure is determined by measuring the pressure changes in the arteries. The left ventricle receives blood, **contracts,** and forces blood into the arteries to circulate throughout the body. The heart's contraction phase is called **systole.** When measured, the blood pumped into the system of arteries is called the **systolic** (sis-TOL-ik) blood pressure. It is affected by the force of the heart's pumping action, the resistance and elasticity of the arteries, blood volume (blood loss means lower pressure), blood thickness, and the amount of other fluids in the cells.

After the left ventricle of the heart contracts, it **relaxes** and refills. This relaxation phase is called **diastole.** During diastole, the pressure in the arteries falls. When measured, this pressure is called the **diastolic** (di-as-TOL-ik) blood pressure.

Blood pressure is measured in specific units called millimeters of mercury (mmHg). These are the units on the blood pressure gauge. Since this system of measurement is standard and known to the people receiving patient information from First Responders, you will not have to say "millimeters of mercury" after each reading. Report the systolic pressure first and then the diastolic, as in 120 over 80 (120/80). The reading of 120/80 is considered a normal blood pressure reading, which represents the average blood pressure obtained from a large sampling of healthy adults. There is a wide range of "normal" for adults and children. Blood pressures are not usually measured in the field for children under three years of age because it is difficult to get accurate measurements.

You will not know the normal blood pressure for a patient unless the person is alert, knows the information, and can tell you what it is. Blood pressure varies greatly among individuals. However, there is a general rule for estimating what a patient's blood pressure should be. This rule works for adults up to the age of 40. To estimate the systolic blood pressure of an adult male at rest, add his age to 100. To estimate the systolic blood pressure of an adult female at rest, add her age to 90.

Since you will not know the normal reading for a particular patient, you will take several readings in order to identify a trend in the patient's condition. One blood pressure reading is of little use. The first reading may be high because of the effects of stress produced by the emergency. Taking several readings, and comparing them is called **trending.** An initial measurement may show that a patient has a blood pressure within normal range, but the condition may worsen. For example, a patient going into shock (hypoperfusion) may have a rapid pulse and a normal blood pressure reading when you first arrive at the scene. A few minutes later, the blood pressure may fall dramatically. Taking several readings while you are providing care is a way of identifying changes in the patient's status. Changes in blood pressure are significant and let you know that additional care is needed and transport is a priority.

A systolic blood pressure reading below 90 mmHg is considered lower than normal in most adults. Some small adult females and small-build athletes may have a normal systolic blood pressure of 90 mmHg. But usually any systolic blood pressure measurement of 90 or less or a measurement that drops to 90/60 or below may be an indication that the patient is going into shock.

A reading above 140/90 is typically considered high blood pressure. But many patients will show a short-term initial rise in blood pressure at the emergency scene, usually due to anxiety, fear, and stress. You will need more than one reading to confirm high blood pressure. High blood pressure readings are typical in individuals who are obese or who have a history of high cholesterol. There are many other underlying medical conditions that cause high blood pressure that you will be unable to determine at the emergency scene. Several readings will help you determine patient status and guide your care and transport decisions.

In addition to the patient's overall appearance, use the following general guidelines at the emergency scene to help you make assessment decisions:

Adults
- Systolic above 140—serious.
- Systolic below 90—serious.
- Diastolic above 90—serious.
- Diastolic below 60—serious.

Children: ages 6 to 14
- Systolic above 140—serious.
- Systolic below 80—serious.
- Diastolic above 70—serious.
- Diastolic below 50—serious.

Children: ages 3 to 5
(Blood pressure is not taken in a child under three years of age.)

- Systolic above 120—serious.
- Systolic below 70—serious.
- Diastolic above 70—serious.
- Diastolic below 50—serious.

Note: Normal ranges for children vary among physicians.

MEASURING BLOOD PRESSURE

There are two common techniques used to measure blood pressure in emergency field situations. They are:

- **Auscultation** (os-kul-TAY-shun)—using a blood pressure cuff and a stethoscope (Figure A1.1) to listen for characteristic sounds.
- **Palpation**—using a blood pressure cuff and feeling the patient's radial pulse in the wrist or brachial pulse on the inner arm above the elbow.

DETERMINING BLOOD PRESSURE BY AUSCULTATION

To determine blood pressure using a blood pressure cuff and a stethoscope, you should:

1. Have the patient sit or lie down (Figure A1.2). Cut away or remove clothing over the arm. Support the arm at the level of the heart.

   Warning: Do not move the patient's arm if there is any possibility of spinal injury. Check to be sure the arm to be used has not been injured.

2. Select the correct-size blood pressure cuff. Do not try to use an adult-size cuff on a child. The cuff should be two-thirds the width of the upper arm.

3. Wrap the cuff around the patient's upper arm. The lower border of the cuff should be about one

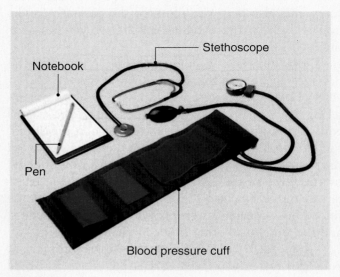

FIGURE A1.1
Blood pressure determination equipment.

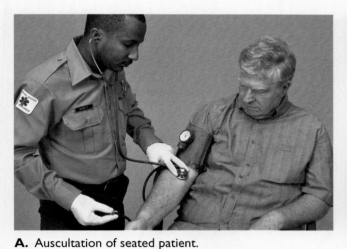

A. Auscultation of seated patient.

FIGURE A1.2
Positions for taking blood pressure.

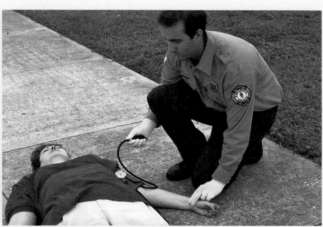

B. Palpation of supine patient.

inch above the crease in the patient's elbow. The center of the bladder inside the cuff must be placed over the brachial artery in the upper arm (Figure A1.3).

Note: Some cuffs have a marker to tell you how to line up the cuff over the brachial artery. Know your equipment. Some cuffs have no markers, while others have inaccurate markers. The tubes entering the bladder in the cuff may not be in the correct location. The AHA recommends that you find the bladder center and line up the center of the bladder over the brachial artery.

4. Apply the cuff securely but not too tightly (Figure A1.4). You should be able to place one finger under the bottom edge of the cuff.
5. Place the ends of the stethoscope in your ears.

   Note: If you are using a dual head stethoscope, one with both a bell and a diaphragm, make certain to check that the appropriate side is activated before placing it on the patient.

6. Use your fingertips to locate the brachial artery at the crease in the elbow.
7. Position the diaphragm or bell of the stethoscope over the brachial artery pulse site. Do not let the

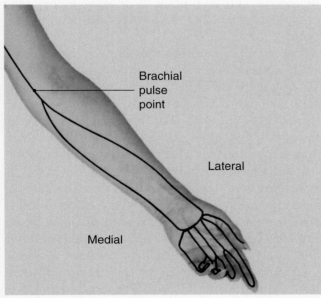

FIGURE A1.3
Brachial pulse point.

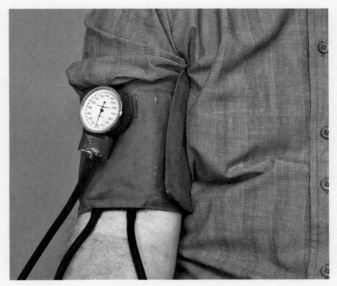

FIGURE A1.4
Positioning of the blood pressure cuff.

head of the stethoscope touch the cuff. If it touches the cuff, the stethoscope rubs against it during inflation and deflation. You will hear the rubbing sounds, which may cause you to record a false reading.

8. Close the bulb valve and inflate the cuff. As you do this, listen to the pulse sounds through the stethoscope. At a certain point, you will not be able to hear the pulse sounds.

   Note: The AHA preferred technique is to place your fingertips over the radial pulse as you inflate the cuff (explained below). When you can no longer feel the pulse, pump up the cuff pressure 30 more mmHg. Then slowly release the pressure as you listen for the systolic pressure sounds.

9. Keep inflating the cuff to a point 30 mmHg higher than the point where the pulse sounds stopped.

10. Open the bulb valve slowly to release pressure from the cuff. It should fall at a smooth rate of 2 to 3 mmHg per second or a little faster than the second hand on a watch.

11. Listen carefully for and note when you begin to hear the sound of the pulse in the stethoscope. This is the systolic pressure.

12. Let the cuff continue to deflate. Listen for and note when the sound of the pulse (clicking or tapping) fades (not when they stop). When the sound turns dull or soft, this is the diastolic pressure (Figure A1.5).

    Note: Some EMS systems have First Responders use the point where the sounds stop as the diastolic pressure.

13. Let the rest of the air out of the cuff quickly. If practical, leave the cuff in place so you can take additional readings.

14. Record the time, the arm used, the position of the patient (lying down, sitting), and the patient's pressure. Round off the readings to the next highest number. For example, 145 mmHg should be recorded as 146 mmHg. (The markings on the gauge are in even numbers. You may "see" the first sound in between two markings and want to record it as an odd number—145—but all blood pressure readings are in even numbers.)

Some people cannot find the brachial artery, or they cannot hear the pulse sounds when they inflate the cuff, but they can hear the sounds when they deflate the cuff. If you have this problem, use your fin-

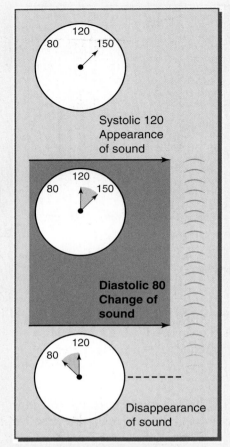

FIGURE A1.5
Example of blood pressure sounds.

gertips to find the radial pulse in the wrist of the arm to which you have applied the cuff. Inflate the cuff until you can no longer feel the radial pulse. Continue to inflate the cuff to a point 30 mmHg higher than where the pulse stopped. The rest of the procedure is the same.

If you are not certain of a reading, be sure the cuff is totally deflated and wait one or two minutes and try again, or use the other arm. Should you try the same arm too soon, you may get false high readings.

Sometimes patients with high systolic readings have sounds that disappear as you deflate the cuff, only to reappear again. This can lead to both false systolic and diastolic readings as you record the high systolic reading and record the first disappearance of sound as the diastolic reading. If you continued to listen, you might find that sounds start up again about 20 mmHg lower. Whenever you have a high diastolic reading, wait one or two minutes and take a second reading and be sure to listen for sounds until all air is deflated from the cuff. On a subsequent reading, feel for the disappearance of the radial pulse as you inflate the cuff (this will ensure that you did not measure a

Measuring Blood Pressure—Auscultation

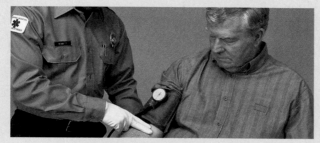

1. Position cuff and find pulse site.

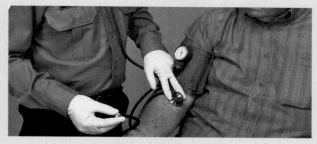

2. Set diaphragm over pulse site.

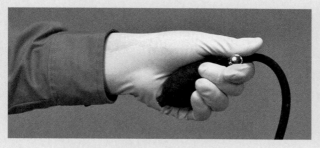

3. Close valve and inflate cuff.

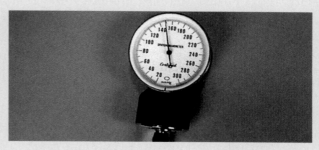

4. Listen for sound to disappear. Inflate 30 mmHg beyond this point.

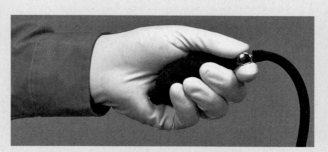

5. Open valve to deflate 2 to 3 mmHg/sec.

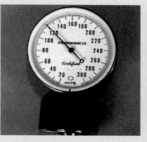

6. Listen for start of sound—systolic. Listen for sound to fade—diastolic.

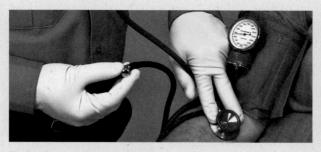

7. Deflate cuff completely.

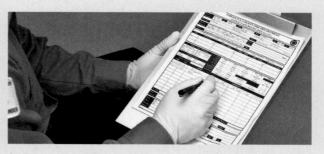

8. Record results.

false systolic pressure) and listen as you deflate the cuff down into the normal range and until all air is released from the cuff. Use the last fade of sound as the diastolic pressure.

See Scan A1-1 for a summary of determining blood pressure by auscultation.

DETERMINING BLOOD PRESSURE BY PALPATION

Using the palpation method (feeling the radial pulse) is not a very accurate method. It will provide you with one reading, an **approximate systolic pressure.** This method is used when there is too much noise around to use a stethoscope, or when there are too many patients for the number of rescuers at the scene. To determine blood pressure by palpation, place the cuff in the same position on the arm as you would for auscultation and:

1. Find the radial pulse on the arm with the cuff (Figure A1.6).
2. Close the valve and inflate the cuff until you can no longer feel the pulse.
3. Continue to inflate the cuff to a point 30 mmHg above the point where the pulse disappeared.

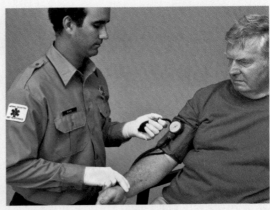

FIGURE A1.6
Measuring blood pressure by palpation.

4. Slowly deflate the cuff and note the reading when you feel the pulse return.
5. Record the time, the arm used, the position of the patient, and the systolic pressure. Note that the reading was by palpation. If you give this information orally to someone, make sure they know the reading was by palpation, as in, "Blood pressure is 146 by palpation."

Appendix 2

Breathing Aids and Oxygen Therapy

FIRST RESPONDER'S ROLE

Some EMS systems do not train First Responders in the use of aids for breathing and oxygen therapy. But in many jurisdictions, supplemental training programs are offered to meet community needs. Learning how to use ventilation aids and how to administer oxygen may be part of your course or may be offered as a special supplement or continuing education program. Your jurisdiction may require this training especially if you are to perform your First Responder duties in an isolated area. You cannot train yourself to use oxygen administration equipment. Do only what you have been trained to do.

Basic life support is possible without equipment and should never be delayed while you locate, retrieve, and set up breathing aids or oxygen. There is no doubt that the prompt and efficient use of certain pieces of equipment can assist you in maintaining an open airway, providing ventilations, and providing oxygen to the patient. But, the patient may suffer if you delay care, use faulty equipment, or use the wrong equipment.

New responsibilities come with the use of equipment in basic life support. You must:

- Be sure that the equipment is clean and operational before it will be needed at an emergency.
- Select the proper equipment for the patient.
- Monitor the patient more closely once you begin to use any device or delivery system.
- Make certain that the equipment is properly discarded, cleaned, refilled, replaced, or tested after its use.
- Practice and maintain the skills needed to use basic life-support equipment in order to provide efficient emergency care.

The administration of oxygen may require orders from the medical director of your jurisdiction. This is because **oxygen is a medication.** As a First Responder, you may be given permission to initiate the use of oxygen by radio communications with a medical facility, or you may be able to begin oxygen administration without oral orders in very specific situations because you are operating under direction of local protocols. You may only be allowed to work with certain devices or administer oxygen while assisting EMTs. Your instructor will give you the guidelines for your jurisdiction.

VENTILATION-ASSIST DEVICES

You may wish to review Chapter 6 at this time. It describes the use of oropharyngeal and nasopharyngeal airways and the pocket face mask with one-way valve and HEPA filter. These devices help you to maintain an open airway and deliver ventilations. The bag-valve-mask (BVM) ventilator is another device that is used to assist with ventilations.

BAG-VALVE-MASK (BVM) VENTILATOR

Note: Most EMS systems recommend that an oropharyngeal airway be inserted before attempting to ventilate the patient with a bag-valve-mask (BVM) ventilator.

The BVM ventilator is one of the most commonly used devices for ventilating a nonbreathing patient. Some EMS systems also use the BVM to ventilate patients with shallow failing respirations (for example, in drug overdose). The BVM is available in sizes for infants, children, and adults. It also acts as an effective infection-control barrier between you and your patient.

The BVM delivers 21% oxygen to the patient when air from the atmosphere (room air) is squeezed through the unit to the patient's lungs. (In contrast, a pocket face mask will deliver 16% oxygen from your exhaled air.) The BVM can be connected to an oxygen supply source to enrich room air and deliver from 50% to nearly 100% oxygen.

Many types of BVMs are available. All have the same basic parts. There is a self-refilling bag, valves that control the flow of air, and a face mask to place on the patient's face. The face mask must have a transparent face piece so that the rescuer can see the patient's mouth in order to monitor for vomiting and lip

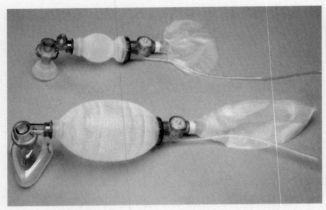

FIGURE A2.1
Disposable BVM ventilators.

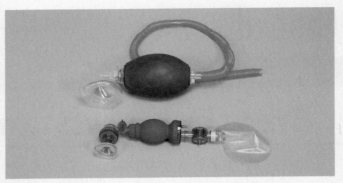

FIGURE A2.2
Pediatric and adult BVM ventilators.

color changes. There is also a standard 15/22 mm respiratory fitting, so a variety of respiratory equipment and face masks can be used with it. The BVM must be made of material that can be easily cleaned and sterilized. Many EMS systems now use disposable units (Figure A2.1).

The principle behind the operation of the BVM is simple. When you squeeze the bag, air is delivered to the patient's airway through a one-way, nonrebreathing valve. When you release the bag, air can flow from the patient's lungs out of another valve and into the atmosphere. The exhaled air does not go back into the bag. While the patient is exhaling, air from the atmosphere refills the bag and delivers a fresh air supply with the next squeeze.

The BVM can be difficult to operate for the single rescuer. This is especially true if you do not use it on a regular basis. You must practice regularly to maintain your skill and effectiveness. If you are assigned a BVM for use in the field, practice using it in the classroom until your technique is well developed. Some EMS systems have decided that skills for this device are poorly maintained, and thus they have selected the pocket face mask as the preferred ventilation assist device for First Responders.

When using the BVM as a single rescuer:

1. Position yourself at the patient's head and provide an open airway. Clear the airway if necessary.

2. Insert an oropharyngeal airway.

3. Use the correct mask size for the patient (Figure A2.2). Place the apex, or top, of the triangular mask over the bridge of the nose (between the eyebrows). Rest the base of the mask between the patient's lower lip and the projection of the chin.

4. Hold the mask firmly in position with (Figure A2.3):

— Thumb holding the upper part of the mask.

— Index finger between the valve and the lower cushion.

— Third, fourth, and fifth fingers on the lower jaw, between the chin and ear.

5. With your other hand, squeeze the bag fully once every 5 seconds delivering each breath over 1.5 seconds to 2 seconds. Make sure the patient's chest rises.

6. Release pressure on the bag and let the patient passively exhale. The bag will refill from the atmosphere.

For trauma patients who must have their airway opened by the jaw-thrust maneuver, the two-rescuer method is more effective. The rescuer holding the mask in place can more easily perform the jaw-thrust maneuver while the other rescuer provides effective ventilations.

The BVM can be used effectively during two-rescuer CPR by a skilled operator. The ventilator squeezes the bag and provides two back-to-back ventilations following each cycle of 15 compressions.

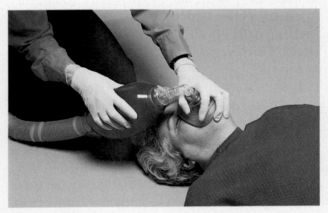

FIGURE A2.3
Hand positioning for using the BVM ventilator with a single rescuer.

There are times when the BVM will not deliver air to the patient's lungs. It is rare for the bag, valves, or mask to be the problem if you have kept the unit clean and in working order. Sometimes the problem is because of an airway obstruction that must be cleared. More often, the problem is caused by an improper seal between the patient's face and mask. If this occurs, you should reposition your fingers and check placement of the mask.

The most difficult part of operation is maintaining an adequate seal with the face mask in the one-rescuer operation. For this reason, it is recommended that ventilating a patient with a BVM should be done by two rescuers when they are available. One rescuer uses two hands to maintain an airway (head-tilt, chin-lift or jaw-thrust maneuver as necessary) and a seal with the mask, while the other rescuer squeezes the bag to ventilate the patient. Two-rescuer BVM ventilation ensures better airway management and ventilation.

To provide ventilations using the two-rescuer BVM technique (Figure A2.4):

1. Position yourself so you can open the airway using the head-tilt, chin-lift or the jaw-thrust maneuver. Clear the airway with a finger sweep (adult) or suction and insert an oropharyngeal or nasopharyngeal airway if necessary.

2. Select the correct BVM size for the patient (adult, child, or infant). If available and you are trained, connect the BVM to an oxygen source. Place the apex (top) of the mask over the bridge of the nose, then lower the mask over the mouth and upper chin. If the mask is the type that has a large, round cuff surrounding the ventilation port, center the port over the patient's mouth.

3. Kneel at the patient's head. For the head-tilt, chin-lift maneuver, place your thumbs over the top half of the mask, index and middle fingers over the bottom half, and your remaining fingers under the chin. For the jaw-thrust maneuver, place your thumbs over the nose portion of the mask, your index and middle fingers on the part of the mask that covers the mouth, and stretch your other fingers behind the jaw.

4. Use your ring and little fingers to bring the patient's jaw up to the mask and maintain the head-tilt, chin-lift; or to bring the jaw upward without tilting the head or neck for the jaw-thrust maneuver.

5. The second rescuer connects the bag to the mask (if not already done) and squeezes the bag with two hands, while you maintain a seal. The second rescuer squeezes the bag once every five seconds for an adult (once every three seconds for a child or an infant). Watch for the patient's chest to rise as the bag is squeezed.

6. The second rescuer releases pressure on the bag, and the patient exhales passively. The bag refills from the oxygen source or from the atmospheric air.

OXYGEN THERAPY

IMPORTANCE OF OXYGEN

A patient may need oxygen for many reasons, including respiratory and cardiac arrest, shock, major blood loss, heart attack or heart failure, lung disease, injury to the lungs or the chest, airway obstruction, and stroke.

The 21% oxygen provided by a BVM is far more than the patient needs and is effective if the airway is open, the exchange surfaces of the lungs are working properly, there is enough oxygen available to be picked up by the blood, and the patient's heart and blood vessels are properly circulating blood to all the body tissues. When any one of these factors is missing or fails, a higher concentration of oxygen must be delivered to the patient so that the required amount reaches the body's tissues.

When performing CPR and using mouth-to-mask ventilations, your exhaled air delivers approximately 16% oxygen to the patient's lungs. This is enough to keep the patient alive for only a short time. CPR is two-thirds less efficient than a healthy, beating heart circulating blood and oxygen. Ventilating by mouth-to-mask provides the patient with only the minimum oxygen required for short-term survival. By providing oxygen from a supply source, nearly 100% oxygen can reach the lungs. With more oxygen in the patient's

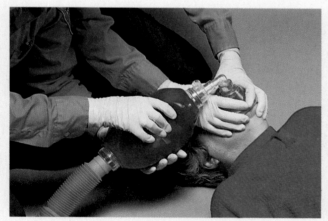

FIGURE A2.4
Two-rescuer BVM technique.

blood, CPR efficiency is improved and the patient has a better chance for survival.

Remember: Oxygen is a medication. Providing oxygen is a special responsibility that can be given only to someone trained in its use.

HAZARDS OF OXYGEN

There are certain hazards associated with oxygen administration including:

- Oxygen used in emergency care is stored under pressure (2,000 pounds per square inch [psi] or greater). If the tank is punctured or if a valve breaks off, the supply tank can become a missile.
- Oxygen supports combustion and causes fire to burn more rapidly. Oxygen can saturate linens and clothing and cause them to ignite quickly.
- Under pressure, oxygen and oil do not mix. When they come into contact with each other, there can be a severe reaction, which may cause an explosion. This can easily occur if you try to lubricate a delivery system or gauge with petroleum products.
- Long-term use of high oxygen concentrations can result in medical dangers. These dangers include lung-tissue destruction (oxygen toxicity), seizure, lung collapse, eye damage in premature infants, and respiratory arrest in patients with chronic obstructive pulmonary disease (COPD), including emphysema, chronic bronchitis, and black lung.

Do not attempt to administer oxygen directly to newborn infants unless ordered to do so by a physician. When oxygen is required (difficult delivery, respiratory distress, very weak infant, premature birth, or other emergency), provide oxygen by blowing it into a foil tent formed over the infant's head, neck, and shoulders. If this is not practical, use a blow-by method by placing the mask near the side of the infant's mouth and nose (Figure A2.5).

Patients with a history of COPD have what is known as a "hypoxic" drive. That is, they have become used to the lower levels of oxygen in their lungs and blood. Prolonged use of high-flow oxygen can lower their drive to breathe, causing respiratory arrest in some patients. This is uncommon in the prehospital setting and is rarely a concern for the First Responder.

Remember: Never withhold the concentration of oxygen that is appropriate for the patient. If you are in

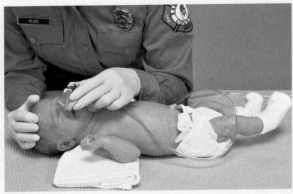

FIGURE A2.5
Blow-by delivery technique.

doubt as to how much oxygen to deliver, contact medical direction for advice.

EQUIPMENT AND SUPPLIES FOR OXYGEN THERAPY

An oxygen delivery system for the breathing patient includes a source (oxygen cylinder), pressure regulator, flowmeter, and a delivery device (face mask or cannula) (Figure A2.6). When possible, a humidifier should be added to provide moisture to the oxygen if the patient will be on the system for more than 30 minutes. (Some EMS systems will not allow the use of humidifiers because of improper storage and potential contamination.) The delivery system is the same for a nonbreathing patient, but a device must be added to allow the rescuer to force oxygen into the patient's lungs. This is known as a *flow-restricted, oxygen-powered ventilation device (FROPVD)* or sometimes called a *demand-valve device.* As a First Responder, you will

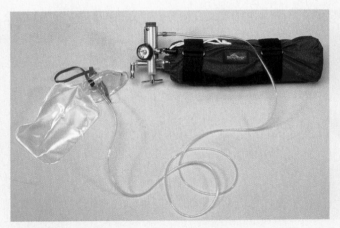

FIGURE A2.6
An oxygen delivery system.

probably use a BVM connected to 100% oxygen when administering oxygen to the nonbreathing patient.

Oxygen Cylinders

When providing oxygen in the field, the standard source of oxygen is a seamless steel or lightweight alloy cylinder filled with pressurized oxygen. The pressure is equal to 2,000 to 2,200 pounds per square inch (psi). Cylinders come in various sizes, identified by letters. The smaller sizes that are practical for the First Responder include (Figure A2.7):

- *D cylinder*—contains about 350 liters of oxygen
- *E cylinder*—contains about 625 liters of oxygen

Part of your duty as a First Responder is to make certain that the oxygen cylinders are full and ready for use before they are needed for patient care. The length of time that you can use an oxygen cylinder depends on the pressure in the cylinder and the flow rate. The method of calculating cylinder duration is shown in Table A2-1. Oxygen cylinders should never be allowed to empty below the safe residual level. The safe residual level for an oxygen cylinder is determined when the pressure gauge reads 200 psi. (You cannot tell if an oxygen cylinder is full, partially full, or empty by lifting or moving the cylinder.) At this point, you must switch to a fresh cylinder; below this point, there is not enough oxygen for proper delivery to the patient.

Safety is of prime importance when working with oxygen cylinders. You should:

- *Never* allow a cylinder to drop or fall against any object. The cylinder must be well secured, preferably in a lying down position. Never let a cylinder stand by itself.
- *Never* allow smoking around oxygen equipment.

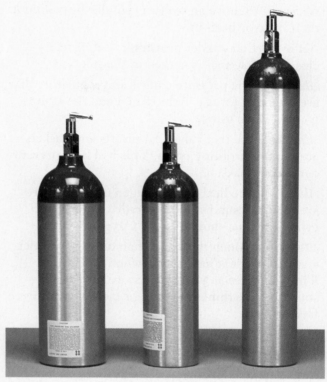

FIGURE A2.7
Various sized portable oxygen cylinders.

- *Never* use oxygen equipment around open flames or sparks.
- *Never* use grease or oil on devices that will be attached to an oxygen supply cylinder. Do not handle these devices when your hands are greasy.
- *Never* put tape on the cylinder outlet or use tape to mark or label any oxygen cylinder or oxygen delivery equipment. The oxygen can react with the adhesive left behind when it is torn from the cylinder and produce a fire.

TABLE A2-1 DURATION OF FLOW FORMULA

SIMPLE FORMULA
$\dfrac{\text{Gauge pressure in psi} - \text{residual pressure} \times \text{constant}}{\text{Flow rate in liters/minute}}$ = Safe duration of flow in minutes

RESIDUAL PRESSURE = 200 PSI CYLINDER CONSTANT

D = 0.16	G = 2.41
E = 0.28	H = 3.14
M = 1.56	K = 3.14

Determine the life of a D cylinder that has a pressure of 2,000 psi and a flow rate of 10 LPM.

$$\frac{(2,000 - 200) \times 0.16}{10} = \frac{288}{10} = 28.8 \text{ minutes}$$

- *Never* try to move an oxygen cylinder by rolling it on its side or bottom.
- *Never* store a cylinder near high heat or in a closed vehicle that is parked in the sun.
- *Always* use the pressure gauges and regulators that are intended for use with oxygen and the equipment you are using.
- *Always* ensure that valve seat inserts and gaskets are in good working order. This will help prevent dangerous leaks.
- *Always* use medical-grade oxygen (USP). There are impurities in industrial-grade oxygen. The cylinder's label should state, "Oxygen USP."
- *Always* fully open the valve of an oxygen cylinder and then close it half a turn, when it is in use. This will serve as a safety measure in the event someone else thinks the valve is closed and tries to force it open.
- *Always* store reserve oxygen cylinders in a cool, ventilated room as approved by your EMS system.
- *Always* have oxygen cylinders hydrostatically tested. This should be done every five years for steel tanks (three years for aluminum cylinders). The date for retesting should be stamped on the top of the cylinder near the valve.

Pressure Regulators

The pressure in an oxygen cylinder is too high to be used directly from the cylinder. A pressure regulator must be connected to the oxygen cylinder before it may be used to deliver oxygen to a patient (Figure A2.8). The safe working pressure for oxygen

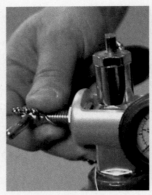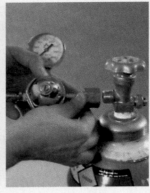

FIGURE A2.8
Common types of portable pressure regulators.

administration is 30 to 70 pounds per square inch (psi).

On cylinders of the "E" size or smaller, a yoke assembly is used to secure the pressure regulator to the cylinder valve assembly. The yoke has pins that must mate with the corresponding holes found in the valve assembly. This is called a *pin-index safety system* (Figure A2.9). The position of the pins varies for different gases to prevent an oxygen delivery system from being connected to a cylinder containing another gas.

Before connecting the pressure regulator to an oxygen supply cylinder, *open the cylinder valve slightly* for just a second to clear dirt and dust out of the delivery port or threaded outlet. This is called "cracking" the cylinder valve. Part of the maintenance of the regulator includes cleaning the inlet filter. Checking the filter for damage and dirt will prevent damage to and contamination of the regulator.

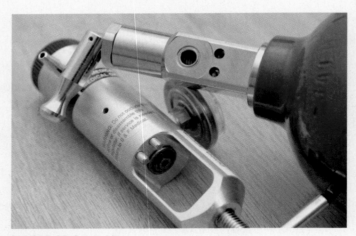

FIGURE A2.9
The PIN safety sytem

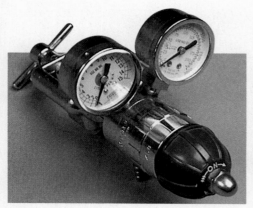

FIGURE A2.10
Bourdon gauge flowmeter (pressure gauge).

Flowmeters

A flowmeter is connected to the pressure regulator to give the user control over the flow of oxygen in liters per minute (LPM). The constant-flow selector valve is one of the most common used in the field today. However, many systems are still using the Bourdon style flowmeter.

- *Bourdon gauge flowmeter* (Figure A2.10). This flowmeter is a pressure gauge calibrated to indicate flow of gas in liters per minute (LPM). It is inaccurate at low flow rates and has been criticized for being unstable. This device will not compensate for back pressure. A partial obstruction (as from a kinked hose) will produce a reading higher than the actual flow. The gauge may read 4 LPM and be delivering only 1 LPM. False high readings also can be produced when the filter in the gauge becomes clogged. The bourdon gauge is fairly sturdy and will operate in any position.
- *Constant-flow selector valve.* This device has no liter flow gauge. (For a photograph of this valve, refer back to Figure A2.9). It allows for the adjustment of flow in liters per minute in stepped increments (2, 4, 6, 8, . . . 15 LPM). When using this type of flowmeter, make certain that it is properly adjusted for the desired flow. Monitor the dial to make certain that it stays properly adjusted. This type of meter should be tested for accuracy as recommended by the manufacturer.

Humidifiers

A humidifier is an unbreakable container of sterile water that can be attached to the flowmeter. As the oxygen from the cylinder passes through the water, it is moisturized and becomes more comfortable for the patient to breathe. Unhumidified oxygen delivered to a patient over a long period of time (usually more than 20 minutes) will dry out the mucous membranes in the airway and lungs. For the short period of time that the patient receives oxygen in the field, this is not usually a problem. A problem does arise, though, when humidifiers are not used appropriately. Too often, the task of changing them between patients is overlooked, or the device is opened but not used, which allows it to become contaminated over time. Because of this infection risk and the fact that they are not required for short transports, many EMS systems no longer use humidifiers.

Oxygen Delivery Devices: Breathing Patients

The nasal cannula and the nonrebreather mask are the main oxygen delivery devices used for the field administration of oxygen to breathing patients (Table A2-2).

The **nasal cannula** delivers oxygen into the patient's nostrils by way of two small plastic prongs (Figure A2.11). Its efficiency is greatly reduced by nasal injuries, colds, and other types of nasal airway obstruction. A flow rate of 2 to 6 LPM will provide the patient with 28% to 44% oxygen. The approximate relationship of oxygen concentration to liter per minute flow is:

1 LPM — 24% oxygen
2 LPM — 28% oxygen
3 LPM — 32% oxygen
4 LPM — 36% oxygen
5 LPM — 40% oxygen
6 LPM — 44% oxygen

TABLE A2-2 OXYGEN DELIVERY DEVICES

OXYGEN DELIVERY DEVICE	FLOW RATE	% OXYGEN DELIVERED	SPECIAL USE
Nasal cannula	1 to 6 LPM	24% to 44%	Most medical and COPD patients at low concentrations
Nonrebreather mask	Start with 10 LPM, practical high is 15 LPM	80% to 95%	Good for patients with respiratory distress and shock. Provides high-oxygen concentrations.

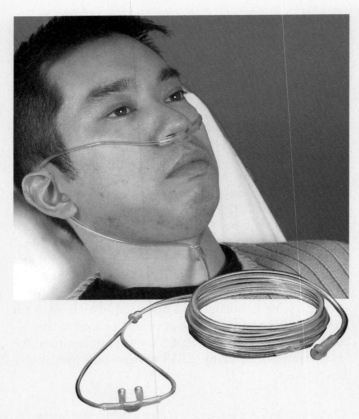

Nasal cannula properly placed on the face of the patient.

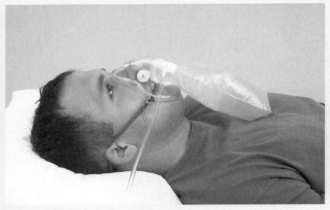

FIGURE A2.12
Example of a nonrebreather mask.

For every one liter per minute increase in oxygen flow, you deliver a 4% increase in the concentration of oxygen. At 4 LPM and above, the patient's breathing patterns may prevent the delivery of the stated percentages. At 5 LPM, rapid drying of the nasal membranes is possible. After 6 LPM, the device does not deliver any higher concentration of oxygen and may be uncomfortable for most patients.

Note: Though the Venturi mask is commonly used for COPD patients in the hospital setting, First Responders should use a nasal cannula. COPD patients often respond well to the lower concentrations of oxygen it provides. A higher concentration can be provided with a nonrebreather mask if the patient does not improve with the nasal cannula. Some patients who need a higher concentration of oxygen from the nonrebreather mask cannot tolerate a mask on the face. In that case, use a nasal cannula set to a higher flow, but keep in mind that a flow rate of 6 LPM may be uncomfortable for the patient. Follow your local guidelines.

A **nonrebreather mask** is used to deliver high concentrations of oxygen. Inflate the reservoir bag before placing the mask on the patient's face (Figure A2.12). This is done by using your finger to cover the one-way valve inside the mask between the mask and the reservoir. Care must be taken to ensure a proper seal with the patient's face. The reservoir must not deflate by more than one-third when the patient takes his deepest inspiration. You can maintain the volume in the bag by adjusting the oxygen flow. The patient's exhaled air does not return to the reservoir; instead, it is vented through the one-way flaps or portholes on the mask. The minimum flow rate when using this mask is 8 LPM, but a higher flow (12–15 LPM) may be required.

ADMINISTERING OXYGEN

Scans A2-1 and A2-2 will take you step by step through the process of preparing the oxygen delivery system, administering oxygen, and discontinuing the administration of oxygen.

Administration of Oxygen to a Nonbreathing Patient

The EMS-approved *pocket face mask* with oxygen inlet and your own breath can be combined to deliver oxygen to a nonbreathing patient. The BVM used alone or with 100% oxygen under pressure and the flow-restricted, oxygen-powered ventilation device (FROPVD) with 100% oxygen under pressure can be used in ventilating the nonbreathing patient. The flow restricted, oxygen-powered ventilation device is considered an EMT-level device. You may receive training with this device so that you can assist EMTs.

Note: When using these devices, an oropharyngeal airway should be inserted.

Warning: BVM and FROPVD devices are not recommended when performing one-rescuer CPR. The preferred device for one-rescuer CPR is a pocket mask with supplemental oxygen.

Preparing the Oxygen Delivery System

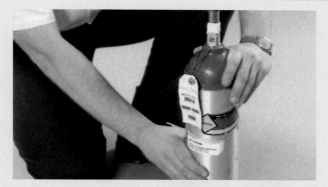

1. Select desired cylinder and check label for "Oxygen USP."

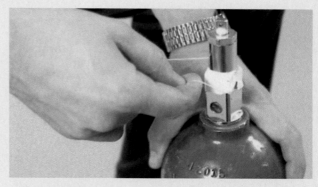

2. Remove the plastic wrapper or cap protecting the cylinder outlet.

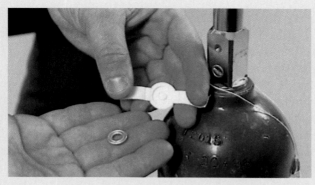

3. Keep the plastic washer that is used in some setups.

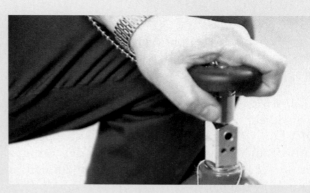

4. "Crack" the main valve for one second.

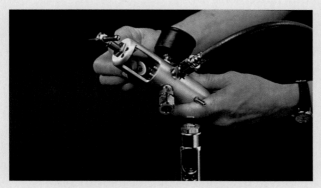

5. Place cylinder valve gasket on regulator oxygen port.

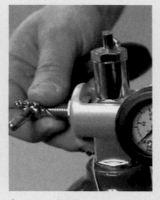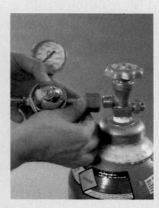

6. Align PINs or thread by hand and . . .

continued...

BVM Ventilator and Oxygen Most BVMs are capable of accepting supplemental oxygen. When available attach it to an oxygen source and adjust the flow to no less than 15 LPM. Many BVMs have an oxygen reservoir (long tube or bag) to increase the oxygen concentration delivered to the patient. Used without a reservoir, it will deliver approximately 50% oxygen. Used with a reservoir, it will deliver nearly 100% oxygen. Maintain an open airway, a tight mask-to-face seal, squeeze the bag to deliver oxygen, and release the bag to allow for a passive expiration. There is no need to remove the mask when the patient exhales.

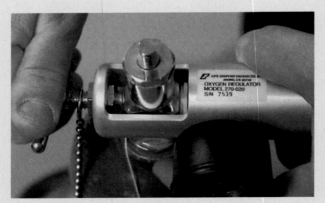

7. Tighten T-screw for PIN index.

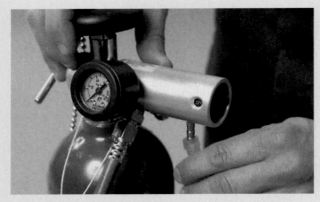

8. Attach tubing and delivery device.

This device can also be used to assist the breathing efforts of a patient who has failing respirations (as in a drug overdose).

Flow-Restricted, Oxygen-Powered Ventilation Device A flow-restricted, oxygen-powered ventilation (FROPVD) device delivers oxygen through a regulator from a pressurized cylinder. By depressing a trigger on the device, the First Responder can deliver ventilations to the patient.

Standard features of this device include:

- Peak flow rate of 100% oxygen delivered at up to 40 LPM.
- Inspiratory pressure relief valve that opens at approximately 60 cm of water pressure.
- Audible alarm that sounds when the relief valve is activated.
- Rugged design and construction.
- Trigger that enables the rescuer to use both hands to maintain a mask seal while activating the device.
- Easy and effective operation during both usual and extreme environmental conditions.

To operate the flow-restricted, oxygen-powered ventilation device, follow the same procedures for placing and sealing the mask as you would for the BVM. Then press the trigger to deliver oxygen until the chest rises and repeat every five seconds. Release the trigger after the chest inflates and allow for passive exhalation. If the chest does not rise, reposition the head or reopen the airway, check for obstructions, reposition the mask, check for a seal, and try again. If the chest still does not rise, consider an alternative ventilation device or procedure.

Monitor your patient carefully when using a flow-restricted, oxygen-powered ventilation device. High pressure caused by the device can force air into the esophagus and fill the stomach. Air distends the stomach, which presses into the lung cavity and reduces expansion of the lungs. To avoid or correct this problem, carefully maintain and monitor airway, mask-to-face seal, and chest rise. Do not continue to provide ventilations after chest rise; allow passive exhalation and reventilate.

If you suspect neck injury, have an assistant stabilize the patient's head or use your knees to prevent head movement. Bring the jaw to the mask without tilting the head or neck and trigger the mask to ventilate the patient.

Warning: The flow-restricted, oxygen-powered ventilation device should be used only on adults.

GENERAL GUIDELINES FOR OXYGEN DOSAGES

The following dosages of oxygen are recommended according to the nature of the patient's problem. The standing orders for oxygen vary slightly in different EMS systems. Follow your local protocols.

Note: In the following scenarios, when the nonrebreather mask is recommended and you only have a nasal cannula or the patient will not tolerate the mask, provide oxygen by cannula at a rate of 6 LPM.

Trauma

Provide oxygen by nonrebreather at 12–15 LPM to deliver 80% to 90% concentration (not necessary for minor scratches, scrapes and cuts, minor extremity injuries [finger or toe], strains, and sprains).

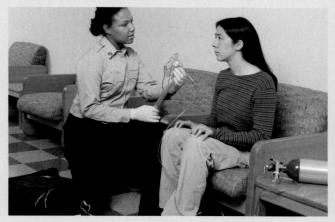

1. Explain the need for oxygen therapy.

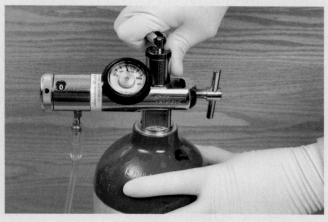

2. Open the main valve.

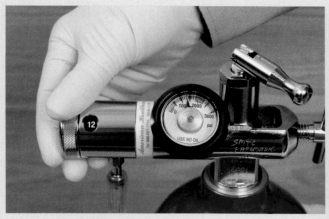

3. Adjust flowmeter.

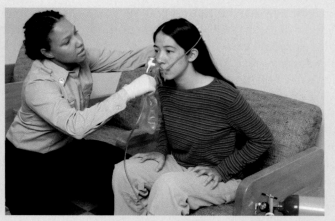

4. Position the oxygen delivery device.

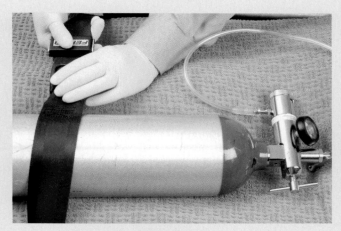

5. Secure the cylinder during transfer.

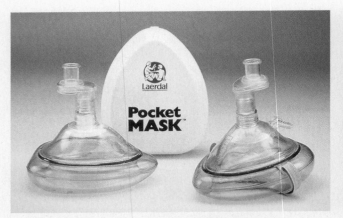

A. One mask without and one with an oxygen inlet.

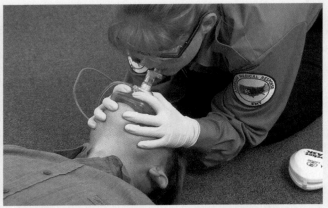

B. Rescuer delivering her own breath through the mask's chimney and oxygen through the inlet.

Childbirth

Provide oxygen by nonrebreather at 12–15 LPM to deliver 80% to 90% concentration for the mother with predelivery bleeding, excessive post-delivery bleeding, breech birth, miscarriage or abortion with excessive bleeding.

For the newborn, provide oxygen into a tent placed over the infant's head and shoulders or by mask and blow-by method to premature infants, difficult breech births, infants with bleeding from the umbilical cord, weak infants, or those who have a lasting blue color (cyanosis) on other than hands and feet.

Environmental Emergencies

Provide oxygen by nonrebreather at 12–15 LPM to deliver 80% to 90% concentration for the following:

- Allergy (anaphylactic) shock.
- Burns.
- Drug overdose.
- Near-drowning.
- Poisoning.
- Scuba incidents.

If the patient is not breathing, provide oxygen through the pocket face mask with oxygen inlet while performing mouth-to-mask ventilations or by BVM attached to an oxygen cylinder. Use a reservoir with the BVM to provide nearly 100% oxygen concentration.

Medical Emergencies

Provide oxygen by nonrebreather at 12–15 LPM to deliver 80% to 90% concentration for the following:

- Chest pain.
- Respiratory disorders and distress or trouble breathing.
- Diabetic emergencies.
- Patients recovering from seizure.
- Abdominal pain or distress.

If the patient is not breathing, provide oxygen through the pocket face mask with oxygen inlet (Figure A2.13) while performing mouth-to-mask ventilations or by BVM attached to an oxygen cylinder (Figure A2.14). Use a reservoir with the BVM to provide nearly 100% oxygen concentration.

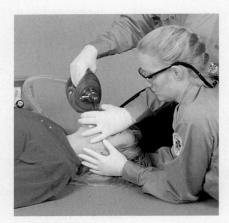

Appendix 3

Pharmacology

INTRODUCTION

Note: This appendix is designed to aid First Responders who are being trained to assist patients in taking specific prescribed medications. This training is meant to be a part of a formal training program that is under the guidance and supervision of a Medical Director. Any provider level in the EMS system that gives or assists patients in taking their own prescribed medications must follow either specific written protocols or oral medical direction. First Responders must not attempt to give any medication without medical direction.

Pharmacology is the study of drugs, their origins, nature, chemistry, effects, and use. First Responders will assess and care for many patients whose histories include the medications they take, and whose problems may be caused by the effects of taking or of not taking those medications properly. This appendix lists and describes the few medications that First Responders may be carrying and the few prescribed medications that you may assist a patient in taking. It also discusses how to give or assist the patient in taking the medications and the effects of these medications on the patients.

Remember: You may only give or assist in giving certain medications under the supervision of medical direction.

MEDICATIONS

There are typically six medications that EMTs and First Responders may be trained to use in the field. Three of the medications are used so commonly—and may be carried by First Responders—that we often do not even consider them medications. They are oxygen, activated charcoal, and oral glucose. Many First Responders are allowed by their EMS medical director to administer these medications under specific conditions and circumstances. Activated charcoal and oral glucose are sold over the counter in most pharmacies and are found in many households.

The other medications described in this appendix must be prescribed by a physician and are usually carried by the patient. They are prescribed inhalers, nitroglycerin, epinephrine, and special transdermal patches sometimes called "transdermal infusion systems." Depending on the specific EMS system, First Responders may be able to assist a patient in taking any one of these medications with the approval of medical direction and under specific conditions and circumstances.

SIDE EFFECTS, INDICATIONS, AND CONTRAINDICATIONS

For every medication there is a desired action. In addition, there are side effects, indications, and contraindications. After a patient has taken any medication, you must monitor him to see how the drug is affecting him. If taken properly, medications will usually ease the ill effects of the medical condition. But if the medications are expired or the patient's condition is beyond the help of the drug, the medication will be ineffective.

Medications sometimes have side effects. A **side effect** is any unwanted action or reaction of the drug other than the desired effect. Some side effects are expected and predictable. Nitroglycerin will dilate vessels, not just in the heart, but also throughout the body. It will cause a drop in blood pressure as the vascular system enlarges, and it will cause a headache as the vessels in the brain expand. You must anticipate side effects and document them when they occur, especially before administering a second dose.

For each drug, there are **indications** for its use. These indications are specific signs or conditions for which it is appropriate to use the drug. For example, nitroglycerin is indicated for patients experiencing cardiac chest pain.

Also, there are **contraindications** for each drug's use. These contraindications are specific signs or conditions for which it is not appropriate to use the drug. For example, giving nitroglycerin is contraindicated in patients experiencing cardiac chest pain and who have a systolic blood pressure below 100. Since nitroglycerin reduces blood pressure, it is possible to cause the blood pressure to drop too low if it is not above 100 systolic before taking the dose.

MEDICATIONS CARRIED ON THE FIRST RESPONDER UNIT

Activated Charcoal (Scan A3-1)

Activated charcoal is not the kind of charcoal you find in the barbecue grill. It is a *slurry*, which is a powder prepared from charred wood and usually premixed with water for use in the prehospital emergency situation. (Some brands require you to add the water.) Activated charcoal is administered to patients who have ingested a poison or who took an overdose of oral drugs or medications. When the patient drinks the activated charcoal slurry, it absorbs some of the poisonous substance and also helps prevent the poison or drug from being absorbed by the body.

Oral Glucose (Scan A3-2)

Glucose is a simple sugar, which is found in foods such as fruit, and is normally present in the blood. It is our chief source of energy and an all-purpose fuel for the body and brain. The brain is very sensitive to low levels of glucose and functions poorly without it. A patient with low glucose levels will have an altered mental status.

Glucose levels can be raised by giving oral glucose, a form of glucose that comes in a gel or chewable tablet and is packaged in different-sized tubes like toothpaste and in plain and flavored tablets. It is indicated for patients with an altered mental status and a history of diabetes. It is taken orally.

Glucose tablets may be colored. If the patient reports having asthma or an allergy to aspirin, note if the tablet is made with FD&C Yellow Dye No. 5. This dye causes the same reaction as aspirin in patients who have allergies to aspirin. It also is believed to set off bronchospasms in some asthma patients.

To assist in the administration of oral glucose, apply some of the gel to a tongue depressor and spread it between the patient's cheek and gum. Continue to apply small doses until the tube is empty. This gum area is rich in blood vessels, which quickly absorb the glucose and carry it through the bloodstream to the brain. Once the level of glucose is elevated in the brain, the patient's condition usually begins to improve.

For tablets, the typical strength is 5.0 grams of D-Glucose (Dextrose). This form of glucose passes through the mucosa (lining) of the mouth, esophagus, and stomach so that no special digestion is needed. It does not have to enter the small intestine to be absorbed. The manufacturer's recommended dosage is three tablets or 15.0 grams of D-Glucose. **DO NOT** try to administer glucose tablets to anyone who is unresponsive and unable to manage his own airway. The patient should respond quickly to the tablets, with profuse sweating becoming controlled and feelings of faintness quickly corrected. Fatigue may remain for various periods of time depending on the patient and how rapidly the blood glucose level fell during the hypoglycemic (low blood sugar) episode. Some patients have feelings of uneasiness that remain for up to one-half hour. Most are able to eat additional foods that help with uneasy feelings. However, do not allow someone to ingest foods if he has been given glucose and reports nausea. The nausea should subside shortly and if the patient requests food and remains alert, most protocols for hypoglycemic events allow it.

Oxygen (Figure A3.1)

Pure oxygen is used as a drug to treat patients who have low oxygen levels in their blood because of medical or traumatic conditions. Oxygen and oxygen therapy is briefly described in Appendix 2. If your First Responder unit carries oxygen and oxygen delivery adjuncts, you must participate in a training program to learn how and when to use them properly. Be sure to follow your jurisdiction's guidelines, protocols, and medical direction.

PRESCRIBED MEDICATIONS

Prescribed Inhalers (Scan A3-3)

Many patients have chronic respiratory diseases—such as asthma, emphysema, or bronchitis—that cause

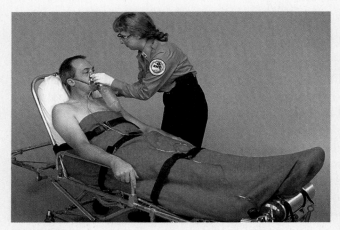

FIGURE A3.1
Oxygen is a powerful drug.

Activated Charcoal

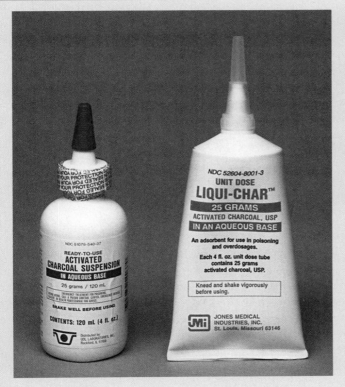

MEDICATION NAME
1. Generic: activated charcoal.
2. Trade: SuperChar, InstaChar, Actidose, Liqui-Char, and others.

INDICATIONS
Poisoning by mouth.

CONTRAINDICATIONS
1. Altered mental status.
2. Ingestion of acids or alkalis.
3. Unable to swallow.

MEDICATION FORM
1. Premixed in water, frequently available in plastic bottle containing 12.5 grams of activated charcoal.
2. Powder—should be avoided in field.

DOSAGE
1. Adults and children: 1 gram activated charcoal/kg of body weight.
2. Usual adult dose: 25–50 grams.
3. Usual pediatric dose: 12.5–25 grams.

STEPS FOR ASSISTING PATIENT
1. Consult medical direction.
2. Shake container vigorously.
3. Since medication looks like mud, patient may need to be persuaded to drink it. Providing a covered container and a straw will prevent the patient from seeing the medication and so may improve patient compliance.
4. If patient does not drink the medication right away, the charcoal will settle. Shake or stir it again before administering.
5. Record the name, dose, route, and time of administration of the medication.

ACTIONS
1. Activated charcoal binds to certain poisons and prevents them from being absorbed into the body.
2. Not all brands of activated charcoal are the same. Some bind much more than others. So consult medical direction about the brand to use.

SIDE EFFECTS
1. Black stools.
2. Some patients, particularly those who have ingested poisons that cause nausea, may vomit. If patient vomits, repeat the dose once.

REASSESSMENT STRATEGIES
Be prepared for the patient to vomit or further deteriorate. If the patient worsens, provide oxygen as you have been trained to do.

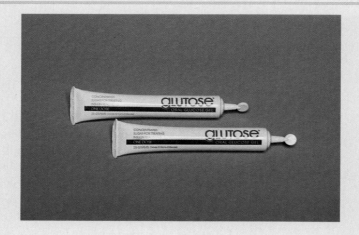

MEDICATION NAME

1. Generic: Glucose, oral.
2. Trade: Glutose, Insta-glucose, BD Glucose Tablets.

INDICATIONS

1. Patients with altered mental status with a known history of diabetes mellitus.
2. Patient has taken insulin but no food recently and may have been very physically active.

CONTRAINDICATIONS

1. Loss of awareness, unresponsiveness.
2. Known diabetic who has not taken insulin for days.
3. Unable to swallow.

MEDICATION FORM

Gel, in toothpaste-type tubes; chewable tablets.

DOSAGE

One tube; three 5.0 gram chewable tablets. This dose can be used for both adults and children.

STEPS FOR ASSISTING PATIENT

1. Ensure signs and symptoms of altered mental status with a known history of diabetes.

2. Ensure patient is alert.
3. Administer glucose.
   a. Place on tongue depressor between cheek and gum.
   b. Self-administered between cheek and gum.
OR –
   c. Have patient chew one to three tablets.
4. Perform ongoing assessment.

ACTIONS

Increases blood sugar.

SIDE EFFECTS

None when given properly. May be aspirated by the patient without a gag reflex.

REASSESSMENT STRATEGIES

If patient experiences an altered mental status or has seizures, remove tongue depressor from mouth. Provide oxygen as you have been trained to do.

SCAN A3-3 Prescribed Inhaler

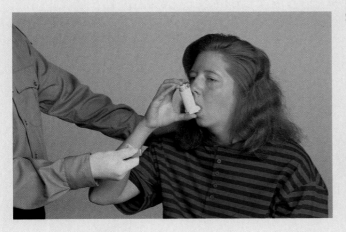

MEDICATION NAME
1. Generic: albuterol, ipratropium, metaproterenol.
2. Trade: Proventil, Ventolin, Atrovent, Alupent, Metaprel.

INDICATIONS
Meets all of the following criteria:
1. Patient exhibits signs and symptoms of respiratory emergency.
2. Patient has physician-prescribed handheld inhaler.
3. Medical direction gives FR specific authorization to use.

CONTRAINDICATIONS
1. Patient is unable to use device (for example, not alert).
2. Inhaler is not prescribed for patient.
3. No permission has been given by medical direction.
4. Patient has already taken maximum prescribed dose prior to rescuer's arrival.

MEDICATION FORM
Handheld metered-dose inhaler

DOSAGE
Number of inhalations based on medical direction's order or physician's order

STEPS FOR ASSISTING PATIENT
1. Obtain order from medical direction either on-line or off-line.
2. Ensure right patient, right medication, right dose, right route, and patient alert enough to use inhaler.
3. Check expiration date of inhaler.
4. Check if patient has already taken any doses.
5. Ensure inhaler is at room temperature or warmer.
6. Shake inhaler vigorously several times.
7. Have patient exhale deeply.
8. Have patient put lips around the opening of the inhaler.
9. Have patient depress the handheld inhaler when beginning to inhale deeply.
10. Instruct patient to hold breath for as long as is comfortable so that medication can be absorbed.
11. Allow patient to breathe a few times and repeat second dose if so ordered by medical direction.
12. If patient has a spacer device for use with the inhaler (device for attachment between inhaler and patient to allow for more effective use of medication), it should be used.
13. Provide oxygen as trained to do.

ACTIONS
Beta agonist bronchodilator dilates bronchioles, reducing airway resistance.

SIDE EFFECTS
1. Increased pulse rate.
2. Tremors.
3. Nervousness.

REASSESSMENT STRATEGIES
1. Take vital signs.
2. Provide oxygen as trained to do.
3. Perform focused reassessment of chest and respiratory function.
4. Observe for deterioration of patient. If breathing becomes inadequate, provide artificial respirations.

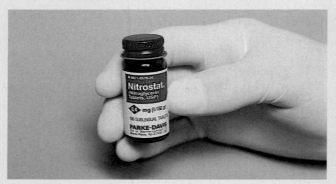

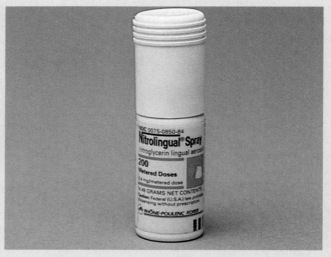

MEDICATION NAME

1. Generic: nitroglycerin.
2. Trade: Nitrostat, NitroTab.

INDICATIONS

All of the following conditions must be met:

1. Patient complains of chest pain.
2. Patient has a history of cardiac problems.
3. Patient's physician has prescribed nitroglycerin.
4. Systolic blood pressure is greater than 100 systolic.
5. Medical direction authorizes administration of the medication.

CONTRAINDICATIONS

1. Patient has hypotension (systolic blood pressure below 100).
2. Patient has a head injury.
3. Patient is an infant or a child.
4. Patient has already taken the maximum prescribed dose.

MEDICATION FORM

Tablet, sublingual (under-the-tongue); or sublingual spray.

DOSAGE

One dose, repeat in 3 to 5 minutes. If no relief, systolic blood pressure remains above 100, and if authorized by medical direction, up to a maximum of three doses. Spray is typically prescribed for one metered spray followed by a second in 15 minutes.

STEPS FOR ASSISTING PATIENT

1. Perform focused assessment for cardiac patient.
2. Take blood pressure. (Systolic pressure must be above 100.)
3. Contact medical direction if no standing orders.

4. Ensure right medication, right patient, right dose, right route. Check expiration date.
5. Ensure patient is alert.
6. Question patient on last dose taken and effects. Ensure understanding of route of administration.
7. Ask patient to lift tongue and place tablet or spray dose on or under tongue (while you are wearing gloves) or have patient place tablet or spray under tongue.
8. Have patient keep mouth closed with tablet under tongue (without swallowing) until dissolved and absorbed.
9. Recheck blood pressure within two minutes.
10. Record administration, route, and time.
11. Perform reassessment.

ACTIONS

1. Relaxes blood vessels.
2. Decreases workload of heart.

SIDE EFFECTS

1. Hypotension (lowers blood pressure).
2. Headache.
3. Pulse rate changes.

REASSESSMENT STRATEGIES

1. Monitor blood pressure.
2. Ask patient about effect on pain relief.
3. Seek medical direction before re-administering.
4. Record assessments.
5. Provide oxygen as trained to do.

the airway passages in the lungs to narrow, or become constricted. Such patients usually carry a device called a **metered dose inhaler.** It typically contains medication called a *bronchodilator.* This medication enlarges, or dilates, the airway passages so the patient can breathe easier. The inhaler device holds the medication in an aerosol form, which can be sprayed into the mouth and inhaled. You must have medical direction to help a patient self-administer this medication. You must also make sure that this medication belongs to the patient and was not lent to him by a well-meaning family member or friend with a similar problem. Also, checking for an expiration date is important since expired medication is less effective.

Warning: Many inhalers contain medications known as beta adrenergic bronchodilators. An example is the commonly prescribed medication albuterol sulfate as found in Proventil and other prescribed bronchodilator inhalants. These compounds affect blood pressure and heart function.

It is essential that you do not let onlookers volunteer medications for your patients and that you do not let couples share a single prescription. Patients should only take their own medications as directed by their physicians. They should not mix over the counter (OTC) drugs in with prescribed medications unless told to do so by their physician, and they should not be taking natural supplements, such as herbal medications, without consent of their physician.

Nitroglycerin (Scan A3-4)

Nitroglycerin is a chemical that is well known as an explosive, but it also has medical uses. It dilates blood vessels and relieves certain types of pain, particularly the type caused by a heart condition called *angina pectoris.* Patients who have heart conditions that cause re-curring chest pain or who have a history of heart attack may have a prescription for nitroglycerin. Nitroglycerin dilates, or enlarges, the constricted vessels in the heart muscle so it can receive blood and oxygen, which help ease the pain.

Often, First Responders will arrive at the scene to find out during the focused assessment that the patient with chest pain has taken a dose of nitroglycerin. Just as often, the patient with chest pain is carrying the medication and has not thought to take it. Patients can usually take up to three tablets—one every five minutes—over a 15-minute period. You will need to consult medical direction to help administer nitroglycerin or to get permission to give more after the patient has taken three doses. As with the inhaler, be sure to check that the nitroglycerin is actually the patient's medication and that it has not reached the expiration date.

The patient may have a bottle of nitroglycerin sublingual spray (e.g., Nitrolingual Pumspray). At the onset of suspected cardiac chest pain, one to two metered sprays may be administered onto or under the tongue within 15 minutes.

The patient may have nitroglycerin transdermal patches (transdermal infusion system). These are for daily application and help prevent angina attacks, but they are not meant to relieve and correct an acute event (Figure A3.2). Contact dispatch and arrange for ALS transport.

Sometimes the medication may not be effective because the patient has not stored it properly or it has expired. Even if the patient's pain diminishes, you should request an EMT response. In fact, you should *arrange for patient transport every time.* Anytime a patient complains of chest pain—whether it persists or not, whether the patient has a history of chest pain or

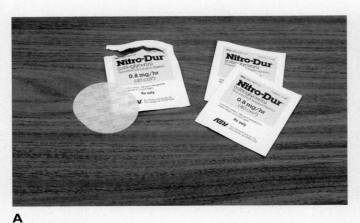

A

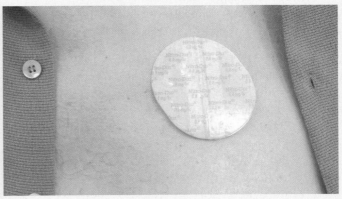

B

FIGURE A3.2
Transdermal nitroglycerine patches may be found applied to the patient's chest, upper arm (usually medially), or upper back.

SCAN A3-5 Epinephrine Auto-Injector

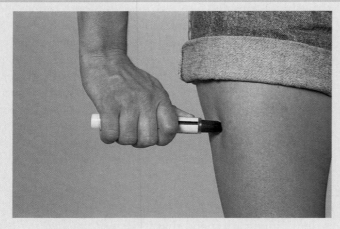

MEDICATION NAME
1. Generic: epinephrine.
2. Trade: Adrenalin, Epi-Pen.

INDICATIONS
Must meet the following three criteria:
1. Patient exhibits signs of a severe allergic reaction, including either respiratory distress or shock.
2. Medication is prescribed for this patient by a physician.
3. Medical direction authorizes use for this patient.

CONTRAINDICATIONS
No contraindications when used in a life-threatening situation.

MEDICATION FORM
Liquid administered by an auto-injector—an automatically injectable needle-and-syringe system.

DOSAGE
Adults—One adult auto-injector (0.3 mg).
Infant and child—One infant/child auto-injector (0.15 mg).

STEPS FOR ASSISTING PATIENT
1. Obtain patient's prescribed auto-injector. Ensure:
   a. Prescription is written for the patient who is experiencing the severe allergic reaction.
   b. Medication is not discolored (if visible).
2. Obtain order from medical direction, either on-line or off-line.
3. Remove cap from auto-injector.
4. Place tip of auto-injector against patient's thigh.
   a. Lateral portion of the thigh.
   b. Midway between waist and knee.
5. Push the injector firmly against the thigh until the injector activates.
6. Hold the injector in place until the medication is injected (at least 10 seconds).
7. Record activity and time.
8. Dispose of injector in biohazard container.

ACTIONS
1. Dilates the bronchioles.
2. Constricts blood vessels.

SIDE EFFECTS
1. Increased heart rate.
2. Pallor.
3. Dizziness.
4. Chest pain.
5. Headache.
6. Nausea.
7. Vomiting.
8. Excitability, anxiety.

REASSESSMENT STRATEGIES
1. Transport.
2. Continue focused assessment of airway, breathing, and circulatory status. If patient's condition continues to worsen (decreasing mental status, increasing breathing difficulty, decreasing blood pressure):
   a. Obtain medical direction for an additional dose of epinephrine.
   b. Provide care for shock, including administration of oxygen as per local protocols.
   c. Prepare to initiate basic life support (CPR, AED).
3. If patient's condition improves, provide supportive care:
   a. Continue oxygen.
   b. Provide care for shock.

not—arrange for immediate transport to a medical facility.

Epinephrine Auto-Injectors (Scan A3-5)

Many people have allergies and will react severely to certain foods, medicines, or the poisons of insect stings or snakebites. Those reactions may be life-threatening when they cause the airway to become swollen and blood vessels to dilate. Epinephrine is a medication that can reverse those reactions. It dilates the air passages so breathing becomes easier, and it constricts the enlarged blood vessels. Reactions to allergies can have a very sudden onset, and any reaction that causes breathing and circulation problems must be recognized and treated quickly. The patient must take his prescribed epinephrine immediately.

Those patients who are aware of their allergies and expect severe reactions generally carry a prescription with them in a device called an **auto-injector.** This is a syringe with a spring-loaded needle that will release and inject epinephrine into a muscle when the patient presses it against his skin (usually in the thigh). If you need to assist the patient in taking epinephrine, first check to see if the injector is prescribed for that patient and get permission from medical direction. Also, check the expiration date.

Remember: An expired medication will be ineffective, but an allergic reaction may not be the reason for the patient's problem. Even when a patient reports that he feels better, he must be transported to a hospital as soon as possible by EMTs.

Note: In recent years the use of aspirin for the treatment of suspected heart attack has become commonplace in most hospitals and EMS systems. In fact, several pharmaceutical companies have created television and radio commercials encouraging the use of aspirin for this purpose. As a First Responder, you may encounter patients who have recently taken aspirin or who may want to take some while in your care. You must follow your local protocols when assisting any patient with the administration of medication.

RULES TO FOLLOW WHEN ADMINISTERING MEDICATIONS

Before you give any of the three medications you may carry (activated charcoal, oral glucose, or oxygen), or before you assist a patient in taking any of the three prescribed medications (bronchodilator, nitroglycerin, or epinephrine), there are a few more things you need to know.

You will check the four "rights" that are rules for giving any medication. Often you will have to rely on the patient's word. Ask the following questions:

- *Right patient?* Is this the right patient for this medication? (Read aloud the name written on the medication bottle: "Is your name Henry Smith?" If the patient does not have a labeled box or bottle, simply ask if this is his own medication. If he says yes, you may believe him.)
- *Right medication?* Is this the right medication for this patient? (The patient is having chest pain but hands you a bottle of penicillin; or the patient has strep throat but hands you a bottle of nitroglycerin.)
- *Right dose?* Is this the right dose for this patient? (The dosage is usually written on the label, but the patient does not always carry the original box or bottle the medication came in.)
- *Right route?* Is this the right route for taking the medication? (Different types of medications, such as tablets, powders, sprays, gels, slurries, and pastes are given by different routes—swallowed by mouth, inhaled by mouth, dissolved under the tongue, injected into or absorbed through the skin.)

ROUTES FOR ADMINISTERING MEDICATIONS

The way a patient takes a medication has an effect on how quickly the medication enters the bloodstream and begins to relieve the medical condition. Medications are administered by the following routes:

- *Oral* or swallowed, usually in some solid form (a tablet or pill), or in some liquid form (powder dissolved in or mixed with a liquid such as the activated charcoal slurry).
- *Intramuscular,* or injected into a muscle, like the epinephrine auto-injector.
- *Sublingual,* or dissolved under the tongue, like the nitroglycerin tablets.
- *Inhaled,* or breathed into the lungs, from an inhaler or oxygen delivery device such as the medication given for chronic respiratory problems or the oxygen gas given for respiratory distress and for most medical and trauma patients.
- *Endotracheal,* or sprayed into a tube inserted into the trachea (windpipe), so it can more directly reach the lungs and be absorbed quickly. (First Responders will not administer medication in this form.)
- *Transdermal patches* or *transdermal infusion systems,* affixed to the skin by an adhesive backing on one

side of the patch. Another chemical is mixed in with the medication, usually a form of alcohol that will carry the medication or drug through the patient's skin into the blood stream. These patches are slow to react and are not meant for acute attacks such as the onset of chest pain. They are meant to stay in place for one to three days or longer, depending on the type of medication. Be careful not to remove a patch, and do not leave a patch at the scene. Some can stop children from breathing. Some patches contain high enough

doses to be poisons if ingested by children and animals.

You can see there is a lot to know and understand about medications. Once you do, you will become more confident in giving the ones that you carry and the prescribed ones you can assist patients in taking. Remember, you may only administer or assist with specific medications and then only with medical direction.

Appendix 4

Swimming and Diving Incidents

Note: The amount of time spent on this subject in your First Responder course will depend upon the area in which you live and the length of your course. There are very few new procedures to learn about caring for patients who have had swimming or diving emergencies. Of key importance to you will be learning the types of injuries associated with water incidents and knowing the care skills used when the patient is a near-drowning victim.

Warning: Do not attempt a water rescue unless you have been trained to do so, you are a good swimmer, and others are on hand to help. Never attempt a water rescue by yourself. A **personal flotation device (PFD)** should be worn by all those involved in a water rescue. Except for shallow pools and open, shallow waters with uniform bottoms, the problems faced in water rescue are too great and too dangerous for the poor swimmer or untrained person to attempt. If not being able to help bothers you, take a course in water safety and rescue. Otherwise, you will probably become a victim yourself, rather than the person who rescues and provides care.

Note: Mouth-to-mask techniques and CPR are not practical while the patient is in the water. Follow your EMS system guidelines.

WATER-RELATED INCIDENTS

Most people, when they think of water-related incidents, tend to think only of drowning. There is no doubt that drowning must be the number one consideration, even when the first problem faced by a person in the water is an injury or a medical emergency.

Injuries occur on, in, and near the water. Boating, water-skiing, and diving incidents produce airway obstructions, fractures, bleeding, and soft-tissue injuries. Other types of incidents, such as falls from bridges and motor-vehicle collisions, also may involve the water. In these cases, the victims suffer injuries normally associated with the underlying mechanism of injury plus the effects of the water hazard (drowning,

hypothermia, delayed care because of complicated rescue, and so on).

Sometimes, the mishap or drowning may have been caused by a medical emergency that took place while the patient was in the water or on a boat. Knowing how the incident occurred may give you clues to detecting the medical emergency. As with all aspects of First Responder care, consider the mechanism of injury or nature of illness and perform a thorough patient assessment. They may be critical in deciding the procedures to be followed when caring for a patient.

Learn to associate the problems of drowning with scenes other than swimming pools and beaches. Remember, bathtub drownings do occur. Only a few inches of water are needed for an adult to drown. Even less is required for an infant.

Note: The U.S. Government Consumer Product Safety Division reports that over 275 children have drowned in five gallon buckets since 1984.

As a First Responder, take particular care to look for the following when your patient is the victim of a water-related mishap:

- *Airway obstruction*—This may be from water, foreign matter in the airway, or a swollen airway (often seen if the neck is injured in a dive). Spasms along the airway are common in cases of near-drowning.
- *Cardiac arrest*—This is usually related to respiratory arrest.
- *Signs of heart attack*—Through overexertion, the patient may have greater problems than the obvious near-drowning. Often, inexperienced rescuers are fooled into thinking that chest pains reported by the patient are due to muscle cramps produced during swimming or the panic of a near-drowning situation.
- *Injuries to the head and neck*—These are to be expected in boating, water-skiing, and diving incidents, but they also occur in cases of near-drowning.

- *Internal injuries*—While doing the patient assessment, be on the alert for suspected fractures or dislocations, soft-tissue injuries, and internal bleeding. The fact that the patient is suffering from internal bleeding is often missed during the first stages of care because of the concern for other problems associated with near-drowning. Constantly monitor patients for the signs and symptoms of shock.

- *Hypothermia*—The water does not have to be very cold and the length of stay in the water does not have to be very long for hypothermia to occur.

REACHING THE VICTIM

The U.S. Coast Guard, the American Red Cross, and the YMCA offer water safety and rescue courses. Unless you are a good swimmer and have been trained in water rescue, do not go into the water to save someone.

Reach, Throw, Then Go

Reach   If the patient is close to shore or poolside, attempt to reach and pull the patient from the water. If unable to reach the victim with your hand, attempt to use a branch, a fishing pole, an oar, a stick, or other such object. A towel, a shirt, or an article of your own clothing may work as well. In cases where there is no object near at hand or conditions are such that you may only have one opportunity to grab the person (for example, strong currents), lie down flat on your stomach and extend your arm or leg (not recommended for the nonswimmer). In all cases, make sure that your position is secure and that you will not be pulled into the water. This is critical if you are extending an arm or leg to the person. If the victim is some distance away from the shore or edge, attempt to throw something to him. In this case, it is best to use a rope (line).

Throw   If the person is alert but too far away to be pulled from the water, then you must carefully throw an object that will float. A personal flotation device (PFD), life jacket, or ring buoy (life preserver) is ideal, but these objects may not be at the scene. If that is the case, then the best course of action is to throw anything that will float and to do this as soon as possible (Figure A4.1). Objects you might use include inflated automobile tubes, foam cushions, plastic jugs, logs, boards, plastic picnic containers, surfboards, pieces of wood, large balls, and plastic toys. Two empty, capped plastic milk jugs can keep an adult afloat for hours. It is best to tie rope to the objects so

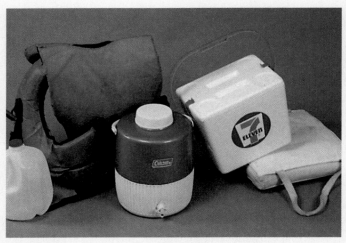

FIGURE A4.1
Throw the patient anything that will float.

that they can be retrieved if they do not land near the patient. You may have to add some water to lightweight plastic jugs so that you can throw them the required distance.

Once you are sure that the person has a flotation device or floating object to hold on to, try to find a way to tow the patient to shore. Throw the patient a line or another flotation device attached to a line. Make sure that your own position is a safe one. If conditions are safe and you are a strong swimmer, wade no deeper than your waist, if you must reduce the distance for throwing the line.

Then Go   You may find that the near-drowning victim is too far from shore to allow for throwing and towing, or the victim may be unresponsive and unable to react to your efforts. In such cases, if there is a boat at the scene, you may be able to take the boat to the patient. Do not go to the patient if you cannot swim. Even if you are a swimmer, you must wear a personal flotation device while you are in the boat. In cases where the patient is alert, try to have the patient grab an oar or the rear of the boat. Take great care in helping the person into the boat. This is a very tricky process in a canoe. Should the canoe or boat tip over, stay with the vessel, holding onto its bottom or side. It will almost certainly stay afloat.

If you take a boat out and find that the patient is unresponsive, assume that the patient has neck or spine injury.

Again, in water-rescue situations (Figure A4.2), begin by trying to pull the patient from the water. If this cannot be done, throw objects that will float and try to tow the patient from the water. Do not try to take a boat to the victim if you cannot swim. Wear a

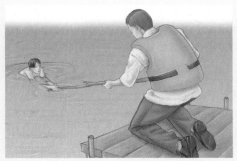

Reach

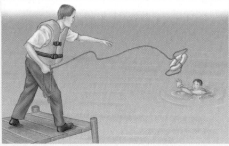

Throw

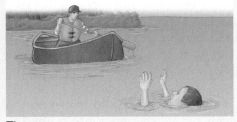

Then go

FIGURE A4.2
Pull the patient from the water, throw an object that will float, and try to tow or, if necessary and you are properly equipped and trained, go to the patient.

personal flotation device while in the boat. Unless you are a good swimmer and trained in water rescue and life-saving, do not swim to the patient. Even so, have on a personal flotation device.

CARE FOR THE PATIENT

Patient with No Neck or Spine Injuries

In all cases of shallow-water incidents, assume that the unresponsive patient has neck and spine injuries. If the patient can be removed quickly from the water using a cervical collar and spine board or if the patient is out of the water when you arrive, you should:

1. Start your initial assessment of the patient.
2. If needed, provide mouth-to-mask resuscitation as quickly as possible. Check for airway obstruction.

Note: Mouth-to-mask techniques are usually not practical when the patient is in the water, since much

of your effort will be in keeping the patient's face above the surface. It is most practical to use the mouth-to-mouth procedure, but know that this might expose you to potentially infectious body fluids. FOLLOW YOUR LOCAL EMS GUIDELINES.

3. Once the patient is out of the water, provide CPR, if needed. As in all such cases, make certain that someone has activated the EMS system.
4. If the patient is breathing and has a pulse, check for bleeding and attempt to control any serious bleeding that you find.
5. If there is breathing and a pulse, perform a patient assessment. But first cover the patient to conserve body heat. Also be sure to put something under the patient to prevent heat loss. Uncover only those areas of the patient's body involved in assessment. Care for any problems you may find. Remove wet clothing if there are no injuries that must first be stabilized.
6. If the patient can be moved, take him to a warm place. Do not allow the near-drowning patient to walk. Handle the patient gently at all times.
7. Provide care for shock and check again to make certain that the EMS system has been activated.

You may find more resistance than expected to your efforts to provide breaths to someone with water in the airway. Apply more force, if necessary, once you are certain that no foreign objects are obstructing the airway. Watch the patient's chest rise and fall. Adjust your ventilations as needed to help prevent gastric distention. Remember, you must not delay ventilating the patient.

Many times, a patient with water in the airway will also have water in the stomach. This may provide resistance to your efforts to resuscitate the patient. When this happens, you may find that some of the air from your breaths will go into the patient's stomach, even when you adjust your ventilations. Current American Heart Association and American Red Cross guidelines indicate that you should not attempt to relieve water or air from the patient's stomach (unless immediate suctioning is available) due to the risk of forcing material from the stomach to enter the patient's airway, even to the point of entering the lungs. When gastric distention occurs, reposition the airway and continue with resuscitation, making sure the breaths are slow and full.

Note: Drowning victims who are resuscitated are very likely to vomit. Rescuers should have suction ready and be prepared to clear the airway when this occurs.

Human beings have a reaction in cold water that is similar to other mammals. This reaction is called the **mammalian diving reflex.** When the face of a person or other mammal is submerged in cold water, the mammalian diving reflex slows down the body's metabolism, which results in a decrease in oxygen consumption. At the same time, the reflex causes a redistribution of blood to more vital organs—the brain, heart, and lungs. The diving reflex is more pronounced in infants and children, and they may fare better in cold-water drowning than adults. Start CPR on all drowning victims as soon as they are pulled from the water. CPR should continue while en route to the hospital. Cases have been reported in which cold-water drowning victims, especially children, were revived and fully recovered after being in the water for longer than 30 minutes. Never believe that a person has drowned; rather, consider the victim to be a *near-drowning* patient.

As a First Responder, you must be realistic when dealing with drownings. Many patients cannot be successfully resuscitated. The effects of water in the airway and the lack of oxygen to the brain may be too harsh for the body to endure. You may resuscitate some patients only to find out that they died within 48 hours due to pneumonia, lung damage, or brain damage. Even when you provide the best of care, some patients will die. However, you must give patients every opportunity for survival. You will not be able to tell which patient will survive. Provide resuscitation for all drowning victims.

Patient with Neck or Spine Injuries

Injuries to the neck (cervical spine) and the rest of the spinal column occur during many water-related incidents. In First Responder care, you will not be expected to know how to use long spine boards and other floating, rigid devices for rescue situations. This does not mean that you cannot take certain actions to protect a patient's neck and spine during both rescue and care.

If a patient is unresponsive, neck and spine injuries may not be easily detected. In such a situation, assume that the patient has them and provide care accordingly. Also assume neck and spine injuries whenever you assess a water-emergency patient and find head injuries. Learn to quickly evaluate the patient for possible neck and spine injuries. Remember, you will not have time to do a complete test for such injuries in patients who are in the water. Likewise, a complete assessment will not be possible for any patient you find in respiratory or cardiac arrest.

When a patient with possible neck and spine injuries is responsive and you are in shallow warm water, stabilize the patient until the EMS system responds with personnel trained to remove the patient from the water. Simply keep the patient floating in a face-up position while you support the back and stabilize the head and neck (Scan A4-1). However, seldom will this be the case. Too often, the water will be too cold or too deep, or there will be dangerous tides or currents. Often in those conditions, the patient will need resuscitation and will have to be removed from the water as quickly as possible. Even so, it is better to wait for trained, equipped rescue personnel to help remove a breathing patient from the water rather than risk injuring the patient's spine by doing it yourself.

Should you arrive at the scene and find the unresponsive patient has already been removed from the water, have someone activate the EMS system and begin your initial assessment. Provide life-support care as needed, using the jaw-thrust maneuver rather than the head-tilt, chin-lift maneuver. After breathing and circulation are ensured, and bleeding is cared for, perform a patient assessment, providing care as needed. Keep the patient warm and provide care for shock. Unless absolutely necessary, do not move the patient if there is any chance of neck or spine injuries.

If the patient is still in the water, do not attempt a rescue unless you are a good swimmer, are trained to do so, and have others on hand who can help you. Make certain that someone activates the EMS system. This should be done immediately. Do not wait until after the rescue is attempted. Valuable time will be lost should the rescue fail. Providing care for a possible spinal injury patient still in the water requires you to:

1. Turn the patient face up in the water. This should be done while you are in the water and wearing a personal flotation device. To turn the patient, you should:
   a. Position yourself at patient's side, as shown in Scan A4-1. Grasp the patient's arms midway between the elbow and shoulder and gently float them above the patient's head.
   b. Clasp the patient's arms firmly against his head to brace the neck and keep the head in line. Move forward in the water to bring the patient's body to the surface and in line.
   c. Rotate the patient by pushing down on the near arm and pulling the far arm toward you, making sure you brace the patient's head firmly with his arms. Do not lift the patient.

Water Rescue

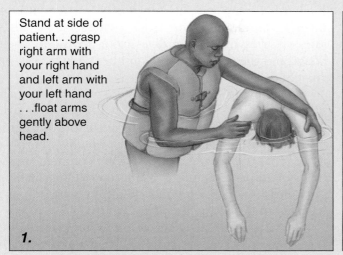

Stand at side of patient. . .grasp right arm with your right hand and left arm with your left hand . . .float arms gently above head.

1.

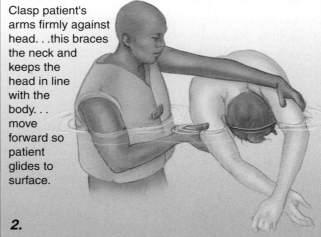

Clasp patient's arms firmly against head. . .this braces the neck and keeps the head in line with the body. . . move forward so patient glides to surface.

2.

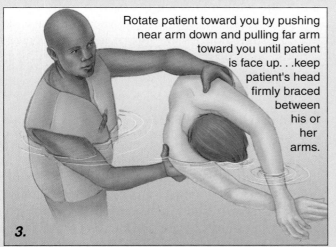

Rotate patient toward you by pushing near arm down and pulling far arm toward you until patient is face up. . .keep patient's head firmly braced between his or her arms.

3.

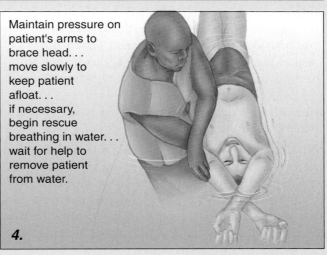

Maintain pressure on patient's arms to brace head. . . move slowly to keep patient afloat. . . if necessary, begin rescue breathing in water. . . wait for help to remove patient from water.

4.

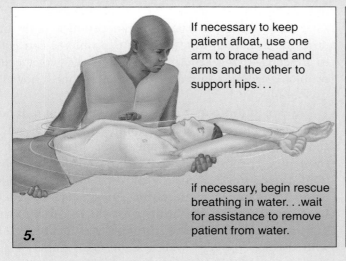

If necessary to keep patient afloat, use one arm to brace head and arms and the other to support hips. . .

if necessary, begin rescue breathing in water. . .wait for assistance to remove patient from water.

5.

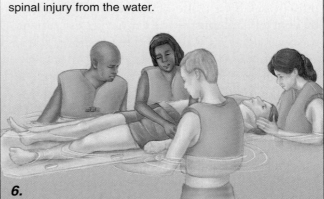

Only specially trained personnel, using a backboard and cervical collar, should remove a patient with a neck or spinal injury from the water.

6.

Adapted from American Red Cross *Swimming and Diving*.

d. Once the patient is face up, maintain pressure on the patient's arms to brace the head.

e. In shallow water, you can hold the patient's arms with one hand and support the hips with the other.

f. In deeper water, continue to move toward shallow water where you can stand or can be supported by someone else.

2. If necessary, begin your initial assessment while the patient is still in the water. Do not delay the detection of respiratory arrest.

3. If needed, provide rescue breathing as soon as possible. Use the jaw-thrust maneuver to protect the patient's neck and spine. Check for airway obstruction. CPR and mouth-to-mask resuscitation will not be effective while the patient is in the water. Give priority to removing the patient from the water.

4. If someone is there to help you, have him support the patient along the midline of the back while you provide support to the patient's head and neck. Float the patient to shore and continue to provide back and neck support as shown in Scan A4-1. Wait for trained rescue personnel equipped with a backboard and cervical collar to remove the patient from the water.

   Note: Attempt to remove the patient from the water yourself ONLY if trained rescue personnel will not arrive soon and the patient has no heartbeat. You must make every effort to maintain in-line stabilization of the patient's body. Support the patient's head and neck while those helping you lift the patient from the water.

5. Once the patient is out of the water, attempts at respiratory resuscitation can begin. Check for a pulse to see if CPR should be started. If you are by yourself and must row a cardiac-arrest patient to shore, delay CPR until you reach shore. You cannot row a boat and perform CPR. Also, CPR will be more effective on shore. In some cases, depending on the boat's stability and water conditions, you may be able to provide effective CPR in the boat until other rescuers arrive.

6. If the patient is breathing, check for and control all serious bleeding. Cover the patient to conserve body heat and perform a patient assessment, caring for any injuries you may find. Do not move the patient if there are any signs of possible neck or spine injuries.

7. Give care for shock and make sure the EMS system has been activated.

DIVING INCIDENTS

DIVING-BOARD INCIDENTS

Each year, many people are injured as they attempt dives or enter the water from diving boards. These same injuries are seen in dives from poolsides, docks, boats, and the shore. A large number of such cases involve teenagers.

Most diving-board incidents involve the head and neck. As a First Responder, you will also see injuries to the spine, hands, feet, and ribs occurring with great frequency. Any part of the body can be injured in these types of emergencies, requiring complete assessment of all patients unless you are providing life-support measures. Remember, a medical emergency may have led to the diving incident.

Once the patient is out of the water, care will be the same as for any victim of trauma. Care in the water and while removing the patient from the water is the same as for any patient who may have skull, neck, or spine injuries. Be sure to look for delayed reactions, particularly weakness, tingling sensations, or numbness in the limbs.

SCUBA-DIVING INCIDENTS

The word *scuba* is short for self-contained underwater breathing apparatus. Scuba-diving emergencies have increased with the popularity of the sport and with inexperienced divers going into the water without the benefit of proper training. There are over two million people who scuba dive for sport or as part of their industrial or military employment. This number has been increasing at a rate of over 200,000 people each year.

Scuba-diving emergencies can produce body injuries or near-drownings. Medical problems can lead to a scuba-diving emergency. However, two special problems are seen in scuba-diving incidents. They are gas bubbles in the diver's blood and the "bends."

An **air embolism,** or gas bubbles in the blood, occurs when gases leave a diver's injured lung and enter the bloodstream. This happens for many reasons, though it is most often associated with divers who hold their breath because of inadequate training, equipment failure, underwater emergency, or when trying to conserve air during a long dive. An air embolism can develop in the automobile-collision victim who is trapped below water, as he takes gulps of air from air bubbles held inside the vehicle.

Air embolism can develop in both shallow and deep waters. The onset is rapid, with signs of personality changes and distorted senses sometimes giving the impression of drunkenness. The patient may have convulsions and rapidly become unresponsive. There may be signs of air outside of the lungs being trapped in the chest cavity.

You should suspect possible air embolism when the patient has any of the following signs or symptoms:

- Personality changes.
- Distorted senses. Blurred vision is most common.
- Chest pains.
- Numbness and tingling sensations in the arms and/or legs.
- Total body weakness, or weakness of one or more limbs.
- Frothy blood in the mouth or nose.
- Convulsions.

Warning: Do not assume air embolism without first considering possible head injury or stroke.

The bends are really part of what is called **decompression sickness.** Patients with decompression sickness usually are those individuals who have come up too quickly from a deep, prolonged dive. When they do this, nitrogen gas is trapped in their tissues and may find its way into the bloodstream. The onset of the bends is usually slow for scuba divers, taking from 1 to 48 hours to appear. Because of this delay, the patient interview and reports from the patient's family and friends may be your only clue to relate the patient's problems to a dive.

Note: Scuba divers increase the risk of decompression sickness if they fly within 12 hours following a dive.

The signs and symptoms of decompression sickness include:

- Fatigue.
- Pain to the muscles and joints (the bends).
- Numbness or paralysis.
- Choking, coughing, and/or labored breathing.
- Chest pains.
- Collapse and unresponsiveness.
- Blotches on the skin (mottling). Sometimes, these rashes keep changing appearance.

If you think a patient has gas bubbles in the blood or decompression sickness due to a dive, be certain that the dispatcher is aware of the problem. The patient will need EMT transport to a medical facility as soon as possible. Dispatch may wish to direct the EMTs to take the patient to a special facility (hyperbaric trauma center) where a patient is exposed to oxygen under greatly increased pressure conditions. This procedure is done in a sealed hyperbaric chamber.

While waiting for the EMTs to arrive, provide care for shock and constantly monitor the patient. Respiratory and cardiac arrest are possible. Positioning of the patient is critical in order to avoid gas bubbles in the blood damaging the brain. Place the patient on the left side. The patient may be placed in a slight head-down position, but for no more than 10 minutes and only if it can be maintained without impairing breathing or other resuscitative measures (Figure A4.3). Provide oxygen as per local protocols.

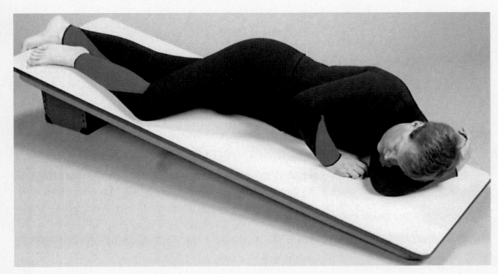

FIGURE A4.3

Position the patient after a scuba-diving incident. He may be placed in a head-down tilt but for no more than 10 minutes.

ICE-RELATED INCIDENTS

Ice rescues require special training. Unless you are trained specifically to work on ice, do not attempt a rescue. If you cannot swim, you have no business going out onto the ice. You may walk on an undetected thin spot, fall through the ice, and quickly drown. All rescuers who are on or at the edge of the ice must wear personal flotation devices.

The major problem faced in ice rescue is reaching the victim. Never walk out to the person or attempt to enter the water through a hole in the ice in order to find the victim. Never attempt an ice rescue by yourself unless you have some basic equipment, such as a personal flotation device and a ladder, and you are specifically trained in one-rescuer techniques. Never go onto ice that is rapidly breaking up. Your best course of action will be to work with others from a safe ice surface or the shore (Figure A4.4).

As the first choice of action, throw a line to the victim or reach out with a stick or a pole. If the victim is not holding onto the ice, but trying to keep afloat in open water, throw anything that will float. Do not try to go onto the ice to rescue the victim. Call for help immediately. *Ice rescues require special training, protective clothing, and rescue equipment.*

If you have had specialized training and the necessary equipment and personnel and you have to go onto the ice to get the patient, it is strongly recommended that you work with other trained help. Pushing a long ladder out onto the ice and then crawling along the ladder is a very effective method of safe rescue, providing someone is holding the ladder from a safe position. If enough people are on hand, a human chain can be formed to reach the patient; however, these people should be trained and wearing PFDs.

One of the few methods of ice rescue that can be tried by the single rescuer is the use of a light boat. This craft can be moved along the ice by riding inside of the boat and pushing the ice with your hands or with a stick or an oar. This is often a very slow and awkward method, but if the ice cracks, at least you are safe in a boat.

Expect to find injuries with any patient who has fallen through the ice. Broken leg bones are common. Hypothermia is often a problem and should always be considered. *Do not attempt to rewarm the severely hypothermic patient.*

Activate the EMS system for all patients who have had incidents on ice or have been in cold water. There may be injuries that are difficult to detect and problems because of the cold that may be delayed.

ASSISTING THE EMTs

You may be the first on the scene of a water or an ice rescue and have the EMTs arrive during rescue or care. At other times, you may arrive at the scene after the EMTs. Some of the things you can do to help, if directed to do so, might be to:

- *Interview bystanders*—Information gained could indicate the number of victims, a hidden medical emergency, or the cause of the incident.
- *Crowd control*—Both the curiosity seeker and those wishing to help may come to the scene. Unless controlled, they may hinder rescue, fall into the water, or place too much weight on the ice surface.
- *Find additional help*—This is usual in emergencies involving ice.
- *Find items used in rescue*—You may have to look for a ladder or a boat.
- *Help provide care*—Two-rescuer CPR, positioning the patient, and splinting the patient may require your aid.
- *Helping with a spine board*—If you are a good swimmer and have been trained in water rescue, the EMTs may need you in the water. Remember, a spine board will float and will pop up very easily from below the surface of the water. If you are called upon to help place a spine board under a patient who is still in the water, make sure of your position so as not to slip, and keep a firm grip on the board. If you have any doubts as to what the EMTs want you to do, ask questions.

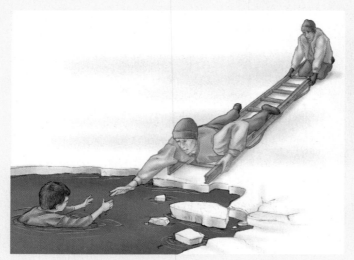

FIGURE A4.4
A safe ice rescue requires teamwork between specially trained First Responders.

Appendix 5

Response to Terrorism and Weapons of Mass Destruction

TERRORISM

The U.S. government defines **terrorism** as "the use of force or violence against persons or property to intimidate or coerce a government, the civilian population, or any segment thereof to further political or social objectives." For years the people of the U.S. remained somewhat insulated from the effects of terrorists and terrorism, since they only viewed such events on the nightly news. However, terrorism is no longer something that only happens in distant countries.

In recent years the effects of terrorism have hit home with incidents such as the bombing of the Federal Building in Oklahoma City, the spread of anthrax through the U.S. Postal Service, and the events of September 11, 2001, in New York, Washington D.C., and Pennsylvania. Terrorism is no longer something that only happens in distant countries.

INCIDENTS INVOLVING NUCLEAR/ RADIOLOGICAL AGENTS

Until recently, the potential for a terrorist organization to obtain or develop nuclear devices was thought to be minimal. With the growing supply of nuclear waste on a worldwide scale and the developing technology of third-world countries, the likelihood of a nuclear threat by a terrorist organization is ever increasing.

There are two types of potential nuclear incidents. One is the possible detonation of a nuclear device, and the other is the detonation of a conventional explosive incorporating nuclear material. A plausible scenario involves the detonation of a **radiological dispersal device (RDD),** which would spread radioactive material for a wide area surrounding the blast site. Another scenario involves the detonation of a large explosive device (such as a truck bomb) near a nuclear power plant or radiological cargo transport.

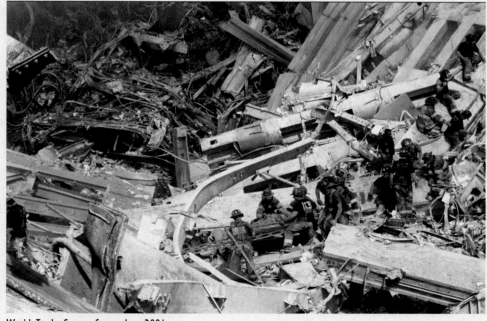

World Trade Center, September, 2001.

Nuclear incidents emit three main types of radioactive particles: alpha, beta, and gamma.

- **Alpha particles** are the heaviest and most highly charged of the nuclear particles. They are easily stopped by human skin but can become a serious hazard if ingested or inhaled.

- **Beta particles** are smaller and travel much faster and farther than alpha particles. Beta particles can penetrate through the skin but rarely reach the vital organs. While they can cause burns to the skin if exposure lasts long enough, the biggest threat occurs when they are ingested or inhaled into the body. Beta particles also can enter the body through unprotected open wounds.

- **Gamma rays** are a type of radiation that travels through the air in the form of waves. They can travel great distances and penetrate most materials, including the human body. Acute radiation sickness occurs when someone is exposed to large doses of gamma radiation over a short period of time and can cause symptoms such as skin irritation, burns, nausea, vomiting, high fever, and hair loss.

INCIDENTS INVOLVING BIOLOGICAL AGENTS

Biological agents pose one of the most serious threats due to their accessibility and ability to spread rapidly. The potential is also very high for widespread casualties. Biological agents are most dangerous when either inhaled (spread through the air) or ingested (through contaminated food or water supplies).

There are four common types of biological agents: bacteria, rickettsia, viruses, and toxins:

- **Bacteria** are single-celled organisms that can quickly cause disease in humans. Some of the more common bacteria used for terrorist activities are anthrax, cholera, the plague, and tularemia.

- **Rickettsia** are smaller than bacteria cells and live inside individual host cells. An example of rickettsia is Q fever.

- **Viruses** are the simplest of microorganisms and cannot survive without a living host. The most common viruses that have served as biological agents include smallpox, Venezuelan equine encephalitis, and Ebola, among others.

- **Toxins** are substances that occur naturally in the environment and can be produced by an animal, plant, or microbe. They differ from biological agents in that they are not manufactured. The four common toxins with a history of use as terrorist weapons are botulism, SEB (staphylococcal enterotoxin), ricin, and mycotoxins. Ricin has been used in several well-publicized incidents in the U.S. and Japan. It is a toxin made from the castor bean plant, which is grown all over the world.

INCIDENTS INVOLVING CHEMICAL AGENTS

The primary routes of exposure for chemical agents are inhalation, ingestion, and absorption or contact with the skin, with inhalation being the most common. The five classifications of chemical agents are: **nerve agents, vesicant (blister) agents, cyanogens agents, pulmonary agents,** and **riot-control agents.**

Nerve Agents

Nerve agents disrupt the nerve impulse transmissions throughout the body and are extremely toxic in very small quantities. In some cases, a single small drop can be fatal to an average human being. Nerve agents include sarin (GB), which has been used against Japanese and Iraqi civilians, soman (GD), tabun (GA), and V agent (VX). These are liquid agents that are typically spread in the form of an aerosol spray.

In the case of GA, GB, and GD, the first letter "G" stands for the country (Germany) that developed the agent. The second letter indicates the order in which the agent was developed. In the case of VX, the "V" stands for venom and the "X" represents one of the chemicals that make up the compound. These agents resemble water or clear oil in their purest form and possess no odor. Sometimes small explosives are used to spread them, which can cause widespread death. Many dead animals at the scene of an incident may be an outward warning sign or detection clue.

Early signs of nerve agent exposure are:

- Uncontrolled salivation.
- Urination.
- Defecation.
- Tearing.

Other later signs and symptoms include:

- Blurred vision.
- Excessive sweating.
- Muscle tremors.
- Difficulty breathing.
- Nausea, vomiting.
- Abdominal pain.

Vesicant Agents

Vesicant agents are more commonly referred to as blister or mustard agents due to their unique smell. They can easily penetrate several layers of clothing and are quickly absorbed into the skin. Mustard (H, HD, HN) and Lewisite (L, HL) are common vesicants. Although less toxic than nerve agents, it takes only a few drops on the skin to cause severe injury.

The signs and symptoms of vesicant exposure include:

- Reddening, swelling, and tearing of the eyes.
- Tenderness and burning of the skin followed by the development of fluid-filled blisters.
- Nausea, vomiting.
- Severe abdominal pain.
- After about two hours, victims will experience runny nose, burning in the throat, and shortness of breath.

Cyanogens

Cyanogens are agents that interfere with the ability of the blood to carry oxygen and can cause asphyxiation in victims of exposure. Common cyanogens are hydrogen cyanide (AC) and cyanogens chloride (CK). All cyanogens are very toxic in high concentrations and can lead to rapid death. Under pressure, these agents are in liquid form. In their pure form, they are a gas. Cyanogens are common industrial chemicals used in a variety of processes and all have an aroma similar to bitter almonds or peach blossoms.

Signs and symptoms of cyanogens exposure include:

- Severe respiratory distress.
- Vomiting.
- Diarrhea.
- Dizziness, headache.
- Seizures, coma.

It is essential that victims of exposure be quickly moved to fresh air and treated for respiratory distress.

Pulmonary Agents

Pulmonary agents are sometimes called choking agents. They directly effect the respiratory system, causing fluid build up (edema) in the lungs, which in turn causes asphyxiation similar to that seen in drowning victims. Chlorine and phosgene are two of the most common of these agents and are commonly found in industrial settings. Chlorine is a familiar smell to most people. Phosgene has an aroma of freshly cut hay. Both of these chemicals are in a gaseous state in their pure form and are stored in bottles or cylinders.

Signs and symptoms include:

- Severe eye irritation.
- Coughing.
- Choking.
- Severe respiratory distress.

Riot-Control Agents

Riot-control agents include both irritating and psychedelic agents, both of which are designed to incapacitate the victim. For the most part, they are non-lethal. However, under certain circumstances irritating agents have been known to cause asphyxiation. In some individuals, psychedelic agents have been known to cause behavior that can lead to death.

Common irritating agents include mace, tear gas, and pepper spray. These agents will typically cause severe pain when they come in contact with the skin, especially moist areas such as the nose, mouth, and eyes.

Signs and symptoms of exposure to irritating agents include:

- Burning and irritation in the eyes and throat.
- Coughing, choking.
- Respiratory distress.
- Nausea.
- Vomiting.

Psychedelic agents include lysergic acid diethylamide (LSD), 3-quinuclidinyl benzilate (BZ), and benctyzine. These agents alter the nervous system causing visual and aural hallucinations and severe changes in thought processes and behavior. The effects of these agents can be unpredictable, ranging from overwhelming fear to extreme belligerence.

ROLE OF THE FIRST RESPONDER

Terrorist attacks are meant to cause fear, and they are likely to occur when they are least expected. Having a high index of suspicion and recognizing the outward warning signs of a possible terrorist attack is of utmost importance for the first units on scene. Donning the appropriate personal protective equipment (PPE) early will minimize the chances of all emergency responders becoming victims themselves.

Firefighters are probably the best prepared of all First Responders because of the wide range of duties they are trained and expected to perform. Ambulance personnel are probably the least equipped to respond to a terrorist attack because their PPE is used to minimize exposure to body fluids and aerosolized droplets from coughing patients.

Without the proper training and equipment, First Responders are likely to become victims if they enter the scene too quickly. In most cases the best action will be to recognize the danger as soon as possible and retreat to a safe distance from the scene. Requesting appropriate resources such as specialized hazardous-materials teams will be important.

DECONTAMINATION

Decontamination is the process by which chemical, biological, and/or radiological agents are removed from exposed victims, equipment, and the environment. Regardless if the incident is a hazardous-materials one or an intentional terrorist act, prompt decontamination can be the single most important aspect of the operation to minimize exposure and limit casualties.

Depending on the size and scope of the incident, First Responders may be asked to assist with the decontamination process. If not a part of the decontamination process, they will certainly play an important role in the emergency care given to patients after coming out of decontamination. It will be important for First Responders assisting at such an event to continue to wear the appropriate PPE even after a victim has been decontaminated. This will minimize any contamination from residual agents remaining on the victim or equipment.

Appendix 6

First Responder Roles and Responsibilities

First Responders are a part of the EMS system, responding to emergencies, usually arriving first on the scene, providing initial care for patients, and working with other emergency care providers to assess, make care decisions, and transport. Each individual on an emergency scene works as a member of a team, whether performing as a First Responder or EMT. The team's actions and interactions are what make the EMS system work effectively.

The following table provides a matrix of how the levels of EMS responders work together to perform the steps of scene safety, patient assessment and care, and transport. You will find that you will work in one or several areas of the matrix as you arrive on the scene and begin assessment and care.

Team actions and interactions make the EMS system work effectively. This course of instruction will provide the knowledge, skills, and practice opportunities for performing the roles and responsibilities of a First Responder.

Remember: One of the most important of your roles is to take appropriate safety precautions. Once personal and scene safety are ensured, First Responders may begin to perform numerous patient-related duties.

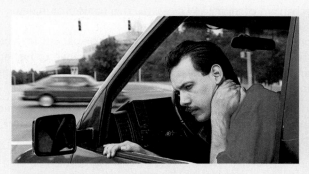

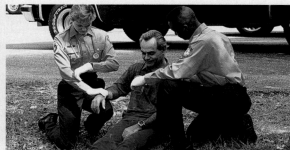

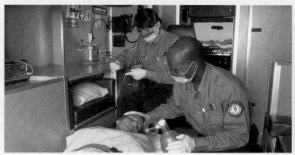

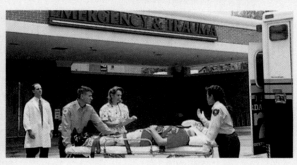

TABLE A6-1 EMS ROLES AND RESPONSIBILITIES

PHASE	FIRST RESPONDER	EMTS	PARAMEDIC
Preparation (Green-Go)	Check unit; restock emergency care supplies; get dispatch information and respond to call.	Check unit; restock emergency care supplies; get dispatch information and respond to call.	Check unit; restock emergency care supplies; get dispatch information and respond to call.
Size-up (Yellow-Caution)	Arrive; perform scene size-up.	Arrive; perform scene size-up.	Arrive; perform scene size-up.
	Determine need for EMTs, paramedics, medevac, rescue, and specialty units.	Determine need for paramedics, medevac, rescue, and specialty units.	Determine need for medevac, rescue, and specialty units.
	Contact medical direction or communications as needed.	Contact medical direction or . communications as needed.	Contact medical direction or communications as needed.
Initial assessment (Orange-Alert)	Perform initial assessment (impression, AVPU, ABCs, priority).	Perform initial assessment (impression, AVPU, ABCs, priority).	Perform initial assessment (impression, AVPU, ABCs, priority).
Assessment (Red-Action)	Perform rapid or focused assessment; perform or assist EMTs and paramedics with assessment and history, vital signs, stabilization, splinting, medications per protocols and medical direction.	Perform rapid or focused assessment; assist paramedics with assessment and history, vital signs, stabilization, splinting, medications per protocols and medical direction.	Perform rapid or focused assessment; perform BLS and ALS procedures per protocols and medical direction.
Care and transport (Orange-Alert)	Arrange for transport; report patient history, vital signs, and nature of illness or mechanism of injury.	Transport or arrange for transport; report patient history, vital signs, and nature of illness or mechanism of injury.	Transport or arrange for transport; report patient history, vital signs, and nature of illness or mechanism of injury.
	Monitor patient for change in status; notify EMTs or paramedics; change to higher or lower priority as needed.	Monitor patient for change in status; notify paramedics; change to higher or lower priority as needed.	Monitor patient for change in status; change to higher or lower priority as needed.
Detailed exam and ongoing assessment (Yellow-Caution)	Perform detailed physical exam or assist EMTs or paramedics during transport.	Perform detailed physical exam or assist paramedics during transport.	Perform detailed physical exam during transport.
	Perform interventions (patient care) or assist during assessment and transport.	Perform interventions (patient care) or assist during assessment and transport.	Perform interventions (patient care) during assessment and transport.
	Perform ongoing assessment or assess en route.	Perform ongoing assessment or assist en route.	Perform ongoing assessment en route.
Wrap-up, report, and preparation (Green-Go)	Hand-off patient to EMTs; complete patient report; restock and return to service.	Hand-off patient to ED; complete patient report; restock and return to service.	Hand-off patient to ED; complete patient report; restock and return to service.

Glossary

A

Abandonment   to leave a sick or an injured patient before equal or more highly trained EMS personnel can assume responsibility for care.

ABCs   short for the words airway, breathing, and circulation.

Abdomen (AB-do-men)   the region of the body between the diaphragm and pelvis.

Abdominal cavity   the anterior body cavity that extends from the diaphragm to the region protected by the pelvic bones. It houses and protects the abdominal organs, glands, major blood vessels, and nerves.

Abdominal quadrants   four divisions of the abdomen used to pinpoint the location of a pain or an injury: the right upper quadrant, the left upper quadrant, the right lower quadrant, and the left lower quadrant.

Abdominal thrusts   manual thrusts that are delivered to the midline of the abdomen, between the xiphoid process and the navel, to create pressure that can help to expel an airway obstruction. See *manual thrusts*.

Abdominopelvic (ab-DOM-i-no-PEL-vik) **cavity**   the front (anterior) cavity below (inferior to) the diaphragm.

Abortion (ah-BOR-shun)   spontaneous miscarriage or induced loss of an embryo or fetus. See *miscarriage*.

Abrasion (ab-RAY-zhun)   the simplest form of open wound that damages the skin surface but does not break all the layers of the skin; scratch or scrape.

Abscess (AB-ses)   a contained or otherwise limited structure that collects pus associated with tissue death and infection.

Acetone breath   a sweet breath with a fruitlike odor. This is a sign of diabetic coma.

Achilles (ah-KEL-ez) **tendon**   the common term for the tendon that connects the posterior leg muscles to the heel; the calcaneal (kal-KA-ne-al) tendon.

Acid   being acidic, as opposed to being neutral or basic (alkaline); associated with free hydrogen ions.

ACLS   See *advanced cardiac life support*.

Acquired immune deficiency syndrome (AIDS)   a contagious, usually fatal disease that suppresses the immune system and allows infections and malignancies to invade the body. The infectious agent is HIV, which may be passed from person to person by sexual contact, blood transfusion, sharing needles, or across the placenta from mother to fetus (unborn child). The virus is found in blood, body fluids, and wastes. It is also associated with mucous membranes. Even though it is found in saliva, there is no clear evidence of the disease being transmitted in this substance.

Activated charcoal   a very fine, treated charcoal powder that is available in premixed form or ready to mix with water. When taken by mouth, it may absorb some forms of ingested poisons, thus preventing or reducing absorption by the patient's body.

Acute   to have a rapid onset; severe.

Acute abdomen   the sudden onset of severe abdominal pain related to a medical condition or specific injury to the abdomen.

Acute myocardial infarction (AMI) (my-o-KARD-e-al in-FARK-shun)   a heart attack; the sudden death of heart muscle due to oxygen starvation. Usually caused by a narrowing or blockage of one of the blood vessels (coronary arteries) supplying the heart muscle.

Advanced cardiac life support (ACLS)   prehospital emergency care that involves the use of intravenous fluids, drug infusions, cardiac monitoring, defibrillation, intubations, and other advanced procedures. See *basic life support (BLS)*.

Afterbirth   the placenta, part of the umbilical cord, and some tissues of the womb's lining, which are delivered after the birth of the baby.

Agonal respirations   sporadic noises from the patient's airway, without chest movement, occurring just prior to death.

AIDS   See *acquired immune deficiency syndrome (AIDS)*.

Air embolism   gas bubbles in the bloodstream.

Air sacs   the microscopic parts of the lung where gas exchange takes place. The medical term is *alveoli* (al-VE-o-li).

Air splint   See *inflatable splint*.

Airway   the passageway for air from the nose and mouth to the exchange levels of the lungs. Also may refer to an artificial airway or airway adjunct.

Airway adjunct   a device that is placed in the patient's mouth or nose to help maintain an open airway. Oral airway adjuncts may help to hold the tongue clear of the airway.

Alkali   a substance that is basic, as opposed to being acid or neutral.

Allergen (AL-er-jin)   any substance that can cause an allergic response.

Allergy shock   See *anaphylactic shock*.

Alveoli (al-VE-o-li)   See *air sacs*.

Amnesia   the short- or long-term loss of memory, which usually has a sudden onset.

Amniotic (am-ne-OT-ik) **sac**   the fluid-filled sac that surrounds the developing embryo or fetus. Also called *bag of waters*.

Amputation   soft-tissue injury that involves the cutting or tearing off of a limb or one of its parts. Often, hard tissues are also injured.

Analgesic   a pain reliever.

Anaphylactic (an-ah-fi-LAK-tik) **shock**   the most severe type of allergic reaction, in which a person goes into shock when he comes into contact with a substance to which he is allergic. Also called *allergy shock*.

Anatomical (AN-ah-TOM-I-kal) **position**   the standard reference position for the body in the study of anatomy. The body is standing erect, facing the observer. The arms are down at the sides, and the palms of the hands are forward.

Anatomy   the study of body structure.

Anesthetic to be free of pain and feeling. Commonly used to mean a substance that will block pain or feeling.

Aneurysm (AN-u-RIZ-m) the dilated or weakened section of an arterial wall. A blood-filled sac formed by the localized dilation of an artery or a vein.

Angina pectoris (an-JI-nah PEK-to-ris) the chest pain often caused by an insufficient blood supply to the heart muscle. Also called *angina*.

Angulation the angle formed above and below a break in a bone. Also may be called *deformed injury*.

Anterior the front of the body or body part. See *posterior*.

Antiseptic a substance that will stop the growth of or prevent the activities of germs (microorganisms).

Anus (A-nus) the outlet of the large intestine.

Aorta (a-OR-tah) the major artery that carries blood from the heart out to the body.

Apical pulse the pulse felt or heard over the lower part of the heart.

Apnea (AP-ne-ah) the temporary cessation of breathing.

Appendicular (ap-en-DIK-u-ler) **skeleton** bones and joints that form the upper and lower extremities. See *axial skeleton*.

Arrhythmia (ah-RITH-me-ah) absence of rhythm; disturbance of heart rate and rhythm. Sometimes the term *dysrhythmia* is used to mean the same thing.

Arterial bleeding the loss of bright red blood from an artery. The flow may be rapid, spurting as the heart beats. See *capillary bleeding* and *venous bleeding*.

Arteriole (ar-TE-re-ol) the smallest of the arteries that typically lead into capillary beds. See *venule*.

Arteriosclerosis (ar-TE-re-o-skle-RO-sis) hardening of the arteries caused by calcium deposits. See also *atherosclerosis*.

Artery any blood vessel that carries blood away from the heart.

Articulate to join together; to unite to form a joint.

Artificial breathing See *artificial respiration*.

Artificial respiration the process of forcing air or oxygen into the lungs of a patient who is in respiratory arrest or who does not have adequate breathing. Also called *artificial ventilation* and *artificial breathing*.

Artificial ventilation See *artificial respiration*.

Aseptic clean, free of most particles of dirt and debris.

Asphyxia (as-FIK-si-ah) suffocation resulting in the loss of responsiveness caused by too little oxygen reaching the brain.

Aspiration to inhale materials into the lungs. Often used to describe the breathing of vomitus.

Asthma (AS-mah) the condition in which the bronchioles constrict, causing a reduction of airflow and creating congestion. Air usually will enter to the level of the air sacs (alveoli), but it cannot be exhaled easily.

Asystole (a-SIS-to-le) when the heart stops beating; cardiac standstill.

Atherosclerosis (ATH-er-o-skle-RO-sis) the buildup of fatty deposits on the inner wall of an artery. This buildup is called *plaque*. If calcium is deposited in the plaque, the arterial wall will become hard and stiff. See *arteriosclerosis*.

Atrium (A-tree-um) one of two (left and right) superior chambers of the heart. Plural *atria*.

Auscultation (os-kul-TAY-shun) listening to sounds that occur within the body.

Automated external defibrillator (AED) an electrical apparatus that can detect certain irregular heartbeats (fibrillations) and deliver a shock through the patient's chest. This shock may allow the heart to resume a normal pattern of beating. See *defibrillation*.

AVPU a memory aid for classifying a patient's level of responsiveness. The letters stand for *alert*, *verbal response*, *painful response*, *unresponsive*.

Avulsion (ah-VUL-shun) a soft-tissue injury in which flaps of skin are torn loose or torn off.

Axial (AK-se-al) **skeleton** bones and joints that form the center, or upright, axis of the body. It includes the skull, spine, breastbone, and ribs. See *appendicular skeleton*.

Axilla (ak-SIL-ah) the armpit.

B

Bag-valve-mask (BVM) ventilator an aid for artificial ventilation, which has a face mask, a self-inflating bag, and a valve that allows the bag to refill while the patient exhales. It can be attached to an oxygen line.

Bandage any material that is used to hold a dressing in place.

Basic life support (BLS) externally supporting the circulation and respiration of a patient in respiratory or cardiac arrest through CPR.

Baseline vital signs the first determination of vital signs; used to compare with all repeated readings of vital signs in order to identify trends.

Battle's sign discoloration behind the ear that suggests a fracture at the base of the skull (late sign).

Behavioral emergency a situation in which a patient exhibits abnormal behavior that is unacceptable or intolerable to the patient, family, or community.

Bilateral existing on both sides of the body.

Bile fluid formed in the liver and sent to the small intestine; may be stored in the gallbladder. It has many functions, including changing the speed at which the intestine moves things along (intestinal motility) and helping to digest fatty foods.

Biological death occurs when the brain cells die; this is usually within 10 minutes of respiratory arrest. See *clinical death*.

Bladder usually refers to the urinary bladder located in the pelvic cavity.

Blanch to become pale or to turn white.

Blood pressure the pressure caused by blood exerting a force on the walls of blood vessels. Usually, arterial blood pressure is measured.

BLS See *basic life support*.

Blunt trauma an injury caused by an object that was not sharp enough to penetrate the skin.

Body mechanics the proper use of the body to facilitate lifting and moving and prevent injury.

Body substance isolation (BSI) a method of infection control based on the presumption that all body fluids are infectious; practice of using specific barriers to minimize contact with a patient's blood and body fluids.

Bones the living tissues of the skeletal system that have a matrix of calcium (for hardness) and protein fibers (for limited flexibility).

Bones provide attachment points for skeletal muscles, and in some cases bone marrow makes blood cells.

Bourdon (bor-DON) **gauge** a gauged flowmeter that indicates the flow of a gas in liters per minute.

Bowel the intestine.

Brachial (BRAY-ke-al) **pulse** the pulse found on the inside (medial) upper arm of the patient between elbow and shoulder; used to evaluate circulation in an infant.

Bradycardia (bray-de-KAR-de-ah) an abnormal condition in which the heart rate is slow.

Breastbone the sternum.

Breech birth a birth in which the buttocks or both legs of the baby are delivered first.

Bronchiole (BRONG-ke-ol) the small branches of the airway that carry air to and from the air sacs of the lungs.

Bronchus (BRON-kus) the portion of the airway connecting the trachea to the lungs. Plural *bronchi*.

Bruise simple closed wound in which blood flows between soft tissues, causing a discoloration; a contusion.

BSI See *body substance isolation*.

Bulky dressing a thick, single dressing or a buildup of thin dressings used to help control profuse bleeding, stabilize impaled objects, or cover large open wounds.

BVM See *bag-valve-mask ventilator*.

C

Capillary a microscopic blood vessel that connects an artery to a vein; where exchange takes place between the bloodstream and the body tissues.

Capillary bleeding the slow oozing of blood from a capillary bed. See *arterial bleeding* and *venous bleeding*.

Capillary refill the return (refill) of capillaries after blood has been forced out by fingertip pressure applied by the rescuer to the patient's nail bed. Normal refill time is two seconds or less.

Cardiac (KAR-de-ak) in reference to the heart.

Cardiac arrest when the heart stops beating. Also, the sudden end of effective circulation caused by erratic muscle activity in the lower chambers of the heart (ventricular fibrillation).

Cardiogenic (KAR-de-o-JEN-ik) **shock** See *heart shock*.

Cardiopulmonary resuscitation (KAR-de-o-PUL-mo-ner-e re-SUS-ci-TA-shun) **(CPR)** heart-lung resuscitation. Combined compression and breathing techniques that maintain circulation and breathing.

Carotid (kah-ROT-id) **pulse** the pulse that can be felt on each side of the neck.

Carpals (KAR-pals) the wrist bones.

Catheter a flexible tube passed through a body channel (such as the urethra or a blood vessel) to allow for drainage or the withdrawal of fluids.

Central nervous system (CNS) the brain and spinal cord.

Cerebrospinal (ser-e-bro-SPI-nal) **fluid (CSF)** the clear, watery fluid that helps to protect the brain and spinal cord.

Cerebrovascular (SER-e-bro-VAS-cu-ler) **accident (CVA)** See *stroke*.

Cervical (SER-vi-kal) **spine** the neck bones.

Cervix (SUR-viks) the neck of the uterus; the lower portion of the uterus where it enters the vagina.

CHEMTREC the Chemical Transportation Emergency Center that provides immediate expert information to emergency personnel at the scene of a hazardous materials incident.

Chief complaint the reason EMS was called, usually in the patient's own words.

Child For the purpose of CPR, a person 1 to 8 years of age.

Child abuse assault of an infant or a child that produces physical and/or emotional injuries. Sexual assault is included as a form of child abuse.

Chronic long and drawn out or recurring.

Chronic obstructive pulmonary disease (COPD) a variety of lung problems related to diseases of the airway passages or exchange levels. The patient will suffer difficulties in breathing.

Circulatory system the heart, blood vessels, and blood; system that moves blood, carrying oxygen and nutrients to the body's cells and removing wastes and carbon dioxide from these cells.

Clavicle (KLAV-i-kul) the collarbone.

Clinical death the moment when breathing and heart actions stop. See *biological death*.

Closed fracture a simple fracture in which the skin is not broken by the broken bones.

Closed injury an injury with no associated opening of the skin. Also called *closed wound*.

Clot a formation composed of fibrin and entangled blood cells that acts to help stop the bleeding from a wound.

Coccyx (KOK-siks) the lowermost bones of the spinal column. They are fused into one bone in the adult.

Collarbone the clavicle (KLAV-i-kul).

Coma the state of complete unresponsiveness.

Compensated shock when a patient's body is still able to maintain perfusion even though shock is developing. See *decompensated shock*, *hypoperfusion*, *perfusion*, and *shock*.

Concussion (kon-KUSH-un) injury to the brain that results from a blow or impact from an object but does not cause permanent neurological damage.

Confidentiality refers to the privacy of patient information (except for medical reporting, medical records, and certain court subpoenas), including the details of the patient and the patient's behavior during the rendering of all aspects of care.

Congestive heart failure (CHF) the condition in which the heart cannot properly circulate the blood, causing a backup of fluids in the lungs and other organs.

Consent oral or written permission from the patient for emergency medical care. See *expressed consent* and *implied consent*.

Constant flow sector valve a meterless device that allows the user to adjust the flow of supplemental oxygen by selecting the flow in stepped increments (2, 4, 6, 8, . . . 15 liters per minute).

Contraction time the period of time a contraction of the womb lasts during labor. It is measured from the start of the uterus contracting until it releases. See *interval time*.

Contraindication any condition, sign, symptom, or existing treatment that makes a particular course of treatment or care procedure inadvisable.

Contusion (kun-TU-zhun) a bruise; in the case of the brain, caused by a force of a blow great enough to rupture blood vessels on the surface of or deep within the brain.

Convulsion uncontrolled skeletal muscle spasm, often violent.

COPD See *chronic obstructive pulmonary disease (COPD)*.

Core temperature the body temperature measured at a central point, such as within the rectum.

Cornea (KOR-ne-ah) the transparent tissue covering that lies over the top of the iris and the pupil of the eye.

Coronary artery disease the narrowing of one or more places in the coronary arteries brought about by atherosclerosis. Blockage (occlusion) will eventually occur in many cases.

CPR cardiopulmonary resuscitation.

Cranial (KRAY-ne-al) **cavity** braincase of the skull that houses the brain and its specialized membranes.

Cranium (KRAY-ne-um) the bones that form the forehead and the floor, back, top, and upper sides of the skull.

Cravat a piece of cloth that can be used to secure a dressing; a triangular bandage that is folded to a width of three or four inches and used to tie soft or rigid splints in place.

Crepitus (KREP-i-tus) a grating noise or the sensation felt when broken bone ends rub together.

Critical incident stress debriefing (CISD) part of critical incident stress management; process in which teams of professional and peer counselors provide emotional and psychological support to rescue personnel who are or have been involved in a highly stressful incident.

Critical incident stress management (CISM) an in-depth, broad plan designed to help rescue personnel cope with the stress resulting from a highly stressful incident.

Croup (kroop) acute respiratory condition found in infants and children; characterized by a barking type of cough or stridor.

Crowing an atypical sound made when a patient breathes; usually indicates airway obstruction.

Crowning during childbirth, the bulging out of the vagina caused by exposure of the baby's head or other presenting part during contractions.

Crush injury soft-tissue injury produced by crushing forces. Soft tissues and internal organs are crushed, and hard tissues are usually damaged.

Cut soft-tissue injury in which all the layers of skin are opened and the tissues immediately below the skin are damaged. Smooth cuts are *incisions* and jagged cuts are *lacerations*.

Cyanosis (si-ah-NO-sis) bluish discoloration of the skin and mucous membranes; a sign that body tissues are not receiving enough oxygen.

D

Danger zone the area around an emergency event in which special safety procedures must be followed. The size and type of zone is often dependent on the type of incident and environmental conditions.

DCAP-BTLS a memory aid for patient assessment factors. The letters stand for deformities, contusions, abrasions, punctures/penetrations, burns, tenderness, lacerations, and swelling.

Decompensated shock takes place when the patient's body can no longer maintain perfusion as shock develops. Usually there is a pronounced fall in blood pressure. See *compensated shock*, *hypoperfusion*, *perfusion*, and *shock*.

Decompression sickness the bends. In most cases, this involves scuba divers who have surfaced too rapidly. Nitrogen is trapped in body tissues and may find its way into the diver's bloodstream.

Deep frostbite See *freezing*.

Defibrillation to apply an electric shock to a patient's heart in an attempt to disrupt a lethal rhythm and allow the heart to spontaneously reestablish a normal rhythm. This is done with a defibrillator. See *automated external defibrillator (AED)*.

Deformed injury an injury that causes a bone or joint to take on an unnatural shape or bend. Also may be called *angulated injury*.

Dehydration excessive loss of body water (fluids).

Delirium tremens (DTs) a severe, possibly life-threatening reaction related to alcohol withdrawal. The patient's hands tremble, hallucinations may be present, behavior may be unusual, and convulsions may occur.

Dermis (DER-mis) the inner (second) layer of the skin. It is the layer that is rich in blood vessels and nerves found below the epidermis.

Detailed physical exam an assessment used for unresponsive patients or those who may be severely injured. The assessment is done more slowly than a rapid trauma assessment and includes a complete head-to-toe examination.

Diabetes (di-ah-BE-teez) usually refers to diabetes mellitus, a disease that prevents individuals from producing enough insulin or from using insulin effectively. See *hyperglycemia* and *hypoglycemia*.

Diabetic coma severe hyperglycemia. The result of an inadequate insulin supply that leads to unresponsiveness, coma, and eventually death unless treated.

Diaphragm (DI-ah-fram) the muscular structure that divides the chest cavity (thorax) from the abdominal cavity (abdominopelvic cavity). It is the major muscle used in breathing.

Diaphragmatic (DI-ah-FRAG-mat-ik) **breathing** weak and rapid respirations with little or no chest movement. There may be slight movement of the abdomen. The patient's attempt to breathe with the diaphragm alone.

Diastolic (di-as-TOL-ik) **blood pressure** the pressure exerted on the internal walls of the arteries when the heart is relaxing. See *systolic blood pressure*.

Digestive system stores and digests food, eliminates waste, and utilizes nutrients.

Dilate to enlarge; expand in diameter.

Direct pressure the quickest, most effective way to control most forms of external bleeding. Pressure is applied directly over the wound site.

Dislocation the pulling or pushing of a bone end partially or completely free of a joint.

Distal farther away from the torso. See *proximal*.

Distal pulse a pulse measured at the distal end of an extremity. Usually, this is the radial pulse for the upper extremity and the dorsalis pedis pulse for the lower extremity. See *radial pulse* and *dorsalis pedis pulse*.

Distended inflated, stretched, or swollen.

Dorsalis pedis (dor-SAL-is PED-is) **pulse** a foot pulse. See *pedal pulse.*

Downer a depressant drug that affects the central nervous system to relax the user.

Dressing any material used to cover a wound that will help control bleeding and reduce contamination.

Drowning death caused by water reaching the lungs and either causing lung tissue damage or spasms of the airway that prevent the inhalation of air. See *near-drowning.*

Duty to act requirement that First Responders in the police and fire service, at least while on duty, must provide care according to their agency's standard operating procedures.

Dyspnea (disp-NE-ah) difficult or labored breathing.

E

Eclampsia (e-KLAM-se-ah) a life-threatening complication of pregnancy that produces convulsions and may result in coma or death.

-ectomy (EK-toe-me) a word ending meaning surgical removal.

Edema (e-DE-mah) swelling due to the accumulation of fluids in the tissues.

Embolism (EM-bo-liz-m) movement and lodgment of a blood clot or foreign body (fat or air bubble) inside a blood vessel. The clot or foreign body is called an *embolus.*

Emergency care the prehospital assessment and care of a sick or injured patient, in which the physical and emotional needs of the patient are considered and attended to.

Emergency medical services (EMS) system the chain of human resources and services linked together to provide continuous emergency care from the prehospital scene, through transport, and arrival at the medical facility.

Emergency medical technician (EMT) a professional-level provider of emergency care, trained above the level of the First Responder. According to the DOT, three levels of EMT are: EMT-Basic, EMT-Intermediate, and EMT-Paramedic.

Emergency move a patient move that is carried out quickly when the scene is hazardous, care of the patient requires repositioning, or you must reach another patient needing life-saving care.

Emesis (EM-e-sis) vomiting.

Emotional emergency when a patient's behavior is not considered typical for the occasion. Often this behavior is not socially acceptable. The patient's emotions are strongly evident, interfering with his thoughts and behavior.

Emphysema (EM-fi-SEE-mah) a chronic disease in which the lungs suffer a progressive loss of elasticity. See *chronic obstructive pulmonary disease (COPD).*

Endocrine (EN-do-krin) **system** the system that produces chemicals called hormones, which help regulate most body activities and functions.

Enhanced 9-1-1 service that allows for caller information (for example, phone number and address) to be received electronically.

Epidermis (ep-i-DER-mis) the outer layer of skin.

Epiglottis (EP-i-GLOT-is) a flap of cartilage and other tissues that is located above the voice box (larynx). It helps to close off the airway when a person swallows.

Epiglottitis (ep-i-glot-I-tis) swelling of the epiglottis that can be caused by bacterial infection. It can obstruct the airway and can be potentially life-threatening.

Epilepsy (EP-i-lep-see) a medical disorder characterized by attacks of unresponsiveness, with or without convulsions.

Epinephrine medicine used to treat severe allergic reactions; relaxes the air passages and constricts enlarged blood vessels.

Episodic a medical problem that affects the patient at regular intervals.

Epistaxis (ep-e-STAK-sis) a nosebleed.

Esophagus (e-SOF-ah-gus) the muscular food tube leading from the throat to the stomach.

Evisceration (e-VIS-er-a-shun) usually applies to the intestine protruding through an incision or a wound.

Expiration the passive process of breathing out. See *inspiration.*

Expire to exhale air.

Expressed consent permission for EMS personnel to provide emergency care; given by a competent adult who has made an informed decision.

External auditory canal the opening of the external ear and its pathway to the middle ear.

External chest compressions measured compressions performed during CPR at a set rate over the CPR compression site. These compressions are applied to help create circulation of the blood.

Extrication any actions that disentangle and free from entrapment.

F

Fainting the simplest form of shock, occurring when the patient has a temporary, self-correcting loss of responsiveness caused by a reduced supply of blood to the brain. Also called *psychogenic shock.*

Febrile feverish.

Femoral (FEM-o-ral) **artery** the main artery of the upper leg (thigh). It is a major pulse location and pressure point site.

Femur (FE-mer) the thigh bone.

Fetus (FE-tus) a developing unborn baby. The fertilized egg is an embryo until the eighth week after fertilization, when it becomes a fetus.

Fibrillation uncoordinated contractions of the heart muscle (myocardium) that are produced from independent individual muscle fiber activity; the totally disorganized activity of heart muscle. See *ventricular fibrillation* and *defibrillation.*

Fibula (FIB-yo-lah) the lateral lower leg bone.

Finger sweeps a procedure used to clear the mouth of visible airway obstructions.

First-degree burn See *superficial burn.*

First Responder a member of the EMS system who has been trained to render first care for a patient and to assist EMTs at the emergency scene.

Flail chest the condition that results when there are two or more ribs fractured in two or more places, or the breastbone separates from the chest and produces a loose segment of chest wall. This segment will move in the opposite direction of the chest during breathing.

Flexion to lessen an angle of a joint; to bend, as in bending the knee or bending at the elbow.

Flowmeter a Bourdon, pressure-compensated, or constant-flow selector-valve device used to indicate supplemental oxygen flow in liters per minute.

Flow-restricted, oxygen-powered ventilation device (FROPVD) a device that delivers oxygen through a regulator from a pressurized cylinder.

Focused history and physical exam the step of patient assessment that follows the initial assessment and includes the patient history, physical exam, and vital signs.

Focused medical exam an examination of the medical patient's problem areas.

Focused trauma assessment an examination of the area that patient tells you is injured.

Fontanelles areas in the infant skull where bones have not yet fused; soft spots.

Foot bones the metatarsals (meta-TAR-sals).

Forearm bones the ulna and radius.

Fracture any break, crack, split, chip, or splintering of a bone.

Freezing an injury due to cold involving the skin and the layers below the skin. Deep structures such as bone and muscle may be involved. See *late or deep local cold injury.*

FROPVD See *flow-restricted, oxygen-powered ventilation device.*

Frostbite localized cold injury, in which the skin is frozen, but the layers below it are still soft and have their normal bounce. See *freezing* and *late or deep local cold injury.*

Full-thickness burn a burn that damages all the layers of skin. Muscle and bone may also be burned. Also called *third-degree burn.*

G

Gag reflex a retching action, hacking, or vomiting that is induced when something touches a certain level of the patient's throat.

Gallbladder an organ attached to the lower back of the liver. It stores bile.

Gastric distention inflation of the stomach.

Gastro- (GAS-tro) used as a beginning of words in reference to the stomach.

Genitalia (jen-i-TA-le-ah) the external reproductive organs.

Genitourinary (jen-eh-to-U-reh-NER-e) **system** reproductive and urinary systems.

Glucose (GLU-kohs) a simple sugar that is the primary source of energy for the body's tissues.

Good Samaritan laws a series of state laws designed to protect certain care providers if they deliver the standard of care in good faith, to the level of their training, and to the best of their abilities.

Grand mal a severe epileptic seizure. Also called *tonic-clonic seizures.*

Gurgling an atypical sound of breathing made by patients having airway obstruction, lung disease, or lung injury due to heat.

H

Hallucinogen a mind-altering drug that acts on the central nervous system to excite the user or to distort his or her perception of the surroundings.

Hand-off the orderly transfer of the patient, patient information, and patient valuables to more highly trained personnel.

Hazardous materials incident the release of a harmful substance into the environment. Also called *hazmat incident.*

HBV hepatitis B virus. See *hepatitis.*

Head-tilt, chin-lift maneuver a procedure for use on patients who do not have neck or spine injury. It opens the mouth, moves the tongue away from the throat, and provides for an open airway in most cases. See *jaw-thrust maneuver.*

Heart attack a general term used to indicate a failure of circulation to the heart muscle that damages or destroys a portion of the heart.

Heat cramps common term for muscle cramps in the lower limbs and abdomen associated with the loss of fluids and possibly salts while active in a hot environment. See *heat emergencies.*

Heat emergencies patients with moist, pale, normal-to-cool skin and hot and dry or moist skin due to exposure to excessive heat that leads to fluid and salt loss. The extreme case is the development of shock or the loss of the body's heat-regulating mechanisms.

Heat exhaustion prolonged exposure to heat, which creates moist, pale skin that may feel normal or cool to the touch. See *heat emergencies.*

Heat stroke prolonged exposure to heat, which creates dry or moist skin that may feel warm or hot to the touch; associated with elevation of core body temperature. See *heat emergencies.*

Hematoma (hem-ah-TO-mah) the collection of blood under the skin or in tissues as a result of an injured blood vessel.

Hemorrhage (HEM-o-rej) internal or external bleeding.

Hemorrhagic shock caused by a significant amount of internal or external bleeding.

Hemothorax (he-mo-THO-raks) the accumulation of blood in the area between the lungs and the walls of the chest cavity.

HEPA respirator short for high-efficiency particulate air respirator.

Hepatitis a disease that inflames and damages the liver; hepatitis viruses may be very infectious and can lead to life-long illness or death. It is a real danger to rescuers who fail to take appropriate BSI precautions.

Hip the joint made between the pelvis and the thigh bone (femur); may refer to the upper portion of the thigh bone.

HIV human immunodeficiency virus. See *acquired immune deficiency syndrome.*

Hives slightly elevated red or pale areas of the skin that may be produced as a reaction to certain foods, drugs, infections, or stress. Often there is an itching sensation associated with hives. See *wheal.*

Human immunodeficiency virus (HIV) virus that causes AIDS. See *acquired immune deficiency syndrome (AIDS).*

Humerus (HU-mer-us) the upper arm bone.

Humidifier a device that is attached to a supplemental oxygen delivery system to add moisture to the dry oxygen coming from the cylinder.

Hyperextension the overextension of a limb or body part.

Hyperglycemia (hi-per-gli-SE-me-ah) a condition in which the sugar (glucose) level increases in the blood and decreases in tissue cells. The problem can be serious enough to produce a coma. See *diabetic coma*.

Hyperthermia (HI-per-THUR-me-ah) an increase in body core temperature above its normal temperature.

Hyperventilation uncontrolled rapid, deep breathing that is usually self-correcting; may occur by itself or as a sign of a more serious problem.

Hypoglycemia (hi-po-gli-SE-me-ah) too little sugar in the blood. See *insulin shock*.

Hypoperfusion the failure of the body to provide adequate circulation to all its vital parts. The development of shock is actually the development of the state of hypoperfusion. See *compensated shock*, *decompensated shock*, *perfusion*, and *shock*.

Hypothermia a general cooling of the body. Also called *generalized cold emergency*.

Hypovolemic (HI-po-vo-LE-mik) **shock** the state of shock that develops due to excessive loss of whole blood or plasma.

Hypoxia (hi-POK-se-ah) an inadequate supply of oxygen to the body tissues.

I

Ileum (IL-e-um) the upper portions of the pelvis that form the wings of the pelvis; also last portion of the small intestine.

Iliac (IL-e-ak) **crest** the upper, curved boundary of the wings of the pelvis. See *ileum*.

Immobilize to fix or hold a body part in place in order to greatly reduce or eliminate motion.

Implied consent a legal position that assumes that an unresponsive or incompetent adult would consent to receiving emergency care. This form of consent may apply to other types of patients (for example, the mentally ill).

Incident management system a system designed to manage all phases of a multiple-casualty incident. It must include provisions for command at different stages, safety, assessment, care, and transport.

Incision a laceration with smooth edges, usually caused by very sharp objects such as a razor blade, knife, or broken glass.

Indication specific sign or condition for which it is appropriate to use a procedure or medication.

Infant for the purpose of CPR, includes the neonate period through one year of age.

Infarction (in-FARK-shun) localized tissue death due to the discontinuation of its blood supply. Sometimes used to mean a myocardial (heart muscle) infarction.

Infectious disease any disease produced by an infectious agent such as a bacterium or virus.

Inferior away from the head; usually compared with another structure that is closer to the head (for example, the lips are inferior to the nose). See *superior*.

Inflammation the pain, heat, redness, and swelling of tissues as they react to infection, irritation, or injury.

Inflatable splint a soft plastic splint that can be inflated with air to become rigid enough to help immobilize a fractured extremity.

Informed consent expressed consent given by a rational adult patient after being informed of the provider's training and what care procedures are to be done. Risks and options may have to be discussed.

Initial assessment the part of a patient assessment that is used to detect and immediately correct life-threatening problems involving the airway, breathing, and circulation.

Inspiration the process of breathing in. See *expiration*.

Inspire to inhale air. See *expire*.

Insulin (IN-su-lin) a hormone produced in the pancreas that is needed to move sugar (glucose) from the blood into the cells.

Insulin shock severe hypoglycemia. A state of shock usually caused by too high a level of insulin in the blood, producing a sudden drop in blood sugar.

Intercostal (in-ter-KOS-tal) **muscles** the muscles found between the ribs. These muscles contract during an inspiration, lifting the ribs. This helps to increase the volume of the chest (thoracic) cavity.

Interval time during labor, the time from the start of one contraction until the beginning of the next. See *contraction time*.

Interventions actions taken to correct or stabilize a patient's illness or injury.

Intravenous (IV) into a vein.

Iris the colored portion of the anterior eye. It adjusts the size of the pupil.

Ischium (IS-ke-em) the lower, posterior portions of the pelvis.

-itis (I-tis) a word ending used to mean inflammation.

IV See *intravenous*.

J

Jaundice (JON-dis) the yellowing of the skin; usually associated with liver or bile apparatus (gallbladder and bile ducts) injury or disease.

Jaw-thrust maneuver a method of opening the airway without lifting the neck or tilting the head. See *head-tilt, chin-lift maneuver*.

K

Ketoacidosis (KE-to-as-i-DO-sis) a condition that occurs when a diabetic breaks down too many fats trying to obtain energy. Toxic ketone bodies form in the blood and the blood becomes acid.

Kidneys excretory organs located high in the back of the abdominal region. They are behind the abdominal cavity.

Kneecap the patella (pah-TEL-lah).

L

L See *liter*.

Labor the three stages of childbirth, including the beginning of contractions, delivery of the infant, and delivery of the afterbirth.

Laceration a jagged cut with rough edges; a soft-tissue injury in which all the layers of skin are opened and the tissues immediately below the skin are damaged.

Laryngectomy (lar-in-JEK-to-me) the total or partial removal of the voice box (larynx). The patient may be called a *neck breather* or a *laryngectomee*.

Larynx (LAR-inks) the airway between the throat and the windpipe. It contains the voice box.

Lateral to the side, away from the midline of the body. See *medial*.

Lateral recumbent position the patient is lying on either his left or right side.

Leukocytes (LU-co-sites) See *white blood cells.*

Level of responsiveness mental status. See *AVPU.*

Ligament fibrous tissue that connects bone to bone.

Liter (LE-ter) the metric measurement of liquid volume that is equal to 1.057 quarts. One pint is almost equal to one-half liter. Also spelled *litre.*

Liver the largest gland in the body, having many functions. Located in the upper-right abdominal region, extending over to the central abdominal region.

Localized cold injury freezing or near freezing of a body part.

Log roll a procedure for moving a patient while keeping the patient's head, neck, and spine aligned.

LPM liters per minute.

Lumbar (LUM-bar) **spine** the five bones (vertebrae) of the lower back.

M

Major burn any full-thickness burn; a partial-thickness burn involving an entire body area or crucial area; a superficial burn that covers a large area; any burn to the face, hands, feet, neck, or genitals; any burn that involves the respiratory system. See *minor burn.*

Mammalian diving reflex a reaction that occurs when a drowning person's face submerges in cold water. The cold water causes a slow heart rate, and blood flow is directed to the heart, lungs, and brain. Oxygen is diverted to the brain.

Mandible (MAN-di-bl) the lower jawbone.

Manual stabilization restricting the movement of an injured person or body part with your hands.

Manual thrusts abdominal or chest thrusts provided to expel an object causing an airway obstruction.

Manual traction the process of drawing or pulling; a stabilizing procedure that precedes the application of a rigid splint.

Mechanism of injury (MOI) the force or forces that may have caused injury.

Meconium staining amniotic fluid that has a green or brownish-yellow color due to fetal fecal contamination.

Medial toward the midline of the body. See *lateral.*

Medical patient one who has signs of or describes symptoms of an illness.

Medical Practices Act requiring an individual to be licensed or certified in order to practice medicine or to provide certain levels of care.

Meninges (me-NIN-jez) the three membranes surrounding the brain and spinal cord.

Meningitis inflammation or infection of the lining of the brain and spinal cord.

Metabolic shock See *body fluid shock.*

Metacarpals (meta-KAR-pals) hand bones.

Metatarsals (meta-TAR-sals) foot bones.

Midline an imaginary vertical line drawn down the center of the body, dividing it into right and left halves.

Minor burn a superficial or partial-thickness burn involving a small portion of the body with no damage to the respiratory system, face, hands, feet, groin, medial thigh, buttocks, or major joints. It does not circle or cover an entire body part. See *major burn.*

Minor's consent a form of implied consent used when a minor is seriously ill or injured and the parents or guardians cannot be reached quickly.

Miscarriage the natural loss of the embryo or fetus before the twenty-eighth week of pregnancy. Also called a *spontaneous abortion.*

MOI See *mechanism of injury.*

Moves a general term used to describe any organized procedure that is employed to reposition or move a sick or an injured person from one location to another. See *emergency move* and *nonemergency move.*

Multiple-casualty incident (MCI) an emergency that involves more than one victim and overwhelms the first responding units.

Musculoskeletal system all the muscles, bones, joints, and related structures such as tendons and ligaments that enable the body and its parts to move and function.

Myocardium (mi-o-KAR-de-um) heart muscle; the cardiac muscle that makes up the walls of the heart.

N

Nasal airway a nasal airway adjunct; nasopharyngeal airway.

Nasal cannula an oxygen delivery device characterized by two soft plastic prongs, which are inserted a short distance into the nostrils.

Narcotic a class of drugs that affects the central nervous system for the relief of pain. Illicit use is to provide an intense state of relaxation.

Nasogastric (NA-zo-GAZ-trik) **tube** a flexible tube inserted through the nose to reach the stomach in order to allow drainage and/or feeding. Also called *NG tube.*

Nasopharyngeal (na-zo-fah-RIN-je-al) **airway (NPA)** a flexible plastic tube that is lubricated and then inserted into a patient's nose down to the level of the nasopharynx (back of the throat) to allow for an open upper airway. Supplemental oxygen may be delivered through this tube. Also may be called *nasal airway.*

Nature of illness (NOI) what is medically wrong with a patient; a complaint not related to an injury.

Near-drowning when the process of drowning is stopped and is reversible. See *drowning.*

Neglect failure of parents or caregivers to provide for a child's basic physical, social, emotional, and/or medical needs.

Negligence failure to provide the expected standard of care.

Neonate for the purpose of CPR, an infant during the first 28 days of life.

Nervous system the system of brain, spinal cord, and nerves that governs sensation, movement, and thought.

Neurogenic (NU-ro-jen-ic) **shock** caused when the nervous system fails to control the diameter of the blood vessels. The vessels remain widely dilated, providing too great a volume to be filled by available blood. Also called *nerve shock.*

Newborn For the purpose of CPR, an infant in the first minutes to hours after birth.

NOI See *nature of illness.*

Nonemergency move a patient move that is carried out if there are other factors at the scene causing the patient to decline, you must reach other patients, part of the care required forces you to move the patient, or the patient insists on being moved.

Nonrebreather mask an oxygen delivery device mask that has an oxygen reservoir bag; delivers a high concentration of oxygen and expels all of the patient's expired air.

NPA a nasal airway adjunct; nasopharyngeal airway.

O

Occlusion a blockage.

Occlusive dressing a dressing used to create an airtight seal or to close an open wound of a body cavity.

Off-line medical direction standing orders and protocols developed by an EMS system that authorize rescuers to perform particular skills in certain situations without actually speaking to the Medical Director. Also called *indirect medical direction*.

Ongoing assessment last step in patient assessment, used to detect changes in a patient's condition; performed every 5 minutes for critical patients and every 15 minutes for stable patients, includes repeating initial assessment, reassessing and recording vital signs, and checking interventions.

On-line medical direction orders to perform a skill or administer care from the on-duty physician given by radio or phone to the rescuer. Also called *direct medical direction*.

OPA an oral airway adjunct; oropharyngeal airway.

Open fracture when a bone is broken and bone ends or fragments cut through the skin. Also called *compound fracture*.

Open injury an injury with an associated opening of the skin.

Open wound an injury to the body in which the skin or its outer layers are opened. Also called *open injury*.

Oral airway an oral airway adjunct; oropharyngeal airway.

Oral glucose a form of glucose that can be administered by way of the mouth.

Orbits eye sockets.

Oropharyngeal (or-o-fah-RIN-je-al) **airway (OPA)** a curved breathing tube inserted into the patient's mouth. It will hold the base of the tongue forward. Also may be called *oral airway*.

P

Packaging part of the procedure of preparation for removal of the patient from an emergency scene. It may involve applying splints and dressings, neck and spine immobilization, and stabilizing impaled objects.

Palpate to feel; to sense by touch.

Pancreas (PAN-cre-as) the gland in the back of the upper portion of the abdominal cavity, behind the stomach. It produces insulin and digestive juices.

Paradoxical motion when a loose segment of an injured chest wall moves in the opposite direction to the rest of the wall during breathing movements; associated with flail chest. Also called *paradoxical movement*.

Paralysis complete or partial loss of the ability to move a body part. Sensation in the area may also be lost.

Partial-thickness burn a burn in which the outer layer of skin is burned through and the second layer (dermis) is damaged. Also called *second-degree burn*.

PASG See *pneumatic anti-shock garment*.

Patella (pah-TEL-ah) the kneecap.

Pathogens organisms, such as viruses and bacteria, that cause infection and disease.

Patient assessment the gathering of information to determine a possible illness or injury. It includes interviews and physical examination.

Pedal pulse a foot pulse.

Pelvic cavity the anterior body cavity surrounded by the bones of the pelvis.

Penetrating wound a puncture with only an entrance wound.

Perforating wound a puncture that has both an entrance wound and an exit wound.

Perfusion the constant flow of blood through the capillaries. See *hypoperfusion*.

Pericardium (per-e-KAR-de-um) the sac that surrounds the heart.

Perineum (per-i-NE-um) the region of the body located between the genitalia and the anus.

Peritoneum (per-i-to-NE-um) the membrane that lines the abdominal cavity.

Personal protective equipment (PPE) equipment such as eyewear, mask, gloves, gown, turnout gear, and helmet, which protect the rescuers from infection and/or from exposure to hazardous materials and the dangers of rescue operations.

Petit mal the minor epileptic attack that is noted by a momentary loss of awareness, with no major convulsive seizures. Also called *partial complex seizure*.

Phalanges (fah-LAN-jez) the bones of the toes and fingers.

Pharmacology the study of drugs, their origins, nature, chemistry, effects, and use.

Pharynx (FAR-inks) the throat.

Physical abuse inflicting any type of physical injury or performing any physical act that harms or disfigures a child.

Placenta (plah-SEN-tah) an organ of pregnancy that is composed of maternal and fetal tissues. Exchange between the circulatory systems of the mother and fetus can take place without the mixing of their blood. It is the main component of the afterbirth.

Plasma (PLAZ-mah) the fluid portion of the blood; the blood minus the blood cells and other structures.

Platelet (PLAT-let) element of the blood that releases factors needed to produce blood clots.

Pleura (PLOOR-ah) a double-membrane sac. The outer layer lines the chest wall, and the inner layer covers the outside of the lungs.

Pleural (PLOOR-al) **cavities** the right and left portions of the chest cavity (thorax), which contain the lungs and the pleura membranes.

Pneumatic anti-shock garment (PASG) garment similar to the air splint that can be used to control bleeding from the lower extremities by direct pressure.

Pneumothorax (NU-mo-THO-raks) the collection of air in the chest cavity to the outside of the lungs; caused by punctures to the chest wall or the lungs.

Pocket face mask a device used to help provide ventilations. It has a chimney with a one-way valve and HEPA filter. Some have an inlet for supplemental oxygen.

Position of function the natural position of a body part; the hand, slightly flexed; the foot, slightly extended.

Posterior the back of the body or body part. See *anterior*.

PPE See *personal protective equipment*.

Premature baby a baby that is born before the thirty-seventh week (prior to the ninth month) of pregnancy; any baby with a birth weight of less than 5.5 pounds.

Prescribed inhaler a device that holds medication in an aerosol form, which can be sprayed into the mouth and inhaled in order to dilate (enlarge) the air passages of someone with a chronic respiratory disease, such as asthma.

Pressure regulator a device that is connected to an oxygen cylinder to reduce the cylinder pressure to a safe working level, thus providing a safe pressure for delivery to the patient.

Priapism (PRI-ah-pizm) persistent erection associated with spinal damage in the male patient.

Prolapsed cord umbilical cord that presents through the vaginal opening before the baby's head during delivery.

Prone lying face down.

Protocols a specific set of steps developed by the EMS system's medical director; part of an EMS system's guidelines for safety, assessment, care, transport, and transfer.

Proximal closer to the torso. See *distal*.

Psychogenic (SI-ko-JEN-ic) **shock** See *fainting*.

Psychological abuse persistent emotional or verbal abuse that affects a child's positive emotional development, self-esteem, and emotional well-being.

Pubic (PYOO-bik) refers to the middle, anterior region of the pelvis. The region associated with the external genitalia.

Pubis (PYOO-bis) bone of the groin.

Pulmonary (PUL-mo-ner-e) refers to the lungs.

Pulmonary resuscitation (PUL-mo-ner-e re-SUS-ci-TAY-shun) to provide breaths to a patient in an attempt to artificially maintain lung function.

Pulse the alternate expansion and contraction of artery walls as the heart pumps blood.

Puncture an open wound that tears through the skin and damages tissues in a straight line.

R

Radial pulse the wrist pulse, which can be felt on the thumb side of the wrist.

Radius the lateral forearm bone.

Rapid physical exam a quick, safe head-to-toe exam of the medical patient.

Rapid trauma assessment a quick, safe head-to-toe exam of the trauma patient.

Rectum (REK-tum) the lower portion of the large intestine, ending with the anus.

Red blood cells (RBCs) the circulating blood cells that carry oxygen to the tissues and return carbon dioxide to the lungs; the erythrocytes (e-RITH-ro-sites).

Referred pain the pain felt in a region of the body other than where the source or cause of the pain is located. For example, pain in the gallbladder may be felt over the right shoulder blade (scapula).

Relative skin temperature an assessment of skin temperature obtained by touching the patient's skin.

Reproductive system produces all structures and hormones needed for sexual reproduction.

Respiration the act of breathing; the exchange of oxygen and carbon dioxide that takes place in the lungs.

Respiratory arrest the cessation of breathing.

Respiratory distress any difficulty in breathing.

Respiratory shock See *lung shock*.

Respiratory system exchanges air to bring in oxygen and expel carbon dioxide; includes the nose, mouth, structures in the throat, lungs, and associated muscles.

Resuscitation (re-SUS-eh-TA-shun) any effort to restore or provide normal heart and/or lung function artificially.

Rigid splint a stiff device made of a material with very little flexibility (such as metal, plastic, or wood) that is long enough to immobilize an extremity and the joints above and below the injury site.

Roller bandage a long strip of soft, self-adherent gauze, a few inches wide and some yards long, rolled on its short axis; used to secure dressings in place.

Rule of nines a system used for estimating the amount of skin surface that is burned. The body is divided into 12 regions. Each of 11 regions equals 9% of the body surface and the genital section is classified as 1%.

S

Sacrum (SA-krum) the fused bones (vertebrae) of the lower back that are immediately inferior to the lumbar spine.

SAMPLE history a system of information gathering that allows the rescuer to ask questions about past or present medical or injury problems. Letters stand for *signs/symptoms, allergies, medications, pertinent past history, last oral intake,* and *events leading to the injury or illness.*

Sanitize a rigid standard of cleaning, often to the point of practical sterilization.

Scapula (SKAP-u-lah) the shoulder blade.

Scene size-up steps taken when approaching the scene of an emergency, which consist of determining the safety of the scene, taking BSI precautions, identifying the mechanism of injury or nature of illness, determining the number of patients, and identifying additional resources needed.

Sclera (SKLE-rah) the whites of the eyes.

Scope of care the level at which a particular individual has been trained to provide emergency medical care. Also called *scope of practice*.

Scope of practice set of responsibilities and ethical considerations that define the extent or limits of the care provider.

Second-degree burn See *partial-thickness burn*.

Seizure   irregular electrical activity in the brain that can cause a sudden change in behavior or movement.

Septic shock   caused by infection-producing poisons. Also called *bloodstream shock*.

Septum   a structure that divides two chambers, such as the septum in the nose that separates the two nostrils.

Sexual abuse   physical sexual contact with or exposure to children and sexual exploitation of children by exposing, displaying, or photographing them for sexual purposes or with sexual intent.

Shock   the reaction of the body to the failure of the circulatory system to provide enough blood to the vital organs.

Shoulder blade   the scapula.

Side effect   any unwanted action or reaction of a medication other than the desired effect.

SIDS   See *sudden infant death syndrome*.

Sign   objective indications of illness or injury that can be seen, heard, felt, and smelled by another person.

Skeletal system   all the bones and joints of the body. The skeletal system provides body support and organ protection, enables movement, and produces blood cells.

Sling   a large triangular bandage or other cloth device that is applied as a soft splint to immobilize possible injuries to the shoulder girdle and upper extremity.

Soft splint   a device, such as a sling and swathe or a pillow secured with cravats, which can be applied to immobilize a painful extremity.

Soft tissues   the tissues of the body that make up the skin, muscles, nerves, blood vessels, fatty tissues, and the cells that line and cover organs and glands.

Sphygmomanometer   (SFIG-mo-mah-NOM-eh-ter)   an instrument used to measure blood pressure. Commonly called *blood pressure cuff*.

Spinal cavity   the area within the spinal column that contains the spinal cord and its coverings, the meninges (me-NIN-jez).

Spleen   an organ located to the left of the upper abdominal cavity behind the stomach. It stores blood and destroys old blood cells.

Splinting   applying a device that will immobilize an injured extremity. See *soft splint* and *rigid splint*.

Sprain   a partial or complete tearing of a ligament.

Stable   refers to the scene or a patient when conditions have a steady quality; remaining steady or the same.

Stabilize   to steady a body part in order to help reduce involuntary movement caused by pain or muscle spasm.

Standard of care   the care provided based on local laws, administrative orders, and guidelines and protocols established by the local EMS system.

START triage system   a system that uses respirations, perfusion, and mental status assessments to categorize patients into one of four treatment categories; letters stand for *Simple Triage and Rapid Treatment*.

Sterile   free of all life forms.

Sternum   (STER-num)   the breastbone.

Stethoscope   an instrument used to amplify body sounds.

Stillborn   infant who is born dead or who dies shortly after birth.

Stoma   (STO-mah)   any permanent opening that has been surgically made; the opening in the neck of a neck breather.

Strain   the overstretching or tearing of a muscle.

Stress   the emotional strain placed on an individual by a situation or a specific element of a situation.

Stressor   a situation or a part of the situation that causes stress; any factor that causes wear and tear on the body's physical or mental resources.

Stroke   the blocking or bursting of a vessel that supplies blood to the brain. A portion of the brain is damaged or destroyed by this event. Also called *cerebrovascular accident (CVA)*.

Subcutaneous   (SUB-ku-TA-ne-us)   beneath the skin. It refers to the fats and connective tissues found immediately below the dermis.

Substernal notch   referring to the area of the lower breastbone to which the ribs attach.

Sucking chest wound   an open chest wound in which air is sucked through the wound opening and into the chest cavity each time the patient breathes.

Sudden infant death syndrome (SIDS)   sudden unexplained death during sleep of an apparently healthy baby in his or her first year of life.

Superficial burn   a involving only the outer layer of skin (epidermis). Also called *first-degree burn*.

Superficial frostbite   See *frostbite*.

Superior   toward the head (for example, the chest is superior to the abdomen). See *inferior*.

Supine   lying face up, flat on the back.

Swathe   a large cravat, usually made of cloth, used to secure a sling or rigid splint and sling to the body. It also may be used to hold an upper limb to the chest.

Sympathetic eye movement   the coordinated movement of both eyes in the same direction. If one eye moves, the other eye will carry out the same movement.

Symptom   subjective indication of illness or injury that cannot be observed by another person but is felt and reported by the patient.

Syrup of ipecac   (IP-eh-kak)   a compound used to induce vomiting in certain responsive poisoning patients. Its use must be approved by the EMS system medical advisory board and be directed by the poison control center or medical direction for each case unless otherwise stated in very special local protocols. Generally, it is considered to be a medication and is not used by civilian First Responders.

Systemic   (sis-TEM-ik)   referring to the entire body.

Systolic   (sis-TOL-ik)   blood pressure; the force exerted on the artery walls when the heart is contracting. See *diastolic blood pressure*.

T

Tachycardia   (tak-e-KAR-de-ah)   rapid heartbeat.

Tarsals   (TAR-sals)   the foot bones.

TB   See *tuberculosis*.

Tendon   fibrous tissue that connects muscle to bone.

Terrorism   the use of force or violence against persons or property to intimidate or coerce a government, the civilian population, or any segment thereof to further political or social objectives.

Third-degree burn See *full-thickness burn*.

Thoracic (tho-RAS-ik) **cavity** the anterior body cavity that is above (superior to) the diaphragm; the thorax. Also called *chest cavity*.

Thorax (THO-raks) the chest.

Tibia (TIB-e-ah) the medial lower leg bone.

Tongue-jaw lift a procedure used to open the mouth of an unresponsive patient.

Tourniquet the last resort used to control bleeding from an extremity; a wide, flat band or belt used to constrict blood vessels to help stop the flow of blood from an extremity.

Trachea (TRAY-ke-ah) the windpipe.

Tracheostomy (TRA-ke-OS-to-me) a surgical opening made in the anterior neck that enters into the windpipe (trachea).

Traction a part of the action taken to pull gently along the length of a limb to stabilize a broken bone. See *manual traction*.

Trauma physical injury caused by an external force. See *blunt trauma*.

Trauma patient one who has a physical injury caused by an external force.

Trendelenburg (trend-EL-un-berg) **position** a position in which the spine-stable patient's feet and legs are higher than the head and shoulders.

Triage a method of sorting patients for care and transport based on the severity of their injuries or illnesses.

Triangular bandage a piece of triangular cloth about 50 to 60 inches long at its base and 36 to 40 inches long on each side. It can be folded and used as a sling, swathe, or cravat.

Tuberculosis (TB) a lung infection that can be transmitted by airborne aerosolized droplets.

Tympanic (tim-PAN-ik) membrane; the eardrum.

U

Ulna (UL-nah) the medial lower arm bone.

Umbilical (um-BIL-i-kal) **cord** the structure that connects the body of the fetus to the placenta.

Umbilicus (um-BIL-i-kus or um-bi-LIK-us) the navel.

Unresponsive no reaction to verbal or painful stimuli; previously referred to as *unconscious*.

Unstable refers to the scene or a patient when conditions do not have a steady quality; unsteady or not remaining the same.

Upper a stimulant drug that affect the central nervous system to excite the user.

Urinary system removes chemical wastes from the blood and helps balance water and salt levels of the blood; includes the bladder, ureters, and kidneys.

Uterus (U-ter-us) the womb; the muscular structure in which the fetus develops.

V

Vagina (vah-JI-nah) the birth canal.

Vascular refers to the blood vessels.

Vein any blood vessel that returns blood to the heart.

Venae cavae (VE-ne KA-ve) the two major veins that return blood from the body into the heart; the superior and inferior vena cava.

Venous bleeding the loss of blood from a vein. It is dark red to maroon in color. The bleeding is a steady flow and can be very heavy.

Ventilation supplying air to the lungs.

Ventral front of the body. See *anterior*.

Ventricle one of the two lower chambers of the heart. Ventricles pump blood from the heart.

Ventricular fibrillation (ven-TRIK-u-ler fib-ri-LAY-shun) the totally disorganized contractions of the myocardium of the lower heart chambers. See *defibrillation*.

Ventricular tachycardia (ven-TRIK-u-ler tak-e-KAR-de-ah) a very fast heart rate in the heart's lower chambers.

Venule (VEN-yul) typically the smallest of veins that begin at the end of capillary beds and return blood to the larger veins. See *arterioles* and *capillaries*.

Vertebra (VER-te-brah) each individual bone of the spinal column.

Vial of Life a program designed to aid emergency care personnel by having certain patients place information and medications in special vials in their refrigerators. A "Vial of Life" sticker is placed on the main outside door, closest window to the main door, or refrigerator door.

Viscera (VIS-er-ah) the internal organs; usually refers to the abdominal organs.

Vital signs objectives signs that include the pulse, respiration, skin, blood pressure, and pupils.

Vitreous (VIT-re-us) **fluid** transparent, jelly-like substance that fills the posterior cavity of the eye.

Volatile chemicals vaporizing chemicals that will cause excitement or produce a "high" when they are inhaled by the abuser.

Vomitus (VOM-i-tus) material ejected from the stomach by vomiting.

Vulva (VUL-vah) the external female genitalia.

W

Wheeze a whistling breathing sound; often associated with asthma when air is trapped in the air sacs and cannot be expired easily.

White blood cells (WBCs) the blood cells that destroy microorganisms and produce antibodies to help fight off infection; the leukocytes (LU-co-sites).

Womb See *uterus*.

X

Xiphoid (ZI-foyd) **process** the inferior portion of the sternum.

Z

Zygomatic (zi-go-MAT-ik) **bone** the cheek bone. Also called the *malar* (MA-lar).

Index

Abandonment, 27–28
ABCs of emergency care, 153
  assessing in infants and children, 467
Abdomen, 58
  abdominal quadrants, 60–61
  acute, 250–253
  caring for injuries to, 337–338
  pain in, 250–253
  rapid assessment of, 162
  rapid trauma assessment of, 174
Abdominal cavity, 59
Abdominal thrusts, 115–116
Abdominopelvic cavity, 59
Abortion, 442
Abrasions, 171, 316
Abuse
  burns in, 347
  genital injuries, 339
  of infants and children, 487, 490–494
  physical, 492–494
  psychological, 490–491
  as reportable event, 28–29
  stress of dealing with, 37
  suspected, 487, 490–494
Access, 494–523
  to buildings, 512–513
  complex, 506
  electrical wires/transformers and, 515–516
  fire and, 513–514
  gas and, 514–515
  hazardous materials and, 516–520
  hazards and, 513–520
  to motor vehicle collisions, 503–512
  safety and, 499
  simple, 506
Acute abdomen, 250–253
  defined, 250
  emergency care for, 252–253
  signs and symptoms of, 251–252
Adolescents
  definition of, 461
  developmental characteristics of, 463
Advance directives, 23–25
Advanced life support
  alerting dispatch and, 158
  early, in chain of survival, 184
Advocacy, 10
AEDs. See Automated external defibrillators (AEDs)
Afterbirth, 423, 432, 439
AIDS, risk of contracting, 43, 45
Airborne pathogens, 45–46
Air medical transport, 520–521
Airway
  in ABCs of emergency care, 153
  burns and, 343
  circulation and, 156–157
  in infants and children, 463–464
  initial assessment of, 153, 156–157
  swelling of, 331
  in triage, 530
Airway management, 93–134
  aids to, 124–129
  airway obstructions and, 112–124
  in children and infants, 211–212
  CPR and, 194, 211–212
  in infants and children, 458, 459, 467–469

opening the airway in, 101–103
positioning the head in, 101–103
pulmonary resuscitation, 101–112
recovery position and, 80
rescue breathing and, 103–112
suction systems in, 129–131
Airway obstruction, 112–124
  abdominal thrusts for, 115–116
  AHA procedure for, 120–124
  back blows for infants and, 114–115
  causes of, 112–114
  chest thrusts for, 116–119
  chest thrusts for infants and, 118, 119
  finger sweeps and, 119–120
  foreign body removal, 114–120
  pregnant women and, 118
  resuscitation aids and, 124–129
  signs of complete, 114
  signs of partial, 113–114
  unresponsive patients and, 117, 121–122, 124
Alcohol abuse, 273–274
  brain injury signs and, 397
  emergency care for, 274
  signs and symptoms of, 273–274
Allergies
  anaphylactic shock and, 261–262, 308
  patient history and, 164–165
Altered mental status, 243–250
  AVPU scale for, 244
  in children, 475–476
  seizures and, 246–247
  in shock, 309, 311
  stroke and, 243–246
American College of Sports Medicine, 406
American Heart Association, 120, 186, 193
Amniotic sac, 423
Amputations, 317
  caring for, 322–323
Anaphylactic shock, 261–262, 308
  defined, 261
  emergency care for, 262
  signs and symptoms of, 262
Anatomical position, 55
Anatomy, 53–66
  abdominal quadrants, 60–61
  body cavities in, 59
  body regions in, 57–58
  of body systems, 61–62
  defined, 54
  overview of, 54–61
  positional/directional terms in, 55–57
  relating structures to the body in, 62–65
  respiratory system, 99–100
Angina pectoris, 236. See also Heart attacks
Anterior, 55
Anterior body cavities, 59
Aorta, 285
  locating, 60–61
Apical pulse, 187
Apnea, 472
Appendicular skeleton, 357–365
  bones in, 357–358
  causes of injury to, 359
  defined, 356
  injury management, 374–391
    lower extremity, 383–391

upper extremity, 376–383
signs and symptoms of injury to, 360, 362–364
splinting, 365–374
total patient care and, 364–365
types of injury to, 359–360
Arrhythmias, 200
Arrival at the scene, 502
Arterial bleeding, 287
Arteries, 286
  CPR and, 186
  pulmonary, 285
  serious bleeding from, 156–157
Arterioles, 286
Assessment
  of behavioral emergencies, 270–271
  of breathing, 100–101
  of burns, 341–342, 343
  in childbirth, 426–427
  of children, 459, 466–470
  of extremity injuries, 364–365
  of infants, 458, 466–470
  in medical emergencies, 231, 232
  of newborns, 433–434
  for shock, 309–312
  of soft-tissue injuries, 319
  triage, 528–538
  in triage, 536–538
Assists, 73, 74
Asthma, 473–474
Asystole, 204
Atrium, 284–285
Automated external defibrillators (AEDs), 184, 200, 203–211
  access time and, 204
  assessment of, 211
  attaching, 207
  children and, 206
  dispatch time and, 205
  First Responder care and, 206–207
  internal defibrillators and, 203
  operating, 208–209
  potential problems with, 210
  quality assurance with, 210–211
  response time and, 205
  semi-, 209–210
  shock time and, 205
  two rescuers and, 197
  using, 206–211
  warnings about, 206–211
AVPU (alert, verbal, painful, unresponsive), 154, 244
Avulsions, 317
  caring for, 322–323
  ear, 330
  eye, 326, 330
Axial skeleton, 391–415
  chest injuries, 411–415
  defined, 356
  head injuries, 396–401
  mechanisms of injury to, 395
  spinal injuries, 401–411
  structures of, 391–395

Babies. See Infants; Newborns
Back blows for infants, 114–115
Bacteria, 43–44